Y. Shch

D1293188

Appendix

Infectious
and Tropical
Diseases

A HANDBOOK FOR
PRIMARY CARE

The Authors

Tao Sheng Kwan-Gett is a pediatrician who has worked in refugee and immigrant health for 9 years overseas and in the United States. He is on the clinical faculty of the University of Washington and practices in Seattle.

Charles Kemp is a nurse practitioner who has worked in refugee and immigrant health for 25 years overseas and in the United States. He has written extensively on cross-cultural healthcare and teaches community health at Baylor University.

Carrie Kovarik recently completed a dermatology residency at the University of Texas Southwestern Medical Center and is currently a dermatopathology fellow at Stanford University Medical Center. She has worked in refugee and immigrant health for 8 years, particularly in the missions field.

Infectious and Tropical Diseases

A HANDBOOK FOR PRIMARY CARE

Tao Sheng Clifford Kwan-Gett, MD, MPH
Clinical Associate Professor of Pediatrics
University of Washington
Virginia Mason Sand Point Pediatrics
Seattle, Washington

Charles Kemp, FNP, FAAN
Senior Lecturer and Clinical Instructor
Baylor University School of Nursing
Waco, Texas

Carrie Kovarik, MD
Stanford University Medical Center
Stanford, California

ELSEVIER
MOSBY

ELSEVIER
MOSBY

11830 Westline Industrial Drive
St. Louis, Missouri 63146

INFECTIOUS AND TROPICAL DISEASES: 978-0-323-02711-3
A HANDBOOK FOR PRIMARY CARE   0-323-02711-3

Copyright © 2006, Mosby Inc.

International Standard Book Number 0-323-02711-3

Executive Publisher: Barbara Nelson Cullen
Publishing Services Manager: John Rogers
Senior Project Manager: Cheryl A. Abbott
Design Direction: Mark Oberkrom

Working together to grow
libraries in developing countries
www.elsevier.com | www.bookaid.org | www.sabre.org

ELSEVIER   BOOK AID International   Sabre Foundation

Printed in the United States of America

Last digit is the print number: 9   8   7   6   5   4   3   2   1

To my wife *Paula* and daughter *Tia* for their infinite support and love and to the refugees and displaced peoples of Burma for opening my eyes and heart to global health.
Tao Sheng Kwan-Gett

This book is dedicated to my wife, *Leslie*, and my son, *David*. It is dedicated also to the many physicians, nurses, and others whose lives are committed to refugees, immigrants, and missions worldwide.
To the USMC: Semper Fidelis, Charles Kemp

This book is dedicated to my *family*, who has encouraged me to challenge myself throughout my life, and to the generous and kind-hearted volunteers who have inspired me during my work with medical missions and refugees.
Carrie Kovarik

PREFACE

Welcome to the first edition of *Infectious and Tropical Diseases: A Handbook for Primary Care*. This book was written by primary care providers for primary care providers—physicians, nurse practitioners, physicians' assistants, as well as those in training in domestic or overseas settings—to aid in the diagnosis and treatment of patients with conditions that are likely to be unfamiliar to Western providers. There are many general medical handbooks that contain reviews of commonly encountered illnesses in the domestic setting but have little on the types of diseases encountered in developing countries. For information on tropical and emerging infectious diseases, one often must turn to thick specialty texts whose depth and detail can be difficult to navigate during a busy clinic. Our goal with this book was to create a reference that would have concise, practical and easy-to-find information that primary care providers and trainees could use when seeing their immigrant, refugee, and traveler patients.

Diseases and conditions covered in this book are presented in several ways:

- The first section of the book examines general approaches to clinical syndromes and problems such as fever, diarrhea, the emergent potential bioterrorism victim, and primary care screening of the newly arrived immigrant or refugee.
- The second section contains individual entries for diseases organized alphabetically. Each entry (chapter) in this section of the book has information on the organism's geographic distribution, agent and vector, incubation, signs and symptoms, complications, laboratory findings, diagnosis, differential diagnosis, treatment, prevention, notification status (see appendixes and references).

- The appendixes contain (1) tables of diseases organized by area of the world from which the patient comes or has traveled and differential diagnoses organized by major presenting signs and symptoms, (2) a separate table on diarrhea, (3) information on notifiable diseases, (4) guidelines on controlling insect and rodent vectors, and (5) a section on the diagnosis and treatment of HIV/AIDS in resource poor settings.

— This format incorporates most of the variables that should be considered in the approach to the immigrant, refugee, or traveler patient.

— A note on the differential diagnoses offered in this book: because we focus on diseases and conditions of immigrants, refugees, and travelers, for the sake of brevity and relevance we omit common general medical conditions about which primary care providers will already be familiar. Thus for the patient with anemia, we might discuss malaria and hookworm while leaving it to the reader to consider malignancy, cirrhosis, pregnancy, and other diseases and conditions.

Tao Sheng Kwan-Gett
Charles Kemp
Carrie Kovarik

REVIEWERS

Maureen B. Boardman, MSN, RNC, FNP
Dartmouth Hitchcock Medical Center
Dartmouth Medical School
Department of Family and Community Medicine
Lebanon/Hanover, New Hampshire

Sheila A. Dunn, RN, MSN, C-ANP
Belleville Veterans Clinic
Bellville, Illinois
St. Louis University
St. Louis, Missouri

Karen Fenstermacher, RN, CS, FNP
Freeman Hospital System
Carthage, Missouri

Joy Laramie, MSN, CNP
Veterans' Affairs Medical Center
Washington, District of Columbia

Susan L. F. McLellan, MD
Infectious Diseases Section
School of Medicine
Department of Tropical Medicine
Tulane University
New Orleans, Louisiana

Kenneth J. Neuburger, MD
Emergency Medicine
Thomas Jefferson University and Hospital
Philadelphia, Pennsylvania

Denise L. Robinson, PhD, RN, FNP
HealthPoint Family Care
Covington, Kentucky;
Northern Kentucky University
Highland Heights, Kentucky

Scott W. Shiffer, MSN, FNP
Department of Family Practice
Naval Hospital
Rota, Spain

CONTENTS

Appendix

CHAPTER

1 INTRODUCTION TO INFECTIOUS DISEASES OF IMMIGRANTS, REFUGEES, AND TRAVELERS

In the last half of the 1900s, important advances in medicine gave hope that infectious diseases might someday be conquered. Vaccines reigned in some of the major killers of children such as measles and *Haemophilus influenzae* type B, and new synthetic antibiotics became powerful weapons against an increasingly broad spectrum of bacteria. But in the past few decades, a series of events shattered this complacency, for example:

- HIV/AIDS exploded into a global scourge.
- Ebola hemorrhagic fever terrorized the African continent in small but deadly epidemics.
- Multiple-drug resistance (MDR) arose in tuberculosis and other bacterial diseases.
- Diseases such as dengue fever expanded from limited geographic areas to far broader ranges.

Today the infectious disease burden in the developing world is showing little decline (Desselberger, 2000; Mairuhu, Wagenaar, Brandjes, & Van Gorp, 2004; Mayer, 2000; Shears, 2000; Wilkins, 2000). In fact, infectious diseases are the second leading cause of death worldwide, account for 30% of years of healthy life lost to disability, and are responsible for more than 25% of the global disease toll (Fauci, 2001; Hotez et al., 2004; World Health Organization, 2002).

"Emerging infectious diseases can be defined as infections that have newly appeared in a population or have existed but are rapidly increasing in incidence or geographic range" (Morse, 1995, p. 7). As globalization increases the flow of people and resources among continents, those in developed countries need to become familiar with emerging infectious disease threats from around the world. This is not just the responsibility of infectious diseases specialists. Primary care providers often treat immigrants and refugees fleeing war-torn lands. They also counsel and prepare businesspeople for assignments overseas; evaluate rashes and fevers in vacationers returning from the tropics; and volunteer on medical missions to complex humanitarian emergencies such as war and natural disasters.

Why are emerging infectious diseases such a hot topic now? Haven't new organisms always evolved as a result of changes in existing organisms? The answers are complex and involve many interrelated factors unique to today's world (Centers for Disease Control and Prevention, 2003; Dedet & Pratlong, 2000; Martens & Hall, 2000; Mayer, 2000; Morse, 1995; Pinner, Rebmann, Schuchat, & Hughes, 2003):

• *Known infections increasingly spread to new geographic areas or populations.* For example, the dengue fever pandemic began in Southeast Asia after World War II and has since spread to more than 100 countries. The spread of infections has since accelerated with the growth of air travel and international trade. Mass movement of refugees, immigrants, nomads, and travelers across the globe exposes both immigrant and native populations to new diseases. More than 70 million immigrants are estimated to be on the move at any one time (Cohen, 2000; Hotez et al., 2004).

• *Ecological transformation (e.g., deforestation, reforestation, climate change, and dam construction) combined with growing population centers increases the contact between humans and animals harboring potentially infectious organisms.* An example is the emergence of Lyme disease in the United States and Europe.

- *Insufficient public health measures permit treatable infections to persist and expand.* Population density, poor hygiene, and poor access to health care have allowed tuberculosis to remain endemic in both the developed and developing worlds despite the existence of effective therapy. Malaria is another example of a disease that is virtually nonexistent in developed countries, but continues to afflict developing countries because they are too poor to purchase and distribute effective medicines (Hotez et al., 2004).

- *The inappropriate use of antibiotics causes some organisms to develop antimicrobial resistance.* Sometimes this results from incomplete antibiotic therapy, as is the case with MDR tuberculosis. At other times, it is caused by the unnecessary use of antibiotics. For example, the use of penicillins to treat viral upper respiratory infections or self-limited ear infections has increased the prevalence of penicillin-resistant *Streptococcus pneumoniae*.

- *Increased numbers of people who have become immunodeficient either from diseases such as HIV/AIDS or medical interventions such as steroids and cancer chemotherapy have greater susceptibility to both common infections and rare opportunistic infections.* The HIV/AIDS epidemic, for example, played a critical role in the reemergence of tuberculosis as a public health threat.

- *Rare but virulent organisms have been made into weapons of war and bioterrorism.* Anthrax is a good example: In its naturally occurring state it is rare and presents in cutaneous form among those who process animal products. But as an aerosolized weapon, it could theoretically kill millions of people in a single attack.

If there is one bright side to the rise of emerging infectious diseases, it is that it forces us to realize how interconnected the world is. Many of the factors just mentioned are the result of human actions on the environment. Others are a result of social forces worsened by war and economic disparity. Perhaps by recognizing the common threat of emerging infectious diseases, we will be stimulated to close the gap in health between "us" in the industrialized world and "them" in the developing world. After all, each of us is descended from ancestors who fled war, survived famines and plagues, and moved their families across continents or oceans in search of a better life.

References

Centers for Disease Control and Prevention. (2003). Emergency preparedness and response: Biological agents and diseases. Retrieved September 27, 2003, from *www.bt.cdc.gov/agent/agentlist-category.asp*

Cohen, R. (2000). Europe tries to turn a tide of migrants chasing dreams. *New York Times*. Retrieved July 2, 2000, from *www.nytimes.com*

Dedet, J.-P., & Pratlong, F. (2000). Leishmania, trypanosoma, and monoxenous trypanosomatids as emerging opportunistic agents. *Journal of Eukaryotic Microbiology, 47,* 37-39.

Desselberger, U. (2000). Emerging and re-emerging infectious diseases. *Journal of Infection, 40,* 3-15.

Fauci, A.S. (2001). Infectious diseases: Considerations for the 21st century. *Clinical Infectious Diseases, 32,* 675-685.

Hotez, P.J., Remme, J.H.F., Buss, P., Alleyne, G., Morel, C., & Breman, J.G. (2004). Combating tropical infectious diseases: Report of the Disease Control Priorities in Developing Countries Project. *Clinical Infectious Diseases, 38,* 871-878.

Mairuhu, A.T., Wagenaar, J., Brandjes, D.P., & Van Gorp, E.C. (2004). Dengue: An arthropod-borne disease of global importance. *European Journal of Clinical Microbiology & Infectious Diseases, 23,* 425-433.

Martens, P., & Hall, L. (2000). Malaria on the move: Human population movement and malaria transmission. *Emerging Infectious Diseases, 6,* 103-109.

Mayer, J.D. (2000). Geography, ecology and emerging infectious diseases. *Social Science and Medicine, 50,* 937-952.

Morse, S.S. (1995). Factors in the emergence of infectious diseases. *Emerging Infectious Diseases, 1,* 7-15.

Pinner, R.W., Rebmann, C.A., Schuchat, A., & Hughes, J.M. (2003). Disease surveillance and the academic, clinical, and public health communities. *Emerging Infectious Diseases, 9,* 781-787.

Shears, P. (2000). Emerging and re-emerging infections in Africa: The need for improved laboratory services and disease surveillance. *Microbes and Infection, 2,* 489-495.

Wilkins, E. (2000). Introduction to the mini-series on emerging infectious diseases. *Journal of Infection, 40,* 2.

World Health Organization. (2002). *World health report 2002.* Retrieved August 28, 2003, from *www.who.int/infectious-disease-report/pages/grfindx.html*

2 CLASSIFICATION OF INFECTIOUS DISEASES

TERMS TO DESCRIBE INFECTIOUS DISEASES

Before reviewing the classification of infectious diseases, it is useful to clarify the terms we use to describe them and their actions. An *infection* occurs when an organism is able to multiply within a *host*. When an infection kills, damages, or alters the host's physiology, it is an *infectious disease*. Organisms that have the ability to cause disease are called *pathogens*; those that do not are *nonpathogenic*. A measure of the likelihood that a particular organism will cause disease is *virulence*. Some symptoms of a disease are caused by *virulence factors* such as toxins that are produced by an organism to increase its ability to multiply in a host and cause disease (Relman & Falkow, 2000). Other symptoms such as fever are not from direct effects of the organism but from the human body's inflammatory response to infection.

Often infections in humans cause no symptoms and no disease (Relman & Falkow, 2000). In fact, the presence of a community of microbes *colonizing* the human body is a normal state of good health. The *normal flora* protect against pathogens and stimulate the immune system. In turn, the immune system plays a regulating role by patrolling the microbial community for pathogens and making sure that the community itself does not get too big or unruly. When the immune system is compromised, diseases from *opportunistic infections* can result from either organisms that are part of the normal flora or from potentially pathogenic organisms that are normally only transient members of the body's microbial community. Antibiotic use can sometimes disrupt the body's normal ecology of microbes and allow pathogens to take hold.

The classic example of this is pseudomembranous colitis, in which the killing of normal intestinal flora allows the *Clostridium difficile* bacteria to multiply in the large intestine and cause inflammation and diarrhea. At other times, antibiotic use will kill most microbes except those that have the ability to survive the presence of antibiotics. These *antibiotic-resistant* (or *drug-resistant*) organisms can then multiply and cause disease in the host or be passed on to another host. When drug-resistant organisms cause disease, larger doses or stronger more expensive antibiotics are usually needed to treat them. Incomplete or inappropriate antibiotic use contributes to the development of drug-resistant organisms.

MECHANISMS FOR THE SPREAD OF INFECTIOUS DISEASES

Infectious diseases can be transmitted both directly and indirectly (Osterholm, Hedberg, & Moore, 2000). Direct mechanisms include contact with another person with the infection (this includes droplet spread less than 1 meter from a cough or sneeze); contact with an animal (e.g., rabies transmitted through a dog bite) or object (e.g., *Clostridium tetani* in soil) that has the infectious organism; and *vertical transmission* in which an infected mother passes the organism to an infant either transplacentally during pregnancy (e.g., cytomegalovirus) or through the birth canal during delivery (e.g., neonatal herpes simplex virus).

There are also three forms of indirect infection: vehicle-borne, vector-borne, and aerosol infections. Vehicle-borne infection occurs when a person is exposed to some contaminated material (water, food, blood, toys, medical instruments) containing the agent. Vector-borne illnesses are transmitted by insect. The insect may have acquired an infection from a contaminated object (e.g., a fly that has landed on feces) or from an infected animal *reservoir* (e.g., a tick that has acquired Lyme disease from biting an infected deer). An organism that primarily infects animals and only occasionally arises to cause disease in humans is called a *zoonosis*. Because some infectious organisms have a greater chance of continuing their life cycle if their presence does not quickly kill the host, many zoonoses that have a high fatality rate in humans often cause no symptoms or only mild disease in their natural reservoir hosts. The third type of indirect infection is transmission from an aerosolized agent, for example, as seen with tuberculosis.

CLASSIFICATION OF INFECTIOUS DISEASES

Infectious agents are often classified based on their level of structural complexity, but recent molecular and DNA sequencing techniques have changed the taxonomy of all life on earth into one of three domains (Gold & Eisenstein, 2000; Tree of Life Project, 2004):

1. *Bacteria*, including typical bacteria, chlamydiae, mycoplasmas, rickettsiae, acinetobacter, and *Nocardia* species
2. *Archaea*, which are prokaryotes like bacteria but do not contain any known agents of human disease
3. *Eucarya*, which are distinguished by the presence of membrane-enclosed nuclei and organelles. This domain includes the three familiar kingdoms of plants, animals, and fungi, as well as a fourth group called protists—a disparate group of organisms including protozoa, algae, and slime molds that do not fit into any of the other three *eucarya* kingdoms.

Prions and viruses are not part of this tree of life but are important infectious agents. Prions are the cause of transmissible, slowly progressive, and ultimately fatal neurogenerative diseases characterized by the buildup of prion protein. Examples include bovine spongiform encephalopathy (BSE or "mad cow disease") in cattle and Creutzfeldt-Jakob disease in humans. Prions do not contain detectable DNA or RNA.

— Viruses are particles containing nucleic acid that require a host cell to replicate. They can be thought of as payloads of RNA or DNA surrounded by a delivery system (Dermody & Tyler, 2000). The current classification system is based on (1) the presence of RNA or DNA, (2) whether the viral capsid or shell is helical or icosahedral, and (3) whether the virus has a lipid envelope. Those without lipid envelopes are better able to survive environmental conditions outside the host and are often transmitted through the fecal-oral route. Table 2-1 summarizes the current classification system with examples of viruses in each family.

— Typical bacteria are single-celled organisms that have a cell wall. They contain DNA and RNA, but unlike eukaryotes they do not have a nuclear membrane or other membrane-enclosed organelles. Bacteria are classified in many ways:

- Color on Gram stain may be negative or positive.
- Morphology varies as follows: round cocci, which occur in pairs, clusters, or chains; bacilli, which are cylindrical, rod shaped, curved, or pleomorphic (i.e., having different shapes at different stages of their life cycle); spirochetes, which are spiral; and branched forms.
- Metabolic properties include aerobic (oxygen metabolizing) vs. anaerobic vs. facultative; for gram-negative bacteria, lactose fermenting vs. nonlactose fermenting.
- Molecular or genetic properties vary widely.

— *Chlamydia* are organisms that are morphologically similar to gram-negative bacteria but are intracellular parasites with a biphasic life cycle. First, a spore-like elementary body (EB) attaches to and enters an epithelial cell. Once inside, it transforms into a reticulate body (RB), which

TABLE 2–1 Classification of Viruses

Family	Example	Type of Nucleic Acid	Genome Size (Kilobases or Kilobase Pairs)	Envelope	Capsid Symmetry
RNA-containing viruses					
Picornaviridae	Poliovirus	SS (+)RNA	7.2–8.4	No	I
Caliciviridae	Norwalk virus	SS (+)RNA	7.4–7.7	No	I
Astroviridae	Astrovirus	SS (+)RNA	7.2–7.9	No	I
Togaviridae	Rubella virus	SS (+)RNA	10–12	Yes	I
Flaviviridae	Yellow fever virus	SS (+)RNA	9.5–13	Yes	Unk
Coronaviridae	Coronavirus	SS (+)RNA	20–30	Yes	H
Rhabdoviridae	Rabies virus	SS (−)RNA	13–16	Yes	H
Filoviridae	Ebola virus	SS (−)RNA	19	Yes	H
Paramyxoviridae	Measles virus	SS (−)RNA	16–20	Yes	H

Orthomyxoviridae	Influenza virus	8 SS (−)RNA segments*	10–14	Yes	H
Bunyaviridae	California encephalitis virus	3 circular SS (ambisense) RNA segments	11–21	Yes	H
Arenaviridae	Lymphocytic choriomeningitis virus	2 circular SS (ambisense) RNA segments	10–14	Yes	H
Reoviridae	Rotavirus	10–12 DS RNA segments†	16–27	No	I
Retroviridae	Human immunodeficiency virus type 1	2 identical SS (+)RNA segments	7–11	Yes	I-capsid H-nucleocapsid
DNA-containing viruses					
Hepadnaviridae	Hepatitis B virus	Circular DS DNA with SS portions	3.2	Yes	I

*Influenza C virus: 7 segments.

†Reovirus, mammalian reovirus and orbivirus: 10 segments; rotavirus: 11 segments; Colorado tick fever virus: 12 segments.

Abbreviations: DS, Double stranded; H, helical; I, icosahedral; SS, single stranded; Unk, unknown; (+), message sense; (−), complement of message sense.

continued

Table 2–1 continued

Family	Example	Type of Nucleic Acid	Genome Size (Kilobases or Kilobase Pairs)	Envelope	Capsid Symmetry
Parvoviridae	Human parvovirus B-19	SS (+) or (−)DNA	5	No	I
Papoviridae	Human papillomavirus	Circular DS DNA	5–8	No	I
Adenoviridae	Adenovirus	Linear DS DNA	36–38	No	I
Herpesviridae	Herpes simplex virus	Linear DS DNA	120–240	Yes	I
Poxviridae	Vaccinia virus	Linear DS DNA with covalently closed ends	130–380	Yes	Complex

Source: From Dermody, T.S., & Tyler, K.I. (2000). Introduction to viruses and viral diseases. In G. Mandell, J. Bennett, & R. Dolin (Eds.), *Principles and practice of infectious diseases* (5th ed., pp. 1536–1552). New York: Churchill Livingstone.

Abbreviations: DS, Double stranded; H, helical; I, icosahedral; SS, single stranded; Unk, unknown; (+), message sense; (−), complement of message sense.

multiplies inside the host cell. The RBs then condense into EBs, which are released from the host cell, sometimes by cell lysis. The EBs then go on to propagate the life cycle. Examples of diseases caused by *Chlamydia* species are ocular trachoma, an important cause of vision loss in the developing world caused by *C. trachomatis,* and psittacosis, a pneumonia caused by *C. psittaci* that is transmitted by birds.

— *Mycoplasma* are the smallest free-living organisms (prions and viruses are smaller, but are not able to live outside a host cell). But mycoplasma are distinct from bacteria in that they lack a cell wall. *Mycoplasma* species are part of the normal flora for plants and animals, but many cause disease. One of the most commonly identified human mycoplasmal diseases is *M. pneumoniae,* which causes upper respiratory infections and pneumonia.

— *Rickettsiae* are pleomorphic coccobacilli that are obligate intracellular organisms. They are almost exclusively zoonoses that, with the exception of louse-born typhus, rely on nonhuman mammal reservoirs for their life cycle. All are transmitted through arthropod vectors. Rocky Mountain spotted fever (RMSF, caused by *R. rickettsii*) and scrub typhus (*Orientia tsutsugamushi*) are examples of rickettsial infectious diseases. *Ehrlichiae* are closely related to rickettsiae and are the causative agents of ehrlichiosis, a tick-borne illness similar to RMSF but with no rash.

— *Fungi* or *mycoses* have rigid cell walls and can appear as either yeasts (round, reproducing by budding) or molds (tubular, reproducing by branching and extension). Some dimorphic fungi can assume either form depending on the environment: Histoplasmosis, blastomycosis, sporotrichosis, and coccidioidomycosis, for example, grow as yeasts when they infect the body, but as molds in the laboratory (Bennett, 2000).

— Protozoa are mostly free-living, unicellular organisms that can classified on the basis of locomotion.

The Sarcodina include organisms such as *Entamoeba histolytica* that move using ameboid pseudopods. Mastigophora move with the use of whip-like flagellae, and include *Giardia lamblia*, *Trypanosoma* species, and *Leishmania* species. Ciliophora such as *Balantidium coli* use cilia for locomotion. Finally, there are the sporozoa with no locomotor organs; examples include the *Plasmodium*, *Toxoplasma*, and *Cryptosporidium* species. The helminths are worms and include nematodes (roundworms), trematodes (flukes), and cestodes (tapeworms); they are summarized in Table 2-2. They have complex life cycles involving eggs or larvae that

TABLE 2–2

Major Helminth Infections of Humans

Group or Class	Infection	Organism	Mode of Transmission to Humans
Nematodes (roundworms)	Trichuriasis	*Trichuris trichiura*	Ingestion of embryonated eggs
	Enterobiasis	*Enterobius vermicularis*	Ingestion of eggs
	Ascariasis	*Ascaris lumbricoides*	Ingestion of embryonated eggs
	Hookworm	*Ancylostoma duodenale, Necator americanus*	Skin penetration by larvae
	Strongyloidiasis	*Strongyloides stercoralis*	Larva penetration of skin or colon
	Trichinosis	*Trichinella spiralis*	Ingestion of muscle larvae

Table 2–2 continued

Group or Class	Infection	Organism	Mode of Transmission to Humans
Nematodes (roundworms)—cont'd	Lymphatic filariasis	*Wuchereria bancrofti, Brugia malayi*	Injection of larvae during mosquito bite
	Onchocerciasis	*Onchocerca volvulus*	Injection of larvae during blackfly bite
Trematodes (flukes)	Schistosomiasis	*Schistosoma haematobium, Schistosoma mansoni, Schistosoma japonicum, Schistosoma intercalcatum, Schistosoma mekongi*	Penetration of intact human skin by cercariae
	Clonorchiasis	*Clonorchis sinensis*	Ingestion of metacercariae in freshwater fish
	Fascioliasis	*Fasciola hepatica*	Ingestion of metacercariae on aquatic plants
	Paragonimiasis	*Paragonimus westermani*	Ingestion of metacercariae in crayfish or freshwater crabs
Cestodes (tapeworms)	Echinococcosis	*Echinococcus granulosus, Echinococcus multilocularis*	Ingestion of eggs

continued ➡

Table 2–2 continued

Group or Class	Infection	Organism	Mode of Transmission to Humans
Cestodes (tapeworms)—cont'd	Taeniasis saginata	*Taenia sagniata*	Ingestion of cysticerci in beef
	Taeniasis solium	*Taenia solium*	Ingestion of cysticerci in pork
	Cysticercosis	*Taenia solium*	Ingestion of eggs
	Diphyllobothriasis	*Diphyllobothrium latum*	Ingestion of cysts in freshwater fish

Source: From Mahmoud, A.A. (2000). Introduction to helminth infections. In G. Mandell, J. Bennett, & R. Dolin (Eds.), *Principles and practice of infectious diseases* (5th ed., pp. 2937-2938). New York: Churchill Livingstone.

transmit the disease outside the human host. Some involve intermediate animal such as snails or fish. *Ectoparasites* are insects that primarily interact with the skin. They include ticks and mosquitoes that serve as vectors for microbial parasites, as well as burrowing flea infections such as tungiasis.

References

Bennett, J.E. (2000). Introduction to mycoses. In G. Mandell, J. Bennett, & R. Dolin (Eds.), *Principles and practice of infectious diseases* (5th ed., pp. 2655-2656). New York: Churchill Livingstone.

Dermody, T.S., & Tyler, K.I. (2000). Introduction to viruses and viral diseases. In G. Mandell, J. Bennett, & R. Dolin (Eds.), *Principles and practice of infectious diseases* (5th ed., pp. 1536-1552). New York: Churchill Livingstone.

Gold, H.S., & Eisenstein, B.I. (2000) Introduction to bacterial diseases. In G. Mandell, J. Bennett, & R. Dolin (Eds.), *Principles and practice of infectious diseases* (5th ed., pp. 2065-2068). New York: Churchill Livingstone.

Mahmoud, A.A. (2000). Introduction to helminth infections. In G. Mandell, J. Bennett, & R. Dolin (Eds.), *Principles and practice of infectious diseases* (5th ed., pp. 2937-2938). New York: Churchill Livingstone.

Murphy, F.A., & Kingsbury, D.W. (1996). Virus taxonomy. In B.N. Fields, D.M. Knipe, & P.M. Howley (Eds.), *Fields virology* (3rd ed., pp. 15-57). Philadelphia: Lippincott-Raven.

Osterholm, M.T., Hedberg C.W., & Moore, K.A. (2000). Epidemiology of infectious diseases. In G. Mandell, J. Bennett, & R. Dolin (Eds.), *Principles and practice of infectious diseases* (5th ed., pp. 156-167). New York: Churchill Livingstone.

Relman, D.A., & Falkow, S. (2000). A molecular perspective of microbial pathogenicity. In G. Mandell, J. Bennett, & R. Dolin (Eds.), *Principles and practice of infectious diseases* (5th ed., pp. 2-12). New York: Churchill Livingstone.

Tree of Life Project (2004). *Life on earth*. Retrieved June 9, 2004, from *http://tolweb.org/tree?group=Life_on_Earth*.

3 DIAGNOSIS AND APPROACHES TO PATIENTS

OVERVIEW OF PHYSICAL DIAGNOSIS: INFECTIOUS DISEASES IN IMMIGRANTS, REFUGEES, AND TRAVELERS

— Although some of the most important information that leads to a diagnosis is to be found in the history of present illness and past medical history, and although advanced rapid antibody tests and polymerase chain reaction (PCR) technology may offer hope for faster laboratory diagnosis, the physical examination remains an important part of evaluating and treating infectious diseases in immigrants, refugees, and returned travelers. Not only does the physical exam provide the clinician with sensory clues, it also strengthens the clinician-patient relationship, which is both therapeutic and diagnostic. Rarely does the acquisition of information follow the rigid traditional sequence of the history, physical examination, laboratory tests, and assessment and plan. Rather, the physical exam starts the moment the clinician makes eye contact with the patient, and the history may extend itself over time as the patient gains trust in the clinician during the encounter. This blurring of information boundaries may be more so for people from cultures in which patients often first seek medical care not from hospitals or clinics, but from family members, village elders, religious leaders, or the local pharmacist.

— Clinicians spend years honing a sense of whether a patient is "sick" or "not sick." Relying too much on this sense can be misleading when treating patients who have traveled from distant lands, not only because we are unfamiliar with the illnesses, but also because some illnesses present with few symptoms that may herald a rapid life-threatening deterioration within hours or days (e.g., *Plasmodium falciparum* malaria, which may present with just fever). Other illnesses might present with seemingly minor symptoms that, untreated, may over months and years lead to permanent disability (e.g., *Mycobacterium leprae,* also called Hansen's disease or leprosy). Finally, immigrants who were born and/or raised in the country of potential disease exposure may present with a less acute picture than travelers. For example, a newly arrived refugee with malaria who grew up in an endemic area likely has partial immunity from repeated bouts of malaria during childhood. As a result, he or she will probably have a less acute presentation than a tourist from a developed country who had never been exposed to malaria.

The purpose of this section is to give an overview and approach to physical diagnosis. Subsequent sections in this chapter integrate important components of the history, physical exam, and laboratory studies for approaches to the common clinical entities of fever, diarrhea, the emergent patient, and refugee screening. For the sake of brevity we highlight unusual findings that might trigger the consideration of diseases specific to immigrants, refugees, and travelers:

• *General.* Assess the patient's general health by looking for stunting, a sign of chronic malnutrition, or wasting, which could point to either chronic infection (such as HIV and tuberculosis) or malignancy. The patient's interaction should also be noted. A flat affect and apathy can be not only a sign of depression, but also be present in African trypanosomiasis, new variant Creutzfeldt-Jakob disease, and HIV encephalopathy.

• *Vital signs.* The next section of this chapter provides an in-depth discussion of fever. Relative bradycardia in a

febrile patient has been observed in many
infections such as typhoid fever and paratyphoid,
chlamydia or mycoplasma pneumonia, tularemia,
legionella (in elderly patients), arenaviruses (Lassa fever,
South American hemorrhagic fever, lymphocytic
choriomeningitis virus), and arboviruses (yellow fever,
dengue fever). Bradycardia secondary to increased
intracranial pressure could also be a sign of a mass
effect caused by a parasite (see Neurologic entry at the
end of this list). Noninfectious causes of relative
bradycardia include fish or shellfish poisoning and
mefloquine therapy. Relative tachycardia with fever is
sometimes present in rheumatic fever.

• *Head, eyes, ears, nose, and throat.* Eyelid edema can be
present in loa loa, which can also present itself as a
worm in the subconjunctivae visible with the naked
eye. Unilateral orbital edema (Romaña's sign) may be
the presenting sign of South American trypanosomiasis
(Chagas' disease). More generalized facial edema is
present in a minority of patients in the early stages of
African trypanosomiasis. Examine the cornea for
diffuse opacities that might suggest trachoma; if they
are present, also look at the inside of the upper lid for
accompanying fibrosis. In refugees, signs of vitamin A
deficiency (especially important to identify in patients
with respiratory illnesses) may be present such as
corneal ulcers, Bitot's spots (dry, foamy-appearing areas
on the scleral conjunctivae), and wrinkling of the
conjunctivae. Conjunctival pallor could be a sign of
anemia caused by malaria or iron deficiency secondary
to hookworm. The hemolytic anemia of malaria can
also cause scleral icterus, which may also be present in
hepatitis or yellow fever. Decreased conjunctival
sensation, lagophthalmus, ectropion (lower lid turned
out), or entropion may be signs of Hansen's disease.
In newly arrived refugees, dentition is often poor and
should be examined.

- *Lymph nodes.* Many acute and chronic infectious diseases cause diffuse adenopathy including HIV, Epstein-Barr virus, tuberculosis, and Hansen's disease. *Winterbottom's sign* of bilateral swollen posterior cervical lymph nodes is a classic finding in African trypanosomiasis. An enlarged, painful firm lymph node with purplish discoloration could signify a bubo of *Yersinia pestis.* Inguinal lymphadenopathy may be a sign of sexually transmitted infections, such as lymphogranuloma venereum (LGV) caused by *Chlamydia trachomatis,* or chancroid caused by *Haemophilus ducreyi.*
- *Chest.* In addition to reactive airway disease and common lower respiratory tract infections, wheezing can be a sign of parasitic infections that involve the lung as part of their life cycle such as ascariasis, hookworm, toxocariasis (visceral larva migrans), paragonimiasis, and strongyloidiasis. The rupture of an echinococcal cyst may also induce wheezing. Right-sided intercostal tenderness on deep palpation can be a sign of a subdiaphragmatic amebic liver abscess.
- *Heart.* Consider rheumatic fever if a valvular murmur is present. Tachycardia and a gallop may be present in a patient with cardiomyopathy caused by Chagas' disease.
- *Abdomen.* Hepatomegaly and splenomegaly can be present in many diseases such as viral hepatitis, malaria, visceral larva migrans, and schistosomiasis. Liver tenderness and hepatomegaly in a febrile patient should stimulate consideration of an amebic liver abscess, typhoid, or brucellosis. A large, smooth hepatic mass may be an echinococcal cyst. Rectal examination may reveal the characteristic rectal strictures of LGV or the itchy erythematous perianal lesions of strongyloidiasis.
- *Genitourinary.* Lymphatic filariasis can sometimes present with scrotal swelling or hydroceles. Ulcers on

the genitalia may signify sexually transmitted infections, such as syphilis, herpes, or chancroid.

- *Extremities.* Localized transient, nonerythematous swelling could represent lymphedema secondary to lymphatic filariasis, especially if the swelling is unilateral. Transient wrist or ankle swelling (also called *Calabar swelling*) is a classic sign of loa loa. Transient edema of hands and feet may be a sign of African trypanosomiasis. Scarred, lost digits are a common sequelae of Hansen's disease. Patchy depigmentation of the extremities may be associated with pinta, caused by *Treponema carateum*, or late stage onchocerciasis. Unilateral swelling of the foot, with draining sinuses, pustules, or nodules, may signify a mycetoma, or Madura foot, which is caused by direct inoculation of fungus or bacteria into the skin.

- *Skin.* Look for petechiae, which may be present in rickettsial diseases, meningococcemia, dengue, yellow fever, typhus, or one of the viral hemorrhagic fevers. Rose spots, which appear as blanching pink macules on the chest and abdomen, are seen with typhoid. Subcutaneous nodules in a patient with a seizure disorder may be associated with cysticercosis, the larval stage of *Taenia solium*. A painful, solitary chancre is present at the inoculation site of African trypanosomiasis. A painless eschar, which appears as a black ulcer with surrounding erythema, may be an inoculation site of tick or scrub typhus. Chronic ulcers may be the sign of many different infections, including cutaneous leishmaniasis, diphtheria, tertiary syphilis, *Mycobacterium tuberculosis* (cutaneous tuberculosis), Hansen's disease, *Mycobacterium ulcerans* (Buruli ulcer), deep fungal infections such as histoplasmosis, or tropical ulcers caused by mixed infections. Excoriations from severe pruritus may be present in parasitic infections such as trypanosomiasis or cutaneous larva migrans, scabies, insect bites, eczema, dry skin, or may be a manifestation of liver or kidney disease. Refugees and asylum seekers may also have scars of past torture such as burns, rope marks, whipping, and lacerations.

• *Neurologic.* A patient with findings suggesting increased intracranial pressure, spinal cord syndrome, or myeloradiculopathy may be suffering from the mass effect secondary to the cysts of a parasite such as *Taenia solium*, schistosomiasis, paragonimiasis, and echinococcosis. Examine the patient for meningeal signs signifying bacterial or viral meningitis. Mental status changes such as decreased levels of consciousness, behavior changes, memory loss, and even hallucinations may accompany one of the viral encephalitides. Hansen's disease can cause enlarged peripheral nerves, claw hand, wrist drop or foot drop, or facial palsy; a classic sign is a hypopigmented or erythematous macule, papule, or nodule with reduced sensation.

APPROACH TO THE PATIENT WITH FEVER

Fever is an elevation in body temperature in which cytokines change the thermoregulatory set point of the hypothalamus. It is different from hyperthermia, which is an elevation in body temperature caused by an imbalance of heat generation and heat dissipation independent of the body's thermoregulatory set point (Root, 1999). Examples of hyperthermia include temperature elevation due to heat stroke and hyperthyroidism.

Fever is a presenting symptom in many infectious diseases of travelers, immigrants, and refugees. It is a challenge for primary care providers to discern those patients with common, self-limiting illness from those with tropical diseases or serious emerging infections.

Because the differential diagnosis can seem overwhelming, it is useful to have an approach to evaluating the patient with fever (Humar & Keystone, 1996; McLellan, 2002; Ryan, Wilson, & Kain, 2002). This section contains an overview of one approach to fever, while Appendix A contains listings of differential diagnoses that include fever.

- *Review the patient's travel history and the incubation period of potential exposures.* The details of when and where a possible exposure occurred combined with the knowledge of the incubation period of different pathogens can be extremely helpful in the diagnosis of fever. Many viral infections have an incubation period of days. Dengue fever, for example, causes fever 5 to 8 days after being bitten by an infected mosquito. A patient who presents with fever 4 weeks after leaving an dengue endemic area is therefore unlikely to have the disease (McLellan, 2002). Bacterial infections (e.g., typhoid fever) and malaria can have incubation periods of several days to months. *P. falciparum* typically causes fever within a few weeks following exposure, whereas *P. vivax* can cause symptoms months after exposure. Chagas' disease, caused by the protozoa *Trypanosoma cruzi*, results in fever 1 to 2 weeks after the bite of an infected Reduviid insect (a species of blood-sucking bugs). Symptoms from some parasitic infections may occur many months or even years after exposure. It is therefore important to review the patient's travel history, taking into account the mode of travel, whether the destinations were urban or rural, the type and quality of food and water the patient consumed, and whether the patient used preventive measures (e.g., vaccinations, antibiotic prophylaxis against traveler's diarrhea, antimalarials, insect repellent). Also ask the patient about his or her activities and specific exposures such as hunting (which increases exposure to arboviral diseases, zoonoses), swimming in freshwater (schistosomiasis), backpacking (arboviral disease, malaria, parasites), sexual activity (sexually transmitted infections, HIV), or medical volunteer work. Altitude is also an important consideration, because mosquito-borne diseases such as malaria are unlikely at altitudes greater than 3000 meters (approximately 10,000 ft) (McLellan, 2002).

- *Determine the fever's pattern and duration.* High, acute fevers may be a sign of infections requiring immediate action such as *P. falciparum* malaria, typhoid fever, viral hemorrhagic fevers, rickettsioses, meningococcemia, and other bacteremias. Classic fever patterns can suggest certain diseases, though the lack of a pattern does not rule out a disease (Cunha, 1996). For example, malaria can produce a periodic fever that peaks every third day (*P. malaria*) or every other day (*P. vivax*). A saddle-back fever pattern in which a fever returns after several days is sometimes seen in patients with dengue. Relapsing fevers can be a sign of leptospirosis, borreliosis, trypanosomiasis, visceral leishmaniasis, and brucellosis. Chronic fever lasting more than 2 weeks can be seen in many infection such as tuberculosis, HIV, typhoid fever, secondary syphilis, and abscesses (e.g., amebic liver abscess).

- *Look for localizing signs and symptoms.* For a discussion of the physical examination, refer back to the beginning of this chapter, and for listings with differential diagnoses organized by presenting signs and symptoms, see Appendix A.

- *Consider possible diagnoses that require urgent or emergent treatment.* Some diseases may cause severe complications or death if not identified and treated rapidly (McLellan, 2002). In the patient population we are considering, malaria is one of the more common diseases of this type presenting with fever. **A febrile patient who has recently been in a malaria endemic area should be considered to have malaria until proven otherwise.** Obtain blood smears for diagnosis as soon as possible, and begin empiric treatment if the results are not available immediately. There are also bacterial infections for which it may be wise to begin empiric treatment while waiting for the results of definitive tests, such as meningococcemia, rickettsiosis, or leptospirosis (McLellan, 2002). Other diseases for which early therapy could be lifesaving include typhoid and amebiasis. Ribavirin may reduce morbidity and mortality for some viral hemorrhagic fevers. For discussion of other severe infections requiring supportive treatment, see the section on the emergent patient later in this chapter.

- *Be aware of possible diagnoses that require rapid public health intervention.* Isolation precautions, personal protective measures for health care personnel, and notification of public health authorities are extremely important for the control of potentially life-threatening diseases that are highly communicable. The possibility of bioterrorism, though remote, should always be considered. For further discussion, see the section on the emergent patient later in this chapter.

APPROACH TO THE PATIENT WITH DIARRHEA

The definition of diarrhea is more than three loose stools in a 24-hour period, or any frequency of loose stools containing blood. There are two basic mechanisms of diarrhea: osmotic diarrhea from malabsorption caused by tissue injury to the lumen of the intestine, or secretory diarrhea from toxins produced by pathogens. Some pathogens cause diarrhea by a combination of these two mechanisms.

Diarrhea is a common illness for refugees, immigrants, and travelers, with a broad spectrum of severity. Though it may be mere nuisance for a family on holiday, worldwide it is a leading cause of death for children less than 5 years old. The exact etiology of diarrhea, particularly travelers' diarrhea, cannot be identified 25% to 50% of the time (Ryan et al., 2002). But because there are many treatable causes of diarrhea, some with substantial morbidity if left untreated, it is important to have a systematic approach to diagnosis. As with fever, a history of recent travel and activities can help narrow the differential diagnosis. Travel and activities more than a month before the onset of diarrhea are unlikely to be relevant. An example of a stepwise approach to evaluating diarrhea follows (also see Appendix A).

• *Determine if there are symptoms and signs suggestive of an invasive pathogen.* Some pathogens disrupt the mucosal surfaces of the intestine and cause fever, blood in the stool, or peritoneal signs. These include *Campylobacter jejuni, Shigella, Escherichia coli* O157:H7, *Clostridium difficile, Entamoeba histolytica, Yersinia enterocolitica,* and sometimes *Salmonella.* Often the symptoms caused by an invasive pathogen have an abrupt onset. Patients with these symptoms should have a diagnostic workup initiated regardless of the duration of their diarrhea (Kolars & Fischer, 2002). Standard bacterial stool cultures in many institutions test only for the presence of *Campylobacter, Salmonella,* and *Shigella.* Additional testing may be suggested by the history and physical examination. If the patient has a history of eating incompletely cooked hamburger or food that was potentially contaminated with manure, consider asking the laboratory to look specifically for *E. coli* O157:H7. A history of recent antibiotic use increases the risk of *C. difficile,* for which a stool toxin test is available. Reactive arthropathy, which can sometimes

occur late in the illness or after the diarrhea has
resolved, suggests the possibility of *Shigella*,
Campylobacter, *Yersinia*, or *Salmonella* (Kolars &
Fischer, 2002). If the patient has right upper
quadrant abdominal pain or right shoulder pain
suggestive of a liver abscess, consider the possibility
of amebic dysentery and investigate with a stool
ova & parasites (O&P) test.

- *If there are no signs of an invasive pathogen and the
diarrhea is not prolonged, treat conservatively.*
Fortunately, most episodes of diarrhea are self-limited
and do not require any treatment other than good
hydration, especially for children and the elderly
(Ryan et al., 2002). Viral gastroenteritis, food
poisoning, and common traveler's diarrhea from
enterotoxigenic *E. coli* usually resolve within a few
days. Oral rehydration is always preferable to
intravenous hydration, especially for children. The
patient's regular diet should be continued as
long as tolerated. Some patients may have improved
symptoms on a lactose-free diet. If vomiting
interferes with solid and liquid intake, frequent
sips of oral rehydration solution will help prevent
dehydration. A commercially available solution may be
used, or a homemade solution can be mixed using 1
quart of drinking water and 2 tablespoons of sugar,
plus either 1/4 teaspoon each of salt and baking soda,
or 1/2 teaspoon of salt (Solutions Made at Home,
2002). Presumptive antibiotic therapy for noninvasive
diarrhea with a fluoroquinolone may be helpful for
adults and adolescents. But because fluoroquinolones
have been associated with arthropathy in laboratory
experiments with growing animals, they should not be
used in children unless the benefits outweigh the
theoretical risk (e.g., in severe illnesses such as typhoid
fever). Azithromycin is a commonly used alternative
for children. However, evidence regarding antibiotic

therapy for traveler's diarrhea in children is lacking, and antibiotics in children possibly infected with *E. coli* O157:H7 may increase the risk for hemolytic uremic syndrome (Ryan et al., 2002). Antimotility agents are not recommended for children though they may alleviate symptoms in adults with noninvasive pathogens (Ryan et al., 2002).

- *Investigate prolonged diarrhea with laboratory studies.* The generally accepted definition of prolonged diarrhea is 2 weeks for children and 4 weeks for adults. Often there may be signs of malabsorption such as weight loss (or for children, decreased weight velocity) and an oily film with bowel movements. If not already done, obtain a stool culture and stool O&P. The latter test may uncover a protozoal infection such as *Giardia, Cyclospora, Cryptosporidium* or *Entamoeba*; specific stool enzyme-linked immunosorbent assay (ELISA) and antigen detection tests are also available for these pathogens. Finding parasites on stool microscopy is not necessarily diagnostic, however, because refugees and travelers may also be infected with organisms such as *Ascaris* and hookworm that are not related to their symptoms. If the initial stool tests are nondiagnostic, consider repeating the O&P test two more times at least 48 hours apart. Other tests that might be helpful (Kolars & Fischer, 2002) include fecal leukocytes and occult blood to detect evidence of an invasive pathogen; a complete blood count to look for anemia, eosinophilia, or leukocytosis; and serum ELISA tests for specific pathogens such as *E. histolytica*, schistosomiasis, and *Strongyloides*. For patients with continued diarrhea and weight loss, consider referral to a gastroenterologist for further evaluation and possible endoscopy. Some patients with chronic diarrhea presumed to be from an infection may actually have a noninfectious illness such as

inflammatory bowel disease, celiac sprue,
tropical sprue, or irritable bowel syndrome (Kolars
& Fischer, 2002).

APPROACH TO THE EMERGENT PATIENT WITH CONSIDERATION OF BIOTERRORISM

An organized approach to the patient who presents
emergently with shock, respiratory distress, or severe
neurologic symptoms is essential. This is especially true
for refugees, immigrants, or travelers for whom unusual
diseases must be considered. Unfortunately, clinicians
also have to be aware of the possibility that their patients
may be victims of bioterrorism. Because there is some
overlap between bioterrorism agents and infectious
diseases of the developing world, we present them here
together.

Three categories of bioterrorism agents are described as
follows on the Centers for Disease Control and
Prevention (CDC) website (CDC, 2003):

- *Category A diseases/agents* are organisms that pose a
  threat to national security because they can be easily
  disseminated or transmitted from person to person;
  result in high mortality rates and have the potential
  for major public health impact; might cause public
  panic and social disruption; and require special action
  for public health preparedness. Examples of Category
  A diseases include anthrax, botulism, plague,
  smallpox, tularemia, and viral hemorrhagic fevers.
- *Category B diseases/agents* are organisms that are
  moderately easy to disseminate; result in moderate
  morbidity rates and low mortality rates; and require
  specific enhancements of CDC's diagnostic capacity
  and enhanced disease surveillance. Examples include
  brucellosis; food safety threats such as *Salmonella*,
  E. coli O157:H7, and *Shigella*; psittacosis; Q fever;

viral encephalitides; and water safety threats such as cholera and cryptosporidium.

- *Category C diseases/agents* are emerging pathogens such as hantavirus that could be engineered for mass dissemination in the future because of availability; ease of production and dissemination; and potential for high morbidity and mortality rates and major health impact.

A useful conceptual framework to approach the potential bioterrorism victim (Henretig, Cieslak, Kortepeter, & Fleisher, 2002) is an extension of advanced trauma life support (ATLS). Before beginning resuscitation, team members should wear protective clothing against blood and body fluids, including eye protection. If an inhalational biological agent is suspected, HEPA filter masks should also be worn. The first step is a primary survey that builds on the ABCs of life support with the three E's of epidemiology:

- **A:** Airway—Using cervical spine precautions if necessary, establish an airway using positioning, suction, or artificial airways.
- **B:** Breathing—Assess oxygenation and ventilation, giving supplemental oxygen and assisted ventilation as needed.
- **C:** Circulation—Assess heart rate, blood pressure, and perfusion. Obtain vascular access. Give fluids, medications, and chest compressions as appropriate.
- **D:** Disability—Evaluate the patient's neurologic status.
- **E:** Expose/environment—Undress the patient, assess for hypo- or hyperthermia, and treat accordingly.
- **E:** Epidemiology:

  Exposure history—Was the patient near an explosion, a visible cloud, some other delivery device, or known threat?

  Epidemic—Are there a number of patients with similar presentation clustered in space or time?

Exotic—Are there signs of unusual diseases or clinical syndromes?

- The primary survey is then quickly followed by a secondary survey as summarized in Table 3-1.
- To narrow the diagnosis, in each survey it is useful to think about whether the patient's findings fit a syndrome: acute respiratory distress with fever, neurologic

TABLE 3–1

Biological Attack Secondary Survey

Step	Mnemonic	Interpretation/Assessment and Action
1	A	Anticipate biological weapons incident (pattern recognition, multiple casualties, etc.)
2	B	Be careful (personal protection issues)
		• Standard precautions for most scenarios
		• When in doubt, use a mask and protect mucous membranes. If known plague, VHF, or smallpox, see specific measures in entry E1 and in text
3	C	Continue life support prn
4	D	Decontaminate, isolate patient as warranted
5	D2	Diagnosis
		• Succinct history: acuity of onset, exposure history, multiple patients, febrile prodrome, respiratory, neurologic, or dermatologic symptoms?
		• Focused physical examination: vital signs; cardiorespiratory, neurologic, and dermatologic findings?
		• Laboratory testing: chest radiograph; CBC, coagulation Studies
		• Diagnostic impressions

Table 3-1 continued

Step	Mnemonic	Interpretation/Assessment and Action
6	D3	(Drugs) treatment
7	E1	Epidemic infection control
		• Plague: droplet precautions
		• VHFs: contact droplet (consider airborne) precautions
		• Smallpox: airborne contact precautions
		• All others: standard precautions
8	E2	Epidemic reporting to law enforcement, public health
9	E3	Epidemiologic investigation
10	E4	Educate others

Source: From Henretig, F.M., Cieslak, T.J., Kortepeter, M.G., & Fleisher, G.R. (2002). Medical management of the suspected victim of bioterrorism: An algorithmic approach to the undifferentiated patient. *Emergency Medical Clinics of North America, 20,* 351-364. Abbreviations: CBC, Complete blood count; VHFs, viral hemorrhagic fevers.

syndrome, acute rash with fever, or influenza-like illness (Patt & Feigin, 2002). Respiratory distress or flu-like symptoms may be presenting signs of SARS, legionella, anthrax, tularemia, brucellosis, Q fever, or plague. Signs of a neurologic syndrome include flaccid paralysis (botulism) or encephalitis-like symptoms of fever, headache, myalgias, and altered levels of consciousness (Venezuelan equine encephalitis, Eastern equine encephalitis, and Western equine encephalitis). Dermatologic syndromes often present with rashes that clinicians should learn to readily identify, such as measles, meningococcemia, rickettsial diseases, hemorrhagic fevers, and smallpox. A syndromic diagnosis might not be possible immediately, because many of the preceding entities might present as an undifferentiated fever, especially early in the illness. In such cases, laboratory data might be the key to diagnosis.

Approach to Laboratory Diagnosis

In Table 3-2 we expand on the syndromic approach described in the previous section with more detailed information about laboratory and imaging studies. The table is adapted from one produced by the California State and Local Health Department Bioterrorism Surveillance and Epidemiology Working Group (2001), to which we have added information on nonbioterrorism diseases. Our intent here is not to encourage "fishing expeditions," but to summarize possible next steps toward establishing a diagnosis in an acutely ill patient after thoughtful application of an organized approach. Additional information about laboratory diagnosis may be found in the entries for individual diseases in later chapters.

Screening, Examination, and Immunizations for Newly Arrived Refugees

There are three common arrival points for refugees who flee their homeland during war or other crisis (Box 3-1). The first is a border camp in the country of first asylum where only the most basic health issues (life-threatening infectious diseases, sanitation, rudimentary shelter, and food and water) are addressed. The second arrival point or place of refuge is a more developed camp, usually a safe distance from the border and conflict. These camps generally have primary care clinics and only the most essential hospital services. The third arrival point is the country of second asylum, where a fortunate few refugees are resettled in a permanent new home. The huge majority of refugees never get past the first or second step. Among those who do find a permanent place of refuge, there are variations on this three-step process, such as people

TABLE 3-2 Laboratory and Imaging Studies for Possible Bioterrorism Syndromes

Syndrome	Differential Diagnoses	Laboratory, Imaging Studies*
Acute Respiratory Distress with Fever	Potential bioterrorism diseases	
	Inhalational anthrax	Chest x-ray with widened mediastinum; possible pleural effusion; gram-positive bacilli in sputum or blood
	Pneumonic plague	Gram-negative bacilli or coccobaccilli in sputum, blood, or lymph node; safety-pin appearance with Wright or Giemsa Stain
	Ricin (aerosolized)	Chest x-ray with pulmonary edema
	Staphylococcal enterotoxin B	Primarily clinical diagnosis; normal chest x-ray
	Other infectious diseases	
	Hantavirus pulmonary syndrome	ELISA for anti-Sin Nombre virus IgM; leukocytosis with atypical lymphocytes, left shift, and thrombocytopenia; chest x-ray with pulmonary edema
	SARS	RT-PCR for SARS coronavirus available, but low positive predictive value for patients without epidemiologic risk factors; serologic tests most accurate after 28 days from onset of illness

*For potential bioterrorism agents, consult your local public health laboratory for available tests and specimen collection procedures.

continued

Table 3–2 continued

Syndrome		Differential Diagnoses	Laboratory, Imaging Studies*
Acute Rash with Fever	Potential bioterrorism diseases	Smallpox	Clinical diagnosis; definitive tests (electron microscopy, gel diffusion, PCR) done on scabs or swabs of vesicular or pustular fluid
	Other infectious diseases	Viral hemorrhagic fevers (e.g., Ebola)	ELISA, PCR, viral culture; CBC may show profound lymphopenia followed by neutrophilia; thrombocytopenia
		Meningococcemia	Gram-negative cocci in Gram stain of CSF, scrapings from petechial or purpural lesion
		Rickettsiosis	Serologic tests useful after second week of illness; empiric therapy therefore started on basis of clinical diagnosis
		Leptospirosis	Dark-field microscopy of blood, CSF, and urine culture; serologic and DNA studies available
		Vaccinia	Rash following smallpox vaccination; PCR
		Monkeypox	Electron microscopy or gel diffusion done on vesicular scrapings
		Typhus	PCR; antibody tests cannot distinguish rickettsial species; CBC shows early leukopenia followed by leukocytosis

Neurologic Syndromes		
	Potential bioterrorism diseases	Botulism	CSF protein normal; EMG with repetitive nerve stimulation shows augmentation of muscle action potential; toxin assays of serum, feces, or gastric aspirate available.
	Other infectious diseases	Arboviral encephalitis (Venezuelan, Eastern equine, Western equine)	Serologic testing available at local public health laboratory
		Other viral encephalitides (e.g., HSV, enterovirus)	For HSV encephalitis, MRI and EEG may show temporal lobe involvement; PCR of CSF is sensitive and specific, brain biopsy is gold standard
		Lyme meningoencephalitis	ELISA for antibodies to *Borrelia burgdorferi*, with confirmation by Western immunoblot

*For potential bioterrorism agents, consult your local public health laboratory for available tests and specimen collection procedures.

continued

Table 3-2 continued

Syndrome		Differential Diagnoses	Laboratory, Imaging Studies*
Influenza-Like Illnesses	Potential bioterrorism diseases	Brucellosis	Tiny, slow-growing faintly staining gram-negative coccobacilli in blood or bone marrow culture. Leukocyte count normal or low. Anemia, thrombocytopenia possible. Chest x-ray nonspecific: normal, bronchopneumonia, abscesses, single or miliary nodules, enlarged hilar nodes, effusions. Serologic testing and culture available at local public health laboratory
		Tularemia	Small, faintly staining, slow-growing gram-negative coccobacilli in smears or cultures of sputum, blood. Chest x-ray may show infiltrate, hilar adenopathy, effusion. Definitive testing available at local public health laboratory
	Other infectious diseases	Influenza	Rapid serologic tests and fluorescent antibody tests
		Malaria	Microscopy of thick and thin blood smears; new rapid diagnostic tests available
		SARS	(See above.)

Source: Adapted from a table created by the California State and Local Health Department Bioterrorism Surveillance and Epidemiology Working Group, 2001.

*For potential bioterrorism agents, consult your local public health laboratory for available tests and specimen collection procedures.

DEFINITION OF THE TERM *REFUGEE*   BOX 3–1

A refugee is "any person who is outside any country of such person's nationality ... and who is unwilling or unable to return ... because of persecution or a well-founded fear of persecution on account of race, religion, nationality, membership in a particular social group, or political opinion" (United Nations High Commissioner for Refugees, 1992).

---

flying directly from their homeland to the new home. However, for most refugees who are resettled overseas, the process is similar to that just described.

Refugee health screening in the country of second asylum or new home is focused on identification of communicable diseases that pose public health risks. Countries that accept documented refugees and immigrants for permanent residency require a medical examination before or immediately after the person arrives. Persons admitted to the United States are screened before entry for communicable diseases of public health significance, documentation of immunizations, physical or mental disorders that may result in harm to self or others, and for drug addiction (American Public Health Association, 2002). Communicable diseases of public health significance in the United States include:

- Tuberculosis (note that negative chest X-rays and health documents are available for sale overseas, so that critical testing is best repeated in the domestic setting)
- HIV infection
- Syphilis
- Chancroid
- Gonorrhea
- Granuloma inguinale

- Lymphogranuloma venereum
- Hansen's disease.

Vaccine-preventable diseases are listed next, with vaccination for these required prior to entry or by the time of adjustment to permanent residence (CDC, 2002):

- Mumps
- Measles
- Rubella
- Polio
- Tetanus and diphtheria toxoids
- Pertussis
- Influenza type B
- Hepatitis B.

Depending on findings, a person may be granted entry, denied entry, or given a waiver for entry despite having a significant health condition (CDC, 2002).

In many cases, screening in the United States is rudimentary, consisting of a short history, vital signs, and testing for tuberculosis, sexually transmitted infections (STIs), and gastrointestinal parasites. Treatment for tuberculosis and STIs is commonly done through the local health department, while other health problems are referred to other facilities. Follow-up to monitor treatment for noninfectious diseases is uncommon. The net result of refugee screening in the United States is identification of a limited number of infectious diseases and ensuring that immunizations are current. In countries of second asylum, positive tuberculin skin tests are found in 42% to 53% of new arrivals, positive hepatitis B surface antigen in 5% to 15%, and gastrointestinal parasites in 19% to 36% (Hawn & Jong, 2003).

HEALTH RISKS AND SCREENING PARAMETERS

The following are general guidelines for health screening of refugees and immigrants. A more complete picture of

risks and screening parameters emerges when the following
"global" risks and screening parameters are examined, as
well as any current health issues globally or in the
countries of origin and asylum. The CDC website
(*www.cdc.gov/*) has an up-to-date section on worldwide
disease outbreaks and risks that should be consulted
when making decisions about refugee health issues.
Global risks and screening and laboratory
recommendations (Ackerman, 1997; CDC, 2002;
Gavagan & Brodyaga, 1998; Kemp, 2002; Minnesota
Department of Health, 2001) are as follows:

Health Risks: Global

- Malnutrition
- Intestinal parasites (especially amebiasis, giardiasis,
  ascariasis, strongyloidiasis, hookworm, trichuriasis,
  enterobiasis)
- Hepatitis B
- Tuberculosis
- Missed or incomplete immunizations rate (risk for
  measles, mumps, rubella, diphtheria, pertussis, tetanus)
- Dental caries
- Malaria
- STIs, including cervical cancer, HIV/AIDS, chancroid,
  chlamydia, gonorrhea, granuloma inguinale, LGV,
  syphilis
- Diarrheal illnesses
- Long-term effects of trauma, rape, torture (PTSD)
- Neonatal tetanus
- Rheumatic heart disease
- Among children, high lead levels are increasingly
  being seen worldwide.

Screening and Laboratory Recommendations (Global)

- Tuberculosis (purified protein derivative [PPD])
- Intestinal parasites (stool for O&P ×3)

- Hepatitis (including blood for hepatitis surface antigen [HBsAg], hepatitis B surface antibody [anti-HBs], and hepatitis B core antibody [anti-HBc])
- HIV (blood for ELISA and Western blot)
- Venereal Disease Research Laboratory/rapid plasma reagin (VDRL/RPR) for syphilis
- CBC with differential
- Urine analysis (UA) (if abnormal, consider urine culture, urine staining for acid-fast bacilli [AFB], or microscopic examination for ova & parasites)
- Other STIs (chancroid, gonorrhea, granuloma inguinale, LGV)
- Biopsy for AFB staining of skin lesions suspicious for Hansen's disease
- Immunization status
- Nutritional status.

Consider the following, based on history and findings:
- Malaria (thick and thin blood smears)
- Pregnancy test
- Varicella titer.

References

Ackerman, L.K. (1997). Health problems of refugees. *Journal of the American Board of Family Practice*, 10, 337-348.

American Public Health Association. (2002). Understanding the health culture of recent immigrants to the United States: A cross-cultural maternal health information catalog. Retrieved November 5, 2002, from *www.apha.org/ppp/red/index.htm*

California State and Local Health Department Bioterrorism Surveillance and Epidemiology Working Group. (2001). California bioterrorism surveillance and epidemiologic response plan Appendix E: Clinical descriptions for syndromes caused by priority biological and chemical threat agents. Retrieved September 29, 2003, from *www.dhs.cahwnet.gov/ps/dcdc/bt/*

Centers for Disease Control and Prevention. (2002). Medical examinations of aliens (refugees and immigrants). Retrieved November 11, 2002, from *www.cdc.gov/ncidod/dq/health.htm*

Centers for Disease Control and Prevention. (2003). Emergency preparedness and response: Biological agents and diseases. Retrieved September 27, 2003, from *www.bt.cdc.gov/agent/agentlist-category.asp*

Cunha, B. (1996). The clinical significance of fever patterns. *Infectious Disease Clinics of North America, 10,* 33-44.

Gavagan, T., & Brodyaga, L. (1998). Medical care for immigrants and refugees. *American Family Physician, 57,* 1061-1068.

Hawn, T.R., & Jong, E.C. (2003). Health screening in immigrants, refugees, and internationally adopted orphans. In E.C. Jong & R. McMullen (Eds.), *The travel and tropical medicine manual* (3rd ed., pp. 255-265). Philadelphia: W.B. Saunders Company.

Henretig, F.M., Cieslak, T.J., Kortepeter, M.G., & Fleisher, G.R. (2002). Medical management of the suspected victim of bioterrorism: An algorithmic approach to the undifferentiated patient. *Emergency Medical Clinics of North America, 20,* 351-364.

Humar, A., & Keystone, J. (1996). Evaluating fever in travellers returning from tropical countries. *British Medical Journal, 312,* 953-956.

Kemp, C. (2002). Infectious diseases: Bioterrorism & infectious diseases of refugees & immigrants. Retrieved November 20, 2002, from *www3.baylor.edu/~Charles_Kemp/Infectious_Disease.htm*

Kolars, J.C., & Fischer, P.R. (2002). Evaluation of diarrhea in the returned traveler. *Primary Care Clinics in Office Practice, 29,* 931-945.

McLellan, S.L. (2002). Evaluation of fever in the returned traveler. *Primary Care, 29,* 47-69.

Minnesota Department of Health. (2001). *Minnesota refugee health provider guide*. Minneapolis: Author.

Patt, H.A., & Feigin R.D. (2002). Diagnosis and management of suspected cases of bioterrorism: A pediatric perspective. *Pediatrics, 109,* 685-692.

Root, R. (1999). Host responses to infection: Fever, hyperthermia, and hypothermia. In R.K. Root, F. Waldvogel, L. Corey, & W. Stamm (Eds.), *Clinical infectious diseases, a practical approach* (pp. 71-81). Oxford: Oxford University Press.

Ryan, E.T., Wilson, M.E., & Kain, K.E. (2002). Illness after international travel. *New England Journal of Medicine, 347,* 505-516.

Solutions Made at Home. (2002). *Rehydration project.* Retrieved September 29, 2003, from *www.rehydrate.org/solutions/homemade.htm*

United Nations High Commissioner for Refugees. (1992). *Handbook on procedures and criteria for determining refugee status under the 1951 Convention and the 1967 Protocol relating to the status of refugees.* Retrieved September 22, 2003, from *www.unhcr.ch/cgi-bin/texis/vtx/home*

4

ACTINOMYCOSIS

Geographic Distribution

Actinomycosis is found worldwide but rarely.

Agent and Vector

The agents that cause actinomycosis are *Actinomyces israelii,* a gram-positive anaerobic bacterium (most common), other *Actinomyces* species, and *Arachnia propionica.* These are normal flora of the oropharynx, gastrointestinal tract, and female genitourinary tract. Infection is endogenous, usually related to disruption of the mucosa, as can happen with a dental procedure, poor dentition, or trauma (Chin, 2000; Scott, 2003).

Incubation

The incubation period is unknown and may be days to months after trauma (Chin, 2000).

Clinical Findings and Treatment

Signs and Symptoms

Common features include the following:
- Indurated, fibrotic lesions crossing tissue planes (fascia)
- Abscesses and tissue destruction
- Sinus tracts with purulent discharge containing yellow or white sulfur granules (Felz & Smith, 2003).

The most common sites of actinomycosis are as follows (Felz & Smith, 2003; Hay & Smego, 2000; Tedeschi et al., 2003):
- *Cervicofacial (especially mandibular).* Infection begins with one or more soft, slightly swollen lesions that

become inflamed, with overlying mucous membranes developing an uneven texture. The lesions become indurated and then suppurate through one or more sinus tracts in the cervicofacial area, including the scalp in some cases.

- *Thoracic.* The thorax, including lungs, pleura, mediastinum, or chest wall, is usually a secondary site with spread via aspiration or extension from the cervicofacial area or the abdomen.
- *Abdominal.* Abdominal actinomycosis is associated with abdominal surgery, especially surgery for acute appendicitis, and with trauma. The most common early manifestation is a tender mass in the lower right quadrant. Because the infection is difficult to diagnose, it may have spread throughout the abdomen and involve multiple systems and multiple fistulae by the time of diagnosis.
- *Pelvic.* Pelvic actinomycosis is associated with long-term use of an intrauterine device (IUD), although the risk of infection is not a contraindication for an IUD. As with other actinomycosis infections, the development of sinus tracts or fistulae is common.

Actinomycosis may appear at other sites as well, such as skin, central nervous system (CNS), bone, and pericardium.

Complications

The infection may extend to the CNS or the thorax (Scott, 2003). Bowel obstruction may occur with abdominal actinomycosis.

Common Laboratory Findings

Laboratory findings are limited to isolation of gram-positive anaerobic branching filamentous rods of the genus *Actinomyces* or *Arachnia*.

Diagnosis

The presence of sulfur granule–containing sinus exudates strongly suggests actinomycosis. Confirmation is through microscopic examination of pus and granules, as well as anaerobic culture (Scott, 2003).

Differential Diagnosis

Differential diagnoses are according to the site of infection as follows:
- *Cervicofacial.* Dental abscess or other lesions of the oropharynx.
- *Thoracic.* Tuberculosis, cancer.
- *Abdominal.* Amebiasis, appendix mass, enteritis, Crohn's disease, ileocecal tuberculosis, diverticulitis.
- *Other.* Impetigo, nocardiosis, other fungal infection; with orthopedic manifestations, differential may include osteomyelitis, septic arthritis, tuberculosis.

Treatment

Penicillin G is the drug of choice, given IV or IM at 5 to 10 million units/24 hours for 6 weeks. This is followed by PO penicillin (500 mg qid) or amoxicillin (500 mg tid) for 2 to 12 months. Surgical drainage and debridement usually are necessary. Penicillin V is not effective, at least for initial therapy. Other effective antibiotics include sulfonamide, erythromycin, chloramphenicol, ceftriaxone, and tetracycline (Felz & Smith, 2003; Scott, 2003).

Prevention

There are no known means of prevention, except that good dental hygiene may reduce colonization of the oropharynx. IUDs should not be left in place for longer than recommended (Chin, 2000).

Reporting

— The U.S. Centers for Disease Control and Prevention does not consider actinomycosis to be a nationally notifiable disease, nor does the World Health Organization (WHO) classify it as a disease important in public health (Class 5). See Appendix C for details and for upcoming changes in WHO reporting.

References

Chin, J. (2000). Actinomycosis. In J. Chin (Ed.), *Control of communicable diseases manual* (17th ed., pp. 9-11). Washington, DC: American Public Health Association.

Felz, M.W., & Smith, M.R. (2003). Disseminated actinomycosis: Multisystem mimicry in primary care. *Southern Medical Journal, 96,* 294-299.

Hay, R.J., & Smego, R.A. (2000). Actinomycosis. In G.T. Strickland (Ed.), *Hunter's tropical medicine and emerging infectious diseases* (8th ed., pp. 316-317). Philadelphia: W.B. Saunders Company.

Scott, G. (2003). Actinomycosis. In G.C. Cook & A.I. Zumla (Eds.), *Manson's tropical diseases* (21st ed., pp. 1091-1093). Philadelphia: W.B. Saunders Company.

Tedeschi, A., Di Mezza, G., D'Amico, O., Ermann, A., Montone, L., et al. (2003). A case of pelvic actinomycosis presenting as cutaneous fistula. *European Journal of Obstetrics & Gynecology and Reproductive Biology, 108,* 103-105.

5

AMEBIASIS

Amebic dysentery, amoebiasis, hepatic amebiasis

Geographic Distribution

— Amebiasis occurs worldwide.

Agent and Vector

— The cysts of the ameba *Entamoeba histolytica* are ingested via water or food contaminated with human feces. The organisms then excyst and colonize the intestinal lumen as trophozoites, which reproduce asexually. Cysts shed in the stool continue the life cycle. Inflammation occurs when the trophozoites penetrate the intestinal mucosa (Centers for Disease Control and Prevention [CDC], 1999; Farthing, Cevallos, & Kelly, 2003).

Incubation

— The incubation period for amebic dysentery is usually 1 to 4 weeks, but may be shorter or substantially longer. Hepatic amebiasis can present anywhere from 2 to 5 months after exposure (CDC, 1999).

Clinical Findings and Treatment

Signs and Symptoms

— About 90% of infected persons are asymptomatic. There are two basic types of amebiasis, intestinal and extraintestinal disease, which may exist simultaneously. In symptomatic intestinal amebiasis, common signs and symptoms include fever, gradual onset of colicky abdominal pain, increased number of stools (often intermittent, with more than six stools daily, sometimes containing mucus and gross blood),

jaundice, anorexia, weight loss, and tenesmus. Severe
infections may have an acute onset and be characterized
by abdominal pain, frequent and profuse bloody diarrhea
(sometimes containing necrotic tissue), more rapid
weight loss, and greater potential for dehydration. Rarely,
a form of chronic amebic colitis develops that mimics
ulcerative colitis.

— The most common extraintestinal infection is hepatic
amebiasis (amebic liver abscess), which occurs more
commonly in males and is rare in children. Symptoms of
hepatic amebiasis include a gradual or acute onset of
fever, right upper quadrant pain (sometimes radiating to
the right shoulder), hepatomegaly and tenderness, nausea
and vomiting, anorexia, weight loss, and malaise.
Intercostal tenderness is common, and rales may be heard
over the right lung base. Prompt treatment is necessary
to prevent the abscess from rupturing. Other extraintestinal
infections include perianal skin infections and rare
metastatic infections to the brain, lungs, and genitalia
(Chin, 2000; Farthing et al., 2003; Haque, Huston,
Hughes, Houpt, & Petri, 2003; Hughes, 2000).

Complications

— Untreated patients especially in less developed areas of
the world may develop megacolon, vomiting, high fever,
dehydration, and circulatory collapse. Amebomas
(amebic granulomas) can mimic colon carcinoma.
Fulminant necrotizing colitis is rare (less than 0.5% of
cases) but carries a high mortality rate. It presents with
fever, toxic appearance, bloody mucoid stools, and
peritoneal signs. Perforation of hepatic abscesses may
lead to peritonitis, pericarditis, and pleurisy
(Farthing et al., 2003; Haque et al., 2003).

Common Laboratory Findings

— Multiple fresh stool examinations in optimal conditions
will only detect organisms in about 80% of the

infections because the trophozoites (immature amebas, Figure 5-1) rapidly autolyze. If a patient has taken antibiotics, antimalarials, antidiarrheals, laxatives, or mineral oil, specimen collection should be delayed for 10 to 14 days. Three negative fecal ova & parasite (O&P) tests are needed to effectively rule out infection. Stool guaiac is usually positive and eosinophilia is sometimes present. Patients with more than mild dysentery often have a mild to moderate leukocytosis (CDC, 2003; Farthing et al., 2003; Haque et al., 2003).

Diagnosis

Detection of fecal trophozoites containing digested red blood cells is diagnostic. Microscopy however cannot distinguish *E. histolytica* cysts from those of nonpathogenic species such as *E. dispar* and *E. moshkovskii*. For this purpose stool antigen and DNA tests are available that are specific for *E. histolytica*. Endoscopy is used when stools are negative but suspicion is high. Serologic testing is available but is only 70% sensitive for intestinal amebiasis. A positive serum antibody can be a

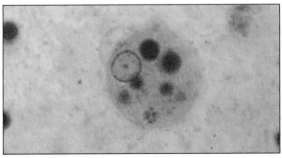

FIGURE 5–1

Trophozoites of intestinal protozoa. (*Source:* From Peters, W. & Pasvol, G. [2002]. *Tropical medicine and parasitology* [5th ed., p. 172]. Chicago: Mosby.)

result of either the avirulent *E. dispar* or *E. histolytica*. The indirect hemagglutination test is sensitive but will not distinguish past from present infections. The agar gel method of serologic testing is less sensitive but is just as specific. For hepatic amebiasis, imaging of the liver and biliary tree is essential. Computed tomography (CT) scans are sensitive but not specific, whereas ultrasound is fast, less expensive but a little less sensitive than CT (CDC, 2003; Farthing et al., 2003; Haque et al., 2003).

Differential Diagnosis

Differentials in diarrheal illness include inflammatory bowel disease (e.g., ulcerative colitis), bacillary dysentery, viral gastroenteritis, diverticulitis, appendicitis, carcinoma, tuberculosis, and irritable bowel syndrome. Because corticosteroid therapy for presumed inflammatory bowel disease can lead to potentially fatal toxic megacolon in a person with intestinal amebiasis, it is important to rule out amebiasis in patients with chronic diarrhea. In hepatic amebiasis, differentials include cholecystitis, cancer, pyogenic abscess, and echinococcal cyst (Farthing et al., 2003; Haque et al., 2003).

Treatment

Pharmacotherapy for *E. histolytica* includes tissue amebicides such as dehydroemetine, emetine, and metronidazole that act on amebas in the bowel wall but not the lumen, and luminal amebicides such as diloxanide furoate, iodoquinol, and paromomycin. Tetracycline inhibits growth in both the bowel wall and lumen. Treatment is indicated for *E. histolytica* even in asymptomatic individuals to reduce the risk of invasive disease and transmission to others, but is usually not needed for nonpathogenic *E. dispar*. Asymptomatic patients are treated with iodoquinol 30 to 40 mg/kg/ 24 hours (maximum: 650 mg/dose) PO tid for 20 days or paromomycin 25 to 35 mg/kg/24 hours PO tid for 7 days. Diloxanide furoate is available only from the CDC for treatment of asymptomatic amebiasis.

— Patients with symptomatic amebiasis should be treated with metronidazole 30 to 50 mg/kg/24 hours (maximum: 500 to 700 mg/dose) PO tid for 10 days. This amount of metronidazole often causes severe nausea, which can be prevented in adults by taking promethazine 1 hour prior to dosing. Patients should also be counseled to avoid alcohol because of metronidazole's disulfiram-like properties. Tinidazole, which is related to metronidazole but has a longer half-life, causes fewer adverse reactions but is not available in the United States. Though metronidazole has a 90% response rate for patients with mild to moderate symptoms, around 50% of patients treated with metronidazole alone will have persistent intraluminal infection and remain at risk for relapse. Therefore, metronidazole should be followed by a luminal agent such as paromomycin or diloxanide furoate. Treat hepatic amebiasis with metronidazole 750 mg PO tid for 10 days or 500 mg IV every 6 hours (35 to 50 mg/kg/24 hours for children) for 10 days followed by paromomycin, iodoquinol, or diloxanide furoate. Chloroquine may be substituted for metronidazole in patients who cannot tolerate or are not responding to therapy.

— Ultrasound or CT-guided aspiration of liver abscesses by percutaneous catheter or needle should be considered for patients who have lesions at increased risk for rupture (i.e., left hepatic lobe involvement or fluid collections greater than 5 cm) or who are not responding to treatment. Antibiotics may also be added to cover the possibility of coexisting bacterial infection. In most cases of amebic liver abscess, clinical improvement occurs within a few days to a week, but complete radiologic resolution may take 3 to 9 months on average; repeated imaging is unnecessary unless symptoms recur. Follow-up care includes confirming cure by examination of stools starting at 4 weeks and up to 3 months after the end of treatment (Farthing et al., 2003; Haque et al., 2003; Hughes, 2000; Rosenblatt, 1999; Weissman & Salata, 2000).

Prevention

Preventive measures (Chin, 2000) include the following:
- Wash hands thoroughly after toileting and before handling or eating food.
- Protect public water supplies from contamination with human waste.
- Boil potentially contaminated water for at least 5 minutes. Iodine crystals or tablets may be used according to packaging instructions to purify small amounts of water. Water treatment tablets containing chlorine are not effective at preventing amebiasis.
- Wash fruits and vegetables in potable water and keep dry. Although washing fruits and vegetables offers incomplete protection, they should nevertheless be washed and kept dry because desiccation does kill cysts. Disinfectant dips are of unproven value.
- Dispose of human feces in a sanitary manner to avoid water supply contamination.
- Treat known carriers and educate on measures to prevent reinfection.
- Educate high-risk groups on the dangers of sexual practices that promote fecal-oral transmission.

Community education regarding the preceding measures should be ongoing in high-risk areas or populations. Chemoprophylaxis is not advised (Chin, 2000).

Reporting

The CDC does not consider amebiasis to be a nationally notifiable disease, nor does the World Health Organization (WHO) classify it as a disease important in public health (Class 3C). However, an outbreak would be classified as an acute diarrheal syndrome outbreak by the WHO and should be reported. See Appendix C for details and for upcoming changes in WHO reporting.

References

Centers for Disease Control and Prevention. (1999). *Amebiasis infection.* Retrieved January 9, 2000, from *www.cdc.gov/ncidod/dpd/amebias.htm*

Centers for Disease Control and Prevention. (2003). *Parasites and health: Amebiasis.* Retrieved July 12, 2003, from *www.dpd.cdc.gov/dpdx/HTML/Amebiasis.htm*

Chin, J. (2000). Amebiasis. In J. Chin (Ed.), *Control of communicable diseases manual* (17th ed., pp. 11-13). Washington, DC: American Public Health Association.

Farthing, M.J.G., Cevallos, A.M., & Kelly, P. (2003). Intestinal protozoa. In G.C. Cook & A. Zumla (Eds.), *Manson's tropical diseases* (21st ed., pp. 1373-1410). Philadelphia: W.B. Saunders Company.

Haque. R., Huston, C.D., Hughes, M., Houpt, E., & Petri, W.A. (2003). Amebiasis. *New England Journal of Medicine, 348,* 1565-73.

Hughes, M.A. (2000). Amebic liver abscess. *Infectious Disease Clinics of North America, 14,* 565-582.

Rosenblatt, J.E. (1999). Antiparasitic agents. *Mayo Clinic Proceedings, 74,* 1161-1175.

Weissman, S., & Salata, R. (2000). Amebiasis. In R. Behrman, R. Kliegman, & H. Jenson (Eds.), *Nelson textbook of pediatrics* (16th ed., pp. 1035-1036). Philadelphia: W.B. Saunders Company

ANISAKIDOSIS

Formerly anisakiasis; also codworm disease, herring worm, whale worm

Geographic Distribution

Anywhere raw fish is eaten, especially Japan, Central and South America, and Europe.

Agent and Vector

Anisakis species and *Pseudoterranova decipiens* are nematodes (roundworms) whose third-stage larvae infect the stomach or intestinal wall of humans. The adult worms live in clusters in the stomachs of marine mammals such as dolphins or whales (or in the case of *Pseudoterranova*, in the stomachs of pinnipedia such as seals or sea lions). The eggs are discharged into cold seawater where they hatch, and second-stage larvae are consumed by small crustaceans in which the larvae develop to the third stage. The crustaceans are consumed by larger fish or squid, which, in turn, are consumed by larger fish. In most fish, the larvae live in the viscera, but in a few (herring, mackerel, cod, salmon, halibut, red snapper, and squid), the larvae are found in the flesh of the fish. When the raw or inadequately cooked flesh (including smoked, salted, or pickled) is eaten by humans, the larvae penetrate the stomach or intestinal wall where hemorrhage and inflammation occur. In severe cases, eosinophilic granulomas form; in chronic cases, abscesses form. The larvae may also migrate up the alimentary tract to the esophagus (Bouree, Paugam, & Petithory, 1995; Chin, 2000).

Incubation

Symptoms of stomach invasion occur a few hours after ingestion of infected fish and symptoms of bowel invasion usually occur 1 to 2 days or longer after infection (Bouree et al., 1995; Chin, 2000).

Clinical Findings and Treatment

Signs and Symptoms

Manifestations vary according to primary site of infection, which is strongly related to geographic area of infection. For example, more than 90% of cases in Japan are gastric; elsewhere, 75% are intestinal, 15% are ectopic, and only 10% are gastric (Sudduth, 2000). Signs and symptoms of anisakidosis (Bouree et al., 1995; Castan et al., 2002; Daschner et al., 1998; McCarthy & Moore, 2000) include:

- *Acute gastric anisakidosis.* A somewhat variable presentation with an acute onset of progressive cramping epigastric pain in about 50% of patients within hours of ingesting infected fish. Less common symptoms include chest pain, indigestion-like pain, allergic symptoms (urticaria and angioedema), and/or melena.
- *Acute intestinal anisakidosis.* Manifests 1 or more days after ingestion of infected fish with sudden-onset colicky lower (or diffuse) abdominal pain, nausea, vomiting, ascites, bowel obstruction, and/or diarrhea.
- *Chronic anisakidosis.* May be indolent, with vague or intermittent symptoms similar to gastritis, peptic ulcer disease, inflammatory bowel disease, and other GI disorders.
- *Ectopic anisakidosis.* Rare and usually involves the gastrointestinal system, with variable symptoms.

In most cases, only one worm is present. In all cases, fever is either slight or absent. The presence of allergic symptoms, especially urticaria and angioedema, is relatively common, and in some cases may be the chief complaint with GI symptoms unnoticed.

Complications

— Bowel obstruction occurs rarely; allergic reaction may be severe. Ectopic anisakidosis is rare and difficult to diagnosis.

Common Laboratory Findings

— Leukocytosis is inconsistent and eosinophilia is uncommon in acute disease. Free peritoneal fluid may be shown on ultrasonography (Castan et al., 2002).

Diagnosis

— Ingestion of raw fish and characteristic symptoms arouse suspicion, which in the case of gastric anisakidosis is confirmed with endoscopy. Diagnosis of intestinal disease is based primarily on history and presentation (acute abdomen preceded by ingestion of raw fish), but given the abdominal presentation, surgery often occurs and the diagnosis then follows. Castan et al. (2002) report diagnosis of intestinal anisakidosis may be made on the basis of presentation and ultrasonography showing free peritoneal fluid, thickened intestinal wall, or intestinal dilatation (McCarthy & Moore, 2000; Suddarth, 2000).

Differential Diagnosis

— Appendicitis, peritonitis, peptic ulcer, cholecystitis, diverticulitis, Crohn's disease, and cancer are among the differentials.

Treatment

— In some cases of gastric anisakidosis, the patient regurgitates the worm and symptoms then resolve. For patients with severe symptoms, removal of the worm during endoscopy early in the illness is the preferred therapy. The disease is usually self-limiting and treatment is supportive, including fasting, fluids, and treatment of symptoms (Castan et al., 2002; Sudduth, 2000).

Prevention

Preventive measures (Chin, 2000) include the following:
- Avoiding consumption of raw or incompletely cooked fish, including that which is smoked, pickled, or salted.
- Freezing at −23° C (−10° F) kills the larvae.
- Eviscerating fish quickly after they are caught minimizes migration from mesentery to flesh.
- Community education regarding the above measures.

Reporting

The U.S. Centers for Disease Control and Prevention does not consider anisakidosis to be a nationally notifiable disease.

References

Bouree, P., Paugam, A., & Petithory, J.C. (1995). Anisakidosis: Report of 25 cases and review of the literature. *Comparative Immunology, Microbiology & Infectious Diseases, 18,* 75-84.

Castan, B., Borda, F., Inarrairaegui, M., Pastor, G., Vila, J., & Zozaya, J.M. (2002). Digestive anisakiasis: Clinical manifestations and diagnosis according to localization. *Revista Espanola de Enfermedadas Digestivas, 94,* 463-472.

Chin, J. (2000). Anisakiasis. In J. Chin (Ed.), *Control of communicable diseases manual* (17th ed., pp. 18-19). Washington, DC: American Public Health Association.

Daschner, A., Alonso-Gomez, A., Caballero, T., Barranco, P., Suarez-De-Parga, J.M., & Lopez-Serrano, M.C. (1998). Gastric anisakiasis: An underestimated cause of acute urticaria and angio-oedema? *British Journal of Dermatology, 139,* 822-828.

McCarthy, J., & Moore, T.A. (2000). Emerging helminth zoonoses. *International Journal for Parasitology, 30,* 1351-1360.

Sudduth, R.H. (2000). Anisakidosis. In G.T. Strickland (Ed.), *Hunter's tropical medicine and emerging infectious diseases* (8th ed., pp. 799-801). Philadelphia: W.B. Saunders Company.

ANTHRAX

Geographic Distribution

Anthrax may occur in any temperate or tropical rural area where animal husbandry is common, including in Latin America, Southern and Eastern Europe, Africa, and Asia (Chin, 2000). Also see later discussion in this chapter of anthrax as a biological weapon.

Agent and Vector

Bacillus anthracis is a hardy gram-positive spore-forming aerobic rod that causes cutaneous or pulmonary infection. Because its skin lesions consist of a black eschar, its name is derived from the Greek *anthrakis,* meaning coal. The vegetative form of *B. anthracis* survives poorly outside a mammalian host, but forms hardy spores when in a nutrient-poor environment and exposed to ambient air (Inglesby et al., 2002). The spores can then survive for decades outside a host, germinating rapidly when reintroduced into a nutrient-rich environment. On microscopy, *B. anthracis* bacilli have a unique "jointed bamboo rod" appearance, and its colonies resemble "curled hair" (Chin, 2000; Dixon, Meselson, Guiillemin, & Hannah, 1999; Inglesby et al., 2002).

ROUTES OF INFECTION

Large epidemics of anthrax have been described among herbivores who contract the disease from spores in the soil. For humans, anthrax may be spread through gastrointestinal, cutaneous, or inhalational routes. Person-to-person transmission is not known to occur. Gastrointestinal spread involves the ingestion of undercooked contaminated meat. Naturally occurring cutaneous anthrax accounts for more than 95% of cases and is contracted primarily through direct inoculation of a break in the skin in contact with an infected animal, often as a part of occupational exposure. It is anthrax's inhalational spread that makes it a potent biological weapon (Box 7-1). Inhaled spores are carried by pulmonary macrophages to tracheobronchial or mediastinal lymph nodes where the *B. anthracis* multiplies and produces at

---

BIOTERRORISM CONSIDERATIONS   BOX 7-1

The CDC categorizes anthrax as a Category A biological warfare agent because it "can be easily disseminated ...; cause high mortality, with potential for major public health impact; might cause public panic and social disruption; and require special action for public health preparedness" (Rotz, Khan, Lillibridge, Ostroff, & Hughes, 2002, p. 226). Potential delivery systems include bombs, disguised cigarette lighters, and, of course, letters. Anthrax has been weaponized by several countries, including the former Soviet Union, the United States, and Iraq (Cieslak & Eitzen, 1999; Shoham, 2000). In a U.S. experiment performed in the 1960s in the South Pacific, sprayed anthrax spores traveled more than 60 miles before losing infectiousness (Inglesby et al., 2002). It has been estimated that release of 100 kg of anthrax spores upwind of Washington, D.C., would result in up to 3,000,000 deaths (U.S. Congress, 1993). It is not known how long aerosolized anthrax spores remain viable in the environment, but experience with accidents in the former Soviet Union indicate a maximum of 45 days (Inglesby et al., 2002 Shoham, 2000). In attacks in 2001 that remain unsolved, 22 cases of anthrax were caused by spores mailed in letters. Because no naturally occurring cases of inhalational anthrax have occurred since 1976, even a single case of anthrax should raise suspicion for a possible attack (Inglesby et al., 2002).

least three proteins: edema factor (or toxin) (EF), lethal factor (LF), and protective antigen (PA), the latter of which is a carrier molecule for EF and LF. These toxins (EF + PA and LF + PA) cause lymphatic tissue necrosis, which releases large numbers of *B. anthracis* that cause overwhelming septicemia and death (Centers for Disease Control and Prevention [CDC], 1999; Dixon et al., 1999; Inglesby et al., 2002; Lew, 2000).

Incubation

The incubation period is usually 1 to 7 days but may be as long as 60 days (Chin, 2000).

Clinical Findings and Treatment

Signs and Symptoms

Cutaneous anthrax lesions begin as a painless pruritic papule that 24 to 36 hours later develops central necrosis, becoming a painless black eschar surrounded by purplish vesicles and moderate to severe edema. Common sites of infection are the head, forearms, and hands. Cutaneous lesions resolve without scarring or complications 80% to 90% of the time (Dixon et al., 1999).

In gastrointestinal anthrax, fever and abdominal pain are sometimes accompanied by either diarrhea or constipation. Stools may be blood tinged or melenic, and vomitus may also have either blood or a "coffee-grounds" appearance. On examination, rebound tenderness is present. Two to 4 days after the onset of symptoms, abdominal pain decreases and ascites develops (Dixon et al., 1999).

Inhalational anthrax is usually biphasic in presentation, beginning with a prodrome of nonspecific febrile flu-like illness with low-grade fever, malaise, headache, nonproductive cough, precordial discomfort or pressure, and myalgia. After 1 to 4 days there is sometimes a brief period of slight improvement, followed by rapid deterioration marked by fever and respiratory distress, including some or all of the following: dyspnea, stridor, cyanosis, increased chest pain, diaphoresis, and sometimes subcutaneous edema of neck and chest. Pneumonia is usually not present, but pleural effusions may be present. Chest X-rays show a pathognomonic widened mediastinum as early as the second day after exposure (Figure 7-1), and effusions may be seen on computed tomography of the chest.

This second phase of respiratory distress is followed by shock and often death. Without treatment the case fatality rate is probably around 90%; treatment started after 48 hours still carries a high fatality rate (Cieslak & Eitzen, 1999; Friedlander, 2000; Inglesby et al., 2002). Experience in treating cases of inhalation anthrax in the attack of fall of 2001 indicates that death rates

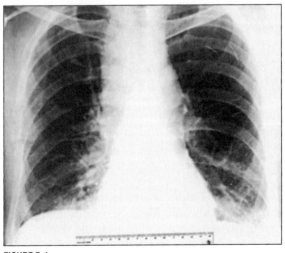

FIGURE 7–1

Chest X-ray showing the widened mediastinum of inhalational anthrax. (*Source:* From Strickland, G.T. [2000]. *Hunter's tropical medicine and emerging infectious diseases* [8th ed.]. Philadelphia: W.B. Saunders Company.)

may be lower than previously thought. If mass exposures occur, yet another story may emerge.

Complications

— Untreated cutaneous anthrax tends to spread to regional lymphatics and progress to overwhelming sepsis with a case fatality rate of around 20% (Chin, 2000). A rare complication is malignant edema with induration, bullae formation, airway obstruction (from neck and thoracic involvement), and shock.

— The bowel ulceration of gastrointestinal anthrax may lead to local necrosis, profound blood loss, shock, and perforation. If these complications do not occur, recovery usually occurs in 10 to 14 days (Dixon et al., 1999).

— Inhalational anthrax is complicated by hemorrhagic meningitis in about 50% of cases. This complication occurs 1 to 6 days after the onset of illness and is almost always fatal.

Common Laboratory Findings

— In the 2001 anthrax attacks, patients had a median white blood cell count of 9800, with most having more than 70% neutrophils. Elevated transaminases were observed, as was metabolic acidosis. Animal models of severe anthrax infection have demonstrated hypocalcemia, hyperkalemia, hypoglycemia, and profound metabolic acidosis with respiratory alkalosis (Inglesby et al., 2002).

Diagnosis

— As we saw in the 2001 anthrax attacks, patients in the first stage of an attack would likely be misdiagnosed as having viral upper respiratory infections, and many people would simply self-medicate. Some would seek care, and the influx of large numbers of otherwise healthy people with the first-stage symptomatology described earlier might arouse suspicion. With large numbers of patients presenting in the second stage of illness, it would be clear that a disaster (either anthrax or pneumonic plague) is unfolding as otherwise healthy people present in a toxic febrile condition with severe respiratory distress and cyanosis without clinical evidence of pneumonia. As mentioned, the widened mediastinum on chest radiography is pathognomic of inhalation anthrax. Gram stain of infected fluid (pleural fluid for inhalational anthrax, peritoneal fluid for gastrointestinal anthrax, cerebrospinal fluid for anthrax meningitis) shows typical gram-positive bacilli. The diagnosis is confirmed by culturing *B. anthracis* from blood or body fluids or on autopsy (Cieslak & Eitzen, 1999; Friedlander, 2000; Inglesby et al., 2002). Suspected cutaneous anthrax lesions can be confirmed by culture and Gram stain of carefully collected vesicular fluid, but specimen collection carries the danger of spreading the infection. Other methods of laboratory diagnosis such as polymerase chain reaction and immunohistochemical staining are only available through the Laboratory Response Network sponsored by the CDC and the Association of Public Health Laboratories (Inglesby et al., 2002).

Differential Diagnosis

When cutaneous anthrax is suspected, other diagnoses to entertain include human orf, staphylococcal lymphadenitis (usually painful), ecthyma gangrenosum, plague, or mycobacterial infection (cutaneous tuberculosis, leprosy, Buruli ulcer). Patients with gastrointestinal anthrax have symptoms that may resemble acute gastroenteritis, peritonitis, obstruction, peptic ulcer, typhoid, or intestinal tularemia. The differential diagnosis for the initial stage of inhalational anthrax includes influenza-like upper respiratory infections, viral pneumonia, mycoplasma pneumonia, and other bacterial pneumonias. For patients presenting with second-stage symptoms, consider the possibilities of ruptured or dissecting aortic aneurysm or pneumonic plague (Chin, 2000; Dixon et al., 1999).

Treatment

Early treatment is essential; obtain specimens for culture and begin empiric antibiotic therapy immediately while waiting for a definitive diagnosis (Table 7-1). Consult an infectious disease specialist if available. Naturally occurring anthrax can be successfully treated with penicillin, but in a biological weapon attack, penicillin resistance is possible. All treatment is for a total of 60 days of therapy to cover the possibility of delayed spore germination. If vaccine is widely available, administration of three doses of anthrax vaccine at 0, 2, and 4 weeks may allow antibiotic treatment to be shortened to 30 to 45 days (Inglesby et al., 2002). Intravenous antibiotics are recommended for gastrointestinal anthrax, inhalational anthrax, and cutaneous anthrax with signs of systemic involvement, extensive edema, or head and neck lesions (Dixon et al., 1999). Though controlled trials are lacking, in the face of life-threatening infection adding 1 or 2 other antimicrobials to the regimens discussed may improve outcomes (Inglesby et al., 2002).

Prevention

See Table 7-1 for postexposure prophylaxis. Person-to-person transmission is not known to occur, hence universal precautions with hospitalized patients are sufficient. Environmental surfaces can be cleaned with standard hospital disinfectants. It is essential that bodies (human and animal) be disposed of quickly. Bodies should not be embalmed. Cremation or deep burial in lime are the ideal means of body disposal. Vaccine is available for persons at high risk. In industrial settings where potentially contaminated materials are handled, for example, raw animal materials processing, the following practices should be followed:

- Ventilation should be adequate to remove dust.

TABLE 7-1

Anthrax Treatment

1. Mass Casualties or Postexposure Treatment	
Adults	Ciprofloxacin 500 mg PO every 12 hours. If the strain of *B. anthracis* is susceptible, amoxicillin 500 mg PO every 8 hours or doxycycline 100 mg PO every 12 hours.
Children	Ciprofloxacin 20 to 30 mg/kg/24 hours PO every 12 hours (not exceeding 1 g/24 hours). Doxycycline may be given if the use of ciprofloxacin is precluded. If the strain of *B. anthracis* is susceptible, children who weigh 20 kg or more can be given amoxicillin 500 mg PO every 8 hours. Children weighing less than 20 kg can be given amoxicillin 40 mg/kg/24 hours divided into three doses taken every 8 hours.
2. Contained Casualties Treatment*	
Adults	Ciprofloxacin 400 mg IV every 12 hours or doxycycline 100 mg IV every 12 hours until the patient's condition improves, at which time ciprofloxacin 500 mg PO or doxycycline 100 mg PO every 12 hours is given.
Children	Ciprofloxacin 20 to 30 mg/kg/24 hours IV divided every 12 hours (not to exceed 1 g/24 hours), changing to PO when clinically indicated. Doxycycline can also be used. Children older than age 8 and over 45 kg receive the adult dose; children age 8 and younger or weighing 45 kg or less receive 2.2 mg/kg IV every 12 hours.

Source: From CDC, 1999; Friedlander, 2000; Inglesby et al., 2002.
*With initial IV therapy, use 1 or 2 additional antimicrobials such as rifampin, vancomycin, penicillin, ampicillin, chloramphenicol, imipenem, clindamycin, or clarithromycin.

- Protective clothing should be worn.
- Facilities for personal hygiene and changing clothes after work should be used and are required by some governments.
- Food should be eaten away from areas where animal products are processed.

- Hair, wool, bone meal, and other feed of animal origin should be disinfected before processing.
- Rendering plants should be controlled and monitored to prevent effluents and wastes from contaminating soil near at-risk industrial settings.
- Suspicious illnesses (especially skin lesions) should be monitored in high-risk employees.
- Animals at risk should be immunized and their immunizations kept current.
- Employees should be educated about disease transmission, prevention, and signs and symptoms of infection (Chin, 2000; Scott, 2003).

Reporting

The CDC considers anthrax to be a nationally notifiable disease, and the World Health Organization (WHO) classifies it as a disease important in public health (Class 2A). See Appendix C for details and for upcoming changes in WHO reporting.

References

Centers for Disease Control and Prevention. (1999). Bioterrorism alleging use of anthrax and interim guidelines for management—United States, 1998. *Morbidity and Mortality Weekly Report, 48,* 69-74.

Chin, J. (Ed.). (2000). *Control of communicable diseases manual* (17th ed.). Washington, DC: American Public Health Association.

Cieslak, T.J., & Eitzen, E.M. (1999). Clinical and epidemiologic principles of anthrax. *Emerging Infectious Diseases, 5,* 552-555.

Dixon, T.C., Meselson, M., Guiillemin, J., & Hannah, P.C. (1999) Anthrax. *New England Journal of Medicine, 341,* 815-826.

Friedlander, A.M. (2000). Anthrax: Clinical features, pathogenesis, and potential biological warfare threat. *Current Clinical Topics in Infectious Diseases, 20,* 335-349.

Inglesby, T.V., O'Toole, T., Henderson, D.A., Bartlett, J.G., Ascher, M.S., et al. (2002). Anthrax as a biological weapon, 2002: Updated recommendations for management. *Journal of the American Medical Association, 287,* 2236-2252.

Lew, D.P. (2000). *Bacillus anthracis* (Anthrax). In G. Mandell, J. Bennett, & R. Dolin (Eds.), *Principles and practice of infectious diseases* (5th ed., pp. 2215-2220). New York: Churchill Livingstone.

Rotz, L.D, Khan, A.S., Lillibridge, S.R., Ostroff, S.M., & Hughes. J.M. (2002). Public health assessment of potential biological terrorism agents. *Emerging Infectious Diseases, 8,* 225-230.

Scott, G. (2003). Anthrax. In G.C. Cook & A.I. Zumla (Eds.), *Manson's tropical diseases* (21st ed., pp. 1115-1117). Philadelphia: W.B. Saunders Company.

Shoham, D. (2000). Iraq's biological warfare agents: A comprehensive analysis. *Critical Reviews in Microbiology, 26,* 179-204.

U.S. Congress, Office of Technology Assessment. (1993). *Proliferation of weapons of mass destruction* (Publication OTA-ISC-559). Washington DC: U.S. Government Printing Office.

8

ARBOVIRUS ENCEPHALITIS

Geographic Distribution

Arboviral encephalitides are arthropod (insect and spider)-borne central nervous system infections found worldwide. Those with the highest case fatality rates are as follows:

- *Japanese encephalitis.* Found throughout Asia and the Pacific. In 2002 Japanese encephalitis caused about 10,000 childhood deaths in south and east Asia (Solomon, 2003a).
- *Murray Valley encephalitis.* Found in Australia and New Guinea. It also causes the clinical syndrome known as Australian encephalitis.
- *Eastern equine encephalomyelitis.* Found in the Americas and Caribbean (Broom, Smith, Hall, Johansen, & Mackenzie, 2003; Chin, 2000; Solomon, 2003a).

Other medically significant arboviruses that cause encephalitis include:

- *West Nile fever.* Found in Africa, Middle East, Europe, Russia and other areas of the former Soviet Union, India, Southeast Asia, and, recently, North America.
- *Dengue fever.* See Chapter 25.
- *Western equine encephalitis.* Found in the Americas.
- *Venezuelan equine encephalitis.* Found in northern areas of South America, Central America, Caribbean Islands, and Southwestern United States.
- *St. Louis encephalitis.* Found in North America and Caribbean.
- *Tick-borne encephalitis.* Found in Russia and other areas of the former Soviet Union and in Europe.
- *Louping ill.* Found in Europe.

- *Kyasanur forest disease.* Found in India. It also causes hemorrhagic fever.
- *Kunjin fever.* Found in Australia and Southeast Asia. It also causes the clinical syndrome known as Australian encephalitis, and it causes polyarthralgic illness.
- *Rift Valley fever.* Found in most of Africa. It also causes hemorrhagic fever.

— It is important to note that the geography of several significant viruses is changing; for example, the West Nile virus has spread from Africa to North America, Japanese encephalitis has spread to Australia, and dengue fever is spreading through much of the world (Broom et al., 2003; Chin, 2000). This chapter contains information generalizable to all arboviral encephalitides, with extra information on those with higher fatality rates: Japanese encephalitis, Murray Valley encephalitis, Eastern equine encephalomyelitis, and West Nile fever.

Agent and Vector

— The three major families of arboviruses are Togaviridae (alphaviruses, e.g., Eastern equine encephalomyelitis), Flaviviridae (flaviviruses, e.g., Japanese encephalitis, West Nile virus, and Murray Valley encephalitis), and Bunyaviridae (bunyaviruses, e.g., Western equine encephalitis). More than 500 arboviruses have been identified worldwide, of which 20 are known to cause encephalitis in humans. In the United States, more than 50 have been isolated but only 6 (Western equine encephalitis, Eastern equine encephalomyelitis, St. Louis encephalitis, Lacross, Powassan encephalitis, and Colorado tick fever) are thought to cause clinically significant illnesses.

— Arboviruses have a complex ecology that centers around a reservoir or maintenance host such as a bird, rodent, or pig. The reservoir host develops viremia and is bitten by an arthropod vector, which then transmits the virus to other animals. The mosquito is the vector for most arboviral encephalitides, though some arboviruses may be spread through ticks (e.g., Powassan encephalitis, Colorado tick fever) and sandflies (e.g., sandfly fever). Humans (and horses in the case of Eastern equine encephalomyelitis) are typically not a significant part of the viral life cycle. Rarely, arboviruses may be transmitted through blood transfusions or organ donation from an infected person (Box 8-1).

Incubation

- Japanese encephalitis: 6 to 16 days.
- Murray Valley encephalitis: 7 to 21 days.
- Eastern equine encephalomyelitis: 7 to 10 days.
- West Nile fever: 2 to 14 days.

Clinical Findings and Treatment

Signs and Symptoms

Most arboviral infections are asymptomatic or cause nonspecific flu-like symptoms that resolve without ever being diagnosed. Populations that have a lower prevalence of background immunity from prior exposure to a particular arbovirus have higher rates of encephalitis (Campbell, Marfin, Lanciotti, & Gubler, 2002). Severe symptoms, which can occur at any age but are more common in young children and in the elderly, include acute onset of fever, vomiting, meningismus (neck ache, back ache, Kernig's sign, stiff neck, Brudzinski's sign), photophobia, tremors, convulsions, mental status changes, and stupor progressing to coma. Specific signs and symptoms (Broom et al., 2003; Solomon, 2003a, 2003b) are discussed next.

JAPANESE ENCEPHALITIS

Although the illness may begin with constitutional symptoms of malaise, fever, headache, myalgia, and

---

BIOTERRORISM CONSIDERATIONS BOX 8–1

The viral encephalitides are designated as nationally notifiable to the CDC's National Notifiable Diseases Surveillance System (NNDSS) and are considered by the CDC to be "critical biologic agents" (Chang, Glynn, & Groseclose, 2003).

---

nausea and vomiting (especially in children), onset is usually abrupt, with fever, headache, change in consciousness, and, often, convulsions. Other features may include ataxia, slurred speech, coarse tremors, involuntary movements, and/or poliomyelitis-like flaccid paralysis. The case fatality rate is around 30%, with 30% of survivors suffering long-term sequelae such as developmental delays in children and neurologic or behavioral abnormalities in adults.

MURRAY VALLEY ENCEPHALITIS

Fever and headache are the presenting signs. The onset of encephalitis is 1 to 2 days after the fever begins. In children, encephalitis is usually accompanied by seizures; and in adults, by confusion. In about one-third of cases, the illness progresses to coma, paralysis, respiratory failure, and then death. Neurologic deficits are sometimes long lasting.

EASTERN EQUINE ENCEPHALOMYELITIS

The illness usually begins with fever, which may last for more than a week. In the few cases (approximately 5%) that progress to encephalitis, the onset of neurologic signs is abrupt, with headache, meningismus, and decreased consciousness. Coma and convulsions commonly follow, with death occurring in more than 50% of patients; and severe neurologic deficits in most survivors, especially among infants.

WEST NILE FEVER

In addition to typical arboviral encephalitis symptoms, a poliomyelitis-like generalized muscle weakness that can lead to respiratory failure is common. Focal neurologic signs and seizures are less common. About 15% of cases progress to coma. In the United States, the case fatality rate of West Nile encephalitis is approximately 20% (Campbell et al., 2002).

Complications

Coma and respiratory failure are ominous signs. Other complications in the early stages include hyponatremia, increased intracranial pressure, and secondary lower respiratory tract infections. Long-term sequelae include neurologic or neuropsychiatric deficits. Extraneurologic complications are uncommon but can include optic neuritis, myocarditis, pancreatitis, and fulminant hepatitis (Campbell et al., 2002).

Common Laboratory Findings

Cerebrospinal fluid (CSF) should be collected as soon as possible from a patient with suspected arboviral encephalitis. Usually the CSF has a normal or slightly raised opening pressure, normal glucose, normal or slightly elevated protein, and pleocytosis with polymorphonuclear leukocyte predominance early in the course evolving into mononuclear cells later. Mild anemia may be observed, as well as either leukocytosis or leukopenia (Campbell et al., 2002). Serum for acute titers should also be drawn, followed 4 to 6 weeks later by convalescent titers. Neuroimaging with computed tomography or magnetic resonance imaging is usually normal, but Japanese encephalitis and Eastern equine encephalomyelitis may show focal lesions in the basal ganglia and thalamus (Roos, 1999).

Diagnosis

To fulfill the Centers for Disease Control and Prevention (CDC) criteria for a confirmed case of arboviral encephalitis, one must have a febrile illness with encephalitis during a time of year when infection is likely, together with one of the following laboratory criteria (CDC, 2003):

- Fourfold or greater change in virus-specific serum antibody titer, *or*
- Isolation of virus from or demonstration of specific viral antigen or genomic sequences (e.g., polymerase chain reaction [PCR]) in tissue, blood, CSF, or other body fluid, *or*
- Virus-specific immunoglobulin M (IgM) antibodies demonstrated in CSF by antibody-capture enzyme immunoassay (EIA), *or*
- Virus-specific IgM antibodies demonstrated in serum by antibody-capture EIA and confirmed by demonstration of virus-specific serum immunoglobulin G (IgG) antibodies in the same or a later specimen by another serologic assay (e.g., neutralization or hemagglutination inhibition).

For a probable case, the laboratory data must consist of either (1) a single or stably elevated titer of virus-specific serum antibodies or (2) serum IgM antibodies detected by antibody-capture EIA but with no available results of a confirmatory test for virus-specific serum IgG antibodies in the same or a later specimen (CDC, 2003). Serum IgM has been observed to persist for more than 12 to 16 months in many West Nile encephalitis patients (Campbell et al., 2002).

Differential Diagnosis

When a patient presents with fever, headache, and neurologic signs, it is extremely important to quickly consider treatable entities such as bacterial meningitis, brain abscesses, and herpes encephalitis. Herpes simplex virus (HSV) is the most common viral encephalitis and the only one that responds to therapy (Steele, 1999). Other disorders to consider include aseptic meningitis (most commonly enteroviral), tick-borne encephalitis, rabies, mumps, meningoencephalitis, and lymphocytic choriomeningitis. Guillain-Barré syndrome and poliomyelitis are possible diagnoses in patients with severe muscle weakness or paralysis. Cerebral malaria should also be considered in patients who have been in malaria-endemic areas.

Treatment

While waiting for a definitive diagnosis of an arboviral encephalitis, clinicians should have a low threshold for starting empiric treatment with acyclovir if HSV encephalitis is suspected and/or antibiotics if meningitis is suspected. There are no specific therapies for any of the arboviral encephalitides. Ribavirin, corticosteroids, and immune globulin have each been proposed, but data supporting their effectiveness in humans is lacking. Though animal models and open clinical trials held hope that interferon alpha might be useful in the treatment of Japanese encephalitis, a recent double-blind placebo-controlled trial showed no difference in outcomes (Solomon, 2003a). Therefore, the mainstays of treatment for the arboviral encephalitides remain supportive: careful attention to fluid and electrolyte management (watching particularly for signs of inappropriate antidiuretic hormone secretion), prevention of secondary bacterial infections, monitoring and treatment of increased intracranial pressure, and seizure control with sedation if necessary (Broom et al., 2003; Solomon, 2003a; Tiroumourougane, Raghava, Srinivasana, & Badrinath, 2003).

Prevention

Japanese encephalitis is the only arbovirus with an effective vaccine. Clinicians should offer the three-dose series to travelers who will spend more than 30 days in endemic areas during seasons when mosquitoes are most active. Also offer the vaccine to travelers who will be spending shorter times but engaging in higher risk outdoor or rural activities. Other preventive measures directed to mosquitoes and other vectors (Lane, 2003; Robert, 2000; Thompson, 2002) include the following:

- Kill adult mosquitoes by spraying inside and outside human habitations and surrounding areas with residual insecticides. The goal is to kill as many female mosquitoes as possible, thus decreasing the likelihood of disease transmission. See Appendix D.
- Kill larvae and eliminate breeding areas as much as possible. Elimination of breeding areas includes draining standing water such as swamps, emptying open water-filled containers and used tires, and reducing the number of plants that hold standing water (e.g., bromeliads).

Personal protection measures include the following:

- Screen living and working quarters.
- Use a residual insecticide inside homes and work areas. See Appendix D.
- Use insecticide-impregnated mosquito netting over beds. Nets must be retreated with insecticide annually. See Appendix D.
- Stay inside as much as possible during hours when mosquitoes are biting, which varies according to species, although dawn to dusk feeding is common.
- Use DEET repellant on skin and permethrin on clothing when outside during biting hours.

Protection against ticks (Powassan encephalitis, Colorado tick fever) includes both community and personal measures as follows:

- Survey birds and livestock (horses in the case of Eastern equine encephalomyelitis) to monitor for sentinel infections.

- Treat infested animals or animals in endemic areas with insecticide washes or dusts intended for animals, especially pyrethroid insecticides. Ultra-low-volume sprays may be used for outdoors spraying. See Appendix D.
- Use DEET repellant on skin and permethrin on clothing when in endemic areas. Keep trousers tucked into boots or socks. Perform a complete inspection of the body for ticks after being in an endemic area.

Protection against sandflies and sandfly fever is similar to measures against mosquitoes and includes both community and personal measures as follows:

- Use DEET repellant on skin and permethrin on clothing when in infested areas, especially at night when sandflies usually bite.
- Use insecticide-impregnated mosquito netting over beds. Sandfly nets have smaller holes than mosquito nets and, hence, are hotter than mosquito nets. Mosquito netting impregnated with insecticide suffices for sandflies. See Appendix D.

Community spraying is not usually effective. Provide ongoing community education regarding the preceding measures.

Reporting

The CDC considers arboviral infections to be nationally notifiable diseases, and the World Health Organization (WHO) classifies them as diseases important in public health (Class 2A). See Appendix C for details and for upcoming changes in WHO reporting.

References

Broom, A.K., Smith, D.W., Hall, R.A., Johansen, C.A., & Mackenzie, J.S. (2003). Arbovirus infections. In G.C. Cook & A.I. Zumla (Eds.), *Manson's tropical diseases* (21st ed., pp. 725-764). Philadelphia: W.B. Saunders Company.

Campbell, G.L., Marfin, A.A., Lanciotti, R.S., & Gubler D.J. (2002) West Nile virus. *The Lancet Infectious Diseases, 9,* 519-29.

Chang, M., Glynn, M.K., & Groseclose, S.L. (2003). Endemic, notifiable bioterrorism-related diseases, United States, 1992-1999. *Emerging Infectious Diseases, 9,* 556-564.

Chin, J. (2000). Arthropod-borne viral encephalitides. In J. Chin (Ed.), *Control of communicable diseases manual* (17th ed., pp. 39-43). Washington, DC: American Public Health Association.

Centers for Disease Control and Prevention, Epidemiology Program Office. (2003). Encephalitis or meningitis, arboviral. Retrieved October 2, 2003, from *www.cdc.gov/epo/dphsi/casedef/encephalitiscurrent.htm*

Lane, R.P. (2003). Phlebotomine sandflies. In G.C. Cook & A.I. Zumla (Eds.), *Manson's tropical diseases* (21st ed., pp. 1733-1741). Philadelphia: W.B. Saunders Company.

Robert, L.L. (2000). Control of arthropods of medical importance. In G.T. Strickland (Ed.), *Hunter's tropical medicine and emerging infectious diseases* (8th ed., pp. 1019-1034). Philadelphia: W.B. Saunders Company.

Roos, KL. (1999). Encephalitis. *Neurology Clinics, 17,* 813-833.

Solomon, T. (2003a). Exotic and emerging viral encephalitides. *Current Opinions in Neurology, 16,* 411-418.

Solomon, T. (2003b). Recent advances in Japanese encephalitis. *Journal of NeuroVirology, 9,* 274-283.

Steele, M.T. (1999). Arboviral infections of the central nervous system— United States, 1996-1997. *Annals of Emergency Medicine, 33,* 366-367.

Thompson, M.J. (2002). Immunizations for international travel. *Primary Care; Clinics in Office Practice, 29,* 787-814.

Tiroumourougane, S.V., Raghava, P., Srinivasana, S., & Badrinath, S. (2003). Management parameters affecting the outcome of Japanese encephalitis. *Journal of Tropical Pediatrics, 49,* 153-156.

9

Ascariasis

Ascaridiasis, roundworm infection

Geographic Distribution

— Ascariasis is found worldwide. With an estimated 1 billion infected persons worldwide, ascariasis is the most common human helminthic infection (Kazura, 2000).

Agent and Vector

— The eggs of *Ascaris lumbricoides* (and other nematodes or roundworms) are ingested via water, food, or hands contaminated with human feces. The *A. lumbricoides* larvae, unlike the ascarids of dogs or cats (*Toxocara* spp.), do not pass through the skin. Once in the intestinal lumen, larvae penetrate the intestinal wall and migrate with the venous return to the heart and lungs. They then break into the alveoli, move up the respiratory tract, are swallowed, and molt in the small intestine. There the mature worms lay eggs, which pass through stool and become infective in 5 to 10 days, remaining so for up to 2 years (Bundy & DeSilva, 2000; Chin, 2000; Gilles, 2003).

Incubation

— *Ascaris* eggs appear in stool 60 to 70 days after ingestion. Pulmonary symptoms may occur 4 to 6 days after ingestion (Gilles, 2003).

Clinical Findings and Treatment

Signs and Symptoms

— *Ascaris* infection is often asymptomatic, with the discovery of a worm in the stool being the presenting complaint (Figure 9-1). Transient respiratory symptoms of productive coughing (sometimes slight hemoptysis),

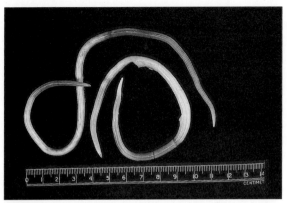

FIGURE 9–1

Adult *Ascaris lumbricoides*. Males reach about 15 to 30 cm and females reach about 20 to 35 cm. (*Source:* From Peters, W., & Pasvol, G. [2002]. *Tropical medicine and parasitology* [5th ed., p. 122]. Chicago: Mosby.)

wheezing, and fever may occur as the larvae travel through the respiratory system. Gastrointestinal symptoms most commonly include vague and/or colicky abdominal pain, nausea, and vomiting. The vomitus is sometimes bile stained and may contain worms. Steatorrhea and diminished vitamin A absorption also may occur. The adult worms can grow to more than 20 cm in length and, hence, are easily seen in stool. Worms may also emerge from the nose or mouth as a result of coughing or vomiting (Chin, 2000; Gilles, 2003; Kazura, 2000).

Complications

Children are more likely than adults to have complications. Heavy worm burdens may cause partial or complete bowel obstruction. Less common complications include intestinal perforation, appendicitis, diverticulitis, pancreatitis, cholecystitis, cholangitis, obstructive jaundice, and invasion of other organ systems. Malnutrition, stunted growth, and cognitive deficits have been observed in infected children in developing countries (Bundy & DeSilva, 2000; Gilles, 2003; Kazura, 2000).

Common Laboratory Findings

Eosinophils are elevated during the pulmonary phase in 30% to 50% of patients, but not in the intestinal phase. Diagnosis of pulmonary ascariasis is primarily on the basis of clinical data. Chest radiographs may show patchy, ill-defined transitory asymmetric infiltrations. The presence of pulmonary infiltrates and eosinophilia is known as Löffler's syndrome. With bowel obstruction, abdominal radiographic examination (with or without barium) may show worms, especially in large air-filled bowel. Ultrasound can be useful in diagnosing biliary or pancreatic involvement (Bundy & DeSilva, 2000; Gilles, 2003; Kazura, 2000).

Diagnosis

Visualization and description of the worms establish diagnosis. Microscopic exam of direct fecal smear shows eggs or ova.

Differential Diagnosis

The pulmonary symptoms may be similar to asthma, pneumonia, aspergillosis, strongyloidiasis, hookworm, or other parasitic infections affecting the lungs. The intestinal phase may resemble a variety of gastrointestinal disorders (see complications listed earlier). Postprandial dyspepsia caused by *Ascaris* may mimic duodenal ulcer, hiatal hernia, or pancreatic or gallbladder disease (Gilles, 2003; Kazura, 2000).

Treatment

There is no effective treatment for the pulmonary phase. The intestinal phase is treated with albendazole 400 mg

PO in a single dose for light infections and a daily dose for 3 days for heavier infections. Pyrantel pamoate 10 mg/kg PO (maximum 1 g) in a single dose OR mebendazole 100 mg PO bid for 3 days OR mebendazole 500 mg PO in one dose are also effective for both children and adults. A benefit of using albendazole or mebendazole is that these also are effective treatments for hookworm and whipworm infections.

— Infections complicated by biliary or intestinal obstruction may be treated with piperazine 50 to 75 mg/kg (maximum 3.5 g for patients older than age 12; 2.5 g for patients ages 2 to 12) by mouth or nasogastric tube each day for 2 days. For severe infections, piperazine treatment may be repeated after 1 week. Rarely, obstruction requires surgery.

— After treatment, stools should be checked in 2 weeks and, if necessary, the patient retreated until there are no more ascarids. There is some disagreement about treatment during pregnancy. Albendazole and mebendazole are Category C drugs and, hence, are not recommended in pregnancy or for nursing mothers. If possible, delay treatment of ascariasis until after the first trimester (Bundy & DeSilva, 2000; Gilles, 2003; Rosenblatt, 1999)

Prevention

— Measures to prevent ascariasis are directed especially at children and include the following:
   - Wash hands thoroughly after toileting and before handling or eating food.
   - Protect public water supplies from contamination with human waste.
   - Protect children's play areas from contamination with human and other waste.
   - Educate the public about prevention of ascariasis.

— When a sanitary water supply is unavailable, periodic deworming of school-age children with mebendazole or albendazole decreases the overall worm burden in the community (Chin, 2000; Gilles, 2003).

Reporting

— The U.S. Centers for Disease Control and Prevention does not consider ascariasis to be a nationally notifiable disease, nor does the World Health Organization (WHO) classify it as a disease important in public health (Class 5). See Appendix C for details and for upcoming changes in WHO reporting.

References

Bundy, D.A.P., & DeSilva, N. (2000). Intestinal nematodes that migrate through lungs (ascariasis). In G.T. Strickland (Ed.), *Hunter's tropical medicine and emerging infectious diseases* (8th ed., pp. 726-730). Philadelphia: W.B. Saunders Company.

Chin, J. (2000). Ascariasis. In J. Chin (Ed.), *Control of communicable diseases manual* (17th ed., pp. 58-60). Washington, DC: American Public Health Association.

Gilles, H.M. (2003). Soil-transmitted helminths (geohelminths). In G.C. Cook & A.I Zumla (Eds.), *Manson's tropical diseases* (21st ed., pp. 1527-1560). Philadelphia: W.B. Saunders Company.

Kazura, J.W. (2000). Ascariasis (*Ascaris lumbricoides*). In R. Behrman, R. Kliegman, & H. Jenson (Eds.). *Nelson textbook of pediatrics* (16th ed., pp. 1064-1065). Philadelphia: W.B. Saunders Company.

Rosenblatt, J.E. (1999). Antiparasitic agents. *Mayo Clinic Proceedings, 74,* 1161-1175.

10

BABESIOSIS
Formerly piroplasmosis
Geographic Distribution

— Babesiosis occurs in the United States (especially north-eastern) and rarely in Europe, Mexico, Asia, and Africa. In North America, most infections are caused by the nymph stage ("seed ticks") of *Babesia microti*; and in Europe by *B. divergens*. There also are more recently discovered forms of babesiosis found in California (CA-1), Washington state (WA-1), and Missouri (MO-1) (Chiodini, 2003; Kjemtrup et al., 2002).

Agent and Vector

— Babesiosis is a tick-borne zoonosis caused by the intraerythrocytic protozoans *B. microti* and other *Babesia* species. They are carried by *Ixodes scapularis* (deer ticks; also known as *Ixodes dammini*), which feed on deer, deer mice, and cattle. These hard-bodied ticks also transmit Lyme disease and ehrlichiosis. After a bite from an infected tick, with attachment lasting more than 24 hours, the *Babesia* sporozoite (infective stage) enters the bloodstream where it invades an erythrocyte and multiplies by asexual budding to form two to four merozoites or daughter cells. Lysis of the erythrocyte releases the merozoites, which then invade other erythrocytes. Less commonly, infection may also occur transplacentally or through blood transfusion (Chiodini, 2003; Krause, 2003).

Incubation

— The illness usually manifests 1 to 6 weeks after a tick bite. The history can be unreliable, however, because the tick nymphs are small (2 mm in length) and attachment may be unnoticed. The incubation for transfusion-transmitted babesiosis may be as long as several months (Chin, 2000; Krause, 2003).

Clinical Findings and Treatment

Signs and Symptoms

Babesiosis ranges from an asymptomatic or mild to moderate flu-like illness to a fulminant malaria-like illness that leads to death. The severity of illness is related more to immune status, asplenia, or advanced age than to parasite load. Fever and hemolytic anemia are the cardinal signs of babesiosis. Other symptoms (in decreasing order of frequency) include gradual onset of fatigue, chills, sweats, headache, myalgia, anorexia, cough, arthralgia, and nausea. Depression and/or emotional lability, hyperesthesias, and dark urine also may occur. Physical exam may be unremarkable, though petechiae, jaundice, and slight hepatosplenomegaly may be found. The illness lasts for several weeks to several months and recovery may take more than a year. Co-infection with ehrlichiosis or Lyme disease may occur with confounding or increased symptoms (Kjemtrup et al., 2002; Krause, 2002, 2003; Weiss, 2002).

Complications

In severe cases patients may experience pulmonary edema and/or acute respiratory distress syndrome. Other complications include disseminated intravascular coagulation, congestive heart failure, myocardial infarction, coma, and renal failure (Krause, 2003; Weiss, 2002).

Common Laboratory Findings

Common findings include evidence of hemolytic anemia (decreased hematocrit and serum haptoglobin; increased reticulocyte count, lactate dehydrogenase, and unconjugated bilirubin), thrombocytopenia, and normal to mildly elevated peripheral leukocytes with a left shift. Increased liver enzymes, proteinuria, and elevations in blood urea nitrogen and creatinine may also occur (Chiodini, 2003; Krause, 2003; Weiss, 2002).

Diagnosis

— Suspect babesiosis in a patient with hemolytic anemia, fever, and either (1) potential exposure in an endemic area during early summer months or (2) blood transfusion. Diagnosis is confirmed by presence of *Babesia* sp. ring forms (similar in appearance to *Plasmodium falciparum*) on Giemsa- or Wright-stained blood smear. (Parasite loads may be small and, hence, difficult to find.) Polymerase chain reaction identifies *Babesia* DNA. Immunofluorescent antibody levels (IFA) shows past exposure or acute illness. Assays for co-infecting agents might be considered depending on severity of illness or resistance to treatment (Herwaldt, 2000; Weiss, 2002).

Differential Diagnosis

— In patients with symptoms suggesting babesiosis, consider other tick-borne diseases, rickettsial diseases, malaria, and influenza (Chiodini, 2003; Herwaldt, 2000).

Treatment

— The standard treatment for babesiosis has been quinine 650 mg PO tid and clindamycin 300 to 600 mg IM or IV qid for 7 to 10 days. Pediatric dosage is quinine 8.3 mg/kg PO tid and clindamycin 5 to 10 mg/kg PO qid. Adverse effects are common.

— An equally effective treatment with significantly fewer side effects is atovaquone 750 mg PO bid and azithromycin 500 mg PO on day 1 and then 250 mg/day for 7 days. Weiss, Wittner, and Tanowitz (2001) reported that a higher daily dosage of azithromycin (600 mg/day) results in more rapid resolution of fever and clearance of parasites from the blood. The use of atovaquone and azithromycin for babesiosis in children has not been studied.

Exchange transfusion may be used for severe cases with high parasite loads (Belman, 1999; Chiodini, 2003; Krause, 2003; Weiss, 2002; Weiss et al., 2001).

Prevention

Preventive measures (Chin, 2000; Chiodini, 2003) include the following:

- Treat tick-infested animals or animals in endemic areas with insecticide washes or dusts intended for animals, especially pyrethroid insecticides. Ultra-low-volume (ULV) sprays may be used for outdoors spraying. See Appendix D.
- Avoid exposure to ticks, especially during May and June; if exposed, limit attachment to less than 24 hours. Because tick nymphs are very small and may match skin color, careful inspection of the entire body in bright light is necessary after potential exposure.
- Use DEET repellant on skin and permethrin on clothing when in endemic areas. Keep trousers tucked into boots or socks. Perform a complete inspection of the body for ticks after being in an endemic area.
- Control rodents (and deer) in areas of human habitation.

Community education regarding the above measures should be ongoing.

Reporting

The U.S. Centers for Disease Control and Prevention does not consider babesiosis to be a nationally notifiable disease, nor does the World Health Organization (WHO) classify it as a disease important in public health (Class 3B). See Appendix C for details and for upcoming changes in WHO reporting.

References

Belman, A.L. (1999). Tick-borne diseases. *Seminars in Pediatric Neurology, 6,* 249-266.

Chin, J. (2000). Babesiosis. In J. Chin (Ed.), *Control of communicable diseases manual* (17th ed., pp. 62-64). Washington, DC: American Public Health Association.

Chiodini, P.L. (2003). Babesiosis. In G.C. Cook & A.I. Zumla (Eds.), *Manson's tropical diseases* (21st ed., pp. 1297-1301). Philadelphia: W.B. Saunders Company.

Herwaldt, B.L. (2000). Babesiosis. In G.T. Strickland (Ed.), *Hunter's tropical medicine and emerging infectious diseases* (8th ed., pp. 688-690). Philadelphia: W.B. Saunders Company.

Kjemtrup, A.M., Lee, B., Fritz, C.L., Evans, C., Chervenak, M., & Conrad, P.A. (2002). Investigation of transfusion transmission of a WA1-type babesial parasite to a premature infant in California. *Transfusion, 42,* 1482-1487.

Krause, P.J. (2002). Babesiosis. *Medical Clinics of North America, 86,* 361-373.

Krause, P.J. (2003). Babesiosis diagnosis and treatment. *Vector-Borne and Zoonotic Diseases, 3,* 45-51.

Weiss, L.M. (2002). Babesiosis in humans: A treatment review. *Expert Opinion on Pharmacotherapy, 3,* 1109-1115.

Weiss, L.M., Wittner, M., & Tanowitz, H.B. (2001). The treatment of babesiosis. *New England Journal of Medicine, 344,* 773.

11

Bartonellosis

Carrión disease, Guaitara fever,
Oroya fever; localized or eruptive stage
known as verruga peruana
Geographic Distribution

Bartonellosis is found primarily in the mountain valleys of Peru, Ecuador, and Columbia. *Bartonella*-like infections have also occurred in Southeast Asia, Africa, the Middle East, and the United States (Chin, 2000; Scott & Wylie, 2003).

Agent and Vector

Bartonellosis is a zoonosis whose agent is *Bartonella bacilliformis*, the only bacteria known to infect human erythrocytes. Other *Bartonella* species that cause disease in humans are *B. henselae*, which causes cat scratch disease (CSD), bacillary angiomatosis, visceral peliosis, bacteremia, endocarditis, and aseptic meningitis; *B. quintana*, which causes trench fever and endocarditis in the immunocompetent, and bacillary angiomatosis, visceral peliosis, bacteremia, endocarditis, and lymphadenopathy in the immunocompromised; and *B. elizabethae*, which causes endocarditis.

B. bacilliformis is a small, aerobic, highly motile pleomorphic bacterium that occurs in two forms: (1) rod-shaped, slightly curved, gram-negative forms that predominate during acute infection and (2) coccoid, oval, or pear-shaped forms containing chromatin granules that are more prevalent during recovery. Vector transmission is believed to be from the bite of the New World sandfly (genus *Lutzomyia*), but this has not been conclusively proven and the natural reservoir is unknown. Transmission also occurs with transfusion from an infected individual. There are two forms of the illness: an acute bacteremic illness marked by hemolysis called Oroya fever and a chronic verrucous disease known as verruga peruana (Chin, 2000). These may be two stages of a single illness, but Oroya fever and verruga peruana sometimes coexist in the same patient and either or both may recur. A chronic asymptomatic bacteremia has also been documented (Laughlin, 2000).

Incubation

The incubation period is 16 to 22 days; and up to 4 months (Chin, 2000; Scott & Wylie, 2003).

Clinical Findings and Treatment

Signs and Symptoms

Oroya fever is usually characterized by the gradual onset of fever and malaise followed by irregular fever, headache, myalgia, and arthralgia. In severe disease, onset is abrupt with high fever, chills, and altered mentation. There may also be weakness, vertigo, nausea and vomiting, syncope, prostration, and, often, delirium. Physical findings may include generalized lymphadenopathy, pallor, and hepatosplenomegaly. Case fatality rates for untreated bartonellosis are around 90%, but fall to less than 5% if the disease is uncomplicated and quickly treated with antibiotics (Olson, 2000).

About 50% of patients with Oroya fever go on to develop verruga peruana; however, about 50% of patients with verrucous disease do not have a clear history of Oroya fever (Laughlin, 2000). Verruga peruana usually begins with a prodrome of myalgia, arthralgia, and constitutional symptoms. These symptoms disappear as crops of skin lesions resembling pyogenic granulomas develop 1 or several months later. Lesions are typically found on the face or on exposed extensor surfaces of the extremities, and less commonly on the scalp, genitalia, or in a generalized distribution. There are three basic types of lesions, sometimes found on the same patient: (1) miliary lesions which are 2- to 3-mm, tender, mobile papules scattered across the body; (2) nodules that begin subcutaneously, are tender, warm, and are usually found over joints; and (3) tumors ("mular" lesions) that usually ulcerate. Mucosal and visceral lesions may also develop, causing localized symptoms. Verrucous lesions bleed easily and are subject to secondary infection.

Complications

Superinfection with salmonella is the most common complication and may occur during convalescence from acute, untreated bartonellosis bacteremia. Invasion of the central nervous system may result in a highly fatal meningoencephalitis or in the formation of spinal or cranial nerve granulomas, causing disability according to their location.

Common Laboratory Findings

The hemolytic anemia of the acute stage is macrocytic or normocytic and usually hypochromic. Sometimes a profound reticulocytosis of more than 50% is seen (Olson, 2000). The white blood cell count is variable, and thrombocytopenia and elevated liver transaminases are common (Edwards, 2002). Cerebrospinal fluid may show pleocytosis.

Diagnosis

Diagnosis is based on fever and pallor in a patient who resides in or has traveled through an endemic region and by the presence of intraerythrocytic bacteria in Giemsa- or Wright-stained thin blood film. The isolation of *B. bacilliformis* in blood culture provides a definitive diagnosis, as does polymerase chain reaction (PCR), but these laboratory studies are difficult to obtain in endemic areas (Chin, 2000; Laughlin, 2000;

Scott & Wylie, 2003). During the chronic verrucous phase, blood smears and cultures are negative but the organism can be identified and cultured from biopsies of skin lesions.

Differential Diagnosis

The differential diagnosis for Oroya fever includes other acute fevers endemic to the region, such as malaria, typhus, and typhoid fever. Consider also other causes of acute hemolytic anemia. Differentials for verruga peruana include yaws (frambesia), bacillary angiomatosis, secondary syphilis, or Kaposi's sarcoma. Single lesion differentials include fibrosarcoma, hemangioma, pyogenic granuloma, molluscum contagiosum, and spindle cell and epithelioid nevus of Spitz (Laughlin, 2000; Scott & Wylie, 2003).

Treatment

Standard treatment is with chloramphenicol 50 mg/kg/day PO or IV qid for at least 3 weeks, longer if bacteremia or organ involvement is present. Pediatric dosage is the same as for adults. Note that chloramphenicol is effective in the treatment of salmonella infection, hence it also serves as a preventive agent for a common complication (Edwards, 2002; Scott & Wylie, 2003). Antibiotic therapy is not very effective for the verrucous stage, although rifampin may reduce the size of large skin lesions (Olson, 2000).

Prevention

The prevention of bartonellosis (Chin, 2000) includes the following:
- Control sandflies with residual-action insecticides; and eliminate or spray open trash heaps, stone walls, and animal shelters. See Appendix D.
- Avoid exposure to sandflies during biting hours (sundown to sun-up) in endemic areas.

Use DEET-formulated insect repellant, and treat clothing with permethrin.

- Avoid locating habitations in areas of heavy sandfly infestation. If such location is unavoidable, practice increased vigilance and other prevention measures. In the New World, sandfly habitats tend to be in forested areas.
- Use of fine-mesh screens in homes is helpful, but they are a luxury (as is insect repellent) in many endemic areas. Sandfly bednets have very fine mesh and are hot in tropical climates. Permethrin-impregnated mosquito nets offer some protection and are more comfortable to sleep under.
- Systematic case identification and prompt treatment help prevent complications and disability.

Community education regarding the preceding measures should be ongoing.

Reporting

The U.S. Centers for Disease Control and Prevention does not consider bartonellosis to be a nationally notifiable disease, nor does the World Health Organization (WHO) classify it as a disease important in public health (Class 3B). See Appendix C for details and for upcoming changes in WHO reporting.

References

Chin, J. (2000). Bartonellosis. In J. Chin (Ed.), *Control of communicable diseases manual* (17th ed., pp. 66-68). Washington, DC: American Public Health Association.

Edwards, B. (2002). Bartonellosis. *EMedicine*. Retrieved July 28, 2003, from *www.emedicine.com/med/topic212.htm*

Laughlin, L.W. (2000). Bartonellosis. In G.T. Strickland (Ed.), *Hunter's tropical medicine and emerging infectious diseases* (8th ed., pp. 394-398). Philadelphia: W.B. Saunders Company.

Olson, J.G. (2000). Bartonella-associated diseases. In G.T. Strickland (Ed.), *Hunter's tropical medicine and emerging infectious diseases* (8th ed., pp. 394-402). Philadelphia: W.B. Saunders Company.

Scott, G.M., & Wylie, S.A. (2003). Bartonellosis, cat scratch disease, trench fever, human ehrlichiosis, Whipple disease. In G.C. Cook & A.I. Zumla (Eds.), *Manson's tropical diseases* (21st ed., pp. 1095-1108). Philadelphia: W.B. Saunders Company.

12

BLASTOMYCOSIS

Gilchrist's disease, North American blastomycosis

Geographic Distribution

— Blastomycosis occurs in North America (especially southeastern, south central, and midwestern states, particularly those that border the Mississippi and Ohio Rivers) and to a lesser extent in Africa, Middle East, and India (Bradsher, 2000; Hay, 2003; Klein, Vergeront, & Davis, 1986).

Agent and Vector

— Blastomycosis is caused by *Blastomyces dermatitidis*, a dimorphic fungus that grows as a mold at room temperature and a yeast at normal human body temperature. *Blastomyces dermatitidis* has been recovered from riverbanks in endemic areas in the United States, but it has not been isolated from these sources in Africa (Hay, 2003; Klein, Vergeront, DiSalvo, Kaufman, & Davis, 1987).

— At least two serotypes of *B. dermatitidis* exist: A-antigen positive and A-antigen negative. Serotypes found in North America seem to contain the A antigen, while most African isolates are A-antigen negative. The organisms found in North America and Africa may be morphologically identical yet antigenically and genetically different (Hay, 2003; Kaufman, Standard, Weeks, & Padhye, 1983).

— Blastomycosis is usually acquired by the inhalation of spores from soil that is in proximity to animals or bodies of water. Cutaneous inoculation blastomycosis is rare, but it is most commonly associated with accidental inoculation in laboratory workers, animal bites

or scratches, and skin trauma during outdoor activities.
Infections in animals such as dogs, cats, and cows have
occurred; however, spread of disseminated disease from
animals to humans has not occurred (Bradsher, 2000;
Gray & Baddour, 2002; Klein et al., 1986).

Unlike other fungal infections, *B. dermatitidis* is
uncommon in HIV patients even where it is endemic.
When it occurs in this setting, the patient usually has
an extremely low CD4 count, and the infection is
disseminated, progressive, and usually fatal (Bradsher,
2000; Marques et al., 2000).

Incubation

The incubation period is 21 to 106 days (median
43 days) after exposure (Klein et al., 1986).

Clinical Findings and Treatment

Signs and Symptoms

There are five primary symptom complexes and other
less common signs and symptoms:

- *Constitutional.* The patient commonly presents with
  nonspecific findings, such as weight loss, fever,
  malaise, and fatigue. These do not offer much help
  with the diagnosis, and the lungs, skin, bones, central
  nervous system (CNS), and genitourinary tract need
  to be thoroughly examined to look for findings
  specific for blastomycosis (Bradsher, Chapman,
  & Pappas, 2003).

- *Pulmonary.* The clinical presentation of most patients
  is pneumonia. The lungs are the most common site
  of infection, and pulmonary involvement is
  demonstrated in 84% to 87% of the cases. Most
  patients with pulmonary disease present with chronic
  illness; however, these patients can also have signs of
  acute pneumonia, multiorgan involvement, or acute
  respiratory distress syndrome. Radiologic findings

in patients with pulmonary disease may reveal airspace consolidation, nodular opacities, air bronchograms, mass-like lesions, or miliary disease. These findings may be confused with pulmonary histoplasmosis, tuberculosis, or lung cancer (Lemos, Guo, & Baliga, 2000; Vasquez, Mehta, Agrawal, & Sarubbi, 1999; Winer-Muram & Rubin, 1992).

- *Cutaneous.* Skin manifestations are the next most common presentation and occur in 20% to 50% of patients. Secondary cutaneous dissemination from a pulmonary site is a common occurrence and may be the first sign of disease. Primary cutaneous blastomycosis from trauma and subsequent inoculation is rare. The most common cutaneous presentations include papulopustules and well-defined verrucous plaques (Figures 12-1A and B). Central ulceration may occur. Healing of the plaques begins centrally, which results in cribriform scarring and annular plaques. Mucous membrane involvement may occur, and the larynx is the most common site. These lesions may resemble well-differentiated squamous cell carcinoma (Bradsher, 2000; Gray & Baddour, 2002; Lemos et al., 2000; Reder & Neel, 1993; Sobera & Elewski, 2003).

- *Skeletal.* Osteomyelitis occurs in 15% to 25% of cases of disseminated blastomycosis. In approximately one-half of these patients, the osseous site does not cause symptoms. The skull, vertebrae, ribs, and metaphyses of long bones are most commonly involved; however, essentially any bone may be involved. The bone may become involved secondary to dissemination or trauma and direct inoculation. Bone deformities and compression fractures may occur, and the involvement of the spine may be confused with vertebral tuberculosis (Bradsher, 2000; Bradsher et al., 2003; Guler et al., 1995; Lemos et al., 2000; MacDonald, Black, & MacKenzie, 1990; Muniz & Evans, 2000).

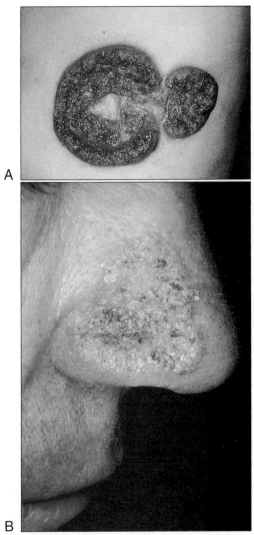

FIGURE 12–1

Cutaneous blastomycosis usually is well-defined and may show central ulceration. (*Source:* **A,** From Bolognia, J.L., Jorizzo, J.L., & Rapini, R.P. [Eds.]. [2003]. *Dermatology* [p. 1191]. Philadelphia: Mosby. **B,** Courtesy of the University of Texas Southwestern Department of Dermatology.)

- *CNS.* Disseminated blastomycosis involves the CNS in 3% to 10% of cases. CNS blastomycosis usually presents as a mass lesion or chronic meningitis (Bradsher et al., 2003; Lemos et al., 2000; Pappas & Dismukes, 2002).
- *Other.* Genitourinary involvement may present as prostatitis and epididymoorchitis. Prostate involvement usually manifests as obstruction and a tender mass on prostate examination. The genitourinary tract of women is less commonly affected, but uterine and adnexal involvement has been described. Virtually any organ can be affected by disseminated blastomycosis. Other sites of involvement that have been described include the adrenals, eyes, sinuses, and liver (Day & Stucker, 1994; Lopez, Mason, Parker, & Pappas, 1994; Pappas & Dismukes, 2002; Rimondi, Bianchini, Barucchello, & Panzavolta, 1995; Ryan, Kirchner, Sell, & Swanson, 1989).

Complications

Life-threatening complications are more common in elderly and immunocompromised patients. Acute respiratory distress syndrome is a relatively uncommon complication (less than 10% of pulmonary cases) that often leads to respiratory failure and death. Other known complications include fractures, spinal cord compression, abscesses of the skin and other organs, adrenal insufficiency, upper airway obstruction, and transplacental infection in pregnancy (Assaly et al., 2003; Chapman et al., 1997; Ebeo et al., 2002; Lagging et al., 1994; Lemos, Baliga, & Guo, 2001; Lemos, Soofi, & Amir, 2002; Rimondi et al., 1995).

Common Laboratory Findings

In patients who develop blastomycosis secondary to HIV infection, severe immunodeficiency is indicated by CD4 counts of less than 200/mm^3 in 85% (Witzig, Hoadley, Greer, Abriola, & Hernandez, 1994).

Diagnosis

— Culture for fungus can be done on sputum, pus, prostatic secretions, urine, or cerebrospinal fluid, depending on the site of involvement. Microscopic examination of infected tissue, pus, exudate, or sputum after digestion with 10% potassium hydroxide is the most rapid and effective means of diagnosis. The organism can also be readily identified on histopathologic examination of infected tissue with special stains, given the characteristic appearance of broad-based budding yeast with a doubly refractile cell wall (Bradsher, 2000; Bradsher et al., 2003; Pappas & Dismukes, 2002).

— Serologic tests for the diagnosis of blastomycosis have had inadequate sensitivity, but results are improved with enzyme immunoassay (EIA) with A-antigen of *Blastomyces dermatitidis*. With newer immunoassays, greater than 80% of patients with culture-proven blastomycosis will have a positive serology.

Cross reactivity is seen with histoplasmosis in one-third of patients. These tests may help to support the diagnosis, but they are still quite unreliable and only available in reference laboratories (Bradsher & Pappas, 1995; Pappas & Dismukes, 2002).

Differential Diagnosis

— Pulmonary mass lesions and abscesses may mimic histoplasmosis, tuberculosis, other fungal pneumonias, or lung cancer. Compression fractures secondary to vertebral involvement may present similarly in tuberculosis or spinal metastases. Nasal and oropharyngeal lesions may resemble paracoccidioidomycosis and leishmaniasis. Verrucous skin lesions can be mistaken for basal cell or squamous cell skin cancer. Skin ulcerations are common in many other infections, including *Mycobacterium ulcerans* (Bradsher, 2000).

Treatment

— Before antifungal therapy, blastomycosis had a chronic progressive course with dissemination and associated mortality of up to 90%. Now, with appropriate treatment, cure rates are greater than 85% and mortality is less than 10% (Chapman, Bradsher, Campbell, Pappas, & Kauffman, 2000).

— Patients with life-threatening pulmonary disease should be treated with amphotericin B (total dose 1.5 to 2.5 g, given at 0.7 to 1 mg/kg/day). Mild to moderate lung involvement can be treated with itraconazole (200 to 400 mg/day for a minimum of 6 months). Some patients with mild disease involving only the lungs have a spontaneous resolution, and these patients may just be monitored.

— Patients with disseminated disease involving the CNS should be treated with amphotericin B (total dose at least 2 g, given at 0.7 to 1 mg/kg/day). Those with life-threatening non-CNS disseminated disease should also be treated with amphotericin B (total dose 1.5 to 2.5 g). Mild to moderate disseminated disease without CNS involvement should be treated with itraconazole (200 to 400 mg/day for a minimum of 6 months). Patients with bone involvement should continue the treatment for 12 months.

— For children with disseminated blastomycosis, amphotericin B (total dose of 30 mg/kg or more) or itraconazole (5 to 7 mg/kg/day) should be used (Chapman et al., 2000).

— Fluconazole and ketoconazole are alternative choices; however, they have lower efficacy than amphotericin B or itraconazole (Bradsher, 2000).

Prevention

— There are no known means of preventing blastomycosis (Bradsher, 2000).

Reporting

The U.S. Centers for Disease Control and Prevention does not consider blastomycosis to be a nationally notifiable disease, nor does the World Health Organization (WHO) classify it as a disease important in public health (Class 5). See Appendix C for details and for upcoming changes in WHO reporting.

References

Assaly, R.A., Hammersley, J.R., Olson, D.E., Farrouk, A., Zaher, A., et al. (2003). Disseminated blastomycosis. *Journal of the American Academy of Dermatology, 48,* 123-127.

Bradsher, R.W., & Pappas, P.G. (1995). Detection of specific antibodies in human blastomycosis by enzyme immunoassay. *Southern Medical Journal, 88,* 1256-1259.

Bradsher, R.W. (2000). Blastomycosis. In G.T. Strickland (Ed.), *Hunter's tropical medicine and emerging infectious diseases* (8th ed., pp. 557-558). Philadelphia: W.B. Saunders Company.

Bradsher, R.W., Chapman, S.W., & Pappas, P.G. (2003). Blastomycosis. *Infectious Disease Clinics of North America, 17,* 21-40.

Chapman, S.W., Lin, A.C., Hendricks, K.A., Nolan, R.L., Currier, M.M., et al. (1997). Endemic blastomycosis in Mississippi: Epidemiological and clinical studies. *Seminars in Respiratory Infections, 12,* 219-228.

Chapman, S.W., Bradsher, R.W. Jr., Campbell, G.D. Jr., Pappas, P.G., & Kauffman, C.A. (2000). Practice guidelines for the management of patients with blastomycosis. *Clinical Infectious Diseases, 30,* 679-683.

Day, T.A., & Stucker, F.J. (1994). Blastomycosis of the paranasal sinuses. *Otolaryngology—Head and Neck Surgery, 110,* 437-440.

Ebeo, C.T., Olive, K., Byrd, R.P., Jr., Mirle, G., Roy, T.M., & Mehta, J.B. (2002). Blastomycosis of the vocal folds with life-threatening upper airway obstruction: A case report. *Ear Nose and Throat Journal, 81,* 852-855.

Gray, N.A., & Baddour, L.M. (2002). Cutaneous inoculation blastomycosis. *Clinical Infectious Disease, 34,* E44-99.

Guler, N., Palanduz, A., Ones, U., Ozturk, A., Somer, A., et al. (1995). Progressive vertebral blastomycosis mimicking tuberculosis. *Pediatric Infectious Disease Journal, 14,* 816-818.

Hay, R.J. (2003). Fungal infections. In G.C. Cook & A.I. Zumla (Eds.), *Manson's tropical diseases* (21st ed., pp. 1173-1194). Philadelphia: W.B. Saunders Company.

Kaufman, L., Standard, P.G., Weeks, R.J., & Padhye, A.A. (1983). Detection of two *Blastomyces dermatitidis* serotypes by exoantigen analysis. *Journal of Clinical Microbiology, 18,* 110-114.

Klein, B.S., Vergeront, J.M., & Davis, J.P. (1986). Epidemiologic aspects of blastomycosis, the enigmatic systemic mycosis. *Seminars in Respiratory Infections, 1,* 29-39.

Klein, B.S., Vergeront, J.M., DiSalvo, A.F., Kaufman, L., & Davis, J.P. (1987). Two outbreaks of blastomycosis along rivers in Wisconsin. Isolation of *Blastomyces dermatitidis* from riverbank soil and evidence of its transmission along waterways. *American Review of Respiratory Disease, 136,* 1333-1338.

Lagging, L.M., Breland, C.M., Kennedy, D.J., Milligan, T.W., Sokol-Anderson, M.L., & Westblom, T.U. (1994). Delayed treatment of pulmonary blastomycosis causing vertebral osteomyelitis, paraspinal abscess, and spinal cord compression. *Scandinavian Journal of Infectious Disease, 26,* 111-115.

Lemos, L.B., Guo, M., & Baliga, M. (2000). Blastomycosis: Organ involvement and etiologic diagnosis. A review of 123 patients from Mississippi. *Annals of Diagnostic Pathology, 4,* 391-406.

Lemos, L.B., Baliga, M., & Guo, M. (2001). Acute respiratory distress syndrome and blastomycosis: Presentation of nine cases and review of the literature. *Annals of Diagnostic Pathology, 5,* 1-9.

Lemos, L.B., Soofi, M., & Amir, E. (2002). Blastomycosis and pregnancy. *Annals of Diagnostic Pathology, 6,* 211-215.

Lopez, R., Mason, J.O., Parker, J.S., & Pappas, P.G. (1994). Intraocular blastomycosis: Case report and review. *Clinical Infectious Disease, 18,* 805-807.

MacDonald, P.B., Black, G.B., & MacKenzie, R. (1990). Orthopaedic manifestations of blastomycosis. *Journal of Bone and Joint Surgery (America), 72,* 860-864.

Marques, S.A., Robles, A.M., Tortorano, A.M., Tuculet, M.A., Negroni, R., & Mendes, R.P. (2000). Mycoses associated with AIDS in the Third World. *Medical Mycology, 38*(Suppl 1), 269-279.

Muniz, A.E., & Evans, T. (2000). Chronic paronychia, osteomyelitis, and paravertebral abscess in a child with blastomycosis. *Journal of Emergency Medicine, 19,* 245-248.

Pappas, P.G., & Dismukes, W.E. (2002). Blastomycosis: Gilchrist's disease revisited. *Current Clinical Topics in Infectious Disease, 22,* 61-77.

Reder, P.A., Neel, H.B. (1993). Blastomycosis in otolaryngology: Review of a large series. *Laryngoscope, 103*(1 Pt 1), 53-58.

Rimondi, A.P., Bianchini, E., Barucchello, G., & Panzavolta, R. (1995). Addison's disease caused by adrenal blastomycosis: A case report with fine needle aspiration (FNA) cytology. *Cytopathology, 6,* 277-279.

Ryan, M.E., Kirchner, J.P., Sell, T., & Swanson, M. (1989). Cholangitis due to *Blastomyces dermatitidis. Gastroenterology, 96*(5 Pt 1), 1346-1349.

Sobera, J.O., & Elewski, B.E. (2003). Fungal diseases. In Bolognia, J.L., Jorizzo, J.L., & Rapini, R.P. (Eds.), *Dermatology* (pp. 1191-1192). Philadelphia: Mosby.

Vasquez, J.E., Mehta, J.B., Agrawal, R., & Sarubbi, F.A. (1999). Blastomycosis in northeast Tennessee. *Chest, 115,* 1224.

Winer-Muram, H.T., & Rubin, S.A. (1992). Pulmonary blastomycosis. *Journal of Thoracic Imaging, 7,* 23-28.

Witzig, R.S., Hoadley, D.J., Greer, D.L., Abriola, K.P., & Hernandez, R.L. (1994). Blastomycosis and human immunodeficiency virus: Three new cases and review. *Southern Medical Journal, 87,* 715-719.

13

Botulism

Geographic Distribution

— Botulism is found worldwide. Even one case is considered a public health emergency because of (1) the virulence of the disease and (2) the potential for bioterrorism (Centers for Disease Control and Prevention [CDC], 2001; Johns Hopkins University, 2002).

Agent and Vector

— Botulism is caused by the neurotoxin produced by the bacillus *Clostridium botulinum*, a spore-forming obligate anaerobe widely found in soil, and rarely by two other *Clostridium* species. *Botulinum* toxin is the most lethal known natural poison. There are seven serologically different *botulinum* toxins, designated A-G. As a naturally occurring disease, botulism appears (CDC, 2001, Chang & Ganguly, 2003; Chin, 2000) in the following forms:

- Food-borne botulism develops from ingesting the preformed neurotoxin, especially from canned foods that were inadequately heated during preservation and inadequately cooked afterward.
- Wound botulism occurs when *C. botulinum* is present in incompletely cleaned wounds, especially when there is ground-in soil; and among subcutaneously injecting drug users.
- Intestinal botulism (formerly *infant botulism*) results when infants ingest *C. botulinum* spores (as opposed to the neurotoxin as in food-borne botulism) from contaminated food (such as honey) or soil. The spores then germinate in the colon and produce neurotoxin.

— Botulism as a bioweapon is discussed in Box 13-1.

BIOTERRORISM CONSIDERATIONS   BOX 13-1

Botulism is considered by the CDC to be a Category
A critical biological agent. Category A agents have the
greatest potential for mass casualties and a moderate to
high potential for large-scale dissemination. As a bioterror
weapon, botulism can be dispersed in aerosol form or
dispensed in food. The aerosol (inhalation) form would
create more casualties, but the food method would also be
disruptive because patients with botulism require lengthy
critical care/ventilator support. Indeed, even a single case
of botulism, especially if there is no obvious source, raises
the possibility of deliberate use. By 2 days after an attack,
aerosolized *botulinum* would likely be degraded to a level
of little danger (Arnon et al., 2001; Chin, 2000; Rotz, Khan,
Lillibridge, Ostroff, & Hughes, 2002). Also see the
Treatment and Prevention sections.

Incubation

The usual incubation period is 12 to 36 hours and
ranges from 2 hours up to 8 days, depending on several
factors (especially the amount of toxin absorbed), with
the shorter period associated with more severe disease.
For infant botulism the incubation period is 2 to
4 weeks (Chin, 2000).

Clinical Findings and Treatment

Signs and Symptoms

Regardless of route of ingestion, all forms of botulism
produce similar neurologic signs (though greater
gastrointestinal distress and visual disturbances tend to
occur from naturally occurring food-borne and wound
botulism). The severity of symptoms varies significantly.
In infants, the classic presentation is the gradual

progression of poor feeding, weakness, and lethargy (Muensterer, 2000). In intestinal botulism, constipation may be one of the first signs and may precede neurologic signs by as much as 1 week. For older children and adults, the classic triad of botulism (Arnon et al., 2001) is:

- Symmetric, descending flaccid paralysis with bulbar palsies
- Afebrile
- Clear sensorium

The initial presentation includes cranial nerve involvement with bulbar palsies, ptosis, diplopia, blurred vision, photophobia, and decreased visual accommodation. The mouth may be dry with pharyngeal injection. Symptoms progress to dysarthria, dysphonia, and dysphagia with loss of gag reflex. Further progression includes a descending and symmetric flaccid paralysis with loss of head control, hypotonia, generalized weakness, and diaphragmatic and respiratory muscle paralysis. There is no change in sensorium and, in the absence of unrelated infection, no fever. Death results from airway obstruction and hypoventilation (Arnon et al., 2001; Cieslak & Eitzen, 2000; Cox & Hinkle, 2002; Robinson & Naharta, 2003).

Complications

Secondary infections may occur, as may prolonged recuperation and, in the case of intestinal botulism, relapse (Cox & Hinkle, 2002).

Common Laboratory Findings

There are no significant or specific laboratory findings in botulism other than diagnostic findings as discussed next. Cerebrospinal fluid is unremarkable. Electromyography of affected muscles may demonstrate increased amplitude with supratetanic rate of nerve stimulation and brief, small, abundant motor unit action potentials (Muensterer, 2000).

Diagnosis

— Initial diagnosis is on clinical grounds and confirmation is through laboratory testing at the Centers for Disease Control and Prevention (CDC) or one of about 20 other laboratories. CDC furnishes instructions for obtaining samples (serum, stool, gastric aspirate, vomitus, and suspect foods). Note that early treatment is critical in preventing further deterioration, hence treatment is initiated without delay on the basis of patient history and clinical presentation (Chang & Ganguly, 2003; Robinson & Nahata, 2003).

Differential Diagnosis

— Differential diagnosis includes Guillain-Barré syndrome, myasthenia gravis, Eaton-Lambert syndrome, tick paralysis, depressant intoxication, and other central nervous system disorders. Differential diagnosis of intestinal botulism in infants includes encephalitis, meningitis, sepsis, dehydration, metabolic diseases, and heavy metal and other poisoning (Cox & Hinkle, 2002; Robinson & Nahata, 2003). Botulism is distinguished from other flaccid paralyses (Arnon et al, 2001) in that prominent cranial nerve palsies are disproportionate to milder weakness, hypotonia is below the neck, paralysis is symmetrical, and there is no sensory nerve damage. A cluster of patients with the classic triad of botulism is highly suspicious for a deliberate attack.

Treatment

— Treatment includes passive immunization with antitoxin and supportive care. If botulism is identified and treated early, the antitoxin decreases the progressive nerve damage and disease severity, but does not reverse existing damage, hence speed is essential. Antitoxin is generally not used in infants because of its low efficacy and risk of adverse reactions (Muensterer, 2000). Botulinum antitoxins are specific to type; that is, type A antitoxin neutralizes only type A and not type B, and so on. The trivalent antitoxin available from state and local health departments and CDC has antibodies effective against the common *botulinum* types A, B, and E. The antitoxins are equine, hence a skin test looking for a wheal and flare reaction is required to minimize the risk of a hypersensitivity reaction. Desensitization (which takes 3 to 4 hours) is necessary in a small percentage of patients. The current recommended dose of antitoxin is 10 mL (7500 international units type A; 5500 international units type B; 8500 international units type E), which is safe for children and in the second and third trimester of pregnancy. Because a negative skin test does not ensure that hypersensitivity and anaphylaxis will not occur, diphenhydramine and epinephrine should be available. For more current information contact CDC at 404.639.2206 during office hours and at 404.639.2888 at other times (Arnon et al., 2001; Cox & Hinkle, 2002; Robinson & Nahata, 2003).

– Supportive care is focused primarily on respiratory support. For isolated severe cases, critical care includes mechanical ventilation, enteral or parenteral feeding, and prevention/treatment of secondary infections. With decreasing respiratory function, anticipatory intubation is indicated. Ventilation may be necessary for more than 6 months. If secondary respiratory infections develop, aminoglycosides and clindamycin are contraindicated due to their exacerbation of neuromuscular blockade (Arnon et al., 2001; Robinson & Nahata, 2003).

– Known weaponized botulinum includes types A, B, E, and F (several strains of A and E) (Shoham, 2000). The U.S. military has a heptavalent antitoxin effective against types A-G. There are currently insufficient critical care beds and/or ventilators or trained staff for a major attack. In the absence of adequate support, positioning at reverse Trendelenburg at 20 to 25 degrees is recommended over

supine or Fowler's position (head of bed raised 45 to
60 degrees with knees slightly elevated). Food should be
given in small amounts; be soft, semisolid, or finely
chopped; nonabrasive and moist; and liquids may be
better tolerated through a straw (Arnon et al., 2001;
Chin, 2000; Cieslak & Eitzen, 2000).

Prevention

Prevention of naturally occurring botulism (Arnon et al.,
2001; Bollinger & Bartlett, 2000; Chin, 2000) includes
the following:

- Monitor commercial canning and food preparation
  facilities.
- Educate people who practice home canning and food
  preservation about how to destroy the spores (heating
  at 120° C for 30 min under pressure), how to destroy
  the neurotoxin (terminal heating at 89° C for 20 min
  or boiling for 1 min), and how to prevent germination
  (refrigeration, freezing, drying, or preserving with
  salt or sodium nitrite).
- Surgically debride wounds when foreign material is
  present.
- Promote the avoidance of parenteral drug use.
- Eliminate honey from the diet of infants younger
  than 12 months of age.

The *botulinum* toxin cannot be absorbed through intact
skin, hence covering the mouth, nose, and eyes provides
some protection in the event of known presence of the
toxin. Aerosolized toxin is significantly degraded after
2 days. Though effective, postexposure prophylaxis is a
problem because of a lack of sufficient doses of antitoxin
and because of the risk of reaction to the antitoxin. The
toxin is destroyed by heat (85° C for at least 5 min).
Clothing and skin can be cleansed with soap and water
and contaminated surfaces with hypochlorite bleach.
Person-to-person transmission is not a danger.

Reporting

The CDC considers botulism to be a nationally notifiable disease. The World Health Organization (WHO) classifies it as a disease important in public health (Class 2A). See Appendix C for details and for upcoming changes in WHO reporting.

References

Arnon, S.S., Schechter, R., Inglesby, T.V., Henderson, D.A., Bartlett, J.G., et al. (2001). Botulinum toxin as a biological weapon: Medical and public health management. *Journal of the American Medical Association, 285,* 1059-1070.

Bollinger, R.C., & Bartlett, J.G. (2000). Botulism. In G.T. Strickland (Ed.), *Hunter's tropical medicine and emerging infectious diseases* (8th ed., pp. 381-383). Philadelphia: W.B. Saunders Company.

Centers for Disease Control and Prevention. (2001). Botulism. Retrieved July 12, 2003, from *www.bt.cdc.gov/agent/botulism/factsheet.asp*

Chang, G.Y., & Ganguly, G. (2003). Early antitoxin treatment in wound botulism results in better outcome. *European Neurology, 49,* 151-153.

Chang, M., Glynn, M.K., & Groseclose, S.L. (2003). Endemic, notifiable bioterrorism-related diseases, United States, 1992-1999. *Emerging Infectious Diseases, 9.* Retrieved August 30, 2003, from *www.cdc.gov/ncidod/EID/vol9no5/02-0477.htm*

Chin, J. (Ed.). (2000). *Control of communicable diseases manual* (17th ed., pp. 70-75). Washington, DC: American Public Health Association.

Cieslak, T.J. & Eitzen, E.M. (2000). Bioterrorism: Agents of concern. *Journal of Public Health Management and Practice, 6,* 19-29.

Cox, N., & Hinkle, R. (2002). Infant botulism. *American Family Physician, 65,* 1388-1392.

Johns Hopkins University Center for Civilian Biodefense Strategies. (2002). Botulinum toxin. Retrieved August 30, 2003, from *www.hopkins-biodefense.org/pages/agents/agentbotox.html*

Muensterer, O.J. (2000). Infant botulism. *Pediatrics in Review, 21,* 427.

Robinson, R.F., & Nahata, M.C. (2003). Management of botulism. *The Annals of Pharmacotherapy, 37,* 127-131.

Rotz, L.D, Khan, A.S., Lillibridge, S.R., Ostroff, S.M., & Hughes. J.M. (2002). Public health assessment of potential biological terrorism agents. *Emerging Infectious Diseases, 8,* 225-230.

Shoham, D. (2000). Iraq's biological warfare agents: A comprehensive analysis. *Critical Reviews in Microbiology, 26,* 179-204.

14

BRUCELLOSIS

Cyprus fever, Gibralter fever, Malta fever, Mediterranean fever, typhomalarial fever, undulant fever

Geographic Distribution

Brucellosis is found worldwide but is a significant problem primarily in the Mediterranean basin, Arabian Gulf, Latin America, Africa, and India. Higher rates are found on the U.S./Mexican border than elsewhere in the United States. The global incidence is estimated to be around 500,000 cases/year, but brucellosis is underreported at a ratio of about 1:26 (1 reported to 26 unreported) (Araj, 1999; Doyle & Bryan, 2000).

Agent and Vector

Brucella species (gram-negative coccobacilli) are transmitted through ingestion of contaminated unpasteurized milk, cheese, and other animal products. The species that tend to cause human disease include *B. melitensis, B. abortus,* and *B. suis.* Persons involved in animal husbandry, slaughtering, or treatment of sick animals can be infected through the respiratory route, skin, mucous membranes, or conjunctiva. Semen, blood transfusions, and organ transplantation are routes of transmission among humans. Laboratory workers are at risk when handling infected body fluids. *Brucella* species, including *B. melitensis* and *B. suis,* are considered to be potential agents of biological terrorism and are classified as Category B agents (Box 14-1) (Centers for Disease Control and Prevention [CDC], 2000a, 2000b; Wright, 2003).

BIOTERRORISM CONSIDERATIONS   BOX 14-1

Brucella species are considered by the CDC to be
Category B biological warfare agents. Category B agents
are moderately easy to disseminate and cause moderate
morbidity and low mortality (CDC, 2000a). Brucellosis has
been documented as one of the agents in Iraq's biological
warfare program and has been produced and/or
investigated by other countries (Shoham, 2000). The
biological warfare route of infection is most likely aerosol.
Treatment of mass casualties would be doxycycline plus
rifampin or streptomycin.

Incubation

The incubation period is usually 1 to 4 weeks, and up to
several months (Araj, 1999; Doyle & Bryan, 2000).

Clinical Findings and Treatment

Signs and Symptoms

Onset may be gradual or sudden. Brucellosis typically
begins as a mild, nonspecific illness with fever, which
may be intermittent. There may be a wide range of
complaints, with common symptoms/signs including
fever, night sweats with a moldy odor, weight loss,
fatigue, headache, nausea and vomiting, hepatosplenomegaly,
myalgia, arthralgia, and lymphadenopathy. Arthritis,
especially of large weight-bearing joints, is common and
may be severe. Vertebral and muscle abscesses, orchitis,
epididymitis, pyelonephritis, and glomerulonephritis can
also occur. Other systems that may be affected (with a
variety of manifestations) include cardiac, respiratory,
gastrointestinal (which may present as an acute
abdomen), ocular, and neurologic. The illness can also
occur in a chronic form, waxing and waning over many
years (Namiduru et al., 2003; Wright, 2000).

Complications

Complications include spinal nerve root compression, cauda equina syndrome, radiculopathy, septic arthritis, disabling arthritis of the peripheral and axial joints, endocarditis, pericarditis, meningoencephalitis, cerebritis, transient ischemic episodes, encephalopathy, and spontaneous abortion (Wright, 2000).

Common Laboratory Findings

Common laboratory findings include leukocytosis or leukopenia, anemia, thrombocytopenia, increased erythrocyte sedimentation rate, and abnormal liver functions (Namiduru et al., 2003).

Diagnosis

Brucella species are found in the blood, urine, cerebrospinal fluid, and bone marrow in the acute phase but often are not detectable in chronic infections. Blood cultures are most commonly used to isolate the organism and are positive in 14% to 50% of cases. Cultures of bone marrow aspirates may have a higher yield. Positive cultures are usually found within 10 to 12 days, but the laboratory should be notified if brucellosis is suspected, because cultures should be retained up to 6 weeks for maximal sensitivity.

The least expensive and most common test is the serum agglutination test (SAT), which has a sensitivity much higher than that of cultures. An increased level of *Brucella* agglutinin (more than 1:160) confirms an acute episode and lower levels indicate earlier infection. Enzyme-linked immunosorbent assay (ELISA) is the test of choice for complicated and chronic cases. With acute brucellosis, elevated titers of *Brucella*-specific immunoglobulin M (IgM) have a high sensitivity and specificity. Patients with chronic brucellosis show elevations of IgG, IgA, and IgE, but not IgM.

In laboratories that do not perform the ELISA, the indirect *Brucella* Coombs' test has been diagnostic after a negative SAT. Advances in polymerase chain reaction assays have resulted in high sensitivity in detecting *Brucella* DNA, but currently these are used primarily in research facilities (Araj, 1999; Schutze & Jacobs, 2000; Wright, 2000, 2003).

Differential Diagnosis

The differential diagnoses include acute febrile illnesses such as influenza, tularemia, malaria, Q fever, mononucleosis, enteric fever, rheumatic fever, typhoid fever, and cat scratch fever. Gastrointestinal symptoms of acute brucellosis may mimic cholecystitis, typhoid, and schistosomiasis. Tuberculosis can cause similar clinical manifestations in the spine and central nervous system. Chronic brucellosis may be confused with lymphoma, tuberculosis, HIV, malaria, and disseminated fungal infections (Wright, 2000).

Treatment

Prognosis is good with treatment. Adults and children greater than 8 years of age may be treated with streptomycin 1 g IM qd for 2 weeks plus either doxycycline 100 mg PO bid for 6 weeks or tetracycline 500 mg qid for 6 weeks. An alternative treatment is doxycycline 100 mg PO bid for 6 weeks plus rifampin 900 mg daily for 6 weeks. If organ-specific complications occur, such as meningitis, osteomyelitis, or endocarditis, treatment is changed by extending the 6-week courses previously mentioned to 12-week courses. Children younger than age 8 may be treated with trimethoprim-sulfamethoxazole (TMP-SMX) 5 mg/kg q12h for 6 weeks (maximum of 480 mg/24 hours) plus gentamicin 2 mg/kg q8h IV or IM for 2 weeks. Some sources recommend at least 8 weeks of therapy, which includes doxycycline 100 mg PO bid plus an aminoglycoside for 4 weeks followed by doxycycline 100 mg PO bid plus rifampin 600 to 900 mg PO daily for 4 to 8 more weeks. Although efficacy has not been established, persons who have been exposed may be given doxycycline 100 mg bid and rifampin 600 to 900 mg daily for 21 days for post-exposure prophylaxis. When inoculation is conjunctival, prophylaxis is maintained for 4 to 6 weeks (Chin, 2000; Gilbert, Moellering, & Sande, 2002; Madkour, 1998; Schutze & Jacobs, 2000; Wright, 2000).

Prevention

‾ The prevention of brucellosis (Chin, 2000; Wright, 2003) includes the following:
- Avoid consuming unpasteurized or untreated milk or milk products, especially in endemic areas.
- Avoid handling carcasses or products (including placental) of potentially infected animals. Butchers and workers who handle meat products are especially at risk. Hunters should wear protective gloves and barrier clothing when handling feral swine. Remains of feral swine should be buried.
- *Brucella* vaccinations should be used to protect uninfected animals.
- Infected animals can be identified through serologic testing. Infected animals should be slaughtered, and in the case of swine, the herd should be destroyed.

‾ There are currently no vaccines for humans.

Reporting

‾ The CDC considers brucellosis to be a nationally notifiable disease. The World Health Organization (WHO) classifies it as a disease important in public health (Class 2B). See Appendix C for details and for upcoming changes in WHO reporting.

References

Araj, G.F. (1999). Human brucellosis: A classical infectious disease with persistent diagnostic challenges. *Clinical Laboratory Science, 12,* 207-212.

Centers for Disease Control and Prevention. (2000a). Biological and chemical terrorism: Strategic plan for preparedness and response. *Morbidity and Mortality Weekly Report, 49*(RR-4), 1-14.

Centers for Disease Control and Prevention. (2000b). Suspected brucellosis case prompts investigation of possible bioterrorism-related activity: New Hampshire and Massachusetts, 1999. *Morbidity and Mortality Weekly Report, 49,* 509-512.

Chin, J. (Ed.). (2000). *Control of communicable diseases manual* (17th ed, pp. 75-78). Washington, DC: American Public Health Association.

Doyle, T.J., & Bryan, R.T. (2000). Infectious disease morbidity in the U.S. region bordering Mexico, 1990-1998. *Journal of Infectious Diseases, 182,* 1503-1510.

Gilbert, D.N., Moellering, R.C., Jr., & Sande, M.A. (2002). *The Sanford guide to antimicrobial therapy* (32nd ed., p. 42). Hyde Park, VT: Antimicrobial Therapy.

Madkour, M.M. (1998). Brucellosis. In A.S. Fauci, E. Braunwald, K.J. Isselbacher, J.D. Wilson, J.B. Martin, et al. (Eds.), *Harrison's principles of internal medicine* (14th ed., pp. 969-971). New York: McGraw-Hill.

Namiduru, M., Gungor, K., Dikensoy, O., Baydar, I., Ekinci, E., et al. (2003) Epidemiological, clinical, and laboratory features of brucellosis: A prospective evaluation of 120 adult patients. *International Journal of Clinical Practice, 57,* 20-24.

Schutze, G., & Jacobs, R. (2000). Brucella. In R. Behrman, R. Kliegman, & H. Jenson (Eds.), *Nelson textbook of pediatrics* (16th ed., pp. 867-869). Philadelphia: W.B. Saunders Company.

Shoham, D. (2000). Iraq's biological warfare agents: A comprehensive analysis. *Critical Reviews in Microbiology, 26,* 179-204.

Wright, S.G. (2000). Brucellosis. In G.T. Strickland (Ed.), *Hunter's tropical medicine* (8th ed., pp. 416-420). Philadelphia: W.B. Saunders Company.

Wright, S.G. (2003). Brucellosis. In G.C. Cook & A.I. Zumla (Eds.), *Manson's tropical diseases* (21st ed., pp. 1173-1194). Philadelphia: W.B. Saunders Company.

15

BURULI ULCER

Geographic Distribution

Buruli ulcer is found with the highest incidence in Uganda and The Congo, but there are also significant numbers of infections in most countries of Central and West Africa, Southeast Asia, Australia, and scattered areas of Latin America. In West Africa, incidence is increasing rapidly (Meyers, 2000).

Agent and Vector

After tuberculosis and leprosy, the Buruli ulcer, caused by *Mycobacterium ulcerans,* is the third most common mycobacterial disease in immunocompetent people. Although individuals of all ages are affected, those in the second and third decades of life have the highest incidence of infection. *M. ulcerans* is a mycobacterium thought to be present in soil, shallow water, vegetation, and in certain aquatic insects. Many believe the *M. ulcerans* infection is acquired from penetrating injuries that transfer the bacterium into the subcutaneous tissue. Person-to-person transmission has rarely been reported (Marsollier et al., 2002; Meyers, 2000; Stienstra et al., 2001; van der Werf, van der Graaf, Tappero, & Asiedu, 1999).

Incubation

Once the initial papule or nodule is present, ulceration occurs within 1 to 2 months (Meyers, 2000).

Clinical Findings and Treatment

Signs and Symptoms

The first stage of disease may be characterized by papules, firm subcutaneous nodules, indurated plaques, or edematous ill-defined plaques that most commonly occur on the limbs, although they can affect the trunk or the face. In the second stage of disease, the primary lesion ulcerates and may be surrounded by extensive edema, which leaves an undermined edge and can involve large areas of the affected limb (Figure 15-1). Ulcers may heal without treatment or spread rapidly to involve an entire limb (van der Werf et al., 1999; Vega-Lopez & Chopera, 2003)

Complications

Most ulcers eventually resolve without treatment. However, without therapy, the affected individual is often left with contractures, severe scarring, lymphedema, and possibly the need for amputation of the affected limb. Edematous forms may progress rapidly and destroy underlying tissues, such as muscle and bone. Osteomyelitis is a rare presentation of *M. ulcerans*. Other complications include sepsis and the loss of other structures such as the

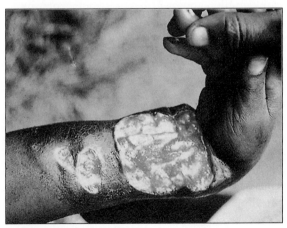

FIGURE 15–1

Buruli ulcer. (*Source:* From Peters, W., & Pasvol, G. [2002]. *Tropical medicine and parasitology* [5th ed., p. 249]. Chicago: Mosby.)

eye or genitalia (Asiedu & Etuaful, 1998; Meyers, 2000; van der Werf et al., 1999; Vega-Lopez & Chopera, 2003).

Common Laboratory Findings

There are no laboratory findings commonly associated with Buruli ulcer.

Diagnosis

In endemic areas, the characteristic clinical presentation is often enough to make the diagnosis. Necrotic slough from the ulcer may reveal acid-fast bacilli (AFB) with Ziehl-Neelsen stain, but a negative test does not rule out the diagnosis. Culture of the organism takes 6 to 8 weeks of incubation at 32° C, and this may be difficult, expensive, and not readily available in endemic areas. Excisional skin biopsy and histopathologic examination of the ulcer can also be helpful, and AFB are often identifiable in areas of necrotic subcutaneous tissues and dermal collagen. Molecular techniques, such as polymerase chain reaction (PCR), can be useful when other techniques yield negative results; however, these tests are expensive and often limited to research facilities (Guarner et al., 2003; Meyers, 2000; van der Werf et al., 1999).

Differential Diagnosis

The differential diagnosis of plaques or edematous lesions includes pyogenic cellulitis secondary to streptococci or staphylococci. These infections may cause fever or systemic symptoms, which rarely occur with a Buruli ulcer. When the ulceration occurs on the face, it may be mistaken for cancrum oris (noma). The characteristic undermined edge of the ulcer resembles that of pyoderma gangrenosum, which is an inflammatory, noninfectious ulceration (van der Werf et al., 1999; van der Werf, Stienstra, & van der Graaf, 2003). Cutaneous anthrax also causes painless ulcers, but with a black eschar.

Treatment

— Surgery is the primary treatment for Buruli ulcers. Complete excision of papules and nodules is curative. When lesions enlarge and ulcerate, surgery is still required. All necrotic tissue needs to be removed in order to prevent persistent infection from residual organisms. Split-thickness skin grafting can be used to cover large defects. Physical therapy or surgery may be needed to release contractures or increase mobility. Antimycobacterial therapy may be helpful in disseminated cases or to prevent osteomyelitis; however, effectiveness for treating extensive ulcerations has been disappointing (van der Werf et al., 1999).

Prevention

— The prevention of Buruli ulcers (Smith, Revill, Lukwago, & Rykushin, 1977; van der Werf et al., 1999) includes the following:
  - The bacille Calmette-Guérin (BCG) vaccination may provide limited, short-lived protection against extensive Buruli ulceration. The protective effect may be confined to those with tuberculin reactions of less than 4 mm before vaccination and is apparent only up to 1 year.
  - Long pants and long-sleeved shirts may provide some protection against inoculation or injuries while farming or working outdoors.

— Until better prevention methods are available, early detection and rapid surgical treatment are the best way to prevent morbidity.

Reporting

— The U.S. Centers for Disease Control and Prevention (CDC) does not consider Buruli ulcer to be a nationally notifiable disease, nor does the World Health Organization (WHO) classify it as a disease important in public health (Class 5). See Appendix C for details and for upcoming changes in WHO reporting.

References

Asiedu, K., & Etuaful, S. (1998). Socioeconomic implications of Buruli ulcer in Ghana: A three-year review. *American Journal of Tropical Medicine and Hygiene, 59,* 1015-1022.

Guarner, J., Bartlett, J., Whitney, E.A., Raghunathan, P.L., Stienstra, Y., et al. (2003). Histopathologic features of *Mycobacterium ulcerans* infection. *Emerging Infectious Diseases, 9,* 651-656.

Marsollier, L., Robert, R., Aubry, J., Saint Andre, J.P., Kouakou, H., et al. (2002). Aquatic insects as a vector for *Mycobacterium ulcerans. Applied and Environmental Microbiology, 68,* 4623-4628.

Meyers, W.M. (2000). Nontuberculous mycobacterial skin infections. In G.T. Strickland (Ed.), *Hunter's tropical medicine* (8th ed., pp. 524-525). Philadelphia: W.B. Saunders Company.

Smith, P.G., Revill, W.D., Lukwago, E., & Rykushin, Y.P. (1977). The protective effect of BCG against *Mycobacterium ulcerans* disease: A controlled trial in an endemic area of Uganda. *Transactions of the Royal Society of Tropical Medicine and Hygiene, 70,* 449-457.

Stienstra, Y., van der Graaf, W.T., te Meerman, G.J., The, T.H., de Leij, L.F., & van der Werf, T.S. (2001). Susceptibility to development of *Mycobacterium ulcerans* disease: Review of possible risk factors. *Tropical Medicine and International Health, 6,* 554-562.

van der Werf, T.S., Stienstra, Y., & van der Graaf, W.T. (2003). Skin ulcers misdiagnosed as pyoderma gangrenosum. *New England Journal of Medicine, 348,* 1064-1066.

van der Werf, T.S., van der Graaf, W.T., Tappero, J.W., & Asiedu, K. (1999). *Mycobacterium ulcerans* infection. *Lancet, 354,* 1013-1018.

Vega-Lopez, F. & Chopera, S. (2003). Dermatologic problems. In G.C. Cook & A.I. Zumla (Eds.), *Manson's tropical diseases* (21st ed., pp. 368-369). Philadelphia: W.B. Saunders Company.

16

Capillariasis

Geographic Distribution

Intestinal capillariasis, the most common *Capillaria* infection, is endemic in the Philippine Islands and Thailand. Rare cases are reported from other Asian and Middle Eastern countries. Pulmonary and hepatic capillariasis (not discussed here) are extremely rare and are reported from various locations around the world (Chin, 2000).

Agent and Vector

Capillaria philippinensis is a small intestinal nematode of the superfamily Trichuroidea. Adults are thread-like and 2 to 4 mm in length. Fish-eating birds are the natural reservoirs of the worm, with freshwater fish serving as intermediate hosts. Humans become infected when they eat raw or incompletely cooked whole fish that have larvae in their intestines. In addition, *Capillaria* are capable of autoinfection in the small intestine (Belizario et al., 2000; Chin, 2000).

Incubation

The incubation period in humans is not known; in animal studies, incubation is approximately 1 month (Chin, 2000).

Clinical Findings and Treatment

Signs and Symptoms

Invasion of the small bowel mucosa causes chronic watery diarrhea, abdominal pain, borborygmi, anorexia, edema, and weight loss. The chronic malabsorption-diarrhea syndrome results in protein loss and electrolyte abnormalities. Without treatment, the infection may result in cachexia, myocardial degeneration, and death from hypokalemia or metabolic cardiomyopathy or secondary infection (Belizario et al., 2000; Bundy & Cooper, 2000; Chin, 2000).

Complications

Autoinfection leading to massive parasite load causes the advanced disease described in the preceding section.

Common Laboratory Findings

In addition to the previously noted electrolyte abnormalities, eosinophilia occurs (Molyneux, 1995).

Diagnosis

Diagnosis of intestinal capillariasis is on the basis of characteristic unembryonated eggs in the stool. Larvae and sometimes adults may also be found in severe infection (Centers for Disease Control and Prevention [CDC], 2003).

Differential Diagnosis

Differential diagnosis would include numerous other causes of chronic diarrhea such as amebiasis, clonorchiasis, cryptosporidiosis, strongyloidiasis, fascioliasis, cysticercosis, trichuriasis, tropical sprue, and others. Geographic location and history of ingestion of small whole fish helps in narrowing the diagnosis.

Treatment

Treatment of capillariasis in children and adults is with mebendazole 100 mg bid or 200 mg daily or bid for 20 days; or albendazole 200 mg bid for 10 days. Treatment should be prompt to reduce autoinfection risk (Bundy & Cooper, 2000; Gal & Reed, 2004).

Prevention

Measures to prevent capillariasis (Chin, 2000) include the following:
- Avoid consumption of raw or incompletely cooked fish, especially small, whole fish.
- Provide sanitary disposal of feces. In particular, defecating in padi (as is common throughout rural Asia) should be avoided.

Community education regarding the preceding measures should be ongoing in endemic areas.

Reporting

The CDC does not consider capillariasis to be a nationally notifiable disease, nor does the World Health Organization (WHO) classify it as a disease important in public health (Class 5). See Appendix C for details and for upcoming changes in WHO reporting.

References

Belizario, V.Y., de Leon, W.U., Esparar, D.G., Galang, J.M., Fantone, J., & Verdadero, C. (2000). Compostela Valley: A new endemic focus for *Capillariasis philippinensis. Southeast Asian Journal of Tropical Medicine and Public Health, 31,* 478-481.

Bundy, D.A.P., & Cooper, E. (2000). Nematodes limited to the intestinal tract. In G.T. Strickland (Ed.), *Hunter's tropical medicine and emerging infectious diseases* (8th ed., pp. 719-726). Philadelphia: W.B. Saunders Company.

Centers for Disease Control and Prevention. (2003). Capillariasis. Retrieved October 1, 2003, from *www.dpd.cdc.gov/dpdx/HTML/Capillariasis.htm*

Chin, J. (Ed.). (2000). *Control of communicable diseases manual* (17th ed, pp. 84-87). Washington, DC: American Public Health Association.

Gal, P. & Reed, M.D. (2004). Medications. In R.E. Behrman, R.M. Kliegman, & H.B. Jenson (Eds.), *Nelson textbook of pediatrics* (17th ed., pp. 2432-2502). Philadelphia: W.B. Saunders Company.

Molyneux, M. (1995). Blood fluke: Schistosomes. In D.R. Bell (Ed.), *Tropical medicine* (4th ed., pp. 221-239). Oxford: Blackwell Science.

17

CHAGAS' DISEASE
American trypanosomiasis
Geographic Distribution

Chagas' disease is endemic to Central and South America, and is an emerging problem in North America. Based on seroprevalence studies in Hispanic blood donors, between 50,000 and 100,000 people in the United States are infected. It is estimated by the World Health Organization (WHO) that 16 to 18 million people are infected worldwide and up to 45,000 die each year. Bolivia currently has the highest rural seroprevalence rate of approximately 20%, but the majority of cases are reported from Brazil (Bonomo & Salata, 2000; Kirchhoff, 2000; Magil & Reed, 2000).

Agent and Vector

The Reduviid insect (triatomine bug) vector is infected with *Trypanosoma cruzi,* a single-celled protozoan parasite, when it ingests blood from mammals with circulating parasites. The ingested organisms multiply in the midgut of the insect and are then transformed in the hindgut to the infective form. When the insect takes a blood meal, the infective form of the parasite is released in its feces and urine, and infection is established in the mammalian host by either crossing mucous membranes or entering through the wound made by the insect bite. Inside the new host, the parasite multiplies intracellularly and invades various tissues (Kirchhoff, 2000; Miles, 2003). Other means of acquiring infection include blood transfusions, congenital transmission, ingestion of food contaminated with infected insect feces, and accidental inoculation of the parasite by laboratory workers (Magil & Reed, 2000).

Incubation

The initial cutaneous lesion (chagoma) that can develop at the port of entry of the organism may occur after 5 to 14 days; however, it may take several months for the acute phase of the infection to begin when the source is a blood transfusion (Kirchhoff, 2000; Miles, 2003).

Clinical Findings and Treatment

Signs and Symptoms

Signs and symptoms depend on whether the infection is acute or chronic.

ACUTE STAGE

The acute stage is often an illness of children but can occur at any age. The clinical severity of acute illness can vary greatly, with 10% to 20% of patients having a mild undifferentiated febrile syndrome. In the acute stage, about 50% of patients develop an edematous nodule (chagoma) at the site of the bite. Conjunctival contamination with the vector's feces results in unilateral painless palpebral and periocular swelling (Romaña's sign) and associated lymphadenopathy (Figure 17-1). Systemic spread of the parasites from the initial site of infection may result in fever, malaise, facial or generalized edema, myalgia, hepatosplenomegaly, and lymphadenopathy. The acute stage lasts 4 to 8 weeks and, in rare cases, may include myocarditis or meningoencephalitis. Most patients experience spontaneous remission of symptoms, followed by a lifelong low-grade parasitemia, which may be exacerbated by HIV infection or other immunocompromised states.

CHRONIC STAGE

In most cases, chronic Chagas' disease is characterized by lifelong low-grade asymptomatic parasitemia, with only

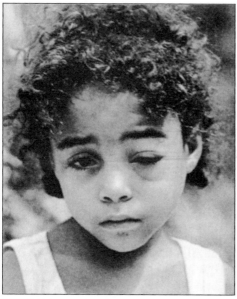

FIGURE 17–1

Romaña's sign. (*Source:* From Peters, W., & Pasvol, G. [2002]. *Tropical medicine and parasitology* [5th ed., p. 58]. Chicago: Mosby.)

10% to 30% of patients developing symptomatic systemic disease. The mean age of onset for symptomatic chronic Chagas' disease is 35 to 45 years of age, which may be decades after the acute illness. The heart is the most commonly affected organ, with manifestations including congestive heart failure (often right sided), thromboembolism, cardiac aneurysms, and rhythm disturbances, which may result in dizziness, syncope, and sudden death. A small proportion of patients develop abnormalities of the gastrointestinal tract, which most commonly include megacolon, constipation, and megaesophagus, leading to dysphagia, odynophagia, chest pain, cough, and regurgitation (Chin, 2000; Goldsmith, 2001; Kirchhoff, 2000; Magill & Reed, 2000; Miles, 2003).

Complications

— Meningoencephalitis and hepatitis are rare complications
   in severe, acute disease. Severe myocarditis may lead to
   chronic cardiomyopathy (in 20% to 30% of patients
   with Chagas' disease), which is characterized by a
   thin-walled, enlarged, flabby heart with a prominent
   right ventricular outflow tract, resulting in right-sided
   heart failure. Ventricular walls are thin and fibrotic,
   which may lead to aneurysms, thrombus development,
   and dysrhythmias. Chronic Chagas' disease causes loss of
   neurons in the gut, which may lead to esophageal
   dilation, megacolon, parotid gland hypertrophy, and
   dilation of the stomach. The resulting symptoms from
   these complications include dysphagia, regurgitation,
   aspiration pneumonia, abdominal distention, delayed
   gastric emptying, intractable constipation, bowel
   obstruction, perforation, and sepsis. Megaesophagus and
   megacolon have not been found north of the equator
   and are most common in Brazil (Hotez et al., 2004;
   Kirchhoff, 2000; Magill & Reed, 2000).
— Congenital transmission occurs in approximately 1% of
   deliveries from seropositive women and may cause
   spontaneous abortion, intrauterine growth retardation, or
   stillbirth. Between 50% and 75% of infected newborns
   are asymptomatic, and 15% to 20% present with
   a mild illness. Rare severe cases may develop
   pneumonitis, meningoencephalitis, hemorrhagic
   symptoms, or die within the first week after birth
   (Magill & Reed, 2000).
— Reactivation of chronic Chagas' disease is a rare
   condition and occurs only in immunosuppressed
   patients, including those with HIV infection.
   The most common presentation in these cases is
   meningoencephalitis (de Oliveira Santos, dos Reis
   Canela, Gomes Moncao, & Guedes Roque, 2002;
   Magill & Reed, 2000).

Common Laboratory Findings

Laboratory findings in the acute phase include lympho-cytosis and elevated transaminases. There may be early electrocardiographic changes including sinus tachycardia, increased P-R interval, T wave changes, and low QRS voltage. In the chronic phase, electrocardiographic changes may include right bundle branch block, left anterior hemiblock, sinus bradycardia, sinoatrial block, and ventricular tachycardia (Miles, 2003).

Diagnosis

A definitive diagnosis can be made by detecting parasites in the blood or tissues. Trypanosomes may be found in peripheral blood when a patient is in the febrile stage of the acute illness by direct examination of wet preparations of anticoagulated blood or buffy coat. Giemsa stain examination of thick or thin blood slides may also be useful. *T. cruzi* may also be detected during the acute phase in other tissues, such as cerebrospinal fluid, pericardial fluid, and organ biopsies, especially in immunocompromised patients. When the patient enters the chronic phase, identifying the parasite may require much more sensitive methods (Magill & Reed, 2000). Antibodies appear in the acute stage and then are present for life. A definitive diagnosis of the acute stage can be made by detecting *T. cruzi*-specific immunoglobulin M (IgM); however, these assays are not standardized or commercially available. There are currently three enzyme-linked immunosorbent assay (ELISA) test kits commercially available to measure *T. cruzi*-specific IgG antibodies in order to diagnose chronic disease. These assays have high sensitivity and specificity (95% to 100%). Other highly sensitive serologic tests used in Latin America include indirect immunofluorescence and complement fixation. In some cases, it is recommended that at least two independent serologic tests be performed, because false positives have been reported in patients with malaria, syphilis, leishmaniasis, or collagen vascular disease. Serologic screening should be considered in high-risk populations, especially pregnant women, organ transplant recipients, and those with immunocompromised conditions such as HIV (Bonomo & Salata, 2000; Kirchhoff, 2000; Magill & Reed, 2000).

— Xenodiagnosis and blood culture may be helpful in the chronic phase. In xenodiagnosis, laboratory-reared triatomine bugs are fed on the patients. Approximately 1 month later, the insects' feces and hindgut contents are examined for parasites. This test is very specific for *T. cruzi*, but the sensitivity may be no greater than 50%. Blood culture using biphasic media can be used to detect parasites, but the sensitivity is not as great as with xenodiagnosis (Magill & Reed, 2000; Miles, 2003).

Differential Diagnosis

— The differential diagnosis includes typhoid fever, schistosomiasis, brucellosis, infectious mononucleosis, African trypanosomiasis, toxoplasmosis, and malaria, as a cause for fever that occurs without a Romaña's sign or chagoma. The edema associated with Romaña's sign lasts for weeks, which will differentiate it from many causes of unilateral palpebral edema, such as periorbital cellulitis or angioedema. Myocarditis due to rheumatic fever or viral causes must be considered when there is cardiac involvement (Magill & Reed, 2000).

Treatment

— No satisfactory treatment currently exists for any stage of Chagas' disease. In the acute stage, medications are effective in reducing the severity and duration of the disease, but cure is only achieved in 50% of patients. Treatment in the chronic stage is controversial, because it is not clear whether it will alter cardiac complications or progression of the disease. Medications used currently for

treatment include nifurtimox or benznidazole. The adult
dose of nifurtimox is 8 to 10 mg/kg/day three times daily
after meals for 30 to 120 days. Nifurtimox is better
tolerated in children than adults, and children can take
up to 15 mg/kg/day three times daily after meals for
90 to 120 days. The frequent side effects include
tremors, insomnia, anorexia, and weight loss.
Benznidazole is the drug of choice in Brazil and South
America because it is more trypanocidal than nifurtimox.
Children also tolerate this drug better than adults, so the
recommended dose for all individuals is 5 to 10 mg/kg/day
twice daily for 30 to 60 days. Common complications of
benznidazole are peripheral neuritis, anorexia, weight
loss, and hematologic alterations, such as neutropenia. In
the United States, nifurtimox is available only from the
Centers for Disease Control and Prevention (CDC), and
benznidazole is not available (Bonomo & Salata, 2000;
Goldsmith, 2001; Magill & Reed, 2000).
Medical management of the chronic complications of
Chagas' disease may be required. Chagasic heart disease
can be managed with restricted salt intake, diuretics,
vasodilatory medications, and antiarrhythmics. The most
effective drug in the management of arrhythmias is
amiodarone. Pacemakers may be required in patients
with intractable bradycardia, complete AV block, or for
atrial fibrillation with a slow ventricular response.
Anticoagulants minimize the risk of thromboembolism.
Referral to a cardiologist is indicated for cardiac
conditions. A light, balanced diet is recommended for
megaesophagus. Nitrates and nifedipine have been used
to lower esophageal sphincter pressure. Megacolon is
initially treated with high dietary fiber and stool
softeners. Acute meningoencephalitis may be managed
with anticonvulsants, sedatives, and intravenous
mannitol (Bonomo & Salata, 2000; Goldsmith, 2001;
Magill & Reed, 2000; Miles, 2003;
Rosenblatt, 1999).

Surgery may be required for megaesophagus or
megacolon. Megaesophagus can be managed with
balloon dilatation of the cardiac sphincter, but more
severe cases may require removal of a section of muscle
from the esophago-gastric junction. Severe megacolon
may need to be managed with resection of the involved
colon (Miles, 2003).

Prevention

Currently, there are no vaccines or chemoprophylaxis to
prevent Chagas' disease. The primary means for control
of the disease involves vector control and serologic
screening of donors at blood banks (Kirchhoff, 2000).
Effective vector control of triatomine bugs is integrated
(Chin, 2000; Hotez et al., 2004; Miles, 2003) and
includes the following:

- When a home with triatomine bugs is identified,
  spray all homes and associated or peridomestic
  structures (e.g., outbuildings, stables, chicken houses)
  in the area with residual insecticide (synthetic
  pyrethroid). See Appendix D. In homes, the insects
  are most commonly found in dark, moist spaces in
  walls (especially bedroom), and also in bedding,
  clothes, behind pictures, and elsewhere. In some
  cases, the insects are found in palm trees and these
  must then be sprayed.
- Plaster or otherwise seal cracks in walls and replace
  thatch roofs with tin or other material inhospitable to
  the triatomine bugs.
- Maintain vigilance for structures with residual
  or new infestations and spray immediately. Vigilance
  also includes serologic testing of all children over
  9 months of age born after the beginning of the
  integrated vector control campaign (except
  children of mothers who were seropositive when
  pregnant).

Community education and involvement is an important aspect of prevention and control.

Reporting

The CDC does not consider Chagas' disease to be a nationally notifiable disease, nor does the WHO classify it as a disease important in public health (Class 3B). However, the expanding geographic range of Chagas' disease into the United States may result in greater public health interest. See Appendix C for details and for upcoming changes in WHO reporting.

References

Bonomo, R., & Salata, R. (2000). American trypanosomiasis (Chagas's disease: *Trypanosoma cruzi*). In R. Behrman, R. Kliegman, & H. Jenson, (Eds.), *Nelson textbook of pediatrics* (16th ed., pp. 1046-1048). Philadelphia: W.B. Saunders Company.

Chin, J. (Ed.). (2000). *Control of communicable diseases manual* (17th ed, pp. 518-520). Washington, DC: American Public Health Association.

de Oliveira Santos, E., dos Reis Canela, J., Gomes Moncao, H.C., & Guedes Roque, M.J. (2002). Reactivation of Chagas' disease leading to the diagnosis of acquired immunodeficiency syndrome. *Brazilian Journal of Infectious Disease, 6,* 317-321.

Goldsmith, R.S. (2001). Infectious diseases: Protozoal and helminthic. In L.M. Tierney, S.J. McPhee, & M.A. Papadakis (Eds.), *Current medical diagnosis & treatment* (40th ed., pp. 1414-1416). Stamford, CT: Appleton & Lange.

Hotez, P.J., Remme, J.H.F., Buss, P., Alleyne, G., Morel, C., & Breman, J.G. (2004). Combating tropical infectious diseases: Report of the Disease Control Priorities in Developing Countries Project. *Clinical Infectious Diseases, 38,* 871-878.

Kirchhoff, L. (2000). Trypanosoma species (American trypanosomiasis, Chagas' disease): Biology of trypanosomes. In G. Mandell, J. Bennett, & R. Dolin (Eds.), *Principles and practice of infectious diseases* (5th ed., pp. 2845-2851). New York: Churchill Livingstone.

Magil, A., & Reed. S. (2000). American trypanosomiasis. In G.T. Strickland (Ed.), *Hunter's tropical medicine* (8th ed., pp. 653-663). Philadelphia: W.B. Saunders Company.

Miles, M.A. (2003). American trypanosomiasis. In G.C. Cook & A.I. Zumla (Eds.), *Manson's tropical diseases* (21st ed., pp. 1325-1337). Philadelphia: W.B. Saunders Company.

Rosenblatt, J.E. (1999). Antiparasitic agents. *Mayo Clinic Proceedings, 74*, 1161-1175.

18

CHIKUNGUNYA FEVER
CHIK
Geographic Distribution

Chikungunya fever occurs in Southeast Asia, India, the Middle East, and Africa (Chin, 2000, Mourya et al., 2001).

Agent and Vector

Chikungunya fever is a dengue-like arthropod-borne viral (arboviral) disease caused by the Chikungunya alphavirus (family Togaviridae, genus *Alphavirus*). The vector is primarily the *Aedes aegypti* mosquito, though other mosquitoes are also involved in transmission. Since the virus was first isolated in the 1950s, a number of epidemics have been identified in Africa and Asia, some of which lasted for several years. In Africa, the virus appears to be maintained in a sylvatic (forest) cycle including monkeys, humans, and other mammals. In Asia, the virus appears to be maintained in an urban cycle. Chikungunya is antigenically related to other viruses, including Semliki Forest (SFV), O'nyong-nyong (ONN), Ross River (RR), and Mayaro (Chin, 2000; Hasebe et al., 2002; Powers, Brault, Tesh, & Weaver, 2000; Tsai, 2000).

Incubation

The incubation period ranges from 2 to 10 days, but most often is 2 to 3 days (Broom, Smith, Hall, Johansen, & Mackenzie, 2003).

Clinical Findings and Treatment

Signs and Symptoms

Chikungunya fever is characterized by the sudden onset of fever, arthropathy, myalgia, conjunctivitis, lymphadenopathy, and, often, pharyngitis. Arthropathy is symmetric, tends to affect the distal extremities more than shoulders or hips, may include effusions, and may be disabling. Back pain is common. These initial manifestations usually improve after several days (except, often, the arthropathy), and are followed by a fine generalized maculopapular rash that spreads centrifugally, including in many cases to the palms and soles. Bleeding from mucous membranes and nausea and vomiting sometimes occur. In some cases the illness is biphasic, and in other cases, is manifested only by fever. The illness tends to be milder in children. Fatalities in adults or children are rare, and in most cases, recovery is complete after several weeks of illness, though arthropathy may continue for years (Broom et al., 2003; Tsai, 2000).

Complications

Serious complications are rare. Gastrointestinal bleeding occasionally occurs and may be severe, leading to shock. Arthropathy lasts for a year or longer in about one-third of patients. There is also evidence of the possibility that infection with chikungunya fever increases the likelihood of contracting endemic Burkitt's lymphoma among children primed with holoendemic malaria and Epstein-Barr virus infection (Broom et al., 2003; van den Bosch & Lloyd, 2000).

Common Laboratory Findings

Erythrocyte sedimentation rate may be increased, as well as C-reactive protein. Rheumatoid factor may be present.

Diagnosis

Arthropathy, myalgia, conjunctivitis, and maculopapular rash are important distinguishing features. A reverse transcription-polymerase chain reaction (RT-PCR) test has been developed for specific identification of chikungunya virus, thus eliminating problems of serologic cross reaction with other alphaviruses such as SFV, ONN, RR, and Mayaro virus (Hasebe et al., 2002). The virus can be isolated from serum. Immunoglobulin M (IgM) can be detected by immunofluorescence assay (IFA) or enzyme immunoassay (EIA), and during acute infection, though the aforementioned cross reactivity somewhat limits these in Africa (Broom et al., 2003).

Differential Diagnosis

Chikungunya closely resembles dengue fever in presentation and distribution in Africa and Asia. Dengue, however, presents with more diffuse musculoskeletal pain as opposed to the marked arthropathy of chikungunya fever. Other differentials include viral infections such as ONN, West Nile, Sindbis, rubella, parvovirus, hepatitis A and B, mumps, Epstein-Barr, and enteroviruses. Reactive arthritis, disseminated gonococcal infection, and rheumatoid arthritis should also be considered (Broom et al., 2003).

Treatment

Treatment is supportive and includes nonsteroidal antiinflammatory drugs and rest (Broom et al., 2003; Tsai, 2000).

Prevention

The prevention of chikungunya (and other arboviral as well as filarial diseases) is directed at community and personal mosquito control in endemic areas (Chin, 2000; Robert, 2000; Thompson, 2002; White, 2003; World Health Organization [WHO], 1998) and includes the following:

- Kill adult mosquitoes by spraying inside and outside human habitations and surrounding areas with

residual insecticides. The goal is to kill as many female mosquitoes as possible, thus decreasing the likelihood of disease transmission. See Appendix D.
- Kill larvae and eliminate breeding areas as much as possible. Elimination of breeding areas includes draining standing water such as swamps, emptying open water-filled containers and used tires, and reducing the number of plants that hold standing water (e.g., bromeliads).

- Personal protection includes the following:
  - Screen living and working quarters.
  - Use a residual insecticide inside homes and work areas. See Appendix D.
  - Use insecticide-impregnated mosquito netting over beds. Nets must be retreated with insecticide annually. See Appendix D.
  - Stay inside as much as possible during hours when mosquitoes are biting, which, in the case of *Aedes* mosquitoes is usually during the day as opposed to *Anopheles,* which feed primarily at dusk to dawn.
  - Use DEET repellant on skin and permethrin on clothing when outside during biting hours.

- Provide ongoing community education regarding the preceding measures.

Reporting

- The Centers for Disease Control and Prevention (CDC) does not consider chikungunya to be a nationally notifiable disease. The WHO classifies it as a disease important in public health (Class 2A). See Appendix C for details and for upcoming changes in WHO reporting.

References

Broom, A.K., Smith, D.W., Hall, R.A., Johansen, C.A. & Mackenzie, J.S. (2003). Arbovirus infections. In G.C. Cook & A.I. Zumla (Eds.), *Manson's tropical diseases* (21st ed., pp. 725-764). Philadelphia: W.B. Saunders Company.

Chin, J. (2000). Arthropod-borne viral diseases. In J. Chin (Ed.), *Control of communicable diseases manual* (17th ed., pp. 28-39). Washington, DC: American Public Health Association.

Hasebe, F., Parquet, M.C., Pandey, B.D., Mathenge, E.G.M., Morita, K., et al. (2002). Combined detection and genotyping of *Chikungunya* virus by a specific reverse transcription-polymerase chain reaction. *Journal of Medical Virology, 67,* 370-374.

Mourya, D.T., Thakare, J.P., Gokhale, M.D., Powers, A.M., Hundekar, S.L., et al. (2001). Isolation of chikungunya virus from *Aedes aegypti* mosquitos collected in the town of Yawat, Pune District, Maharashtra State, India. *Acta Virologica, 45,* 305-309.

Powers, A.M., Brault, A.C., Tesh, R.B., & Weaver, S.C. (2000). Re-emergence of chikungunya and O'nyong nyong viruses: Evidence for distinct geographical lineages and distant evolutionary relationships. *Journal of General Virology, 81,* 471-479.

Robert, L.L. (2000). Control of arthropods of medical importance. In G.T. Strickland (Ed.), *Hunter's tropical medicine and emerging infectious diseases* (8th ed., pp. 1019-1034). Philadelphia: W.B. Saunders Company.

Thompson, M.J. (2002). Immunizations for international travel. *Primary Care; Clinics in Office Practice, 29,* 787-814.

Tsai, T. (2000). Chikungunya fever. In G.T. Strickland (Ed.), *Hunter's tropical medicine and emerging infectious diseases* (8th ed., pp. 246-248). Philadelphia: W.B. Saunders Company.

van den Bosch, C. & Lloyd, G. (2000). Chikungunya fever as a risk factor for endemic Burkitt's lymphoma in Malawi. *Transactions of the Royal Society of Tropical Medicine and Hygiene, 94,* 704-705.

White, G.B. (2003). Mosquitoes. In G.C. Cook & A.I. Zumla (Eds.), *Manson's tropical diseases* (21st ed., pp. 1741-1772). Philadelphia: W.B. Saunders Company.

World Health Organization. (1998). Use of DDT in vector control. WHO Expert Committee on Malaria. Retrieved May 28, 2004, from *http://mosquito.who.int/docs/ecr20_annex1.htm*

19

CHOLERA

Geographic Distribution

Since 1817 there have been seven cholera pandemics with every continent affected by at least one of the pandemics. In the current seventh pandemic, beginning in 1961, cholera entered Southeast Asia, the Indian subcontinent, the Middle East, Africa, and South America. Today most cases are reported in Africa, often in conjunction with refugee crises. The Americas were not affected by the current pandemic until 1991, and since then have shown a steady decline in incidence and mortality: In 1991 there were 396,536 cases and 4093 deaths; and in 2002 there were 23 cases and no deaths (Pan American Health Organization, 2003; World Health Organization [WHO], 2003).

Agent and Vector

Epidemic cholera is caused by serovars of *Vibrio cholerae*, a comma-shaped, aerobic, gram-negative, non–spore-forming bacteria with a characteristic darting movement. Three types of *V. cholerae* cause disease in humans: serogroup O139 and the two biotypes of serogroup O1, classical and El Tor. All three elaborate a pathogenic cholera enterotoxin that causes the characteristic diarrhea. El Tor is responsible for the current seventh pandemic. During epidemics, one type tends to dominate; however, different types may dominate at different times in the same geographic location. Moreover, variations in the same strain may result in different susceptibility to antibiotic treatment in different epidemics. Humans are the only known natural hosts. However, environmental reservoirs exist in brackish water or estuaries. Transmission is via ingestion of feces or vomitus-contaminated water or food, especially shellfish or other inadequately cooked seafood (Chin, 2000; Faruque et al., 2003; Hart & Shears, 2003; WHO, 2000).

Incubation

The incubation period ranges from a few hours to 5 days, and is usually 2 to 3 days (Chin, 2000).

Clinical Findings and Treatment

Signs and Symptoms

Asymptomatic infections are very common, especially with El Tor infection (Box 19-1). Infection often causes nondebilitating diarrhea, most commonly among children. Severe infection occurs in less than 10% of infected persons and is characterized by accumulation of diarrheal fluid in the small intestine followed by the abrupt onset of profuse watery diarrhea and, often, nausea and vomiting. After a few hours diarrhea may take on a "translucent, fishy-smelling, rice water appearance" (Albert & Morris, 2000, p. 327). Brief fever occurs in a few patients as does borborygmi. Severe dehydration, electrolyte loss, metabolic acidosis, and shock may ensue, with death occurring in several days if treatment is not started (Albert & Morris, 2000; Hart & Shears, 2003; WHO, 2000).

Susceptibility and resistance vary according to several factors. Breastfeeding is protective for infants. Resistance to reinfection occurs with *V. cholerae* O1 and O139, but infection with one serogroup does not protect against infection by the other. Within O1 strains, infection with classical type confers resistance to both classical and El Tor cholera, but initial infection with El Tor confers only incomplete protection from El Tor. Achlorhydria (as occurs with pernicious anemia) increases susceptibility, and persons with blood type O have increased risk of severe cholera from O1 and O139 strains (Chin, 2000).

BIOTERRORISM CONSIDERATIONS   BOX 19–1

Cholera is a Category B potential biological terrorism agent. Category B agents have "some potential for large-scale dissemination with resultant illness, but generally cause less illness and death and therefore would be expected to have lower medical and public health impact" than Category A agents, for example, smallpox, anthrax, plague, botulism, tularemia, and certain viral hemorrhagic fevers (Rotz, Khan, Lillibridge, Ostroff, & Hughes, 2002, p. 226).

Complications

Complications of severe cholera (Hart & Shears, 2003) include the following:
- Hypovolemia and hypotension lead to renal failure.
- Hyponatremia and hypokalemia with potassium loss cause ileus, muscle weakness, and cardiac arrhythmias.
- Hypoglycemia (especially among children) sometimes causes brain damage.
- Metabolic acidosis, if left uncorrected, may cause pulmonary edema during rapid rehydration.

Common Laboratory Findings

In addition to the laboratory findings mentioned in the Complications section, look for abnormalities consistent with hemoconcentration from isotonic dehydration. Hyperglycemia is not uncommon. Severe cholera may be accompanied by leukocytosis.

Diagnosis

During an epidemic, diagnosis is on the basis of acute watery diarrhea. Microscopic exam of feces shows the characteristic darting movement of *V. cholerae,* and the diagnosis may be confirmed by culture. When an outbreak occurs, a reference laboratory should perform biotyping and serotyping, and antimicrobial sensitivity should be determined (Hart & Shears, 2003).

Differential Diagnosis

— Differential diagnosis includes any acute-onset diarrheal disease such as amebiasis, bacillus cereus infection, *Campylobacter enteritis, Escherichia coli* infection, rotavirus infection, and others.

Treatment

— Rapid rehydration is the mainstay of treatment of severe cholera and in most cases oral rehydration solution (ORS) is effective. ORS consists of 1 L potable water, 3.5 g sodium chloride, 1.5 g potassium chloride, 22 g glucose monohydrate (or 40 g sucrose or 30 to 50 g rice powder, the latter giving the better taste), and 2.9 g trisodium citrate dehydrate (or 2.5 g sodium bicarbonate). (See Chapter 3 section on approach to diarrhea for a recipe for homemade ORS.) If dehydration is severe (more than 10% body weight lost, lethargy, impaired consciousness, hypovolemic shock, and acidosis), rapid intravenous rehydration with Ringer's lactate, Dhaka solution, or acetate solution is indicated. Restoration of baseline body weight and acid-base balance should be achieved within 2 to 3 hours.

— Antibiotic treatment decreases the severity of symptoms and volume of diarrhea. Depending on the particular outbreak vs. the type of *Vibrio*, antibiotic therapy for adults may include doxycycline 100 mg PO bid for 1 day, then 100 mg PO daily for 3 days; or doxycycline 300 mg PO in one dose; or tetracycline 500 mg PO qid for 3 days; or sulfamethoxazole 800 mg/trimethoprim 160 mg PO bid for 3 days; or erythromycin 500 mg PO qid for 3 days; or ciprofloxacin 250 to 500 mg PO daily for 3 days. For children older than age 8 years, doxycycline is given 2 mg/kg with a maximum of 100 mg/24 hours for 3 days. For children older than age 2 months, 25 to 40 mg/kg/24 hours and trimethoprim/sulfamethoxazole 8 mg/kg/24 hours divided bid is given for 3 days; or erythromycin 10 mg/kg tid for 3 days (Albert & Morris, 2000; Faruque et al., 2003; Hart & Shears, 2003; Rosenblatt, 1999).

Prevention

Cholera vaccines are available outside the United States, but are not recommended for travelers except for those with significant exposure, for example, persons working with refugees in epidemic areas. Current vaccines are effective against classical and El Tor strains, but not O139. One vaccine (Dukoral) also affords protection against traveler's diarrhea caused by enterotoxigenic *E. coli* (Aventis Pasteur, 2003). Vaccination is not recommended during the acute phase of an epidemic. However, in very crowded conditions such as refugee camps, the risk remains high after the acute phase and vaccination of close contacts is recommended by at least some authorities, for example, Albert and Morris (2000). Other preventive measures (Albert & Morris, 2000; Centers for Disease Control and Prevention [CDC], 2003; Chin, 2000; WHO, 2000) include the following:

- Enteric precautions should be taken for persons with cholera, though strict isolation is not necessary.
- Provide surveillance and contact tracing. If secondary transmission is likely, chemoprophylaxis is indicated. If epidemiologic data indicate high rates of secondary transmission, chemoprophylaxis may be indicated.
- Test water supplies. In at least some epidemics, water supplies previously thought to be clean were discovered to be a major source of infection. Chlorination of community supplies and household boiling of water are thus priorities.

- Provide sanitary disposal of human waste. During an epidemic, construction of temporary latrines is indicated, control of flies should be instituted, and adequate supplies of toilet paper should be provided.
- Contaminated clothing, household items, and other objects should be terminally cleaned with disinfectant.
- Enforce careful food handling precautions such as hand washing. Food should be protected from contamination after preparation, for example, from flies and unsanitary handling.
- Avoid raw shellfish; cook all shellfish for at least 10 min.
- Although person-to-person transmission is rare, limit large gatherings during severe outbreaks and improve sanitation in markets.
- Food should not be served at funerals for persons who died from cholera.
- Encourage breastfeeding at all times, especially in endemic areas.

Community education on these measures is essential.

Reporting

The CDC considers cholera to be a nationally notifiable disease. Cholera is one of three diseases that the WHO requires its member states to report (Class 1). See Appendix C for details and for upcoming changes in WHO reporting.

References

Albert, M.J., & Morris, J.G. (2000). Cholera and other *Vibrioses*. In G.T. Strickland (Ed.), *Hunter's tropical medicine* (8th ed., pp. 323-334). Philadelphia: W.B. Saunders Company.

Aventis Pasteur. (2003). Dukoral [Drug information sheet]. Retrieved July 14, 2003, from *www.aventispasteur.com/canada/products/files/DUKORAL_E.pdf*

Centers for Disease Control and Prevention. (2003). *Cholera: Travelers' health*. Retrieved July 24, 2003, from *www.cdc.gov/travel/diseases/cholera.htm*

Chin, J. (Ed.) (2000). *Control of communicable diseases manual* (17th ed., pp. 100-110). Washington, DC: American Public Health Association.

Faruque, S.M., Chowdhury, N., Kamruzzaman, M., Ahmad, Q.S., Faruque, A.S., et al. (2003). Reemergence of epidemic *Vibrio cholerae* O139, Bangladesh. *Emerging Infectious Diseases, 9,* 1116-1122.

Hart, C.A., & Shears, P. (2003). Gastrointestinal bacteria. In G.C. Cook & A.I. Zumla (Eds.), *Manson's tropical diseases* (21st ed., pp. 915-935). Philadelphia: W.B. Saunders Company.

Pan American Health Organization. (2003). Cholera: Number of cases and deaths in the Americas. Retrieved September 2, 2003, from *www.paho.org/English/AD/DPC/CD/cholera-1991-2002.htm*

Rosenblatt, J.E. (1999). Antiparasitic agents. *Mayo Clinic Proceedings, 74,* 1161-1175.

Rotz, L.D., Khan, A.S., Lillibridge, S.R., Ostroff, S.M., & Hughes. J.M. (2002). Public health assessment of potential biological terrorism agents. *Emerging Infectious Diseases, 8,* 225-230.

World Health Organization. (2000). Cholera. Retrieved July 4, 2003, from *www.who.int/inf-fs/en/fact107.html*

World Health Organization. (2003). Disease outbreaks: Cholera. Retrieved October 1, 2003, from *www.who.int/disease-outbreak-news/disease/A00.htm*

20

CHROMOBLASTOMYCOSIS

Chromomycosis, cladosporiosis, dermatitis verrucosa, Fonseca's disease

Geographic Distribution

— Chromoblastomycosis is most commonly found in tropical and subtropical climates, especially in countries with high rainfall. Areas with the highest incidence include Central America, the northern region of South America, the eastern coast of southern Africa (including Madagascar), the Far East, and the West Indies (Hay, 2003).

Agent and Vector

— Chromoblastomycosis is a chronic skin infection caused by several pigmented, or dematiaceous, fungi. The most common organisms to cause this infection are *Cladophialophora carrionii*, *Fonsecaea pedrosoi*, *Fonsecaea compactum*, *Phialophora verrucosa*, and *Rhinocladiella aquaspera*. The predominant isolated organism varies with geographic location. *C. carrionii* is more common in drier climates, such as Madagascar and Africa, and *F. pedrosoi* is often isolated in humid forests, such as Central America and Brazil. Agricultural workers and populations that do not routinely wear shoes are most commonly affected since the organism is found in decaying plants, wood, and soil. Inoculation of the fungus into the skin occurs through puncture wounds, which most commonly occur on the lower extremities (Bonifaz, Carrasco-Gerard, & Saul, 2001; Esterre, Andriantsimahavandy, Ramarcel, & Pecarrere, 1996; Queiroz-Telles, McGinnis, Salkin, & Graybill, 2003; Silva, de Souza, & Rozental, 1998-99; Sobera & Elewski, 2003).

Incubation

In most cases, the patient cannot remember the incident that led to the inoculation and subsequent development of disease. This makes it difficult to determine the incubation period. In a retrospective review of patients with chromoblastomycosis in Brazil, the average time between the appearance of the disease and medical diagnosis was 14 years (Hay, 2000; Minotto, Bernardi, Mallmann, Edelweiss, & Scroferneker, 2001).

Clinical Findings and Treatment

Signs and Symptoms

Although chromoblastomycosis can be caused by several different fungi, the clinical presentation of each is indistinguishable. The initial lesion at the site of inoculation is usually a papule or nodule. These slowly enlarge to form verrucous or multinodular plaques that may appear annular secondary to central scarring (Figure 20-1). Only one limb is typically involved, but autoinoculation from scratching may cause the infection to spread to other sites. The lesions are asymptomatic, but necrosis of the keratin within verrucous plaques may cause an unpleasant odor (Hay, 2003; Sobera & Elewski, 2003).

Complications

Long-standing lesions may lead to limb deformity or, rarely, squamous cell carcinoma. Plaques may become superinfected, which can result in lymph stasis and elephantiasis of the limb. Chromoblastomycosis is primarily an infection of the skin, but it has rarely been isolated from other organ systems, which may be the result of systemic spread (Hay, 2000, 2003).

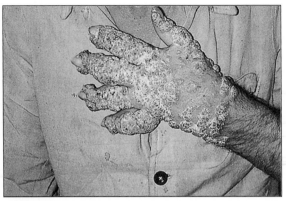

FIGURE 20–1

Chromoblastomycosis of the hand. (*Source:* From Peters, W., & Pasvol, G. [2002]. *Tropical medicine and parasitology* [5th ed., p. 259]. Chicago: Mosby.)

Common Laboratory Findings

There are no known common laboratory findings.

Diagnosis

The clinical manifestation may be diagnostic; however, further studies are often indicated. Skin scrapings taken from the surface of the lesion may be treated with potassium hydroxide and viewed microscopically. A positive scraping will demonstrate hyphae or Medlar bodies, which are round pigmented cells that resemble copper pennies and are 5 to 15 μm in diameter. A biopsy of the plaque is characteristic and will show pseudoepitheliomatous hyperplasia, intraepidermal abscesses, suppurative granuloma formation, and Medlar bodies. Cultures can be performed, but a specialist laboratory may be required for identification of the organism (Hay, 2003; Sobera & Elewski, 2003).

Differential Diagnosis

Few other processes are characterized by plaques similar to chromoblastomycosis; however, other verrucous processes such as tuberculosis verrucosa and papillomaviruses must be considered. Mycetoma may resemble chromoblastomycosis since it is also a fungal infection that is caused by implantation of the organism into the lower extremity. This entity can be distinguished because it creates draining sinus tracts and extrudes characteristic grains. Other infections to consider include blastomycosis, syphilis, and leishmania (Hay, 2000, 2003; Sobera & Elewski, 2003).

Treatment

Local application of heat was widely used before the availability of antifungal medications and may be effective since the organisms cannot grow at high temperature. Systemic treatment with amphotericin B is not often used because of the toxic doses required to kill the organism in the tissue. Intralesional amphotericin is a reasonable alternative; however, its use may be limited by pain and scarring. Itraconazole at a dosage of 200 to 400 mg/day may provide a clinical and mycological cure; however, depending on the severity of the infection, treatment may be required for 6 months to 2 years or more. Poorly responding infections to itraconazole alone may respond well to alternate week or combination therapy with terbinafine (250 mg/day). Other possible treatments include excision of smaller lesions and cryosurgery (Gupta, Taborda, & Sanzovo, 2002; Queiroz-Telles et al., 1992, 2003; Sobera & Elewski, 2003).

Prevention

Protective clothing and shoes may help prevent the initial inoculation from puncture wounds. Diagnosis and treatment of early lesions may help to prevent large plaque formation and possible complications.

Reporting

The U.S. Centers for Disease Control and Prevention (CDC) does not consider chromoblastomycosis to be a nationally notifiable disease, nor does the World Health Organization (WHO) classify it as a disease important in public health (Class 5). See Appendix C for details and for upcoming changes in WHO reporting.

References

Bonifaz, A., Carrasco-Gerard, E., & Saul, A. (2001). Chromoblastomycosis: Clinical and mycologic experience of 51 cases. *Mycoses, 44,* 1-7.

Esterre, P., Andriantsimahavandy, A., Ramarcel, E.R., & Pecarrere, J.L. (1996) Forty years of chromoblastomycosis in Madagascar: A review. *American Journal of Tropical Medicine and Hygiene, 55,* 45-47.

Gupta, A.K., Taborda, P.R., & Sanzovo, A.D. (2002). Alternate week and combination itraconazole and terbinafine therapy for chromoblastomycosis caused by *Fonsecaea pedrosoi* in Brazil. *Medical Mycology, 40,* 529-534.

Hay, R.J. (2000). Chromoblastomycosis. In G.T. Strickland (Ed.), *Hunter's tropical medicine* (8th ed., pp. 542-544). Philadelphia: W.B. Saunders Company.

Hay, R.J. (2003). Fungal infections. In G.C. Cook & A.I. Zumla (Eds.), *Manson's tropical diseases* (21st ed., pp. 1182-1183). Philadelphia: W.B. Saunders Company.

Minotto, R., Bernardi, C.D., Mallmann, L.F., Edelweiss, M.I., & Scroferneker, M.L. (2001). Chromoblastomycosis: A review of 100 cases in the state of Rio Grande do Sul, Brazil. *Journal of the American Academy of Dermatology, 44,* 585-592.

Queiroz-Telles, F., Purim, K.S., Fillus, J.N., Bordignon, G.F., Lameira, R.P., et al. (1992). Itraconazole in the treatment of chromoblastomycosis due to *Fonsecaea pedrosoi. International Journal of Dermatology, 31,* 805-812.

Queiroz-Telles, F., McGinnis, M.R., Salkin, I., & Graybill, J.R. (2003). Subcutaneous mycoses. *Infectious Disease Clinics of North America, 17,* 59-85.

Silva, J.P., de Souza, W., & Rozental, S. (1998-99). Chromoblastomycosis: A retrospective study of 325 cases on Amazonic Region (Brazil). *Mycopathologia, 143,* 171-175.

Sobera, J.O., & Elewski, B.E. (2003). Fungal diseases. In J.L. Bolognia, J.L. Jorizzo, & R.P. Rapini (Eds.), *Dermatology* (pp. 1186-1187). Philadelphia: Mosby.

21

COCCIDIOIDOMYCOSIS

Desert rheumatism, San Joaquin Valley fever

Geographic Distribution

Coccidioidomycosis is found mostly in warm dry climates and is endemic throughout the southwestern United States, northern Mexico, and scattered areas of Central and South America, including Venezuela, Columbia, Argentina, Paraguay, Honduras, and Guatemala. The southern San Joaquin Valley of California and southern Arizona have the highest endemicity, and there has been a massive increase in cases in these areas in recent years (Chiller, Galgiani, & Stevens, 2003; Graybill, 2000; Hay, 2003).

Agent and Vector

Coccidioidomycosis is caused by a dimorphic fungus, *Coccidioides immitis,* which grows as the mycelial form in the soil of endemic areas. Arthroconidia are the infecting form of the fungus, which is inhaled via dust particles from the soil and subsequently transformed into spore-like structures, called spherules. The spherules divide and rupture within the host, releasing small endospores, which can develop further into spores. The populations most at risk include agricultural workers, construction workers, archaeologists, and other occupations where there is exposure to dust and soil. The tissue spherular form is not contagious; therefore, person-to-person transmission is rare. On the other hand, if infected tissue or body fluids are allowed to grow in culture in the laboratory, the fungus may progress to the highly infectious mycelial form.

Laboratory workers are therefore at risk for acquiring the infection if they are exposed to samples containing coccidioidomycosis. Individuals with HIV disease or other causes of suppressed cellular immunity are also at an increased risk of infection (Chiller et al., 2003; Graybill, 2000; Hay, 2003; Kim & Parker, 2002).

Incubation

Once endospores are released from the spherule, maturation takes approximately 3 days, and the replication process continues. The incubation time depends partly on the control of the organism by cell-mediated immunity. Once the primary pneumonia develops, dissemination in susceptible individuals almost always occurs within a few weeks (Graybill, 2000; Kirkland & Fierer, 1996).

Clinical Findings and Treatment

Signs and Symptoms

Approximately 60% of individuals who become infected with *C. immitis* never develop symptoms. When the primary infection is symptomatic, it may present as a flu-like illness with fever, weight loss, cough, and pleuritic chest pain. Other symptoms that may develop with the primary infection include arthralgias, myalgias, conjunctivitis, and skin disease, such as pustules, nodules, abscesses, sinus tracts, ulcerations, erythema nodosum, and erythema multiforme (Figures 21-1A and B). Pneumonia and other symptoms often clear within 2 to 3 weeks, although fatigue may take many months to resolve. In patients with depressed cellular immunity, an extensive pneumonia with chronic pulmonary nodules/cavities or dissemination of the infection may develop (Chiller et al., 2003; Hay, 2003; Sobera & Elewski, 2003).

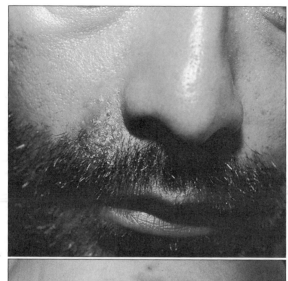

A

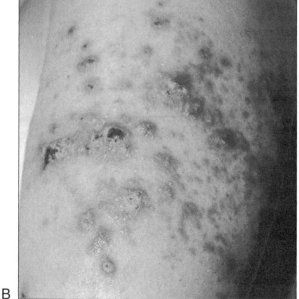

B

FIGURE 21–1

Coccidioidomycosis: **A,** Erythematous plaque. **B,** Papules and suppurative nodules. (*Source:* From Bolognia, J.L., Jorizzo, J.L., & Rapini, R.P. [Eds.]. [2003]. *Dermatology* [p. 1192]. Philadelphia: Mosby.)

Complications

— The skin is the most common site of disseminated disease, and approximately half the patients with symptomatic infections experience cutaneous manifestations. One-third of patients with dissemination develop meningitis, which manifests as meningismus, headache, and characteristic changes in the cerebrospinal fluid, including lymphocytic pleocytosis, elevated protein, and eosinophilia. Mortality from this type of meningitis is greater than 90% if left untreated for 1 year.

— Osteomyelitis is also a complication of disseminated disease, with the vertebral column being the most commonly affected site. Infection of the synovium occurs in approximately 20% of disseminated cases. Most often only a single joint is involved, and the knee is the most commonly affected. Meningitis and focal pulmonary disease often occur in HIV patients with higher CD4 counts and are associated with a lower mortality if treated. Diffuse pulmonary disease is the worst manifestation in patients with AIDS, with median survival of less than 1 month (Al-Abdely & Graybill, 2001; Chiller et. al., 2003; Graybill, 2000; Kim & Parker, 2002).

Common Laboratory Findings

— The primary infection may be associated with eosinophilia, which is sometimes the only manifestation of the disease (Graybill, 2000).

Diagnosis

— Once infection is suspected, the diagnosis of coccidioidomycosis can be made in many ways. The most specific way of making the diagnosis is with culture or histopathology. Tissue biopsies or sputum samples may demonstrate the pathognomonic spherule, which contains endospores and a double-edged thick wall. The organism can also be readily cultured on most media and appears within 7 to 10 days. It may take some time for the spherules to convert to the mycelial form, and during this time the specimens should be handled carefully to avoid accidental infection of laboratory workers. The coccidioidin and spherulin skin tests can be used to test for prior exposure but not active disease. A reaction of greater than 5 mm of induration at 48 to 72 hours indicates prior exposure; however, there is limited usefulness since cross-reaction with histoplasmin and blastomycin has been reported. Some research laboratories have detected specific antibodies in acute and chronic disease; however, the clinical utility of these tests is still being evaluated (Al-Abdely & Graybill, 2001; Graybill, 2000).

Differential Diagnosis

Chronic coccidioidomycosis pneumonia with cavity formation may resemble blastomycosis or tuberculosis. Blastomycosis can also manifest as osteomyelitis of the vertebral bodies, which is a common manifestation of disseminated coccidioidomycosis. Meningitis can be caused by bacteria, viruses, and other fungal infections, such as cryptococcus; a lumbar puncture and demonstration of the organism can distinguish these entities. A wide range of cutaneous manifestations occurs, and many of these may be confused with other deep fungal or bacterial infections.

Treatment

Primary infection and less aggressive disease is treated with itraconazole or fluconazole 400 mg/day orally for several months in order to prevent chronic infection and dissemination. Total eradication of the disease is often very difficult, and treatment may be continued for many years. Itraconazole seems to be associated with lower

relapse rates than fluconazole. Amphotericin B
(0.5 to 1.0 mg/kg/day for the first few weeks, then
decreasing to 50 mg three times per week for a
cumulative dose of 2 to 3 g) can be used in seriously
ill patients, and the response rate is approximately
50% to 75%.

— Fluconazole is an effective treatment for coccidioidal
meningitis and should be given in a loading dose of
800 mg/day for the first 3 days, then lowered to
400 mg/day, and given indefinitely due to the high
relapse rate. Children with pulmonary and
extrapulmonary disease may be treated with
amphotericin B 1.0 mg/kg/day for 4 to 6 weeks; there
is insufficient data on fluconazole in children with
coccidioidomycosis.

— Patients with disseminated disease or AIDS will
need lifelong prophylaxis with azole antifungals
(Al-Abdely & Graybill, 2001; Chiller et. al., 2003;
Graybill, 2000).

Prevention

— Decreasing the amount of airborne dust by planting
grass and paving roads may help lower the risk for
coccidioidomycosis in endemic areas. Research is
currently being conducted to develop a recombinant
vaccine using specific proteins. No practical means of
preventing infection currently exist (Chiller et al., 2003;
Kirkland & Fierer, 1996).

Reporting

— The U.S. Centers for Disease Control and Prevention
considers coccidioidomycosis to be a nationally notifiable
disease, and the World Health Organization (WHO) also
lists it as a disease important in public health (Class 3B).
See Appendix C for details and for upcoming changes in
WHO reporting.

References

Al-Abdely, H., & Graybill, J.R. (2001). Histoplasmosis, blastomycosis, coccidioidomycosis, and cryptococcus. In R.L. Guerrant, D.H. Walker, & P.F. Weller (Eds.), *Essentials of tropical diseases* (pp. 294-302). New York: Churchill Livingstone.

Chiller, T.M., Galgiani, J.N., & Stevens, D.A. (2003). Coccidioidomycosis. *Infectious Disease Clinics of North America, 17,* 41-57.

Graybill, J.R. (2000). Coccidioidomycosis. In G.T. Strickland (Ed.), *Hunter's tropical medicine* (8th ed., pp. 552-556). Philadelphia: W.B. Saunders Company.

Hay, R.J. (2003). Fungal infections. In G.C. Cook & A.I. Zumla (Eds.), *Manson's tropical diseases* (21st ed., pp. 1188-1189). Philadelphia: W.B. Saunders Company.

Kim, A., & Parker, S.S. (2002). Coccidioidomycosis: Case report and update on diagnosis and management. *Journal of the American Academy of Dermatology, 46,* 743-747.

Kirkland, T.N., & Fierer, J. (1996). Coccidioidomycosis: A reemerging infectious disease. *Emerging Infectious Diseases, 2,* 192-199.

Sobera, J.O., & Elewski, B.E. (2003). Fungal diseases. In J.L. Bolognia, J.L., Jorizzo, & R.P. Rapini (Eds.), *Dermatology* (pp. 1192-1193). Philadelphia: Mosby.

22

CRYPTOCOCCOSIS

Geographic Distribution

Cryptococcosis is caused by *Cryptococcus neoformans*, which has two subspecies, *C. neoformans* var. *neoformans* and *C. neoformans* var. *gattii*. The variety *neoformans* is found worldwide, and the variety *gattii* is found in tropical and subtropical areas, including Africa, the Far East, Papua New Guinea, Australia, and Latin and Central America (Al-Abdely & Graybill, 2001; Castanon-Olivares, Arreguin-Espinosa, Ruiz-Palacios y Santos, & Lopez-Martinez, 2000; Hay, 2003; Ohkusu et al., 2002).

Agent and Vector

Cryptococcus neoformans is an encapsulated yeast fungus that can cause serious systemic infections. *C. neoformans* var. *neoformans* can infect both immunocompetent and immunodeficient individuals, including those with AIDS, and is found throughout the world in association with guano from pigeons, canaries, and cockatoos. *C. neoformans* var. *gattii* is associated with several species of eucalyptus trees in subtropical and tropical regions and causes disease in immunocompetent hosts more commonly than in AIDS patients (Al-Abdely & Graybill, 2001; Perfect & Casadevall, 2002).

Incubation

The incubation period for cryptococcosis is variable and heavily depends on the competence of the host's cellular immune system.

Clinical Findings and Treatment

Signs and Symptoms

— The most common initial site of infection is the lung; however, up to one-third of infected immunocompetent hosts are asymptomatic. Those with symptoms may present with cough, chest pain, and fever. Focal infiltrates are a typical sign of infection, and cavity formation is rare. The most common presentation in the non-AIDS patient is meningitis or meningoencephalitis, and possible accompanying symptoms include headache, neck stiffness, confusion, photophobia, and cranial nerve deficits. The interval between the onset of symptoms and presentation to medical facilities varies from days to months. Skin infection is almost always a result of disseminated disease, and a wide variety of lesions have been reported, including acneiform lesions, pustules, nodules, ulcers, and molluscum contagiosum-like papules (Figures 22-1 and 22-2) (Dromer & Dupont, 2000; Hay, 2003; Perfect & Casadevall, 2002).

— AIDS is a major risk factor for cryptococcosis infection, which often occurs when the immune system is severely depressed and CD4 counts fall below 100. Compared with non–HIV-infected patients, those with HIV develop symptoms faster, have more central nervous system (CNS) and extrapulmonary involvement, more positive blood cultures, and fewer inflammatory cells on the cerebrospinal fluid (CSF) examination. AIDS patients may have vague symptoms, with fever being the only manifestation of infection. Almost any organ system can be involved, and other extrapulmonary manifestations include prostatitis, osteolytic bone lesions, arthritis, lymphadenopathy, keratitis, retinitis, endocarditis, peritonitis, and hepatitis (Dromer & Dupont, 2000; Hay, 2003; Perfect & Casadevall, 2002).

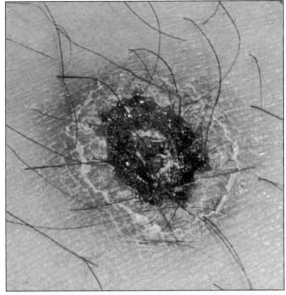

FIGURE 22–1

Cutaneous cryptococcosis: erythematous scaly and crusted plaque. (*Source:* Courtesy of the University of Texas Southwestern Department of Dermatology.)

Complications

Dissemination of disease is a major complication and can lead to involvement of almost any site, as reviewed earlier. Complications specific to pulmonary involvement include acute respiratory distress syndrome, superior vena cava syndrome, and Pancoast's syndrome (shoulder and arm pain, Horner's syndrome, and atrophy of the hand muscles). An immune reconstitution syndrome can occur when highly active antiretroviral therapy (HAART) is initiated and may be due to an inflammatory reaction against a latent cryptococcal infection. These patients may present with acute symptoms of cryptococcal

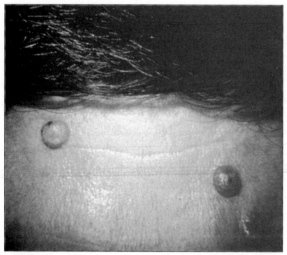

FIGURE 22–2

Cutaneous cryptococcosis: erythematous dome-shaped papules on the forehead. (*Source:* Courtesy of the University of Texas Southwestern Department of Dermatology.)

meningitis or pain and swelling of the involved tissues. Cryptococcal meningitis and cryptococcemia are poor prognostic factors, and the mortality rate of these entities in immunocompromised patients ranges from 36% to 50% (Jean et al., 2002; Perfect & Casadevall, 2002; Wu et al., 2002).

Common Laboratory Findings

Blood cultures are often positive in AIDS patients, and the CD4 count is usually less than 50 when they present with the disease. Imaging of the brain may show edema, hydrocephalus, or mass lesions, which are more common in var. *gattii*. CSF findings are not specific for cryptococcosis, but the most common features include pleocytosis, elevated protein, low glucose, and an elevated opening pressure (Dromer & Dupont, 2000).

Diagnosis

The diagnosis of cryptococcosis can be made using several different methods. The organism and its surrounding capsule may be identified in tissue smears, CSF, urine, pleural fluid, bronchoalveolar lavage fluid, or sputum using India ink staining. Specimens can also be cultured on Sabouraud agar, but 3 to 12 days may be required to identify the organism. Tissue sections, including skin biopsies, can be stained with mucicarmine to allow demonstration of the organism and capsule. Antigen detection tests, such as the enzyme-linked immunosorbent assay, can be used to detect the capsular antigen in serum or CSF, and sensitivity and specificity is more than 95% with commercially available tests (Dromer & Dupont, 2000; Hays, 2003).

Differential Diagnosis

Meningitis and meningoencephalitis can be caused by many other organisms, including bacteria, viruses, tuberculosis, and other fungi. Mass lesions that can occur with cryptococcal CNS infection may resemble toxoplasmosis or a brain tumor. Cryptococcal pneumonia in immunocompromised individuals needs to be distinguished from infection caused by tuberculosis, aspergillosis, pneumocystosis, blastomycosis, and coccidioidomycosis. Skin lesions are nonspecific and may resemble other infections or neoplastic processes (Dromer & Dupont, 2000).

Treatment

Immunocompetent children and adults with CNS disease are often treated with a combination of intravenous amphotericin B, 0.7 to 1.0 mg/kg daily, and flucytosine 100 mg/kg daily. Therapy usually lasts 6 to 10 weeks and is associated with a good response. For immunocompetent hosts with isolated symptomatic pulmonary disease, treatment is with fluconazole 200 to 400 mg daily for 36 months. In patients with AIDS and meningitis, primary therapy is with amphotericin B at 0.7 mg/kg or more daily and flucytosine 100 mg/kg daily for 2 weeks followed by fluconazole at 400 mg or more daily for an additional 8 to 10 weeks. Lifelong maintenance is required in patients with AIDS and consists of fluconazole at 200 mg or more daily. For patients with HIV who have isolated pulmonary or urinary tract disease, treatment is with fluconazole 200 to 400 mg daily (Dromer & Dupont, 2000; Saag et al., 2000).

Prevention

Patients who are at high risk should avoid environments where the yeasts may be aerosolized or there are accumulations of pigeon droppings. Large accumulations of pigeon or other potentially infectious droppings should be decontaminated with iodophor or other means before removal. Complete wetting of the accumulation may prevent aerosolization. Patients with AIDS should receive prophylaxis with fluconazole; small studies suggest that with HAART therapy antifungal prophylaxis can be stopped after 1 year. Research on developing a vaccination against cryptococcus is currently under way. High-risk patients and their families should be educated about prevention (Chin, 2000; Perfect & Casadevall, 2002).

Reporting

The U.S. Centers for Disease Control and Prevention does not consider cryptococcosis to be a nationally notifiable disease. The World Health Organization (WHO) classifies it as a disease important in public health (Class 2B). See Appendix C for details and for upcoming changes in WHO reporting.

References

Al-Abdely, H., & Graybill, J.R. (2001). Histoplasmosis, blastomycosis, coccidioidomycosis, and cryptococcus. In R.L. Guerrant, D.H. Walker, & P.F. Weller (Eds.), *Essentials of tropical diseases* (pp. 294-302). New York: Churchill Livingstone.

Castanon-Olivares, L.R., Arreguin-Espinosa, R., Ruiz-Palacios y Santos, G., & Lopez-Martinez, R. (2000). Frequency of Cryptococcus species and varieties in Mexico and their comparison with some Latin American countries. *Revista Latinoamericana de Microbiologia y Parasitologia, 42,* 35-40.

Chin, J. (Ed.). (2000). *Control of communicable diseases manual* (17th ed.). Washington, DC: American Public Health Association.

Dromer, F., & Dupont, B. (2000). Cryptococcosis. In G.T. Strickland (Ed.), *Hunter's tropical medicine* (8th ed., pp. 561-564). Philadelphia: W.B. Saunders Company.

Hay, R.J. (2003). Fungal infections. In G.C. Cook & A.I. Zumla (Eds.), *Manson's tropical diseases* (21st ed., pp. 1191-1192). Philadelphia: W.B. Saunders Company.

Jean, S.S., Fang, C.T., Shau, W.Y., Chen, Y.C., Chang, S.C., et al. (2002). Cryptococcaemia: Clinical features and prognostic factors. *Quarterly Journal of Medicine, 95,* 511-518.

Ohkusu, M., Tangonan, N., Takeo, K., Kishida, E., Ohkubo, M., et al. (2002). Serotype, mating type and ploidy of Cryptococcus neoformans strains isolated from patients in Brazil. *Revista do Instituto de Medicina Tropical de São Paulo, 44,* 299-302.

Perfect, J.R., & Casadevall, A.C. (2002). Cryptococcosis. *Infectious Disease Clinics of North America, 16,* 837-874.

Saag, M.S., Graybill, R.J., Larsen, R.A., Pappas, P.G., Perfect, J.R., et al. (2000). Practice guidelines for the management of cryptococcal disease, Infectious Diseases Society of America. *Clinical Infectious Diseases, 30,* 710-718.

Wu, G., Vilchez, R.A., Eidelman, B., Fung, J., Kormos, R., & Kusne, S. (2002). Cryptococcal meningitis: An analysis among 5,521 consecutive organ transplant recipients. *Transplant Infectious Disease, 4,* 183-188.

CRYPTOSPORIDIOSIS

Geographic Distribution

Cryptosporidiosis is found worldwide. Prevalence is highest in developing countries and among children less than 2 years of age, travelers, men who have sex with multiple other men, animal handlers, and close personal contacts of infected individuals. The illness also affects mammals, reptiles, birds, and fish (Chin, 2000).

Agent and Vector

Cryptosporidiosis is caused by *Cryptosporidium* species, coccidian protozoa first identified as a cause of human diarrhea in 1976. The most common species in human infection (97%) is *C. parvum*. Transmission occurs with the ingestion (fecal-oral) of oocytes, which are able to survive adverse conditions for long periods of time and are resistant to a variety of chemicals, notably those used to treat drinking water (Box 23-1). *Cryptosporidium* spp. contaminate 65% to 97% of the earth's water and are found in up to 17% of children with diarrhea in the developing world. Although serologic studies show that exposure to *Cryptosporidium* is high, susceptibility to infection and severity of infection is greatest among persons with immune deficiencies (Chappell & Okhuysen, 2002; Chin, 2000; Farthing, Cevallos, & Kelly, 2003).

Incubation

The incubation period is probably 1 to 12 days, with 7 days the likely average (Chin, 2000).

BIOTERRORISM CONSIDERATIONS   BOX 23–1

Cryptosporidiosis is a Category B potential biological
terrorism agent. Category B agents have "some potential
for large-scale dissemination with resultant illness, but
generally cause less illness and death and therefore would
be expected to have lower medical and public health
impact" than Category A agents, such as smallpox,
anthrax, plague, botulism, tularemia, and certain viral
hemorrhagic fevers (Rotz, Khan, Lillibridge, Ostroff, &
Hughes, 2002, p. 226).

Clinical Findings and Treatment

Signs and Symptoms

- Among immunocompetent persons, cryptosporidiosis is
  most commonly a small-bowel disease, characterized by
  self-limiting diarrhea that ranges from mild to profuse
  and watery, with cramping abdominal pain. Mucus is
  sometimes present in stool. Less common symptoms
  include malaise, fever, nausea and vomiting, myalgia,
  arthropathy, and headache. The illness may wax and
  wane, with the duration ranging from 4 days up to
  2 weeks, and oocyte shedding continuing for 1 to
  4 weeks. In children the illness is commonly preceded
  by anorexia and nausea and vomiting.
- Among immunosuppressed persons, cryptosporidiosis is
  often characterized by prolonged and fulminant diarrhea,
  along with abdominal cramping and vomiting, leading in
  some cases to death. In some cases, however, patients
  with HIV-related cryptosporidiosis have remitting
  and relapsing diarrhea (Chappell & Okhuysen,
  2002; Chin, 2000; Farthing et al., 2003;
  Robinson et al., 2003).

Complications

Biliary tract infection leads to symptoms of cholecystitis, especially in patients with chronic diarrhea (Chin, 2000; Farthing et al., 2003).

Common Laboratory Findings

Biliary tract infection may result in increased serum levels of alkaline phosphatase and gamma-glutamyltransferase (GGT).

Diagnosis

Current means of diagnosis are immunofluorescent assay visualization of oocysts in feces and detection of oocysts using an enzyme immunoassay format (Chappell & Okhuysen, 2002). Many laboratories in the United States do not include *Cryptosporidium* in standard testing for ova and parasites. Examination of feces requires an acid-fast stain (Juranek, 2000).

Differential Diagnosis

Most diarrheal diseases can be included in the differential diagnosis.

Treatment

Nitazoxanide is currently the only effective treatment for cryptosporidiosis and is approved only for immunocompetent children. For ages 12 to 47 months, nitazoxanide suspension is given 5 mL (100 mg) PO bid for 3 days. For ages 4 to 11 years, nitazoxanide suspension is given 10 mL (200 mg) PO bid for 3 days (U.S. Food and Drug Administration, 2003a, 2003b; White, 2003). Among AIDS patients, highly active retroviral therapy with serine protease inhibitors (PIs) leading to increased CD4+ T cells results in control of symptoms and, in many cases, elimination of the parasite. The combination of a PI and the aminoglycoside paromomycin shows increased inhibitory effect over PIs alone. Oral rehydration and antimotility medications are mainstays of symptom management (Chappell & Okhuysen, 2002; Hommer, Eicholz, & Petry, 2003; Robinson et al., 2003).

Prevention

— Preventive measures for cryptosporidiosis (Chin, 2000; Preiser, Preiser, & Madeo, 2003; Strachan, Ogden, Smith-Palmer, & Jones, 2003) include the following:

- Provide sanitary disposal of feces and avoid handling human or animal excreta.
- Wash hands thoroughly after contact with persons or animals with diarrhea.
- Isolate animals with diarrhea.
- Boil water supplies for 1 min at a full, rolling boil.
- Filter water with filters capable of removing particles 0.1 to 1.0 μm in size.
- Prevent infected persons from preparing uncooked foods.
- Prevent infected children from attending day care facilities.
- Prevent infected persons from contact with immunosuppressed persons.
- Avoid oral-anal sex.

— Community education on the preceding measures is important in preventing or minimizing outbreaks.

Reporting

— The U.S. Centers for Disease Control and Prevention considers cryptosporidiosis to be a nationally notifiable disease. The World Health Organization (WHO) classifies it as 3B. See Appendix C for details and for upcoming changes in WHO reporting.

References

Chappell, C.L., & Okhuysen, P.C. (2002). Cryptosporidiosis. *Current Opinion in Infectious Diseases, 15,* 523-527.

Chin, J. (2000). Cryptosporidiosis. In J. Chin (Ed.), *Control of communicable diseases manual* (17th ed., pp. 134-137). Washington, DC: American Public Health Association.

Farthing, M.J.G., Cevallos, A.M., & Kelly, P. (2003). Intestinal protozoa. In G.C. Cook & A.I Zumla (Eds.), *Manson's tropical diseases* (21st ed., pp. 1373-1410). Philadelphia: W.B. Saunders Company.

Hommer, V., Eicholz, J., & Petry, F. (2003). Effect of antiretroviral protease inhibitors alone, and in combination with paromomycin, on the excystation, invasion and in vitro development of Cryptosporidium parvum. *Journal of Antimicrobial Chemotherapy, 53,* 359-364.

Juranek, D.D. (2000). Cryptosporidiosis. In G.T. Strickland (Ed.), *Hunter's tropical medicine and emerging infectious diseases* (8th ed., pp. 594-600). Philadelphia: W.B. Saunders Company.

Preiser, G., Preiser, L., & Madeo, L. (2003). An outbreak of cryptosporidiosis among veterinary science students who work with calves. *Journal of American College Health, 51,* 213-215.

Robinson, P., Okhuysen, P.C., Chappell, C.L., Weinstock, J.V., Lewis, D.E., et al. (2003). Substance P expression correlates with severity of diarrhea in cryptosporidiosis. *The Journal of Infectious Diseases, 188,* 290-296.

Rotz, L.D, Khan, A.S., Lillibridge, S.R., Ostroff, S.M., & Hughes. J.M. (2002). Public health assessment of potential biological terrorism agents. *Emerging Infectious Diseases, 8,* 225-230.

Strachan, N.J., Ogden, I.D., Smith-Palmer, A., & Jones, K. (2003). Foot and mouth epidemic reduces cases of human cryptosporidiosis in Scotland. *The Journal of Infectious Diseases, 188,* 783-786.

U.S. Food and Drug Administration. (2003a, May-June). New drug for parasitic infections in children. *FDA Consumer Magazine.* Retrieved September 23, 2003, from *www.fda.gov/fdac/departs/2003/303_upd.html*

U.S. Food and Drug Administration. (2003b). Prescribing information (Alinia). Retrieved September 28, 2003, from *www.fda.gov/cder/foi/label/2002/21498_Alinia_lbl.pdf*

White, A.C. (2003). Nitazoxanide: An important advance in anti-parasitic therapy. *American Journal of Tropical Medicine and Hygiene, 68,* 382-383.

24

CUTANEOUS LARVA MIGRANS

Creeping eruption, dew itch, ground itch, sandworm

Geographic Distribution

— Cutaneous larva migrans occurs worldwide but is most commonly seen in warm tropical and subtropical climates, including Africa, the Caribbean, Southeast Asia, Central and South America, and the southeastern United States along the Gulf of Mexico (Blackwell & Vega-Lopez, 2001; Gilles, 2003).

Agent and Vector

— Cutaneous larva migrans is most often caused by the dog and cat hookworms, *Ancylostoma caninum* and *Ancylostoma braziliense*. The infected animal passes the nematode eggs with its stool, and the larval forms penetrate the skin of humans, who are an accidental host. The larvae are unable to complete their life cycle within the human; therefore, they wander under the skin and die within weeks to months. Humans may contract this eruption after sitting or walking in sand or soil that is contaminated with infected feces (Blackwell & Vega-Lopez, 2001).

Incubation

— The mean period between penetration of the larva and the onset of symptoms ranges from days to weeks (Brenner & Patel, 2003).

Clinical Findings and Treatment

Signs and Symptoms

— The skin lesions of cutaneous larva migrans are erythematous, edematous, and serpiginous tracts.

The site of entry may present as an erythematous papule or vesicle, and the larva migrates millimeters to centimeters each day, leaving linear tracts and occasionally vesicles. Patients experience intense pruritus, and the skin may become secondarily infected. The most common locations include the feet, buttocks, abdomen, and extremities (Figures 24-1A and B). Single or multiple lesions may be present (Blackwell & Vega-Lopez, 2001; Brenner & Patel, 2003; Gilles, 2003).

Complications

The larvae rarely progress to organs other than the skin, and Loeffler's syndrome, which consists of migratory pulmonary infiltrates, peripheral eosinophilia, asthma, fever, and urticaria, is rarely seen. Larvae also rarely migrate to the gastrointestinal tract, causing eosinophilic enterocolitis, which manifests as acute abdominal pain, nausea, and diarrhea. Other more common superficial complications include secondary bacterial infection and urticarial allergic reactions (Brenner & Patel, 2003; Sangüeza, Lu, Sangüeza, & Pereira, 2003).

Common Laboratory Findings

Peripheral blood eosinophilia and elevated immunoglobulin E (IgE) levels are occasionally seen (Brenner & Patel, 2003).

Diagnosis

The diagnosis of cutaneous larva migrans is clinical. The characteristic linear, slow-moving eruption, usually on the feet or buttocks, intense pruritus, and a history of contact with contaminated sand or soil allow the diagnosis to be made. Isolation of the larva within the skin lesions is not possible since it is usually in advance of the visible tract (Gilles, 2003).

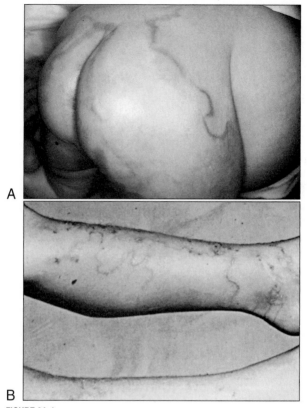

FIGURE 24–1

The linear tracts of cutaneous larva migrans. (*Source:* **A,** Courtesy of the University of Texas Southwestern Department of Dermatology. **B,** From Strickland, G.T. [2000]. *Hunter's tropical medicine and emerging infectious diseases* [8th ed., p. 798]. Philadelphia: W.B. Saunders Company.)

Differential Diagnosis

Strongyloides (larva currens) is also caused by a larva, which moves relatively quickly, and usually causes skin lesions on the buttocks or trunk. This infection can be spread by autoinoculation around the anus and buttocks, where the larva can reenter the skin and cause skin lesions similar to cutaneous larva migrans. *Loa loa* causes transient subcutaneous edema secondary to migrating adult worms, and they appear and disappear within minutes (Gilles, 2003; Sangüeza et al., 2003).

Treatment

Cutaneous larva migrans may resolve spontaneously within weeks to months, but treatment is sometimes required in persistent and symptomatic infections. Topical application of 10% to 15% thiabendazole solution, cream, or ointment to the affected area two to three times per day has a cure rate greater than 90%. Pruritus and track migration usually stops within 48 hours. This treatment is advantageous because of the avoidance of systemic medication and side effects; however, it is not very helpful for multiple lesions. Thiabendazole 50 mg/kg/day can be given in oral form in extensive cases, and many patients can be cured with a single dose. The cure rate increases if it is given for 2 to 4 consecutive days; however, it sometimes causes adverse effects including giddiness, headache, vomiting, and nausea. Alternate regimens that may be better tolerated include albendazole 400 mg/day for 1 to 5 days (adults and children) and ivermectin in a single dose of 12 mg (pediatric dosage 200 mcg/kg/day for 1 to 2 days) (Caumes, 2000).

Prevention

The best way to prevent cutaneous larva migrans is to ban dogs from beaches. This is often impractical, and the most reasonable method of prevention may be to wear shoes and avoid lying in sand (Caumes, 2000).

Reporting

The U.S. Centers for Disease Control and Prevention does not consider cutaneous larva migrans to be a nationally notifiable disease, nor does the World Health Organization (WHO) classify it as a disease important in public health (Class 5). See Appendix C for details and for upcoming changes in WHO reporting.

References

Blackwell, V., & Vega-Lopez, F. (2001). Cutaneous larva migrans: Clinical features and management of 44 cases presenting in the returning traveler. *British Journal of Dermatology, 45,* 434-437.

Brenner, M.A., & Patel, M.B. (2003). Cutaneous larva migrans: The creeping eruption. *Cutis, 72,* 111-115.

Caumes, E. (2000). Treatment of cutaneous larva migrans. *Clinical Infectious Diseases, 30,* 811-814.

Gilles, H.M. (2003). Soil-transmitted helminths (geohelminths). In G.C. Cook & A.I. Zumla (Eds.), *Manson's tropical diseases* (21st ed., pp. 1544-1545). Philadelphia: W.B. Saunders Company.

Sangüeza, O.P., Lu, D., Sangüeza, M., & Pereira C.P. (2003). Protozoa and worms. In J.L. Bolognia, J.L. Jorizzo, & R.P. Rapini (Eds.), *Dermatology* (pp. 1307-1309). Philadelphia: Mosby.

25

Dengue

Breakbone fever, dandy fever, dengue fever

Geographic Distribution

— Dengue is found worldwide but is most prominent in tropical and subtropical areas. It is endemic in Southeast Asia, the Pacific, East and West Africa, the Caribbean, and the Americas. With approximately 150,000 deaths annually, dengue is now the 10th leading infectious disease cause of death worldwide. Approximately 80 to 100 million new cases occur annually worldwide and approximately 40% of the world's population lives in an area of risk (Chin, 2000; Ericsson & Steffen, 2000; Nimmannitya, 2003; World Health Organization [WHO], 1998).

Agent and Vector

— Dengue viruses (DEN) types 1, 2, 3, 4, which are classified as Flaviviridae, are principally transmitted from human to human through the bites of the *Aedes aegypti* mosquitoes (Box 25-1). The female mosquito bites the infected human during the day and can transmit the virus to another host immediately or after 8 to 10 days of incubation within the salivary glands of the mosquito. The mosquito host remains infected for life (Nimmannitya, 2003).

Incubation

— After an individual is bitten by an infective mosquito, the virus undergoes an incubation period of 3 to 14 days (Gubler, 2001).

BIOTERRORISM CONSIDERATIONS   BOX 25-1

Viral hemorrhagic fevers, including Ebola, Marburg, Lassa, Crimean-Congo, and dengue, are considered by the Centers for Disease Control and Prevention (CDC) to be Category A biological warfare agents. Category A agents include organisms that can be easily disseminated or transmitted from person to person, result in high mortality rates, and have the potential for major public health impact. Dengue is transmitted by mosquitoes, while others, such as Ebola, Marburg, Lassa, and Crimean-Congo, can spread from one person to another once an initial person has been infected. The Special Pathogens Branch is required to work with hemorrhagic fever viruses that are classified as biosafety level four (BSL-4) pathogens and include all the above except for dengue fever (CDC, 2003).

Clinical Findings and Treatment

Signs and Symptoms

- Dengue fever is usually a self-limited illness characterized by abrupt onset of high fever accompanied by chills, headache (frontal/retro-orbital), eye pain, bleeding (epistaxis, gums), changes in taste, sore throat, nausea, vomiting, diarrhea, anorexia, depression, severe aching myalgia and arthralgia (hence the term *breakbone fever*), petechiae, and a generalized erythematous flush-like rash on face, neck, and chest.
- In uncomplicated dengue fever, the syndrome usually abates in 48 hours. In other cases, the fever is biphasic with the initial phase lasting 3 to 7 days, followed by a decline in fever and resurgence in 1 to 3 days. The rash is also biphasic, with the second phase beginning during fever remission and lasting several hours to several days. This rash is usually characterized by scarlatiniform and/or purpuric macules beginning on the trunk and

spreading to the extremities, with subsequent desquamation in 1 to 3 days (Gubler, 1998; Rigua-Perez et al., 1998; Tsai, 2000; Vaughn & Green 2000; Weir & Weir, 2002).

Complications

- Unfortunately, there is no durable cross protection between the four dengue viruses. Individuals sensitized to one serotype by past infection may develop non-neutralizing antibodies that can enhance disease by other serotypes, resulting in complement activation and increased vascular permeability, the underlying pathophysiology of dengue hemorrhagic fever (DHF) and dengue shock syndrome (DSS). Ninety percent of cases of DHF and DSS occur during a secondary episode of dengue fever, but due to passive transfer of maternal antibodies, DHF and DSS can also occur with the primary infection in infants born to mothers who are immune to dengue fever.
- After an initial febrile phase similar to classic dengue, patients with DHF enter a second phase characterized by petechiae, ecchymoses, epistaxis, ocular hemorrhage (Figure 25-1), gastrointestinal bleeding, fluid leakage into serosal cavities and tissue spaces, and sometimes disseminated intravascular coagulation (DIC). Approximately 20% to 30% of patients with DHF develop DSS, with increasing vascular permeability and massive plasma leakage. DSS is characterized by shock, hypotension, pleural effusions, ascites, a narrow pulse pressure (less than 20 mm Hg), and potentially circulatory collapse and death.
- Seizures sometimes occur during the febrile phase of dengue. Meningoencephalitis is another complication that occurs in 5% to 10% of children with dengue. Other less common complications include depression, pneumonia, bone marrow failure, iritis, orchitis, and oophoritis (Chin, 2000; Chuansumrit et al.,

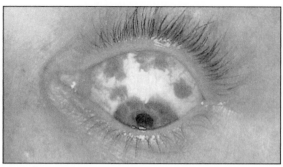

FIGURE 25–1

Scleral hemorrhage in dengue hemorrhagic fever. (*Source:* From Peters, W., & Pasvol, G. [2002]. *Tropical medicine and parasitology* [5th ed., p. 12]. Chicago: Mosby.)

2000; Tsai, 2000; Vaughn & Green, 2000; Weir & Weir, 2002).

Common Laboratory Findings

— Laboratory findings in dengue fever include neutropenia, followed by lymphocytosis, often with atypical lymphocytes. Liver enzymes are usually mildly elevated, but some patients may have extraordinary elevations in their alanine and aspartate transaminases. Thrombocytopenia is common in dengue fever, and often is less than 10,000/µL between the third and eighth day of DHF and DSS. Hemoconcentration is a constant finding in DHF and DSS. Hypoproteinemia and metabolic acidosis are also common. Many patients with DHF have a prolonged partial thromboplastin time (PTT), decreased fibrinogen level, and increased fibrin degradation products.

— The tourniquet test is frequently used to assess capillary integrity. The vasculopathy of DSS and DHF is often first visualized as petechiae. The tourniquet test is performed by inflating a blood pressure cuff on an arm to greater than venous pressure (70 mm Hg) for 5 min and then relieving the pressure. The extremity is inspected for petechiae. If there are greater than two petechiae, the test is positive. This test does not have high specificity, and confounding factors include women who are premenstrual or postmenstrual and not taking hormones, or those with sun-damaged skin leading to increased capillary fragility. Large petechiae are often associated with thrombocytopenia (Gubler, 2001; Pagana & Pagana, 1998; Tsai, 2000).

Diagnosis

Except for the presence of the rash, dengue fever is difficult to distinguish from other febrile illnesses or arboviral diseases with dengue-like courses. For this reason, an initial diagnosis may be "dengue-like disease." When laboratory facilities are limited, DHF may be clinically diagnosed using the following WHO (1997) case definition: fever, minor or major hemorrhagic manifestations, platelet count less than $100,000/mm^3$, and evidence of increased vascular permeability such as pleural effusions, hematocrit greater than 20% above normal, or a drop in hematocrit of more than 20% after volume resuscitation. To fulfill the case definition for DSS, patients must meet the criteria for DHF and have evidence of shock such as rapid, weak pulse, narrow pulse pressure, hypotension, and poor perfusion. Serologic diagnosis is on the basis of a fourfold or greater increase in antibody titer in paired sera by hemagglutination inhibition, complement fixation, enzyme immunoassay, or neutralization test. Typically, paired samples from patients utilize IgM capture enzyme-linked immunosorbent assay (ELISA) and indirect IgG ELISA. Detection of dengue virus-specific IgA serum antibodies by indirect immunofluorescence assay is diagnostic of dengue fever. Viral RNA can be detected by specific complementary DNA probes or by polymerase chain reaction (PCR) (Carlini & Shandera, 2001; Gren et al., 1999; Vaughn & Green, 2000; WHO, 1997).

Differential Diagnosis

— The major differential diagnoses include early stages of malaria, yellow fever, influenza and viral respiratory diseases, viral hepatitis, typhoid, chikungunya infection, rickettsial diseases, and leptospirosis. Four arboviral diseases have a dengue-like course without a rash and include Colorado tick fever, Rift Valley fever, Ross River fever, and sandfly fever (Halstead, 2000; Nimmannitya, 2003).

Treatment

— Treatment of uncomplicated dengue is primarily supportive, and includes pain relief, bed rest, oral fluid replacement, and gradual convalescence. Acetaminophen rather than aspirin is used for fever and pain relief to reduce the risk of bleeding.

— DHF may be treated on an outpatient basis initially but any patient with early signs of shock or a rising hematocrit signifying plasma leakage should be hospitalized. DHF results in death in 40% to 50% of untreated patients who go into shock, but with intensive care, the mortality rate drops to 2%. Children younger than 15 years are the most vulnerable.

— Patients with severe shock, cyanosis or respiratory distress should receive oxygen immediately. In addition to maintenance fluids, patients with signs of moderately decreased intravascular volume should have their fluid deficits replaced with half- to full-strength normal saline in D_5W or Ringer's lactate. For patients in shock, administer a 10 to 20 mL/kg bolus of normal saline or Ringer's lactate rapidly (over less than 20 min), then reassess and repeat if needed. In severe cases of circulatory failure, plasma, plasma substitutes, or 5% albumin may be necessary. Volume status must be closely monitored using physical exam, vital signs, urine output, and hematocrit. Parenteral fluids should be stopped when the hematocrit drops to approximately 40% and clinical signs and urine output improve. This will help to avoid fluid overload, pulmonary edema, and congestive heart failure.

Invasive procedures and instrumentation should be minimized to reduce the risk of bleeding. Electrolytes, blood gases, hematocrit or hemoglobin, platelet count, and coagulation studies (PT, PTT, TT) should be followed closely. Suspect internal bleeding if there is a rapid drop in hematocrit without clinical improvement, and transfuse packed red blood cells if necessary. If there is evidence of DIC or intractable bleeding, platelets or fresh frozen plasma may be given (Chuansumrit et al., 2000; Dung et al., 1999; Ericsson & Steffen, 2000; Tsai, 2000; Vaughn & Green, 2000; WHO, 1997).

Prevention

The prevention of dengue is directed at community and personal mosquito control in endemic areas (Chin, 2000; Robert, 2000; White, 2003; WHO, 1998) and includes the following:

- Kill adult mosquitoes by spraying inside and outside human habitations and surrounding areas with residual insecticides. The goal is to kill as many female mosquitoes as possible, thus decreasing the likelihood of disease transmission. See Appendix D.
- Kill larvae and eliminate breeding areas as much as possible. Elimination of breeding areas includes draining standing water such as swamps, emptying open water-filled containers and used tires, and reducing the number of plants that hold standing water, for example, bromeliads.

– Personal protection includes the following:
  - Screen living and working quarters.
  - Use a residual insecticide inside homes and work areas. See Appendix D.
  - Use insecticide-impregnated mosquito netting over beds. Nets must be retreated with insecticide annually. See Appendix D.
  - Stay inside as much as possible during hours when mosquitoes are biting, which, in the case of *Aedes* mosquitoes, is usually during the day as opposed to *Anopheles,* which feed at dusk to dawn.
  - Use DEET repellant on skin and permethrin-treated clothing when outside during biting hours.
– Provide ongoing community education regarding the preceding measures.

Reporting

– The CDC does not currently consider dengue to be a nationally notifiable disease. The WHO classifies dengue as a disease important in public health. See Appendix C for details and for upcoming changes in WHO reporting.

References

Carlini, M.E., & Shandera, W.X. (2001). Infectious diseases: Viral and rickettsial. In L.M. Tierney, S.J. McPhee, & M.A. Papadakis (Eds.), *Current medical diagnosis & treatment* (40th ed., pp. 1330-1331). Stamford, CT: Appleton & Lange.

Centers for Disease Control and Prevention. (2003). Viral hemorrhagic fevers. Retrieved October 15, 2003, from *www.cdc.gov/ncidod/dvrd/spb/mnpages/dispages/vhf.htm*

Chin, J. (Ed.). (2000). *Control of communicable diseases manual* (17th ed.). Washington, DC: American Public Health Association.

Chuansumrit, A., Phimolthares, V., Tardtong, P., Tapaneya-Olam, C., Tapaneya-Olarn, W., et al. (2000). Transfusion requirements in patients with dengue hemorrhagic fever. *The Southern Asian Journal of Tropical Medicine and Public Health, 31,* 10-14.

Dung, N.M., Day, N.P., Tam, D.T., Chau, H.T., Minh, L.N., et al. (1999). Fluid replacement in dengue shock syndrome: A randomized, double-blind comparison of four intravenous-fluid regimens. *Clinical Infectious Diseases, 29,* 787-794.

Ericsson, C., & Steffen, R. (2000). Dengue fever in international travelers. *Clinical Infectious Diseases, 31,* 144-147.

Gren, J., Velzing, J., Copra, C., Balentien, E., Deubel, V., et al. (1999). Diagnostic value of dengue virus-specific IgA and IgM serum antibody detection. *Microbes Infection, 131,* 1085-1090.

Gubler, D.J. (1998). Dengue and dengue hemorrhagic fever. *Clinical Microbial Review, 11,* 480-496.

Gubler, D.J. (2001). Dengue and dengue hemorrhagic fever. In R.L. Guerrant, D.H. Walker, & P.F. Weller (Eds.), *Essentials of tropical diseases* (pp. 580-583). New York: Churchill Livingstone.

Halstead, S. (2000). Dengue fever/dengue hemorrhagic fever. In W.E. Nelson, R.E. Behrman, R.M. Kliegman, A.M. Arvin (Eds.), *Nelson textbook of pediatrics* (16th ed., pp. 1005-1008). Philadelphia: W.B. Saunders Company.

Nimmannitya, S. (2003). Dengue and dengue haemorrhagic fever. In G.C. Cook & A.I. Zumla (Eds.), *Manson's tropical diseases* (21st ed., pp. 765-772). Philadelphia: W.B. Saunders Company.

Pagana, K., & Pagana, T. (1998). Flaviviruses. *Mosby's manual of diagnostic and laboratory tests.* Philadelphia: Mosby.

Rigau-Perez, J.G., Clark, G.G., Gubler, D.J., Reiter, P., Sanders, E.J., & Vorndam, A.V. (1998). Dengue and dengue haemorrhagic fever. *Lancet, 352,* 971-977.

Robert, L.L. (2000). Control of arthropods of medical importance. In G.T. Strickland (Ed.), *Hunter's tropical medicine and emerging infectious diseases* (8th ed., pp. 1019-1034). Philadelphia: W.B. Saunders Company.

Tsai, T. (2000). Yellow fever, dengue, dengue hemorrhagic fever, Japanese encephalitis, St. Louis encephalitis, tick-born encephalitis. In G. Mandell, J. Bennett, & R. Dolin (Eds.). *Principles and practices of infectious diseases* (5th ed., pp. 1714-1731). New York: Churchill Livingstone.

Vaughn, D., & Green, S. (2000). Dengue and dengue hemorrhagic fever. In G. Strickland (Ed.), *Hunter's tropical medicine and emerging infectious diseases* (8th ed.) (pp. 240-245). Philadelphia: W. B. Saunders Company.

Weir, M.R., & Weir, T.E. (2002). Flaviviridae. In S.K. Tyring (Ed.), *Mucocutaneous manifestations of viral diseases* (pp. 473-480). New York: Marcel Dekker.

White, G.B. (2003). Mosquitoes. In G.C. Cook & A.I. Zumla (Eds.), *Manson's tropical diseases* (21st ed., pp. 1741-1772). Philadelphia: W.B. Saunders Company.

World Health Organization (1997). *Dengue haemorrhagic fever: diagnosis, treatment, prevention and control* (2nd ed.). Geneva: Author.

World Health Organization (1998). *The world report, 1998.* Geneva: Author.

Diphtheria

Geographic Distribution

Diphtheria is endemic in less developed areas of the world where immunizations are not universal. Cutaneous diphtheria may also occur among persons living in unhygienic conditions, for example, homeless people (Gasser & Vitek, 2000; White & Hien, 2003).

Agent and Vector

Diphtheria is caused by several toxin-producing strains of *Corynebacterium diphtheriae*, a pleomorphic, gram-positive, non–acid-fast, nonmotile, slightly curved or club-shaped bacillus. Humans are the only known reservoir for *C. diphtheriae*, with spread occurring person to person, usually from contact with respiratory secretions either by aerosol or droplets, or by contact with exudates. Carriers may be ill or asymptomatic. Epidemics have started from milk contaminated by a carrier (Chin, 2000; White & Hien, 2003).

Incubation

The incubation period for respiratory tract diphtheria is usually 1 to 6 days. Persons who are asymptomatic carriers are usually clear of the organism by 10 days postexposure, but in some cases, carriage lasts for as long as a month (Gasser & Vitek, 2000).

Clinical Findings and Treatment

Signs and Symptoms

Diphtheria most commonly affects children and presents in several forms, according to the location of the characteristic pseudomembranous lesion, which is gray-white, asymmetrical, adherent, surrounded by inflammation, and preceded by regional edema. The lesion usually involves one or both tonsils and may extend to the soft palate, oropharynx, and/or nasopharynx. Lymphadenopathy is significant and the neck may appear enlarged. In some cases there is no visible membrane. Types of diphtheria (Chin, 2000; Gasser & Vitek, 2000; White & Hien, 2003) include the following:

- *Anterior nasal diphtheria.* Most common among infants and is sometimes characterized by unilateral thin nasal discharge, progressing to purulent and often blood-tinged discharge. The illness is usually mild, except when involving other areas as described next.
- *Faucial diphtheria.* Affects the area between the mouth and pharynx. Characterized by insidious onset of sore throat, painful dysphagia, fever, malaise, and sometimes fetid breath and nausea and vomiting.
- *Tracheolaryngeal diphtheria.* Usually secondary to faucial diphtheria, although a faucial lesion is not always present. Onset is relatively rapid (24 hours) with the illness progressing from hoarseness, fever, and cough to dyspnea. If the membrane detaches, respiratory distress follows, manifested by accessory muscle use, retractions, and cyanosis. Obstruction requires tracheostomy.
- *Cutaneous diphtheria.* This type of diphtheria is increasingly found among the homeless who live in unhygienic conditions. The disease is characterized by a cutaneous lesion that ranges from a pustule to a chronic ulcer with a grayish membrane. Coinfection with streptococci and/or *Staphylococcus aureus* is common.
- *Malignant diphtheria.* Characterized by rapid onset of fever, tachycardia, hypotension, cyanosis, and often bleeding from the mouth, nose, and skin. The lesion exhibits rapid and extensive growth.

Lymphadenopathy and regional edema result in a "bull-neck" appearance. Myocarditis with heart block or a wide variety of other rhythm abnormalities develops rapidly and mortality is around 50%.

Complications

— Complications are due to toxin-mediated damage and are related to the extent of pseudomembranous growth and delay in treatment. The most common complications are myocarditis, neuropathy, airway obstruction, and pneumonia (Gasser & Vitek, 2000; White & Hien, 2003).

— Significant myocarditis occurs in about 10% of patients with respiratory diphtheria, and evidence of cardiac involvement may be found in up to 65% of such patients. Onset of myocarditis is usually 3 to 7 days after the onset of the diphtheria. Initial manifestations may include soft heart sounds, angina, syncope, arrhythmia, new or changes in preexisting murmurs, or, sometimes, congestive heart failure. Mortality rates are high with clinically significant cardiac involvement.

— Neuropathy tends to develop late in the illness, from 10 days to 12 weeks after onset, and there is wide variation in frequency in different epidemics. Cranial nerves are usually the first to show dysfunction and peripheral nerves, especially motor, show dysfunction later.

— Airway obstruction occurs when the diphtherial membrane extends into the larynx or tracheobronchial tree, or when the membrane is detached and aspirated. Pneumonia may be due to obstruction or to cranial nerve (IX and/or X) paralysis.

Common Laboratory Findings

— See Diagnosis section.

Diagnosis

Diagnosis is on the basis of characteristic signs and symptoms, including the characteristic pseudomembrane with tonsillitis, pharyngitis, cervical lymphadenopathy, or serosanguineous nasal discharge. When these are present, treatment (see later section) is initiated and continued, even if laboratory results are negative. Confirmation of diphtheria is through isolation and identification of *C. diphtheriae* from *beneath* the membrane at infected sites or polymerase chain reaction testing (Gasser & Vitek, 2000; White & Hien, 2003).

Differential Diagnosis

Differentials include bacterial and viral pharyngitis, acute necrotizing ulcerative gingivitis (trench mouth, Vincent's angina), infectious mononucleosis, oral syphilis, and oral candidiasis. The "bull-neck" of severe diphtheria may be mistaken for mumps. Note that streptococcal pharyngitis is a common co-infection (Chin, 2000; Gasser & Vitek, 2000).

Treatment

Treatment includes maintaining the airway, administration of diphtheria antitoxin and antibiotics, supportive measures, and community health measures. Diphtheria antitoxin is administered IM immediately on the basis of clinical suspicion as follows:

- For suspected faucial diphtheria of less than 48 hours duration or cutaneous diphtheria, give 20,000 to 40,000 units.
- For suspected faucial diphtheria of more than 48 hours duration or laryngeal infection, give 40,000 to 80,000 units.
- For malignant diphtheria, give 80,000 to 100,000 units.

Antibiotics stop toxin production and further spread of the disease. Penicillin G, 50,000 units/kg/24 hours, is given IM qid for 14 days. Alternatively, erythromycin, 5 mg/kg, is given PO or parenterally qid for 14 days. Asymptomatic adult carriers are given a single dose of 1.2 million units of penicillin G IM or erythromycin 250 mg PO qid for 7 to 10 days. Child carriers younger than age 6 are given a single IM dose of 600,000 units of penicillin G. Child carriers older than age 6 are given a single IM dose of 1.2 million units of penicillin G. Alternatively, child carriers may be given erythromycin 40 to 50 mg/kg in divided doses for 7 to 10 days.

Regardless of immunization status, all persons exposed to a patient with diphtheria should (1) have nose and throat cultures taken, (2) receive treatment for carrier state as outlined earlier, and (3) be placed under surveillance for 7 days. In addition, diphtheria toxoid booster is administered if the last dose was taken more than 5 years previously or if the initial series is not complete.

Patients with respiratory diphtheria should be placed in strict isolation until two throat and nose cultures (or skin lesions in the case of cutaneous diphtheria) taken not less than 24 hours apart and not less than 24 hours after cessation of antibiotic therapy are negative. When culture is not available, isolation may be discontinued after 14 days of antibiotic therapy. All articles in contact with the patient should be disinfected (Chin, 2000; Gasser & Vitek, 2000; White & Hien, 2003).

Prevention

Prevention of diphtheria is achieved through population-wide vaccination, booster doses at appropriate intervals, and prompt treatment and isolation of patients and carriers (Gasser & Vitek, 2000).

Reporting

The U.S. Centers for Disease Control and Prevention considers diphtheria a nationally notifiable disease. The World Health Organization (WHO) classifies diphtheria as 2A. See Appendix C for details and for upcoming changes in WHO reporting.

References

Chin, J. (2000). Diphtheria. In J. Chin (Ed.), *Control of communicable diseases manual* (17th ed., pp. 165-170). Washington, DC: American Public Health Association.

Gasser, R.A., & Vitek, C. (2000). Diphtheria. In G.T. Strickland (Ed.), *Hunter's tropical medicine and emerging infectious diseases* (8th ed., pp. 302-306). Philadelphia: W.B. Saunders Company.

White, N.J., & Hien, T.T. (2003). Diphtheria. In G.C. Cook & A.I Zumla (Eds.), *Manson's tropical diseases* (21st ed., pp. 1137-1141). Philadelphia: W.B. Saunders Company.

27

EBOLA AND MARBURG HEMORRHAGIC FEVERS

Geographic Distribution

Ebola hemorrhagic fever is found in the Democratic Republic of Congo, Gabon, Ivory Coast, Sudan, and Uganda. Marburg hemorrhagic fever is found in the Democratic Republic of Congo, Kenya and Uganda (Centers for Disease Control and Prevention [CDC], 2003; Chin, 2000).

Agent and Vector

Ebola and Marburg viruses are the only identified members of the Filoviridae family of RNA viruses. Ebola virus has four subtypes, three of which (Zaire, Sudan, Ivory Coast) are pathogenic in humans and one (Reston) in nonhuman primates. Ebola and Marburg are believed to exist in an unidentified animal host reservoir in African forests, arising sporadically to cause epidemics among humans and nonhuman primates. The highly contagious viruses are passed from human to human through exposure to body fluids, either by direct contact or by handling objects touched by infected persons (Box 27-1). Transmission is increased in the later stages of infection, placing health care workers at particular risk. Humans may also acquire the virus from infected cadavers, animal tissue, and carcasses. The viruses attack primarily endothelial cells, macrophages, monocytes, and hepatocytes, causing focal necrosis of the liver, lymphoid tissue, kidneys, and gonads (CDC, 2003; Chin, 2000; Rollin, Calain, & Ksiazek, 2000; World Health Organization [WHO], 2000).

BIOTERRORISM CONSIDERATIONS   BOX 27–1

Ebola and Marburg hemorrhagic fevers are considered by the CDC to be Category A biological warfare agents, thus posing a risk to national security because they "can be easily disseminated or transmitted from person to person; cause high mortality, with potential for major public health impact; might cause public panic and social disruption; and require special action for public health preparedness" (CDC, 2000, p. 5).

Ebola and Marburg hemorrhagic fevers are stable as aerosols and very readily transmitted human to human. Though the use of Ebola and Marburg hemorrhagic fevers in biological warfare is speculative, their virulence is such that they should not be ignored (Federation of American Scientists, 2000). Treatment is supportive and complex, making treatment of mass casualties difficult (Cieslak & Eitzen, 2000).

Incubation

The incubation period is 4 to 10 days (Solomon, 2003).

Clinical Findings and Treatment

Signs and Symptoms

Ebola and Marburg hemorrhagic fevers are characterized by the sudden onset of fever, chills, severe headache, and myalgia. On about the fifth day of illness, a maculopapular rash may appear, most prominently on the trunk, which sometimes eventually desquamates. Other manifestations appearing at about the same time as the rash can include pharyngitis, chest pain, abdominal pain, nausea, vomiting, diarrhea, and hemorrhagic symptoms (epistaxis, hematemesis, melena, menorrhagia, petechiae, ecchymoses, and bleeding at needle puncture sites).

Symptoms may increase in severity and include jaundice, pancreatic inflammation, rapid weight loss, prostration, delirium, shock, hepatic failure, massive hemorrhaging, and multiple-organ system failure.

Complications

The case fatality rate for Ebola infections in Africa ranges from 50% to 90% and for Marburg infections, about 25%. Death usually occurs 6 to 9 weeks after the onset of illness. For survivors, recovery is marked by fatigue and joint pain and may be complicated by orchitis, hepatitis, transverse myelitis, or uveitis.

Common Laboratory Findings

Early profound lymphopenia has been seen followed by a rapid shift to neutrophilia. Severe thrombocytopenia and abnormal platelet function have been observed. Liver enzymes may be elevated with AST greater than ALT, together with normal to moderately raised bilirubin and alkaline phosphatase.

Diagnosis

Tests include antigen-capture enzyme-linked immunosorbent assay (ELISA), immunoglobulin M (IgM)-capture ELISA, polymerase chain reaction, and viral culture. However, because Ebola and Marburg hemorrhagic fever epidemics have occurred in resource-poor areas without access to sophisticated laboratory facilities, thus far these tests have been used to identify infections retrospectively. In an epidemic situation the diagnosis should be based on the presenting symptoms combined with a history of possible exposure to an infected person or animal. Past experience has shown that the social stigma of infection may lead some people to hide such information, making the history an unreliable tool. Therefore it is recommended that all suspected cases be isolated and observed for the typical symptoms of disease (CDC, 1996, 2003; Solomon, 2003).

Differential Diagnosis

The diagnosis and control of Ebola and Marburg hemorrhagic fevers are complicated by the fact that the early symptoms resemble those of more common infections such as influenza, malaria, and typhoid fever. For persons with severe symptoms, the differential diagnosis expands to include viral encephalitis, dengue and other viral hemorrhagic fevers, and other arboviral infections (Solomon, 2003).

Treatment

There is no specific treatment for Ebola or Marburg hemorrhagic fevers. However, a study released in late 2003 shows reason for optimism about inhibiting the tissue-factor pathway with recombinant nematode anticoagulant protein c2 (rNAPc2) as a means of ameliorating the effects of Ebola. As this is written, studies have been conducted only on rhesus monkeys, but in those subjects, the survival rate was 33% versus about 6% among controls. The treated subjects also survived longer than controls (Geisbert et al., 2003). Supportive care includes maintaining hemodynamic stability, fluid and electrolyte balance, oxygenation, nutrition, and blood and clotting factor replacement. The keys to controlling Ebola and Marburg hemorrhagic fever epidemics are the rapid identification and isolation of index cases, isolation of possible secondary cases, and prevention of nosocomial transmission by ensuring that health care facilities practice strict universal blood and body fluid precautions. Reporting requirements and procedures are given in the 1996 CDC reference at the end of this chapter (CDC, 1996, 2003; Colebunders & Borchert, 2000; Solomon, 2003).

Prevention

To prevent Ebola and Marburg hemorrhagic fevers, travelers should be aware of suspected or confirmed outbreaks and avoid those areas. Those traveling in African forests should avoid contact with ill people and stay away from nonhuman primates and their carcasses. Health care workers in epidemic areas should practice strict blood and body fluid precautions by wearing masks, eye protection, gloves, gowns, and boots. These precautions should also be observed around medical equipment and cadavers. For confirmed or suspected cases the following measures (CDC, 2003; Chin, 2000; Solomon, 2003) should be taken:

- Surveillance, not quarantine, is required.
- Immediate strict barrier isolation is essential. Strict isolation extends to the patient's body fluids and excreta.
- Keep laboratory tests to a minimum and make laboratory staff aware of risks. Ensure that they follow isolation procedures for specimens. Conduct testing in a high containment area; if such an area is not available, use gloves, mask, and a biological safety cabinet. Serum may be disinfected by heating at 140°F or 60°C for 1 hour.
- Place patients in isolation units or, at a minimum, private rooms away from traffic patterns. A negative-pressure room and respiratory protection are preferred.
- Disinfect or incinerate body fluids, excreta, and all objects with which the patient has had contact. Effective disinfectants include 0.5% sodium hypochlorite or 0.5% phenol with detergent. Equipment and other materials with which the patient has had contact may be autoclaved or boiled to disinfect.
- Male patients should abstain from sexual contact for 3 months or until semen is free from virus.

- Upon death, immediately seal deceased patients in a casket or other container and cremate or bury immediately.
- Monitor contacts (close surveillance) twice daily for at least 3 weeks for fever.

Reporting

The CDC considers hemorrhagic fevers to be nationally notifiable diseases. The WHO considers hemorrhagic fevers as diseases important in public health (Class 2A). See Appendix C for details and for upcoming changes in WHO reporting.

References

Centers for Disease Control and Prevention. (1996). Notice to readers update: Management of patients with suspected viral hemorrhagic fever—United States. *Morbidity and Mortality Weekly Report, 44,* 475-479. Retrieved June 18, 2003, from *www.cdc.gov/epo/mmwr/preview/mmwrhtml/00038033.htm*

Centers for Disease Control and Prevention. (2000). Biological and chemical terrorism: Strategic plan for preparedness and response. *MMWR: Morbidity and Mortality Weekly Report, 49(RR-4),* 1-14.

Centers for Disease Control and Prevention. (2003). Marburg hemorrhagic fever. Retrieved July 22, 2003, from *www.cdc.gov/ncidod/dvrd/spb/mnpages/dispages/marburg.htm*

Chin, J. (Ed.). (2000). *Control of communicable diseases manual* (17th ed.). Washington, DC: American Public Health Association.

Cieslak, T.J., & Eitzen, E.M. (2000). Bioterrorism: Agents of concern. *Journal of Public Health Management Practice, 6,* 19-29.

Colebunders, R., & Borchert, M. (2000). Ebola haemorrhagic fever—a review. *Journal of Infection, 40,* 16-20.

Federation of American Scientists. (2000). Biological weapons. Retrieved October 31, 2001, from *www.fas.org/index.html*

Geisbert, T.W., Hensley, L.E., Jahrling, P.B., Larsen, T., Geisbert, J.B., et al. (2003). Treatment of Ebola virus infection with a recombinant inhibitor of factor VIIa/tissue factor: A study in rhesus monkeys. *The Lancet, 362,* 1953-1958.

Rollin, P.E., Calain, P., & Ksiazek, T.G. (2000). Ebola and Marburg virus infections. In G.T. Strickland (Ed.), *Hunter's tropical medicine and emerging infectious diseases* (8th ed., pp. 281-284). Philadelphia: W.B. Saunders Company.

Solomon, T. (2003). Viral haemorrhagic fevers. In G.C. Cook & A.I. Zumla (Eds.), *Manson's tropical diseases* (21st ed., pp. 773-793). Philadelphia: W.B. Saunders Company.

World Health Organization. (2000). Disease outbreak news: Ebola haemorrhagic fever in Uganda. Retrieved October 16, 2000, from *www.who.int/disease-outbreak-news/index.html* (Readers are encouraged to use this site for current and complete information on major infectious diseases.)

28

ECHINOCOCCOSIS
Hydatid disease
Geographic Distribution

— Echinococcosis is distributed throughout most of the world. The geographic distribution of *Echinococcus* subspecies depends on their natural hosts (Table 28-1).

Agent and Vector

— The *Echinococcus* tapeworms infect canines as their definitive hosts, with humans as inadvertent hosts. The disease is transmitted through either direct contact with infected feces or by ingesting fecally contaminated food. Tapeworm eggs remain viable in the feces of infected canines for weeks, allowing transmission to individuals even if they have no direct contact with the vector animal. Once in the intestine, the eggs hatch to form embryos or oncospheres that penetrate the mucosa and enter the circulation. Oncospheres then encyst in host viscera and develop into mature larval cysts. Most patients present with one cyst, which is usually asymptomatic until it reaches a size that causes pain, obstruction, or other dysfunction through mass effect in the target organ. *E. granulosus* creates unilocular cysts (hydatid disease) usually in the liver (50% to 70%) or lung (20% to 30%), but may occur in the brain, heart, or bones (less than 10%). *E. multilocularis* creates more aggressive alveolar cysts, nearly always in the liver (98%). *E. vogeli* causes polycystic hydatid disease primarily in the liver but can also affect the lungs (15%).

Incubation

— The incubation for all the *Echinococcus* parasites varies from one to many years. The average age at diagnosis of

TABLE 28–1

Echinococcus Hosts and Distribution

Echinococcus Species	Definitive Hosts	Intermediate Hosts	Geographic Distribution
E. granulosus	Dogs, foxes, wolves, dingoes	Sheep, cattle, horses, pigs	South America, Mediterranean, central Asia, Australia, Africa
E. multilocularis	Foxes primarily; wolves, coyotes, cats, dogs	Mice, lemmings, shrews, voles	North America (especially central portion of the U.S.-Canadian border), northern Europe, central Asia, northern Asia
E. vogeli	Bush dog	Paca and other rodents	Central and northern South America

Sources: CDC, 1999, 2002; Chin, 2000; Gottstein & Reichen, 2003; King, 2000.

alveolar echinococcosis in Europe is 55 years (Chin, 2000; Gottstein & Reichen, 2003).

Clinical Findings and Treatment

Signs and Symptoms

Most people with *Echinococcus* infections are asymptomatic, especially in the lengthy early stages. *Echinococcus* embryos are trapped in various organs (especially the liver or lungs), and also in muscles, bones, kidneys, brain, heart, and other organs. Embryos that are not destroyed by the body's defenses may develop into hydatid cysts, which grow and eventually cause dysfunction according to the function or area of the involved organ (Figure 28-1).

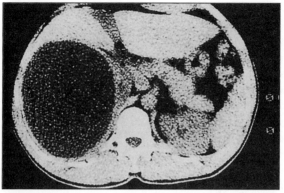

FIGURE 28–1

A hydatid cyst in the liver, shown by computed tomography. (*Source:* From Peters, W., & Pasvol, G. [2002]. *Tropical medicine and parasitology* [5th ed., p. 212]. Chicago: Mosby.)

Cystic echinococcosis from *E. granulosus* infection is most commonly a single cyst 1 to 15 mm in diameter in the liver (62%), lung (20% in adults, higher in children), spleen (6%), bones/muscles (4%), heart/thorax (2%), or kidney (2%), as well as rarely in other sites. Infection manifests after years of silent presence until the cyst (1) grows large enough to affect function or cause pain; (2) ruptures and spills contents, thus causing gastrointestinal symptoms or shock; or (3) becomes superinfected. Hepatic cyst growth causes abdominal pain (not necessarily limited to the right upper quadrant), hepatomegaly with or without palpable mass, nausea and vomiting, biliary duct obstruction, and jaundice. Pulmonary cyst(s) may cause chest pain, chronic cough, hemoptysis, biliptysis (bile in sputum), pneumothorax, pleuritis, abscess, and embolism. Signs and symptoms associated with other organs are according to the site. Rupture of the cyst in the liver, lungs, or other organs may result in fever, urticaria, eosinophilia, anaphylactic shock, and cyst dissemination. Anaphylactic shock is often the first sign of infection. Superinfection may produce sepsis and shock.

Alveolar echinococcosis from *E. multilocularis* infection affects the liver in 98% of cases. Infection usually manifests as a result of cyst growth, leading to nonspecific abdominal pain, hepatomegaly, cholestasis, jaundice, secondary biliary cirrhosis, liver abscess, portal hypertension, fatigue, weight loss, and/or Budd-Chiari syndrome (progressive hepatomegaly, tenderness, ascites, lower extremity edema, abdominal collateral vein distention, mild splenomegaly, and occasionally jaundice and hemorrhage from esophageal varices). Superinfection may produce sepsis and shock.

E. vogeli infection is rare and is found most commonly in the liver, where it grows slowly and may produce secondary cysts. *E. oligarthrus* infection in humans is very rare (Centers for Disease Control and Prevention [CDC], 1999, 2002; Chin, 2000; Gottstein & Reichen, 2003).

Complications

Complications such as cyst rupture and superinfection were discussed earlier. The presence of a cyst in the central nervous system or heart is of grave concern.

Common Laboratory Findings

Eosinophilia is variable, but relatively uncommon.

Diagnosis

The diagnosis is often made by the detection of a cyst by ultrasound, computed tomography (CT), or magnetic resonance imaging (MRI) together with a positive serology. Although immunoblot (Western blot) and enzyme-linked immunosorbent assay (ELISA) are 80% to 100% sensitive for liver cysts they are only 50% to 56% sensitive for lungs and other organs, with a specificity of 25% to 56%. Cysts in bone are more likely to stimulate detectable antibody than cysts in the lung, brain, or spleen. Percutaneous aspiration of cysts may reveal multiple protoscolices in the cyst fluid, but the procedure is difficult to perform safely without cyst spillage. When a cyst ruptures there is an abrupt stimulation of antibodies. However, patients with senescent, calcified, or dead cysts become seronegative. Therefore, if CT or MRI shows a characteristic cyst, the diagnosis should be made regardless of confirmation by serology (CDC, 2002; Gottstein & Reichen, 2003; King, 2000; Wilson & Schantz, 2000).

Differential Diagnosis

Hepatic echinococcal cysts may resemble cystadenomas, tumors, or abscesses. For pulmonary cysts, the differential diagnosis includes tuberculosis or cancer.

Treatment

Cysts that are either symptomatic or affecting vital anatomic structures should be treated. Though no well-designed clinical trials have compared all the different treatment methods, surgical excision is the treatment of choice for most symptomatic cysts. Another technique called PAIR (puncture, aspiration, injection, reaspiration) involves percutaneously aspirating cyst contents, injecting an agent into the cyst to kill the protoscolices, then reaspirating. One prospective randomized trial for the treatment of hepatic echinococcal cysts found PAIR combined with albendazole to be as effective as surgery with shorter hospital stays and fewer complications.
For chemotherapy, albendazole is the drug of choice, given orally at 10 to 15 mg/kg/day or fixed doses of 400 mg bid with meals in adults. Because of toxicity concerns, albendazole has been used with cycles of 4 weeks on and 2 weeks off for at least 3 months. However, recent data suggest that continuous therapy is just as effective with no increase in adverse effects. Mebendazole can be used as a second drug of choice in

higher doses (50 to 70 mg/kg/day divided tid with meals) for 3 months. Praziquantel is used as adjunct therapy because it only kills the inside of the hydatid cyst and not the germinal layer. It is currently being used with albendazole for preoperative and postoperative protection against cyst spillage, although there are concerns that it may potentiate albendazole toxicity. Praziquantel is given in two doses (one dose both preoperative and postoperative) of 5 to 10 mg/kg for both children and adults. Praziquantel causes considerable nausea and abdominal pain, which can be reduced with a dose of promethazine (Phenergan) before administration. Avoid use of praziquantel in pregnancy or in children younger than 4 years of age. Breast-feeding mothers should not breast-feed for 72 hours after treatment (Goldsmith, 2001; King, 2000; McManus, Zhang, Li, & Bartley, 2003; Moro, Gonzales, & Gilman, 2000; Safioeas et al., 1999).

Prevention

In endemic areas, the reservoir of *Echinococcus* may be controlled by treating wild canines with praziquantel-impregnated baits and domestic dogs with arecoline hydrobromide or praziquantel. People can reduce their risk of infection by avoiding contact with dog or fox feces, washing their hands with soap and water after handling these animals, washing and cooking fruits and vegetables picked from the wild, and preventing their pets from capturing wild rodents. Ranchers should be educated not to feed their dogs scraps from butchered animals. Hikers should avoid wild canines and wear gloves when handling their carcasses. Prolonged freezing of meat (lower than 18° C) or thorough cooking of meet (higher than 50° C) kills cysts in tissue. Careful disposal of human sewage limits the spread of parasitic eggs (CDC, 1999; Chin, 2000; King, 2000; McManus et al., 2003; Moro et al., 2000).

Reporting

The CDC does not consider echinococcosis to be a nationally notifiable diseases. The World Health Organization (WHO) considers it a Class 5 disease. See Appendix C for details and for upcoming changes in WHO reporting.

References

Centers for Disease Control and Prevention. (1999). Alveolar hydatid disease. Retrieved August 30, 2003, from *www.cdc.gov/ncidod/dpd/ahd.htm*

Centers for Disease Control and Prevention. (2002). Echinococcosis. Retrieved August 30, 2003, from *www.dpd.cdc.gov/dpdx/html/Echinococcosis.htm*

Chin, J. (Ed.). (2000). *Control of communicable diseases manual* (17th ed.). Washington, DC: American Public Health Association.

Goldsmith, R. (2001). In L.M. Tierney, S.J. McPhee, & M.A. Papadakis (Eds.), *Current medical diagnosis & treatment* (40th ed., pp. 1330-1331). Stamford, CT: Appleton & Lange.

Gottstein, B., & Reichen, J. (2003). Echinococcosis/hydatidosis. In G.C. Cook & A.I. Zumla (Eds.), *Manson's tropical diseases* (21st ed., pp. 1561-1582). Philadelphia: W.B. Saunders Company.

King, C. (2000). Cestodes (tapeworms). In G. Mandell, J. Bennett, & R. Dolin (Eds.) *Principles and practices of infectious diseases* (5th ed., pp. 2956-65). New York: Churchill Livingstone.

McManus, D.P., Zhang, W., Li, J., & Bartley, P. B. (2003). Echinococcosis. *Lancet, 362,* 1295-304.

Moro, P., Gonzales, A., & Gilman, R. (2000). Cystic hydatid disease. In T. Strickland (Ed.), *Hunter's tropical medicine and emerging diseases* (8th ed., pp. 866-875). Philadelphia: W.B. Saunders Company.

Safioeas, M., Misiakos, E.P., Dosios, T., Manti, C., Lambrou, P., & Skalkeas, G. (1999). Surgical treatment for lung hydatid disease. *World Journal of Surgery, 23,* 1181-1185.

Wilson, M., & Schantz, P.M. (2000). Parasitic immunodiagnosis. In T. Strickland (Ed.), *Hunter's tropical medicine and emerging diseases* (8th ed., pp. 1117-1122). Philadelphia: W.B. Saunders Company.

29

ENTEROBIASIS

Enterobius vermicularis, pinworm, threadworm

Geographic Distribution

— Enterobiasis is an infection that occurs worldwide and is most prevalent in school-aged children (ages 5 to 10) in areas of high population density (Bundy & Cooper, 2000).

Agent and Vector

— Enterobiasis is caused by the intestinal nematode *Enterobius vermicularis*, for which humans are the only known host. The adult worms live in the lumen of the ascending colon, and the female migrates down to the anus during the night to deposit her eggs on perianal skin. The female worms and eggs invariably cause perianal pruritus. Scratching the affected area allows transfer of the eggs from the fingers to the mouth of the host. The eggs are then ingested and deposit in the intestine, where they mature over several weeks. Retroinfection may also occur, which involves migration of the newly hatched larvae from the perianal region up into the large intestine. Eggs may be transmitted to others through direct contact or transfer from infected material, such as sheets, clothing, and food (Liu, 2001).

Incubation

— The incubation period from ingestion of the eggs to the deposition of the next generation of eggs on the perianal skin is approximately 3 to 5 weeks (Bundy & Cooper, 2000; Liu, 2001).

Clinical Findings and Treatment

Signs and Symptoms

Enterobiasis results in pruritus ani, which varies from mild to severe itching. The most intense itching usually occurs at night, and excoriations may result in secondary bacterial infections. Vulvovaginitis may also occur when the worms enter the vulva. This results in perineal irritation and occasionally vaginal discharge. Enterobiasis rarely produces changes in the intestine or systemic manifestations. Children can also present with vague symptoms, such as restlessness, insomnia, loss of appetite, and enuresis (Bundy & Cooper, 2000; Gilles, 2003).

Complications

Rarely, the worms gain access to the peritoneal cavity through the female genital tract or a perforation in the bowel. This can result in chronic peritonitis or granulomatous nodules in abdominal organs, which may be confused with tuberculosis or metastatic disease (Bundy & Cooper, 2000; Gilles, 2003).

Common Laboratory Findings

None.

Diagnosis

The diagnosis is made by isolation of eggs or worms from the feces or the perianal area. Eggs are found in the feces in less than 5% of infected patients; therefore, other diagnostic tests are more useful. The cellulose acetate (Scotch tape) test is the most reliable means of finding eggs or worms on the perianal skin. The tape is mounted on a swab and pressed against the perianal skin at night or early in the morning, then placed on a slide. Examination of one smear can detect approximately half

of the infections, and three swabs from separate days
can detect 90% of infections (Bundy & Cooper, 2000;
Gilles, 2003; Liu, 2001).

Differential Diagnosis

Other intestinal worms, such as *Strongyloides*, can cause
perianal itching; however, unlike enterobiasis, there are
often systemic symptoms, such as diarrhea, abdominal
pain, anemia, and eosinophilia. Demonstration of the
presence of eggs using the cellulose acetate test excludes
all other diagnoses.

Treatment

To avoid reinfection, the entire family requires treatment.
Several medications are used to treat enterobiasis.
Albendazole is the treatment of choice and is given as a
single oral dose (400 mg for adults, 10 to 14 mg/kg for
children). Mebendazole is given as a single initial dose
(100 mg repeated 2 to 4 weeks later). Pyrantel pamoate
may also be given as a single oral dose (10 mg/kg) and is
repeated every 4 to 6 weeks until the patient is clear
(Bundy & Cooper, 2000; Gilles, 2003).

Prevention

Hygiene and cleanliness, including hand washing,
wearing clean clothes, changing linens, frequent
vacuuming, and covering food, should be stressed to
decrease the prevalence and transmission of the infection
(Bundy & Cooper, 2000; Gilles, 2003; Liu, 2001).

Reporting

The U.S. Centers for Disease Control and Prevention
does not consider enterobiasis to be a nationally notifiable
disease. The World Health Organization (WHO)
considers it a Class 5 disease. See Appendix C for details
and for upcoming changes in WHO reporting.

References

Bundy, D.A., & Cooper, E. (2000). Nematodes limited to the intestinal tract (*Enterobius vermicularis, Trichuris trichiura,* and *Capillaria philippinensis*). In G. Strickland (Ed.), *Hunter's tropical medicine and emerging infectious diseases* (8th ed., pp. 719-721). Philadelphia: W.B. Saunders Company.

Gilles, H.M. (2003). Soil-transmitted helminths (geohelminths). In G.C. Cook & A.I. Zumla (Eds.), *Manson's tropical diseases* (21st ed., pp. 1527-1529). Philadelphia: W.B. Saunders Company.

Liu, L.X. (2001). Enterobiasis. In R.L. Guerrant, D.H. Walker, & P.F. Weller (Eds.), *Essentials of tropical diseases* (pp. 949-953). New York: Churchill Livingstone.

CHAPTER

30

FILARIASIS: DRACUNCULIASIS
Dracontiasis, Guinea worm disease
Geographic Distribution

In 1986, the World Health Organization (WHO) targeted dracunculiasis as the next disease for eradication. At that time 3.5 million people in 20 countries had the disease; however, by the end of 2002, the annual incidence of the disease had been reduced by greater than 98%. Seven countries where dracunculiasis was formerly endemic (Cameroon, Chad, India, Kenya, Pakistan, Senegal, and Yemen) have been freed of the disease. The Central African Republic, Ethiopia, Mauritania, and Uganda each reported less than 100 cases. Most remaining cases are in Sudan, Nigeria, and Ghana (Centers for Disease Control and Prevention [CDC], 2003; Sarwari, 2000; Simonsen, 2003).

Agent and Vector

Dracunculus medinensis is the only nematode that causes dracunculiasis in humans. The life cycle of this worm is complex and begins as the intermediate host, a copepod microcrustacean of the genus *Cyclops*, ingests the larvae released in water by the female guinea worm. The larvae reach the midintestine of the copepod, break through the wall, and remain in the hemocoelom. The development of third-stage larvae in the copepod takes approximately 2 to 3 weeks. Humans acquire dracunculiasis when they drink water that contains copepods infected with third-stage larvae of the guinea worm. Larvae are released from copepods in the human gastrointestinal tract, penetrate the intestinal wall, and migrate into the abdominal or thoracic cavity, where they mature and mate. During maturation, the female guinea worm migrates to the subcutaneous tissue and forms a blister, typically in the lower extremities. When the affected area is immersed in water, the female worm protrudes and releases thousands of larvae (Sarwari, 2000).

Incubation

Once ingested by the human host, the female worm takes about 1 year to mature. Infection becomes evident when the worm migrates to and protrudes from the subcutaneous tissue (Bell, 1995).

Clinical Findings and Treatment

Signs and Symptoms

Days before the worm exits the skin, a blister develops, and the patient may feel itching or burning of the affected area, which is most often on the foot or lower leg. Many patients also experience systemic symptoms, including generalized urticaria, wheezing, nausea, vomiting, diarrhea, dizziness, and fever. If the patient exposes the affected area to water, the blister ruptures, the worm protrudes, and larvae are released (Figure 30-1). A superficial ulcer remains that heals quickly and leaves a small hole in the center where the worm occasionally protrudes. Sometimes the female worms fail to emerge and die in the body, which can lead to calcification or sterile subcutaneous abscesses. Most often only one or two worms emerge per year (Sarwari, 2000; Simonsen, 2003).

Complications

The most common complication is secondary bacterial infection of the site of emergence, which can lead to abscesses, cellulitis, arthritis, epididymo-orchitis, and chronic ulcerations. Inflammation or calcification of worms near joints can cripple patients to the degree that they cannot work. Worms can also rupture within

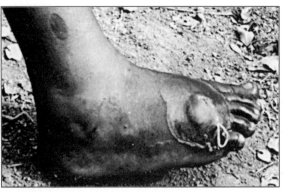

FIGURE 30–1

Dracunculiasis. A female worm extends from the blister. (*Source:* From Strickland, G.T. [2000]. *Hunter's tropical medicine and emerging infectious diseases* [8th ed., p. 110]. Philadelphia: W.B. Saunders Company.)

tissues, leading to the formation of large abscesses. Tetanus infection is a serious complication and is potentially lethal. Rarely, calcified worms or worms within abscess cavities have been found in the pericardium, subconjunctival space, extradural space of the spinal cord, lung parenchyma, and testes. Another rare complication is anaphylactic shock, which has been known to occur in previously sensitized individuals (Marchie, 1999; Pendse, Soni, Omprakash, & Gupta, 1982; Ruiz-Tiben & Gutierrez, 2001; Sarwari, 2000; Simonsen, 2003).

Common Laboratory Findings

— Substantial eosinophilia is common (Simonsen, 2003).

Diagnosis

— The diagnosis is made by demonstration of the guinea worm or larvae from the site of emergence. Cold water or ethyl chloride can be placed on the ulcer, which

results in release of larvae from the female worm.
The larvae can then be examined and characterized
microscopically. Worms that fail to emerge and instead
calcify within the host can be shown radiologically.
Serologic tests are not useful; therefore, diagnosis before
the worm emerges from the soft tissue may not be
possible (Sarwari, 2000).

Differential Diagnosis

A guinea worm that tracks underneath the skin may be
confused with cutaneous larva migrans; however, the
latter are much shorter and do not emerge from a single
ulcer upon contact with water. The characteristic
appearance of the guinea worm, which typically measures
60 to 80 cm long and 2 mm wide, allows for definitive
diagnosis (Sarwari, 2000).

Treatment

The traditional extraction of the guinea worm is effective
and involves attaching the protruding part of the worm
to a small stick and twisting it a few centimeters each day
until the worm is removed. To ease extraction, the
emerging worm may be immersed in cold water, which
releases the larvae and decompresses the engorged uterus.
Sterile dressings and antibiotics are recommended to
prevent secondary infection. Surgical removal of worms
before emergence may prevent the disability that is
sometimes caused by the guinea worm; however, complete removal may be difficult if the worm is adherent to
or wrapped around deep structures. No medications have
been shown to be effective in treating worms that have
yet to emerge. Some medications may be helpful in
facilitating worm removal and reducing inflammation.
They include metronidazole (400 mg/day for 10 to
20 days for adults, 25 mg/kg/24 hours divided tid for
10 days for children), niridazole (25 mg/kg/day for
10 days), thiabendazole (50 mg/kg/day for 3 days),

or mebendazole (400 to 800 mg/day for 6 days for adults) (Sarwari, 2000; Simonsen, 2003).

Prevention

Dracunculiasis is potentially an eradicable disease because it has a relatively simple life cycle with humans as its only reservoir. Prevention/eradication measures (Simonsen, 2003) include the following:

- Provide safe drinking water, preferably though the use of bore-hole wells in endemic areas. Water should be boiled, filtered, or chemically treated before consumption. For filtering nylon filters are ideal, but polyester or tightly woven cotton cloth may suffice.
- People with guinea worm blisters or ulcers should avoid entering water sources.
- Ponds and wells may be treated with the insecticide temephos. See Appendix D on vector control.

Community education on the preceding measures should be ongoing.

Reporting

The CDC does not consider dracunculiasis to be a nationally notifiable disease. The WHO classifies dracunculiasis as Class 2B. See Appendix C for details and for upcoming changes in WHO reporting.

References

Bell, D.R. (1995). *Lecture notes on tropical medicine* (4th ed., pp. 271-276). Malden, MA: Blackwell Science.

Centers for Disease Control and Prevention. (2003). Progress toward global eradication of dracunculiasis, January-June 2003. *Morbidity and Mortality Weekly Report, 52*, 881-883.

Marchie TT. (1999). Guinea worm cause of adult onset asthmatic attack, a radiological diagnosis. *West African Journal of Medicine, 18*, 214-216.

Pendse, A.K., Soni, B.M., Omprakash, R., & Gupta, S.P. (1982). Testicular dracunculosis—a distinct clinical entity. *British Journal of Urology, 54*, 56-58.

Ruiz-Tiben, E., & Gutierrez, Y. (2001). Dracunculiasis. In R.L. Guerrant, D.H. Walker, & P.F. Weller (Eds.), *Essentials of tropical diseases* (pp. 426-428). New York: Churchill Livingstone.

Sarwari, A.R. (2000). Dracunculiasis. In G. Strickland (Ed.), *Hunter's tropical medicine and emerging infectious diseases* (8th ed., pp. 775-780). Philadelphia: W.B. Saunders Company.

Simonsen, P.E. (2003). Filariases. In G.C. Cook & A.I. Zumla (Eds.), *Manson's tropical diseases* (21st ed., pp. 1518-1526). Philadelphia: W.B. Saunders Company.

CHAPTER
31

FILARIASIS: LOIASIS
Eyeworm disease, loa loa
Geographic Distribution

Loiasis is endemic in the tropical rain forests of Central and West Africa, infecting 3 to 13 million people (Klion, 2000).

Agents and Vectors

Loiasis is caused by the nematode *Loa loa* (African eye worm), whose vector is the *Chrysops* red fly (primarily *C. silacea* and *C. dimidiata*). The female *Chrysops* acquires and transmits loa microfilaria larvae during blood meals. In the human host, the larvae mature into thin, transparent adult worms. The adult female worms measure 50 to 70 mm in length and survive for long periods of time (Centers for Disease Control and Prevention [CDC], 2003a; Klion, 2000).

Incubation

Larvae appear in the peripheral blood in 6 or more months after infection. Adult worms live as long as 17 years in humans, shedding microfilariae throughout that time. Symptoms of infection take from 4 months to several years to manifest (Chin, 2000; Simonsen, 2003).

Clinical Findings and Treatment

Signs and Symptoms

Loiasis is often asymptomatic among indigenous people of endemic areas; it causes a stronger immune response and disease in nonindigenous persons. The worms migrate in subcutaneous tissues and cause intermittent localized areas (more than 10 cm) of erythema and edema known as *Calabar swellings,* usually on the face and extremities. Migrating worms are sometimes visible in the eye between the bulbar conjunctiva and sclera (Figure 31-1). Eye worms usually cause lid edema and conjunctival injection. Patients with loiasis often have fatigue, pruritus, myalgias, arthralgias, and malaise (CDC, 2003a; Simonsen, 2003).

Complications

Loiasis may cause meningoencephalitis, glomerulonephritis, or transient pulmonary infiltrates and has been implicated in endomyocardial fibrosis. Hydroceles, arthritis, and lymphangitis are other uncommon manifestations (Klion, 2000; Simonsen, 2003).

Common Laboratory Findings

Eosinophilia (sometimes greater than 70% of peripheral white blood cells), hematuria, and proteinuria often occur. Occasionally, dead calcified worms may be detected in radiographs (Klion, 2000).

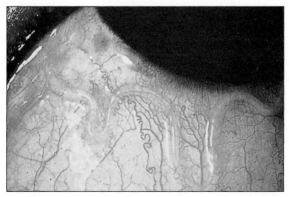

FIGURE 31–1

An adult loa worm in the eye. (*Source:* From Peters, W., & Pasvol, G. [2002]. *Tropical medicine and parasitology* [5th ed., p. 94]. Chicago: Mosby.)

Diagnosis

The presence of a worm in the eye is diagnostic. The diagnosis should also be suspected in a patient who has traveled to an endemic area and has unexplained eosinophilia and Calabar swellings. Serology is also available, but cannot distinguish loiasis from other filarial infections (CDC, 2003a; Simonsen, 2003).

Differential Diagnosis

Lymphatic filariasis and onchocerciasis share many of the same symptoms with loiasis.

Treatment

Diethylcarbamazine (DEC) eliminates microfilariae at a dose of 5 to 10 mg/kg/day tid after meals for 2 to 4 weeks. The Medical Letter (2002) recommends giving increasing doses as follows:
- Day 1: 50 mg after meals
- Day 2: 50 mg tid after meals
- Day 3: 100 mg tid after meals
- Days 4 through 21: 9 mg/kg/day divided tid after meals

Multiple courses may be necessary to eliminate adult worms, and relapses may occur as many as 8 years after treatment. Patients with high numbers of microfilariae are at risk for serious complications of DEC treatment, including meningoencephalitis and renal failure. DEC may also cause the Mazzotti reaction (a systemic and ocular reaction, including intense pruritus, rash, fever, headache, and arthralgia). Neither graduated doses of DEC nor corticosteroids or antihistamines are completely effective in preventing these complications, although both strategies are used. The pediatric dosage recommended by the Medical Letter (2002) is:
- Day 1: 1 mg/kg after meals
- Day 2: 1 mg/kg tid after meals

- Day 3: 1-2 mg/kg tid after meals
- Days 4 through 21: 9 mg/kg/day divided tid

Although DEC remains the drug of choice, albendazole at a dose of 200 mg bid for 3 weeks slowly reduces loa microfilariae without adverse effects (Klion, 2000; Medical Letter, 2002; Simonsen, 2003).

Prevention

Eradication of the *Chrysops* red fly vector for loiasis is impractical; hence, prevention is directed primarily to personal protective measures against biting flies in endemic areas (CDC, 2003b; Chin, 2000; Minter, 2003), including the following:

- Wear light-colored clothing, because the flies are attracted to dark objects, including dark vehicles (and their occupants).
- Impregnate clothing with DEET repellent or permethrin. Long sleeves and long pants are preferable to short sleeves and pants. Headgear should be worn.
- Try to avoid being outdoors in typical fly hunting times and grounds, although this may be difficult because the flies are most active in bright sunlight and their hunting ranges include woodlands, marshlands, and savannas or grasslands. Moreover, a major vector species, *C. silacea*, bites indoors as opposed to most Chrysops, which bite only outdoors.
- Locate dwellings or campgrounds away from forest edge and swamps.
- Chemoprophylaxis using DEC at a dose of 300 mg weekly is an effective option for travelers who will be staying long term in endemic areas.

Community education in endemic areas is important.

Reporting

The CDC does not consider loiasis to be a nationally notifiable disease. The World Health Organization (WHO) considers it a Class 5 disease. See Appendix C for details and for upcoming changes in WHO reporting.

References

Centers for Disease Control and Prevention. (2003a). Filariasis. Retrieved December 1, 2003, from *www.dpd.cdc.gov/dpdx/HTML/Filariasis.htm*

Centers for Disease Control and Prevention. (2003b). Protection against mosquitoes and other arthropods. Retrieved December 1, 2003, from *www.cdc.gov/travel/bugs.htm*

Chin, J. (Ed.) (2000). *Control of communicable diseases manual* (17th ed., pp. 299-301). Washington, DC: American Public Health Association.

Klion, A. (2000). Loiasis. In G.T. Strickland (Ed.), *Hunter's tropical medicine and emerging infectious diseases* (8th ed., pp. 754-756). Philadelphia: W.B. Saunders Company.

Medical Letter. (2002). Drugs for parasitic infections. Retrieved November 26, 2003, from *www.medletter.com/freedocs/parasitic.pdf*

Minter, D.M. (2003). Horse flies, clegs, deer flies. In G.C. Cook & A.I. Zumla (Eds.), *Manson's tropical diseases* (21st ed., pp. 1774-1781). Philadelphia: W.B. Saunders Company.

Simonsen, P.E. (2003). Filariases. In G.C. Cook & A.I. Zumla (Eds.), *Manson's tropical diseases* (21st ed., pp. 1487-1526). Philadelphia: W.B. Saunders Company.

FILARIASIS: LYMPHATIC

Bancroftian filariasis, Malayan filariasis

Geographic Distribution

Lymphatic filariasis is endemic in more than 80 countries in the tropics and subtropics, affecting both urban and rural areas. More than one-third of affected people live in India, another third in Africa, and most of the remainder in southeast Asia, the Pacific islands, and the Americas (The Global Alliance to Eliminate Lymphatic Filariasis [Global Alliance], 2003).

Agent and Vector

The parasites that cause lymphatic filariasis are tissue-dwelling nematodes (roundworms) whose microfilaria larvae are transmitted by mosquitoes and flies. The microfilariae disseminate in the blood and lodge in lymphatic vessels and nodes, where they mature into white, thread-like adult worms measuring up to 100 mm in length. The adult female lives 4 to 6 years, producing millions of microfilariae.

Bancroftian filariasis is caused by the nematode *Wuchereria bancrofti*, transmitted by *Anopheline* mosquitos, and occurs in much of the tropical and subtropical world except western South America and Northern Australia. About 90% of patients with lymphatic filariasis are infected with *W. bancrofti*. Malayan filariasis is caused by the nematode *Brugia malayi*, transmitted by *Mansonia* or *Anopheline* mosquitoes, and occurs primarily in Malaysia, Indonesia, and some nearby Pacific islands, as well as scattered areas of India, Bangladesh, Vietnam, and China.

W. bancrofti and *B. malayi* infections are similar, except that *B. malayi* is less widely distributed and has less severe clinical features. *Brugia timori* infections are similar, confined to Timor and nearby islands, and transmitted by *Anopheles barbirostris,* which also carries malaria (Global Alliance, 2003; Hotez et al., 2004; Simonsen, 2003).

Incubation

Symptoms begin anywhere from 4 to 12 months, but usually more than 6 months, after infection (Chin, 2000; Global Alliance, 2003).

Clinical Findings and Treatment

Signs and Symptoms

About 50% of all infected persons are asymptomatic (Global Alliance, 2003). Symptoms usually begin with localized inflammation in the genitalia or extremities. Lymphadenitis and lymphangitis begin at a single site and spread regionally within hours. Recurrent bouts of acute onset fever, chills, headache, and malaise also occur. Lymphedema may begin accumulating in the first 24 hours of symptoms (Figure 32-1). Acute symptoms of mild attacks resolve within a few days, but lymphedema takes several weeks to resolve. Hydrocele, orchitis, epididymitis, and/or spermatic cord inflammation are common in males and increase in incidence with age. Filarial abscesses are usually found in the groin or axillae, but may also occur in deep fascial spaces of muscles among patients from the Pacific Islands. Chronic disease may lead to obstruction of lymph and serous fluid resulting in permanent (and disabling) elephantiasis of the lower extremities or testes. This occurs less commonly in the arms, breasts, labia, and penis (Global Alliance, 2003; King & Freedman, 2000; Simonsen, 2003).

Complications

Patients with elephantiasis, which includes hyperplasia of the skin and subcutaneous tissue, are predisposed

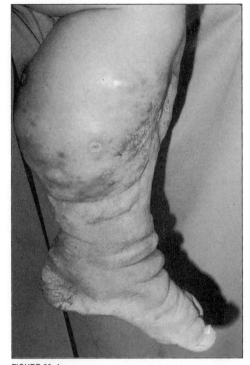

FIGURE 32–1

Lymphatic filariasis. (*Source:* Courtesy of the University of Texas Southwestern Department of Dermatology.)

to ulceration and secondary infection. Chyluria (galacturia) occurs when obstruction between the intestinal lymphatics and the thoracic duct leads to increased pressure and rupture of renal lymphatics into the renal tubules. The chronic urinary loss of chyle (an emulsion of lymph and triglycerides) often causes weight loss and malnutrition (King & Freedman, 2000).

Common Laboratory Findings

Moderate eosinophilia is often found, along with elevation of serum IgE (King & Freedman, 2000).

Diagnosis

Microfilariae are detectable primarily in blood and hydrocele fluid. Giemsa-stained thick blood film is a commonly used test, but sample collection must coincide with the periodicity of the specific microfilariae. *W. bancrofti* and *B. malayi* are nocturnal in most endemic areas, but are subperiodic in others. Polymerase chain reaction-based assays are available for the presence of *W. bancrofti* and *B. malayi* in blood and sputum. Enzyme-linked immunosorbent assay (ELISA), complement fixation, and immunofluorescent tests for serum are also available but cannot distinguish between different species of filaria nor between active and past infection. In endemic regions, most people will have positive serology for filarial parasites. Ultrasound of the scrotum detects adult worms, nodules, or lymphatic dilatation in 80% of affected men (Abbasi et al., 1999; King & Freedman, 2000; Simonsen, 2003).

Differential Diagnosis

Acute filarial adenolymphangitis may resemble acute bacterial lymphangitis, thrombophlebitis, lymphogranuloma inguinale, and other infections. For patients with recurrent attacks, consider other causes of recurrent fever such as tuberculosis or urinary tract infection. The differential diagnosis of filarial orchitis includes gonorrhea, tubercular epididymitis, hernia, and trauma. Other causes of chronic lymphedema include malignancy, heart failure, renal failure, and congenital malformations. Nonfilarial elephantiasis occurs in persons from the Ethiopian highlands with African "bigfoot" disease, in which chronic exposure of bare feet to silica microparticles leads to lymphatic obstruction in the lower extremities but not hydroceles (Abbasi et al., 1999; King & Freedman, 2000; Simonsen, 2003).

Treatment

— Few clinical trials exist to guide chemotherapy. The traditional therapy is to use diethylcarbamazine (DEC) at a dose of 6 mg/kg per day for 12 days in bancroftian filariasis and for 6 days in brugian filariasis. The Medical Letter (2002) recommends giving increasing doses after meals as follows:
  - Day 1: 50 mg after meals
  - Day 2: 50 mg tid after meals
  - Day 3: 100 mg tid after meals
  - Days 4 through 14: 6 mg/kg/day divided tid after meals
— The pediatric dosage recommended by the Medical Letter (2002) is:
  - Day 1: 1 mg/kg after meals
  - Day 2: 1 mg/kg tid after meals
  - Day 3: 1-2 mg/kg tid after meals
  - Days 4 through 21: 6 mg/kg/day divided tid after meals
— Because DEC can cause adverse reactions in those with onchocerciasis or loiasis, patients in endemic areas should be assessed for these conditions before starting therapy. Ivermectin can kill microfilariae but not adult worms. Albendazole can be effective against adult worms if used daily for 2 to 3 weeks (Global Alliance, 2003; Medical Letter, 2002).

Prevention

— The prevention of lymphatic filariasis (and other arboviral diseases) is directed at community and personal mosquito control in endemic areas (Centers for Disease Control and Prevention, 2003; Chin, 2000; Global Alliance, 2003; Robert, 2000; Thompson, 2002; White, 2003) and includes the following:
  - Kill adult mosquitoes by spraying inside and outside human habitations and surrounding areas with residual insecticides. The goal is to kill as many

female mosquitoes as possible, thus decreasing the likelihood of disease transmission. See Appendix D.
- Kill larvae and eliminate breeding areas as much as possible. Elimination of breeding areas includes draining standing water such as swamps, emptying open water-filled containers and used tires, and reducing the number of plants that hold standing water, for example, bromeliads. In the case of *Mansonia* spp., the elimination of floating plants significantly reduces the mosquito population.

Personal protection includes the following:
- Screen living and working quarters.
- Use a residual insecticide inside homes and work areas. See Appendix D.
- Use insecticide-impregnated mosquito netting over beds. Nets must be retreated with insecticide annually. See Appendix D.
- Stay inside as much as possible during hours when mosquitoes are biting, which, in the case of *Anopheles,* is from dusk to dawn. *Mansonia* species are difficult to avoid because they feed throughout the day and night, with increased activity at dusk and dawn.
- Use DEET repellant on skin and permethrin on clothing when outside during biting hours.
- Prophylactic DEC at a dose of 6 mg/kg taken 2 days a month may possibly prevent infection. On a population level, mass treatment with repeated annual doses of a two-drug regimen (albendazole plus DEC or ivermectin) interrupts transmission by reducing microfilariae levels.

Provide ongoing community education regarding the preceding measures.

Reporting

The U.S. Centers for Disease Control and Prevention does not consider lymphatic filariasis to be a nationally notifiable diseases. The World Health Organization (WHO) considers it a Class 3C disease. See Appendix C for details and for upcoming changes in WHO reporting.

References

Abbasi, I., Githure, J., Ochola, J.J., Agure, R., Koech, D.K., Ramzy, R.M., Williams, S.A., & Hamburger, J. (1999). Diagnosis of *Wuchereria bancrofti* infection by the polymerase chain reaction employing patient's sputum. *Parasitology Research, 85,* 844-849.

Centers for Disease Control and Prevention. (2003). Protection against mosquitoes and other arthropods. Retrieved December 1, 2003, from *www.cdc.gov/travel/bugs.htm*

Chin, J. (Ed.) (2000). *Control of communicable diseases manual* (17th ed.). Washington, DC: American Public Health Association.

The Global Alliance to Eliminate Lymphatic Filariasis. (2003). Retrieved December 1, 2003, from *www.filariasis.org*

Hotez, P.J., Remme, J.H.F., Buss, P., Alleyne, G., Morel, C., & Breman, J.G. (2004). Combating tropical infectious diseases: Report of the Disease Control Priorities in Developing Countries Project. *Clinical Infectious Diseases, 38,* 871-878.

King, C.L., & Freedman, D.O. (2000). Filariasis. In G.T. Strickland (Ed.), *Hunter's tropical medicine and emerging infectious diseases* (8th ed., pp. 740-752). Philadelphia: W.B. Saunders Company.

Medical Letter. (2002). Drugs for parasitic infections. Retrieved November 26, 2003, from *www.medletter.com/freedocs/parasitic.pdf*

Robert, L.L. (2000). Control of arthropods of medical importance. In G.T. Strickland (Ed.), *Hunter's tropical medicine and emerging infectious diseases* (8th ed., pp. 1019-1034). Philadelphia: W.B. Saunders Company.

Simonsen, P.E. (2003). Filariases. In G.C. Cook & A.I. Zumla (Eds.), *Manson's tropical diseases* (21st ed., pp. 1487-1526). Philadelphia: W.B. Saunders Company.

Thompson, M.J. (2002). Immunizations for international travel. *Primary Care; Clinics in Office Practice, 29,* 787-814.

White, G.B. (2003). Mosquitoes. In G.C. Cook & A.I. Zumla (Eds.), *Manson's tropical diseases* (21st ed., pp. 1741-1772). Philadelphia: W.B. Saunders Company.

33

FILARIASIS: ONCHOCERCIASIS
River blindness
Geographic Distribution

— Onchocerciasis (river blindness) occurs primarily in equatorial Africa, but it can also be found in the Arabian peninsula and northern parts of South America. Endemicity is near areas with swiftly moving water where the insect vectors breed (Centers for Disease Control and Prevention [CDC], 2003a; Chin, 2000).

Agent and Vector

— Onchocerciasis is caused by the nematode *Onchocerca volvulus*, transmitted by *Simulium* blackflies. Female blackflies receive and transmit *O. volvulus* microfilariae when they take a blood meal, which they require for ovulation. Once in the human host, the microfilariae mature into adult worms over a period of approximately 12 months. The female worms encapsulate in fibrous subcutaneous nodules and are fertilized by adult male worms that migrate between the nodules. The females can then produce thousands of microfilariae daily. Disease is caused by the microfilariae after they disseminate to skin, eyes, and lymph nodes, where they die and degenerate, eliciting severe inflammatory reactions (CDC, 2003a; Cooper & Nutman, 2000).

Incubation

— The earliest symptoms coincide with the production of microfilariae by gravid females, usually 10 to 15 months after infection (Chin, 2000; Cooper & Nutman, 2000).

Clinical Findings and Treatment

Signs and Symptoms

Subcutaneous nodules containing adult worms (onchocercomata), usually located over bony prominences, may be the presenting sign. Intermittent, severe pruritus, with or without papular rash, usually follows and is caused by microfilariae in subcutaneous tissue. In chronic onchocerciasis, the skin may become thickened, wrinkled, lichenified, and hyperpigmented, which is sometimes likened to "lizard" or "elephant" skin (Figure 33-1). Late in the disease, patients may also develop hypopigmentation of the skin, with retained pigment around the follicles. Eczematous changes and secondary infections may result from scratching. Skin involvement among patients in Africa tends to be greatest on the lower extremities, while in Central America, the upper body is more commonly involved. Involvement of the eyes usually is manifested first by conjunctivitis and photophobia. Neovascularization,

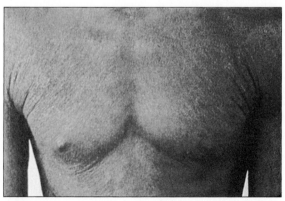

FIGURE 33–1

Diffuse lichenification and hyperpigmentation in onchocerciasis. The patient has intense itching. (*Source:* From Bolognia, J.L., Jorizzo, J.L., & Rapini, R.P. [Eds.]. [2003]. *Dermatology* [p. 1130]. Philadelphia: Mosby.)

keratitis, and corneal scarring leading to blindness occur in a small percentage of patients. Vision loss is more common among populations in the African savanna than South America. Uveitis, chorioretinitis, and optic atrophy also occur, as may secondary glaucoma. Lymphadenopathy in the femoral and inguinal areas may lead to "hanging groin" (CDC, 2003a; Cooper & Nutman, 2000; Hoerauf, Buttner, Adjei, & Pearlman, 2003; Sangueza, Lu, Sansueza, & Paniago Pereira, 2003).

Complications

Cachexia may occur with heavy infestation. Abdominal hernias, gynecomastia, amenorrhea, spontaneous abortion, and infertility have also been described. Arthritis and synovitis may occur with chemotherapy. River blindness is associated with an increased mortality rate, probably due to malnutrition and poverty from the loss of livelihood (CDC, 2003a; Cooper & Nutman, 2000).

Common Laboratory Findings

Eosinophilia may be seen.

Diagnosis

The most common method of diagnosis is "skin snips." A skin biopsy (snip) is incubated in tissue culture medium or saline and, within 2 to 24 hours, microfilariae can be seen with a low-power microscope. There are serologic methods based on homologous native or recombinant diagnostic antigens, but these are not widely available (CDC, 2003a; Cho-Ngwa, Akoachere, & Titanji, 2003).

Differential Diagnosis

The initial dermatitis is often mistaken for eczema, food allergies, contact dermatitis, and scabies. Chronic skin disease may resemble chronic eczema, scleroderma, severe malnutrition, and leprosy. The differential diagnosis for subcutaneous nodules includes lymphadenopathy, lipomas, fibromas, and granulomas (Cooper & Nutman, 2000; Hoerauf et al., 2003).

Treatment

Ivermectin in a single oral dose of 150 mcg/kg (for adults or children) kills microfilariae, but not adult worms. It must be repeated every 3 to 12 months to prevent microfilariae levels from rising again. However, a systematic review of clinical trials failed to find a difference in vision loss for patients treated with ivermectin compared to placebo. In Central America, nodules on the head are sometimes removed to reduce the load of microfilariae in the eyes, although nodulectomy has not been shown to be beneficial in Africa. A promising new target for chemotherapy is *Wolbachia,* an endosymbiotic bacterium that is essential for the fertility of adult female worms and is sensitive to inexpensive antibiotics such as doxycycline (Cooper & Nutman, 2000; Ejere, Schwartz, & Wormald, 2003; Hoerauf et al., 2003; Medical Letter, 2002).

Prevention

The prevention of onchocerciasis is directed at community and personal mosquito control in endemic areas (CDC, 2003b; Chin, 2000; White, 2003) and includes the following:

- Prevent *Simulium* fly bites by using DEET-containing repellent and wearing permethrin-impregnated headgear, long sleeves, and long pants.
- Avoid concentrations of flies during the peak biting hours of daylight. The females do not enter dwellings.
- Large-scale prevention measures include yearly or twice yearly administration of ivermectin

(150 mcg/kg body weight) to people older than age 5 in communities where the disease is endemic.

- Spray blackfly breeding grounds with insecticides (see Appendix D). Females are able to fly long distances (more than 200 km), so insecticide use is an imperfect, but important measure.

The World Health Organization (WHO) and other groups are working in coordinated control programs in West Africa and Latin America. Community education should be ongoing.

Reporting

The CDC does not consider onchocerciasis to be a nationally notifiable disease. The WHO considers it a Class 5 disease. See Appendix C for details and for upcoming changes in WHO reporting.

References

Centers for Disease Control and Prevention. (2003a). Filariasis. Retrieved October 30, 2003, from *www.dpd.cdc.gov/dpdx/HTML/Filariasis.htm*

Centers for Disease Control and Prevention. (2003b). Protection against mosquitoes and other arthropods. *The yellow book*. Retrieved December 1, 2003, from *www.cdc.gov/travel/bugs.htm*

Chin, J. (Ed.) (2000). *Control of communicable diseases manual* (17th ed.). Washington, DC: American Public Health Association.

Cho-Ngwa, F., Akoachere, M., & Titanji, V.P. (2003). Sensitive and specific serodiagnosis of river blindness using *Onchocerca ochengi* antigens. *Acta Tropical, 89,* 25-32.

Cooper, P.J., Nutman, T.B. (2000). Onchocerciasis. In G.T. Strickland (Ed.), *Hunter's tropical medicine and emerging infectious diseases* (8th ed., pp. 756-769). Philadelphia: W.B. Saunders Company.

Ejere, H., Schwartz, E., & Wormald, R. (2003). Ivermectin for onchocercal eye disease (river blindness). Cochrane Collaboration. Retrieved December 1, 2003, from *www.cochrane.org/cochrane/revabstr/AB002219.htm*

Hoerauf, A., Buttner, D.W., Adjei, O., & Pearlman, E. (2003). Onchocerciasis. *British Medical Journal, 326,* 207-210.

Medical Letter. (2002). Drugs for parasitic infections. Retrieved November 26, 2003, from *www.medletter.com/freedocs/parasitic.pdf*

Sangueza, O.P., Lu, D., Sansueza, M., & Paniago Pereira, C. (2003). Protozoa and worms. In Bolognia, J.L., Jorizzo, J.L., & Rapini, R.P. (Eds.), *Dermatology* (pp. 1309-1310). Philadelphia: Mosby.

White, G.B. (2003). Blackflies, buffalo gnats, turkey gnats. In G.C. Cook & A.I. Zumla (Eds.), *Manson's tropical diseases* (21st ed., pp. 1773-1774). Philadelphia: W.B. Saunders Company.

34

GIARDIASIS

Giardia intestinalis, Giardia lamblia

Geographic Distribution

Giardiasis is present worldwide, with higher prevalence in warmer climates. The organism can be detected in 2% to 5% of stool from people in industrialized nations, and 20% to 30% of stool from people in developing countries (Katz & Taylor, 2001).

Agent and Vector

Giardia intestinalis, also known as *Giardia lamblia,* is a protozoan flagellate that is one of the most common pathogenic parasite infections of humans. It is most commonly transmitted by fecally contaminated water or food, and can also be transmitted by anal-oral sex. Approximately 5% of cases of traveler's diarrhea are attributed to *Giardia. Giardia* cysts are somewhat resistant to chlorine and can remain viable for several months in cool, moist environments. The infective dose is approximately 10 to 100 cysts. Once in the gastrointestinal tract, the organism excysts to form two trophozoites, which replicate by binary fission in the mucosal crypts of the small intestine. The trophozoites then encyst to be passed into the environment via stools to continue the life cycle (Centers for Disease Control and Prevention [CDC], 2003; Katz & Taylor, 2001).

Incubation

The incubation period is 1 to 3 weeks or longer (CDC, 2003).

Clinical Findings and Treatment

Signs and Symptoms

— Although many infected persons are asymptomatic, others experience the gradual onset of diarrhea as the primary symptom. Diarrhea ranges from one loose stool per day to frequent copious watery stools; it may be acute or chronic, and continuous or intermittent (with bouts of constipation). When copious, stools often contain mucus, but seldom blood, and are pale, frothy, steatorrheic, and foul smelling. Other common symptoms are abdominal pain (which may be predominant), nausea and vomiting, anorexia, flatulence, fatigue, and weight loss. The acute phase may last days or weeks and usually resolves spontaneously. Some patients develop chronic giardiasis, in which abdominal pain, flatus, and belching are more common than diarrhea (CDC, 2003; Katz & Taylor, 2001; Pickering, 2004).

Complications

— Chronic giardiasis may cause malabsorption with weight loss, dehydration, and in infants and young children, failure to thrive and developmental delays (CDC, 2003; Katz & Taylor, 2001; Pickering, 2004).

Common Laboratory Findings

— Stools are usually heme negative.

Diagnosis

— Microscopic examination of three stool samples taken from different days is 85% sensitive for detecting *Giardia* parasites. Commercial stool antigen tests by enzyme-linked immunosorbent assay (ELISA) and immunofluorescence assay (IFA) are available. For difficult to diagnose cases, duodenal biopsy can sometimes reveal trophozoites (CDC, 2003).

Differential Diagnosis

The acute illness resembles many common causes of diarrhea. For those with chronic diarrhea, consider also cryptosporidium, isospora, and tropical sprue (Katz & Taylor, 2001).

Treatment

In the United States metronidazole 250 mg PO tid for 5 days is standard therapy; for children, metronidazole can be given at a dose of 15 mg/kg/day divided tid. Albendazole is as effective as metronidazole, but has fewer adverse effects and is effective against many helminths, hence is an appropriate choice under most circumstances. Albendazole is given 400 mg PO once daily for 5 days for adults and children. Tinidazole (not available in the United States) given as a single dose of 2 g for adults or 50 mg/kg for children has a comparable parasitologic cure rate but a higher clinical cure rate than metronidazole. Pregnant patients after the first trimester may be treated with either metronidazole or paromomycin at a dose of 500 mg tid for 7 to 10 days (Medical Letter, 2002; Pickering, 2004; Zaat, Mank, & Assendelft, 2005).

Prevention

Measures to prevent giardiasis (Chin, 2000) include the following:
- Wash hands thoroughly after toileting and before handling or eating food.
- Protect public water supplies from contamination with human waste.
- Boil potentially contaminated water for at least 5 min. Iodine crystals or tablets may be used according to packaging instructions to purify small amounts of water.
- Wash fruits and vegetables in potable water.

- Dispose of human feces in a sanitary manner to avoid water supply contamination.
- Educate high-risk groups on the dangers of sexual practices that promote fecal-oral transmission.

Community education regarding the preceding measures should be ongoing in high-risk areas or populations.

Reporting

The CDC lists giardiasis as a nationally notifiable disease. The World Health Organization (WHO) classifies giardiasis as Class 3b, with particular interest in outbreaks. See Appendix C for details and for upcoming changes in WHO reporting.

References

Centers for Disease Control and Prevention. (2003). Giardiasis. Retrieved December 6, 2003, from *www.dpd.cdc.gov/dpdx/HTML/Giardiasis.htm*

Katz, D.E., & Taylor, D.N. (2001). Parasitic infections of the gastrointestinal tract. *Gastroenterology Clinics of North America, 30,* 797-815.

Medical Letter. (2002). Drugs for parasitic infections. Retrieved October 8, 2003, from *www.medletter.com/freedocs/parasitic.pdf*

Pickering, L.K. (2004). Giardiasis and balantidiasis. In R.E. Behrman, R.M. Kliegman, & H.B. Jenson (Eds.), *Nelson textbook of pediatrics* (17th ed., pp. 1125-1127). Philadelphia: W.B. Saunders Company.

Zaat, J.O., Mank, T., & Assendelft, W.J. (2005). Drugs for treating giardiasis. *The Cochrane Library, 1,* 1-39.

35

GNATHOSTOMIASIS

Eosinophilic myeloencephalitis, several folk names according to geographic location

Geographic Distribution

Gnathostomiasis occurs most commonly in Southeast Asia and Japan and is increasingly found in Central and South America. Folk names for the illness include Tau Cheed (Thailand), Yangtze River edema and Shanghai rheumatism (China), Rangoon tumor (Burma), Woodbury bug (Australia), and Chokofishi (Japan) (Moore, McCrodden, DeKumyoy, & Chiodini, 2003).

Agent and Vector

Gnathostomiasis is caused by *Gnathostoma spinigerum*, a nematode for which humans are paratenic or incidental transfer hosts. The adult nematode lives in a tumor mass in the stomach wall of domestic and wild carnivores. Eggs are passed in the feces and hatch 10 to 12 days after reaching water. First-stage larvae are ingested by freshwater copepods (small, freshwater crustaceans), in whom they develop to the second stage. When infected copepods are eaten by an intermediate host such as freshwater fish, amphibians, fowl, or reptiles, the larvae develop into the third stage. Humans acquire infection by ingesting the uncooked or undercooked flesh of an infected intermediate host. Raw or salted and fermented freshwater fish are especially common sources of infection. The nematode is unable to complete its life cycle in humans and begins to migrate within the body, thus causing an inflammatory reaction and the signs and symptoms of the infection (Bunnag, 2000; Moore et al., 2003; Peters & Pasvol, 2002).

Incubation

The incubation period is unknown (Bunnag, 2000).

Clinical Findings and Treatment

Signs and Symptoms

Gnathostomiasis commonly begins with low-grade fever, right upper quadrant abdominal pain, and nausea. Hepatomegaly, pleuritis or pneumonitis, and eosinophilia may also occur. These early signs and symptoms may be followed by intermittent, migratory skin and subcutaneous swellings that are edematous and pruritic, but rarely painful. Swellings may appear as lumps or as localized edema, developing rapidly and lasting about a week, with intervals between swellings ranging from days to months. The eyelid is a common site of swelling and may be accompanied by chemosis or hemorrhage. In a few cases, a worm may be found in the eye itself. A small proportion of patients have transient large pruritic serpiginous tracks appearing on the trunk and extremities (Bunnag, 2000; Moore et al., 2003).

Complications

Rarely, eosinophilic myeloencephalitis may develop. This form of *Gnathostoma* infection is caused by migration of the nematode along a large nerve into the central nervous system and is manifested by painful radiculopathy, followed by paraplegia, urinary retention, and, less commonly, quadriplegia and/or coma. Blindness may occur in untreated ocular infection (Bunnag, 2000).

Common Laboratory Findings

Eosinophilia (eosinophil count exceeding $0.4 \times 10^9/L$) is common, but does not always occur (Moore et al., 2003).

Diagnosis

Characteristic transient migratory swellings, positive dietary history, travel to an area where gnathostomiasis is known to occur, and eosinophilia together are highly suspicious. The diagnosis should also be considered in patients with nonspecific gastrointestinal symptoms and epidemiological risk factors. Serologic tests available for diagnosis of gnathostomiasis include immunoblot to detect the specific 24-kDa band that is diagnostic of *Gnathostoma* infection (Moore et al., 2003).

Differential Diagnosis

The Calabar swellings of loiasis are similar to the swellings of gnathostomiasis, but loiasis occurs in central Africa. Ectopic fascioliasis, paragonimiasis, and sparganosis cause painless migratory subcutaneous swelling and eosinophilic leukocytosis. Hookworm infection may cause smaller creeping eruptions that are nonpruritic. Acute trichinellosis may cause bilateral periorbital edema (Bunnag, 2000).

Treatment

Current treatment for children and adults is albendazole 400 mg bid for 21 days. A second course may be required based on recurrence of symptoms and incomplete resolution of eosinophilia. Surgical removal of the worm may also be indicated (Bunnag, 2000; Moore et al., 2003).

Prevention

To prevent gnathostomiasis, avoid raw, undercooked, or fermented foods in endemic areas. Untreated groundwater may contain infectious copepods (Bunnag, 2000).

Reporting

The U.S. Centers for Disease Control and Prevention does not consider gnathostomiasis to be a nationally notifiable disease. The World Health Organization (WHO) considers it a Class 5 disease. See Appendix C for details and for upcoming changes in WHO reporting.

References

Bunnag, T. (2000). Gnathostomiasis. In G.T. Strickland (Ed.), *Hunter's tropical medicine and emerging infectious diseases* (8th ed., pp. 790-793). Philadelphia: W.B. Saunders Company.

Moore, D.A.J., McCrodden, J., DeKumyoy, P., & Chiodini, P.L. (2003). Gnathostomiasis: An emerging imported disease. *Emerging Infectious Diseases, 19*, 647-650.

Peters, W., & Pasvol, G. (2002). *Tropical medicine and parasitology* (5th ed.). Philadelphia: Mosby.

Granuloma Inguinale

Donovanosis, granuloma venereum

Geographic Distribution

Granuloma inguinale is endemic in several tropical areas, including Papua New Guinea, Brazil, India, and South Africa (Ballard, 2001; Mabey & Richens, 2003).

Agent and Vector

The disease is caused by *Calymmatobacterium granulomatis*, a gram-negative coccobacillus that has recently been reclassified as *Klebsiella*. Low socioeconomic status and prostitution are commonly associated with the disease, and sexual exposure is the primary means of transmission. The risk of transmission is lower than for other sexually transmitted diseases, and some individuals remain disease free even after repeated exposure. Occasionally nonsexual transmission, including congenital infection and possibly fecal contamination with autoinoculation, has been reported (Mabey & Richens, 2003; O'Farrell, 2002; Richens, 2000).

Incubation

The incubation period is between 3 and 40 days (Richens, 2000).

Clinical Findings and Treatment

Signs and Symptoms

The initial lesion is typically a papule or nodule that subsequently becomes ulcerated. The ulcer is painless, beefy-red, friable, and elevated above the surrounding skin with a rolled border (Figure 36-1). The lesions may become painful if secondarily infected. The most common sites of primary infection include the vulva

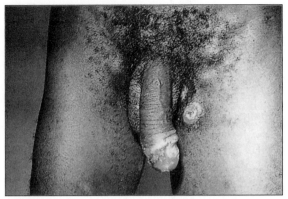

FIGURE 36–1

Granuloma inguinale. (*Source:* From Peters, W., & Pasvol, G. [2002]. *Tropical medicine and parasitology* [5th ed., p. 231]. Chicago: Mosby.)

in women and distal penis in men. Untreated ulcers can progress along skin folds in the groin and toward the anus. Subcutaneous granulomatous tissue may extend into the inguinal folds, mimicking adenitis, and erode through the skin. Autoinoculation is common and may lead to "kissing" lesions on adjacent skin. Extragenital lesions occur in approximately 6% of patients and are found in the oral mucosa, on the neck, legs, and chest (Ballard, 2001; Mabey & Richens, 2003; O'Farrell, 2001, 2002; Richens, 2000; Roest & van der Meijden, 2001).

Complications

Granuloma inguinale can rarely disseminate and may spread to the bone, liver, spleen, bowel, uterus, and/or lungs. When this complication occurs, it is typically associated with cervical infection and/or pregnancy. Other complications include scarring, elephantiasis of the genitalia, and development of squamous cell carcinoma of the skin (Mabey & Richens, 2003; O'Farrell, 2002).

Common Laboratory Findings

— There are no laboratory findings common to granuloma inguinale except as described next.

Diagnosis

— The most common method of diagnosis in endemic areas is through clinical appearance. Definitive diagnosis can be provided through the demonstration of Donovan bodies, which appear as pin-shaped intracytoplasmic inclusion bodies within histiocytes. They can be found on skin biopsies or smears of granulation tissue that has been stained with Giemsa or silver stains. *C. granulomatis* is difficult to culture, and isolation may require a specialty laboratory. Polymerase chain reaction has been developed for *C. granulomatis,* but no serologic tests are available (Mabey & Richens, 2003; Roest & van der Meijden, 2001).

Differential Diagnosis

— Granuloma inguinale must be distinguished from other causes of genital ulcers, including chancroid, syphilis, ulcerating genital warts, amebiasis, and squamous cell carcinoma. Lymphogranuloma venereum causes swelling in the inguinal folds due to true adenitis and may also lead to elephantiasis of the genitalia. Cervical lesions of granuloma inguinale may mimic a tuberculous infection or carcinoma of the cervix. (Ballard, 2001; Richens, 2000).

Treatment

— This infection responds to several oral antibiotics, which should be given for at least 3 weeks or until all of the lesions have completely healed: co-trimoxazole one double-strength tablet (160 mg/800 mg) twice daily or doxycycline 100 mg twice daily; alternatively, ciprofloxacin 750 mg twice daily, or erythromycin base

500 mg four times daily (safe in pregnancy), or azithromycin, 1 g once a week. Gentamicin, 1 mg/kg every 8 hours, may be added to the preceding regimens if the lesions fail to respond in the first few days of treatment (Centers for Disease Control and Prevention [CDC], 2002).

Prevention

Programs have been set up in Papua New Guinea during past epidemics to arrange for medical workers to go house to house, providing examinations and treatment. This type of program may calm the epidemic, but the disease remains in the population. The prevalence of the disease seems to decline with the improvement of hygienic standards, but this is not often attainable in underdeveloped countries. Unprotected sex outside of monogamous relationships, and especially with prostitutes, should be avoided. Sexual contacts should be urged to seek medical attention when their partner is diagnosed with any sexually transmitted disease, including granuloma inguinale (O'Farrell, 2002).

Reporting

The CDC considers granuloma inguinale to be a nationally notifiable disease and in some cases grounds for exclusion from immigration to the United States. The World Health Organization (WHO) considers it a Class 3B disease. See Appendix C for details and for upcoming changes in WHO reporting.

References

Ballard, R.C. (2001). *Calymmatobacterium granulomatis* infection (Donovanosis). In R.L. Guerrant, D.H. Walker, & P.F. Weller (Eds.), *Essentials of tropical diseases* (pp. 397-400). New York: Churchill Livingstone.

Centers for Disease Control and Prevention. (2002). Sexually transmitted diseases treatment guidelines. *MMWR, 51*(No. RR-6), 17-18.

Mabey, D., & Richens, J. (2003). Sexually transmitted infections (excluding HIV). In G.C. Cook & A.I. Zumla (Eds.), *Manson's tropical diseases* (21st ed., pp. 449-451). Philadelphia: W.B. Saunders Company.

O'Farrell, N. (2001). Donovanosis: An update. *International Journal of STD & AIDS*, *12*, 423-427.

O'Farrell, N. (2002). Donovanosis. *Sexually Transmitted Infections*, *78*, 452-457.

Richens, J. (2000). Granuloma inguinale. In G. Strickland (Ed.), *Hunter's tropical medicine and emerging infectious diseases* (8th ed., pp. 369-372). Philadelphia: W.B. Saunders Company.

Roest, R.W., & van der Meijden, W.I. (2001). European guideline for the management of tropical genito-ulcerative diseases. *International Journal of STD & AIDS*, *12*, 78-83.

HANTAVIRUS HEMORRHAGIC FEVER WITH RENAL SYNDROME

Geographic Distribution

Hemorrhagic fever with renal syndrome is an acute zoonotic viral disease occurring primarily in Europe, Russia, East China, and Korea, with serologic evidence of infection found in South America, Africa, and India (Chin, 2000; Khan & Ksiazek, 2000).

Agent and Vector

Hemorrhagic fever with renal syndrome is caused by Old World hantaviruses (family *Bunyaviridae*) carried by Old World field rodents as follows:

- *Hantaan virus and Dobrava-Belgrade virus.* Carried by *Apodemus* species in Asia, the Balkans, and Russia. Hantaan virus disease usually occurs in late fall and early winter and usually among rural populations. Dobrava-Belgrade virus causes severe and rare disease in the Balkans in spring and early summer.
- *Seoul virus.* Carried by *Rattus* species worldwide, but usually causes human disease only in Asia in late fall and early winter, usually among rural populations except that in Korea there is urban occurrence.
- *Puumala virus.* Carried by *Clethrionomys* species in Europe, the Balkans, and Russia. Puumala virus infection, known as nephropathia epidemica, is generally mild and usually occurs in summer, fall, and early winter.

Other, newly discovered (and, surely, undiscovered) hantaviruses and hosts also exist (Box 37-1). Transmission is most often through inhalation of aerosolized dried excreta (urine, feces, and saliva) from infected rodents, and also from inoculation through conjunctiva or entry though broken skin (Chin, 2000; Khan & Ksiazek, 2000; Lokugamage et al., 2002; Scharinghausen, Meyer, Pfeffer, Davis, & Honeycutt, 1999).

Incubation

The incubation period ranges from a few days to 2 months, but is usually 2 to 4 weeks (Chin, 2000; Peters, 2000).

Clinical Findings and Treatment

Signs and Symptoms

The severity of the illness varies, with mild or subclinical infections common. More severe cases are generally caused by Hantaan virus or Dobrava-Belgrade virus and are characterized by five phases as follows:

1. *The febrile (or toxic) phase* lasts 3 to 7 days and begins with abrupt onset of fever, chills, headache, and malaise followed by photophobia, blurred vision, facial flushing (blanching) extending to neck and shoulders, conjunctival injection, periorbital edema, pharyngeal injection and/or petechiae, petechiae (particularly in the axillae and waist), lumbar back pain, and costovertebral angle tenderness. In some cases the illness may gradually resolve after this febrile stage or a hypotensive phase may begin as the temperature falls. About 35% of deaths in hemorrhagic fever with renal syndrome are from shock occurring at the end of this phase and during the following hypotensive phase.

2. *The hypotensive phase* lasts from several hours to several days and is characterized by decreased blood pressure, tachycardia, and sometimes shock and hemorrhagic manifestations.

3. *The oliguric (or renal) phase* features oliguria and, in most cases, decreased symptoms overall except that some patients experience periods of hypertension

---

BIOTERRORISM CONSIDERATIONS BOX 37–1

Agents responsible for hemorrhagic fever with renal syndrome are Category C critical biological agents, unlike other causes of viral hemorrhagic fever, which are Category A agents (Clement, 2003; Rotz, Khan, Lillibridge, Ostroff, & Hughes, 2002).

---

and/or nausea and vomiting. About 15% of patients develop more severe hemorrhagic manifestations, including epistaxis, ecchymosis, mucosal bleeding, and subconjunctival bleeding. In the most severe cases, patients exhibit hemoptysis, gross hematuria, and central nervous system and/or gastrointestinal bleeding with corresponding signs and symptoms. It is during this phase that death is most likely.

4. *The diuretic phase* marks improvement and is characterized by diuresis and decreased symptoms.

5. *The convalescent phase* may include polyuria and inability to concentrate urine. Long-term sequelae may include renal tubular acidosis, renal hypertension, or chronic renal failure (Chin, 2000; Khan & Ksiazek, 2000; Peters, 2000; Vapalahti et al., 2003).

Complications

Disseminated intravascular coagulation may occur relatively early in the course of illness. Hemorrhagic manifestations and/or renal failure are the most significant complications. About 65% of deaths are during the oliguric phase, usually from pulmonary edema or cerebrovascular accident (Peters, 2000).

Common Laboratory Findings

Progressive thrombocytopenia and leukocytosis occur during the febrile and hypotensive phases. Electrolyte abnormalities and evidence of renal failure (elevated serum creatinine, hematuria, and proteinuria) are common during the oliguric phase.

Diagnosis

Diagnosis is on the basis of (1) characteristic signs and symptoms, geographic location, and exposure factors such as agricultural occupation (see earlier section), and (2) enzyme immunoassay or immunofluorescence assay (Hujakka et al., 2003).

Differential Diagnosis

The differential diagnosis includes leptospirosis, scrub typhus, dengue fever, renal vein thrombosis, and, in the case of Puumala virus illness, other mild febrile illnesses (Khan & Ksiazek, 2000).

Treatment

Treatment is supportive and includes maintenance of fluid balance, with focus on preventing fluid overload during early phases and replacing fluid losses during the diuretic phase. Early hospitalization is recommended. Trauma and invasive procedures should be minimized to reduce the risk of bleeding. Dialysis may be necessary for renal failure. Hypotension may require vasopressor support in addition to fluids. Ongoing frequent monitoring of blood pressure, fluid balance, and electrolyte balance help with (essential) immediate identification of progression and complications. A randomized double-blind placebo-controlled trial demonstrated that intravenous ribavirin (33 mg/kg loading dose, followed by 16 mg/kg q6h for 4 days; then 8 mg/kg q8h for 6 days) given within 6 days of fever onset decreases mortality (Peters, 2000).

Prevention

See the following chapter on hantavirus pulmonary syndrome.

Reporting

The U.S. Centers for Disease Control and Prevention considers hemorrhagic fevers to be nationally notifiable diseases. The World Health Organization (WHO) considers hemorrhagic fevers as diseases important in public health (Class 2A). See Appendix C for details and for upcoming changes in WHO reporting.

References

Chin, J. (Ed.). (2000). *Control of communicable diseases manual* (17th ed., pp. 230-234). Washington, DC: American Public Health Association.

Clement, J.P. (2003). Hantavirus. *Antiviral Research, 57*, 121-127.

Hujakka, H., Koistinen, V., Kuronen, I., Eerikainen, P., Parviainen, M., et al. (2003). Diagnostic rapid tests for acute hantavirus infections: Specific tests for Hantaan, Dobrava and Puumala viruses versus a hantavirus combination test. *Journal of Virological Methods, 108*, 117-122.

Khan, A.S., & Ksiazek, T.G. (2000). Diseases caused by hantaviruses. In G.T. Strickland (Ed.), *Hunter's tropical medicine and emerging infectious diseases* (8th ed., pp. 288-293). Philadelphia: W.B. Saunders Company.

Lokugamage, K., Kariwa, H., Hayasaka, D., Cui, B.Z., Iwasaki, T., et al. (2002). Genetic characterization of hantaviruses transmitted by the Korean field mouse (*Apodemus peninsulae*), Far East Russia. *Emerging Infectious Diseases, 8*. Retrieved October 31, 2003, from *www.cdc.gov/ncidod/EID/vol8no8/01-0494.htm*

Peters, C.J. (2000). Bunyaviridae. In G. Mandell, J. Bennett, & R. Dolin (Eds.), *Principles and practice of infectious diseases.* (5th ed., pp 1849-1855). New York: Churchill Livingstone.

Rotz, L.D., Khan, A.S., Lillibridge, S.R., Ostroff, S.M., & Hughes. J.M. (2002). Public health assessment of potential biological terrorism agents. *Emerging Infectious Diseases, 8*, 225-230.

Scharinghausen, J.J., Meyer, H., Pfeffer, M., Davis, D.S. & Honeycutt, R.L. (1999). Genetic evidence of Dobrava virus in *Apodemus agrarius* in Hungary. *Emerging Infectious Diseases, 5*, 468-470.

Vapalahti, O., Mustonen, J., Lundkvist, A., Henttonen, H., Plyusnin, A., & Vaheri, A. (2003). Hantavirus infections in Europe. *Lancet Infectious Diseases, 3*, 653-661.

38

HANTAVIRUS PULMONARY SYNDROME

Geographic Distribution

Hantavirus pulmonary syndrome occurs in the Americas, from Canada to Argentina. Although first identified in 1993, hantavirus pulmonary syndrome existed well before its modern identification (Chin, 2000; Clement, 2003).

Agent and Vector

Hantavirus pulmonary syndrome is a zoonosis caused by New World hantaviruses (family *Bunyaviridae,* genus *Hantavirus*) such as Sin Nombre, Bayou, Black Creek Canal, Laguna Negra, and Juquitiba (Box 38-1). Hantaviruses are carried asymptomatically by rodents such as deer mice, white-footed mice, vesper field mice, and yellow pygmy rice rats. These animals, which also are hosts for *Yersinia pestis* (the agent for plague), are wild rodents not usually associated with urban environments, though in some instances they enter human habitations. Consequently, hantavirus pulmonary syndrome is associated with rural environments and agricultural occupations. Transmission to humans is incompletely understood, but is generally through the inhalation of viral particles shed in rodent feces, urine, and saliva. Rare person-to-person transmission may occur (Chin, 2000; Khan & Ksiazek, 2000; Mills et al., 2002; Pini et al., 2003; Wells et al., 1997).

Incubation

The incubation period is thought to be around 2 weeks, and it may range from several days to 6 weeks (Chin, 2000).

BIOTERRORISM CONSIDERATIONS BOX 38–1

Although hantavirus pulmonary syndrome may be considered a viral hemorrhagic fever in severe forms, it is caused by a Category C critical biological agent, unlike other viral hemorrhagic fevers, which are caused by Category A agents (Clement, 2003; Rotz, Khan, Lillibridge, Ostroff, & Hughes, 2002).

Clinical Findings and Treatment

Signs and Symptoms

Hantavirus pulmonary syndrome begins with a 3- to 5-day prodrome characterized by fever, chills, and myalgias. Other common early signs are malaise, headache, cough, abdominal pain, nausea, vomiting, and diarrhea. Less common signs are dizziness, shortness of breath, back or chest pain, arthralgia, and sweats. These are followed by the abrupt onset of hypotension and pulmonary edema, progressing rapidly to shock and respiratory failure. Those who survive (often with mechanical ventilation assistance) experience rapid improvement. The case fatality rate was originally observed to be 40% to 50%, and remains this high in some locales. However, in some parts of South America, clinical symptoms may be mild and the case fatality rate substantially lower. The reasons for this are not clear, but could possibly include differences in virulence as well as host or environmental factors (Centers for Disease Control and Prevention [CDC], 2002; Chin, 2000; Khan & Ksiazek, 2000; Peters & Khan, 2002; Pini et al., 2003). Signs and symptoms that make hantavirus pulmonary syndrome unlikely include rash, conjunctivitis, pharyngitis, petechiae, and periorbital or peripheral edema (CDC, 2002).

Complications

The usually rapid progression of hantavirus pulmonary syndrome into shock and respiratory failure is an enormous clinical challenge. Patients who die from hantavirus pulmonary syndrome have severe hypotension leading to sinus bradycardia, electromechanical dissociation, ventricular tachycardia, or fibrillation. Severely ill patients may develop disseminated intravenous coagulation; hence, hantavirus pulmonary syndrome has been considered a viral hemorrhagic fever (CDC, 2002; Khan & Ksiazek, 2000).

Common Laboratory Findings

In the early prodromal stages of illness, laboratory findings may include a raised WBC count with a left shift. Circulating immunoblasts appear as large atypical lymphocytes, with the WBC differential showing up to 50% white blood cell precursors. Thrombocytopenia may also be present; a dramatic fall may precede the transition to pulmonary edema (CDC, 2002). Other abnormalities that are seen in the cardiopulmonary phase include a fall in serum albumin and a rise in the hematocrit as fluid shifts into pulmonary interstitial and alveolar spaces. The "combination of atypical lymphocytes, a significant bandemia, and thrombocytopenia in the setting of pulmonary edema is strongly suggestive of a hantavirus infection" (CDC, 2002). The characteristic radiological evolution of hantavirus pulmonary syndrome includes slight changes of interstitial pulmonary edema progressing to alveolar edema with severe bilateral involvement and pleural effusions. Heart size is usually normal (CDC, 2002).

Diagnosis

Currently, CDC and some state health laboratories use an enzyme-linked immunosorbent assay (ELISA) to detect immunoglobulin M (IgM) antibodies to Sin Nombre virus and as a means of diagnosing acute infections with other hantaviruses. A Western blot assay is also in use (CDC, 2002). Immunohistochemistry staining of viral antigens in tissue samples is very sensitive and often used for retrospective diagnosis. Polymerase chain reaction is experimental.

Differential Diagnosis

The differential diagnosis of the prodromal phase of hantavirus pulmonary syndrome includes influenza, leptospirosis, Legionnaire's disease, mycoplasma, Q fever, chlamydia, septicemic plague, tularemia, coccidioidomycosis, histoplasmosis, and Goodpasture's syndrome. In the cardiopulmonary stage of hantavirus pulmonary syndrome, the differential diagnosis includes myocardial infarction, adult respiratory distress syndrome, and advanced stages of the previously noted prodromal differential diagnoses. Among immunocompromised patients, consider also *Pneumocystis carinii* pneumonia, cytomegalovirus, cryptococcus, aspergillus, and graft versus host disease (CDC, 2002; Khan & Ksiazek, 2000).

Treatment

Treatment is supportive because no specific therapy exists. Ribavirin has in vitro activity against Sin Nombre virus, but no clinical benefit in controlled studies (CDC, 2002). Clinicians faced with a patient with possible hantavirus pulmonary syndrome should start broad-spectrum antibiotics, restore and maintain fluid balance, provide respiratory support as needed, and transfer the patient as soon as possible to an intensive care unit. Mechanical ventilation, pulmonary artery catheterization, and administration of vasopressor drugs are often required. Ongoing frequent assessment of blood pressure, pulmonary wedge pressure, fluid balance, and electrolyte balance will help monitor disease progression and complications. Extracorporeal membrane oxygenation has been used in a few patients with some success.

Prevention

The best means of prevention is to reduce risk by deterring home rodent colonization and avoiding contact with rodent waste and nesting materials, especially the inhalation of rodent-related materials. Preventive measures (Mills et al., 2002) include the following, which are discussed in greater detail in the Mills reference:

- Do not occupy previously vacant structures that are actively infested with rodents.
- When cleaning infested areas, wear a properly fitting respirator with an N-100 filter and rubber or plastic gloves. Wash and disinfect these before removing them.
- Avoid disturbing excreta or rodent nests around the home, workplace, campground, or other areas.
- Trap and kill rodents found in vacant, infested structures, and dispose of their carcasses properly.
- Do not handle mice without wearing gloves.
- Do not keep captive wild rodents as pets or research subjects.
- Avoid handling equipment or machinery that has been stored in infested areas. (See respirator and barrier precautions mentioned earlier.)
- Do not sleep on the ground in endemic areas. Other camping precautions include airing out and disinfecting shelters before using them; pitching tents away from rodent droppings, burrows, or possible rodent shelters such as woodpiles or garbage dumps; keeping food in rodent-proof containers; and using only bottled, filtered, boiled, or chemically disinfected water.

Community education in prevention is important.

Reporting

The CDC considers hantavirus pulmonary syndrome to be a nationally notifiable disease. The World Health Organization (WHO) considers hantavirus pulmonary syndrome as important in public health (Class 2A). See Appendix C for details and for upcoming changes in WHO reporting.

References

Centers for Disease Control and Prevention. (2002). Hantavirus pulmonary syndrome. Retrieved October 31, 2003, from *www.cdc.gov/ncidod/diseases/hanta/hantvrus.htm*

Chin, J. (Ed.). (2000). *Control of communicable diseases manual* (17th ed., pp. 234-236). Washington, DC: American Public Health Association.

Clement, J.P. (2003). Hantavirus. *Antiviral Research, 57*, 121-127.

Khan, A.S., & Ksiazek, T.G. (2000). Diseases caused by hantaviruses. In G.T. Strickland (Ed.), *Hunter's tropical medicine and emerging infectious diseases* (8th ed., pp. 288-293). Philadelphia: W.B. Saunders Company.

Mills, J.N., Corneli, A., Young, J.C., Garrison, L.E., Khan, A.S., & Ksiazek, T.G. (2002). Hantavirus pulmonary syndrome—United States: Updated recommendations for risk reduction. *MMWR, 51(RR09)*, 1-12. Retrieved October 28, 2003, from *www.cdc.gov/mmwr/preview/mmwrhtml/rr5109a1.htm*

Peters, C.J., & Khan, A.S. (2002). Hantavirus pulmonary syndrome: The new American hemorrhagic fever. *Clinical Infectious Diseases, 34*, 1224-1231.

Pini, N., Levis, S., Calderon, G., Ramirez, J., Bravo, D., et al. (2003). Hantavirus infection in humans and rodents, northwestern Argentina. *Emerging Infectious Diseases, 9*, 1070-1076.

Rotz, L.D, Khan, A.S., Lillibridge, S.R., Ostroff, S.M., & Hughes. J.M. (2002). Public health assessment of potential biological terrorism agents. *Emerging Infectious Diseases, 8*, 225-230.

Wells, R.M., Estani, S.S., Yadon, Z.E., Enria, D., Padula, P., et al. (1997). An unusual hantavirus outbreak in southern Argentina: Person-to-person transmission? *Emerging Infectious Diseases, 3*, 171-174.

39

HEMORRHAGIC FEVERS, VIRAL

Geographic Distribution

This chapter summarizes the viral hemorrhagic fevers that are not described in detail in their own chapters. (See separate entries for dengue, Ebola and Marburg hemorrhagic fevers, hantavirus pulmonary syndrome, hantavirus hemorrhagic fever with renal syndrome, Lassa fever, and yellow fever.) Viral hemorrhagic fevers are zoonoses found in numerous areas of the world. Each virus is associated with a host reservoir species and therefore limited to the area where the host species is found (Table 39-1). Occasionally, cases occur in other areas when the host species is transported.

TABLE 39–1

Geographic Distribution and Natural Vectors of Viral Hemorrhagic Fevers

Family	Name	Distribution	Host or Vector
Arenaviridae	Lassa fever	Central and West Africa	Rodents
	New World arenaviruses (Guanarito, Junin, Machupo, Sabia)	South America	Rodents
Bunyaviridae	Crimean-Congo hemorrhagic fever	Eastern Europe, Middle East, Asia, and Africa	Ticks
	Rift Valley fever	Middle East and Africa	Mosquitoes

continued ➲

Table 39–1 continued

Family	Name	Distribution	Host or Vector
Bunyaviridae—cont'd	Hantavirus hemorrhagic fever with renal syndrome	Europe, East China, and Korea	Rodents
	Puumala	Scandinavia and Eastern Europe	Rodents
	Hantaan	Northeast Asia	Rodents
	Dobrava-Belgrade	Balkans	Rodents
	Seoul	Worldwide	Rodents
	Hantavirus–Sin Nombre	North America	Rodents
Filoviridae	Ebola, Marburg hemorrhagic fever	Sub-Saharan Africa	Unknown
Flaviviridae	Yellow fever	Sub-Saharan Africa and South America	Mosquitoes
	Dengue	Africa, North and South America, Caribbean, Pacific, Middle East, Australia, and India	Mosquitoes
	Omsk, Kyasanur Forest disease	Asia	Ticks

Sources: Borio et al., 2002; CIDRAP, 2003.

Agent and Vector

The term *viral hemorrhagic fever* describes a syndrome of hemorrhage, vascular damage, and multisystem organ involvement. Viral hemorrhagic fevers are caused by four families of lipid-encapsulated RNA viruses: arenaviruses, filoviruses, bunyaviruses, and flaviviruses. Each is thought to asymptomatically infect a species that serves as an ecological reservoir, although for some viral hemorrhagic fevers such as Ebola and Marburg, the identity of the reservoir species remains a mystery. Historically, viral hemorrhagic fevers sporadically infect other species including humans, causing disease in unpredictable epidemics. Some viral hemorrhagic fevers are transmitted by direct contact, whereas others use an arthropod vector. A few have an unknown mechanism of transmission.

Person-to-person transmission is possible for Ebola, Marburg, Lassa, and Crimean-Congo hemorrhagic fever (Centers for Disease Control and Prevention [CDC], 2002). A case of person-to-person transmission of hantavirus was documented in Argentina, but this is unusual (Wells et al., 1997). Only 1 to 10 organisms are needed to cause disease (Center for Infectious Disease Research and Policy [CIDRAP], 2003). The viruses attack endothelial cells, causing increased vascular permeability and vascular dysregulation (CIDRAP, 2003). This endothelial dysfunction combined with thrombocytopenia and/or severe platelet dysfunction leads to the hemorrhagic manifestations of infection. The viral hemorrhagic fevers are classified by the CDC as Category A biological warfare agents, as discussed in Box 39-1 (CDC, 2000).

Incubation

The range of incubation for viral hemorrhagic fevers is 2 to 35 days (Table 39-2).

Clinical Findings and Treatment

Signs and Symptoms

Depending on the severity of vascular instability and platelet dysfunction, presentation may range from mild to severe illness. Hemorrhagic manifestations are not always apparent. A common course of illness begins with

BIOTERRORISM CONSIDERATIONS

BOX 39-1

The viruses that cause viral hemorrhagic fevers are considered by the CDC to be Category A biological warfare agents because they pose a risk to national security: They can be easily disseminated or transmitted from person to person; cause high mortality, with potential for major public health impact; might cause public panic and social disruption; and require special action for public health preparedness (CDC, 2000, p. 5). All are potentially infectious by the aerosol route and most are stable as respirable aerosols (Cieslak & Eitzen, 2000, p. 28).

Hemorrhagic fever viruses have been weaponized by the former Soviet Union, Russia, and the United States prior to 1969 (Borio et al., 2002). Yellow fever may have been weaponized by North Korea. The Working Group on Civilian Biodefense determined that the following viral hemorrhagic fevers pose a serious threat as biological weapons:

- Ebola
- Marburg
- Lassa fever
- New World arenaviruses
- Rift Valley fever
- Yellow fever
- Omsk hemorrhagic fever
- Kyasanur viral hemorrhagic fever

The absence of vaccines and specific treatments for viral hemorrhagic fevers makes their medical and public health management very challenging in a mass casualty situation (Borio et al., 2002; Varkey, Poland, Cockerill, Smith, & Hagen, 2002).

an abrupt onset of fever, myalgia, cutaneous flushing, and conjunctival suffusion. Relative bradycardia may also be seen. Within several days, the patient's condition worsens to include syncope, photophobia, headache,

TABLE 39-2 Clinical Features of Viral Hemorrhagic Fevers

Family	Name	Incubation (days)	Distinctive Characteristics in Addition to General VHF Signs and Symptoms	Secondary Transmission Possible	Case Fatality Rate	Ribavirin Possibly Beneficial
Arenaviridae	Lassa fever	5-16	Most infections mild or subclinical with severe disease in 5-10%; illness with gradual onset; retrosternal pain and arthralgias by 3rd or 4th day; severe exudative pharyngitis, facial swelling, proteinuria, tremors, encephalitis; sometimes permanent hearing loss	Yes	15-20% of hospitalized patients	Yes
	New World arenaviruses (Guanarito, Junin, Machupo, Sabia)	7-14	Illness with gradual onset; facial and trunk flushing, generalized lymphadenopathy and petechiae often seen early in illness; bleeding manifestations common; tremors of tongue and upper extremities, myoclonic movements, seizures	Yes (Machupo)	15-30%	Yes
Bunyaviridae	Crimean-Congo hemorrhagic	3-12	Sudden onset of symptoms; mood swings and agitation evolve to lassitude; early severe abdominal pain gradually	Yes	30%	Yes

fever		localized to right upper quadrant; hemorrhagic symptoms and hepatitis common			
Rift Valley fever	2-6	Subclinical infection common, hemorrhagic fever affects less than 1%; retro-orbital pain and photophobia common in prodrome; jaundice in 18%; retinitis in 10% sometimes leads to blindness	No	<1% overall, but 50% for hemorrhagic disease	Yes
Hantavirus hemorrhagic fever with renal syndrome	9-35	Back pain; renal failure precedes pulmonary edema and DIC; Hantaan and Dobrava viruses associated with severe disease; Seoul virus causes moderate illness; Puumala infection usually mild without hemorrhage	No	1-15%	Yes
Hantavirus pulmonary syndrome—Sin Nombre	9-33	Febrile prodrome leads to shock and rapid pulmonary edema	Not observed in United States	50%	No

continued

Table 39–2 continued

Family	Name	Incubation (days)	Distinctive Characteristics in Addition to General VHF Signs and Symptoms	Secondary Transmission Possible	Case Fatality Rate	Ribavirin Possibly Beneficial
Filoviridae	Ebola, Marburg hemorrhagic fever	2-21	Severe prostration; diffuse maculopapular rash early in illness; bleeding and DIC common in 2nd week of illness; jaundice and pancreatitis common	Yes	50-90%	No
Flaviviridae	Yellow Fever	3-6	Subclinical infection common; relative bradycardia; biphasic course with jaundice, renal failure, and hemorrhagic complications in 2nd phase; severe disease occurs in about 15%	No	20% for hospitalized patients, 50% for those with jaundice and hemorrhagic manifestations	No
	Omsk, Kyasanur Forest disease	2-9	Papulovesicular palate lesions; hyperemia of face and trunk; lymphadenopathy, splenomegaly, CNS dysfunction; Kyasanur Forest is biphasic with meningoencephalitis common	No	0.5-10%	No

Sources: Borio et al., 2002; CDC, 2002; CIDRAP, 2003.

hyperesthesia, abdominal pain, nausea and vomiting, anorexia, and prostration. Petechiae, ecchymoses, purpura, hematuria, hematemesis, and melena may develop at this time. Those with severe illness progress to hypotension and shock (Borio et al., 2002; CIDRAP, 2003; Tolan & Whitner, 2003). Signs and symptoms of some of the specific viral hemorrhagic fevers are summarized in Table 39-2.

Complications

— Shock, encephalopathy, seizures, convulsions, or coma may occur in more serious infections. Pleural and pericardial effusions may also develop. Disseminated intravascular coagulation may be seen in Ebola, Marburg, Rift Valley fever, and Crimean-Congo hemorrhagic fever, but is not generally seen in other viral hemorrhagic fevers (CIDRAP, 2003). Renal failure is a complication of hantavirus hemorrhagic fever and renal syndrome but is less common with other viral hemorrhagic fevers.

— Case fatality rates vary with the specific virus and level of medical care available. For example, the fatality rate for patients with dengue hemorrhagic fever who receive supportive care is less than 1%, whereas that for patients with Ebola hemorrhagic fever ranges from 50% to 90%. Death typically occurs 1 to 2 weeks following the onset of symptoms. Survivors often have a prolonged convalescence with weakness, fatigue, anorexia, and arthralgias. Other complications include hearing loss (especially for Lassa fever), vision loss (particularly with Rift Valley fever), uveitis, pericarditis, orchitis, parotitis, pancreatitis, and decreased motor coordination (Borio et al., 2002; CDC, 2002, 2003a, 2003b; Tolan & Whitner, 2003).

Common Laboratory Findings

— Most viral hemorrhagic fevers cause thrombocytopenia. Leukopenia is usually present except for Crimean-Congo

hemorrhagic fever and Lassa fever, which cause
leukocytosis. Increased liver enzymes, hematuria,
proteinuria, and hemoconcentration are sometimes seen.
Rift Valley fever and yellow fever typically cause
increased bilirubin levels. Bleeding time, prothrombin
time, and partial thromboplastin time may all be
prolonged; decreased fibrinogen and elevated fibrin
degradation products may be present in patients with
disseminated intravascular coagulation (Borio et al.,
2002; CDC, 2002).

Diagnosis

Naturally occurring viral hemorrhagic fever is diagnosed
on the basis of hemorrhagic manifestations with a history
of travel to an endemic area. Contact with sick animals
or animal carcasses, sick people, or insect bites within
21 days of the onset of illness increases suspicion.
The Working Group on Civilian Biodefense adapted the
following criteria from World Health Organization
(WHO) surveillance standards for hemorrhagic fever to
identify a suspected index case of viral hemorrhagic
fever (Borio et al., 2002):

- Acute onset of temperature above 101° F for less
  than 3 weeks duration,
- Severe illness, no predisposing factors for
  hemorrhagic manifestations,
- No established alternative diagnosis, and
- At least two of the following hemorrhagic symptoms:
  hemorrhagic or purple rash, epistaxis, hematemesis,
  hemoptysis, blood in stools, or other hemorrhagic
  symptom.

This broad definition is intended to detect an outbreak
before an etiologic agent is identified; more specific case
definitions would be developed after the specific viral
hemorrhagic fever is determined.
Specialized laboratories can detect viral hemorrhagic
fevers by antigen-capture enzyme-linked immunosorbent

assay (ELISA), reverse transcriptase polymerase chain reaction (RT-PCR), serology, and viral isolation. RT-PCR is currently available only in research settings, but may be more widely available in the future. Serologic diagnosis is on the basis of immunoglobulin M (IgM) antibodies in acute specimens, or a fourfold or greater increase in antibody titer in paired sera by hemagglutination inhibition, complement fixation, enzyme immunoassay, or neutralization test. Some viral hemorrhagic fevers such as Ebola and Lassa fever have detectable IgM relatively early in the course. In general, however, serology may be of limited utility in the acute setting because antibodies in most viral hemorrhagic fevers do not appear until the recovery phase in the second week of illness. Acute samples should be collected within 7 days of the onset of illness, and convalescent sera 2 to 3 weeks later. Viral isolation by cell culture is very dangerous and should only be done by specialized laboratories. All suspected cases of viral hemorrhagic fever should be reported immediately to local and state health departments (Borio et al., 2002; CDC, 2002; CIDRAP, 2003).

Differential Diagnosis

The differential diagnosis includes rickettsial diseases (typhus, Q fever, trench fever, spotted fevers such as Rocky Mountain or Boutonneuse), meningococcemia, sepsis, toxic shock syndrome, malaria, septicemic plague, hantavirus pulmonary syndrome, malaria, shigellosis, leptospirosis, hemorrhagic smallpox. Noninfectious entities to consider include idiopathic or thrombocytopenic purpura, hemolytic uremic syndrome, and leukemia (Borio et al., 2002; CDC, 2002; CIDRAP, 2003).

Treatment

Treatment is supportive in most cases. Because of the risk of hemorrhage, IM injections should be avoided and invasive procedures such as vascular catheters should be minimized. Use acetaminophen instead of nonsteroidal antiinflammatory drugs for fever and comfort, and do not give anticoagulants. Steroids are not beneficial unless there is adrenal involvement (CIDRAP, 2003).

Intravenous fluids should be used as needed for fluid and electrolyte balance, but given cautiously because many of the viral hemorrhagic fevers can cause rapid pulmonary edema. Therefore clinicians should consider transfer to an intensive care unit for vasopressor support and hemodynamic monitoring early in the course of illness (Borio et al., 2002). Mechanical ventilation and dialysis may also be required.

Ribavirin has been effective in some cases of Lassa fever, the South American hemorrhagic fevers, Crimean-Congo hemorrhagic fever, Rift Valley fever, and hemorrhagic fever and renal syndrome. Because of this, some experts recommend that it be started immediately in suspected viral hemorrhagic fever pending diagnostic confirmation of the specific agent, and discontinued if the infection is determined not to be an arenavirus or bunyavirus. Ribavirin is given as a slow initial intravenous loading dose of 30 mg/kg (maximum 2 g) followed by 16 mg/kg (maximum 1 g) every 6 hours for 4 days, and then 8 mg/kg (maximum 500 mg) every 8 hours for 6 days. In a mass casualty setting, it may be given orally with a loading dose of 2,000 mg, followed by 600 mg twice a day for 10 days; for patients weighing less than 75 kg the dose is 1200 mg followed by 400 mg in the morning and 600 mg in the evening for 10 days. Pregnant women are given the adult dosage; children are given 30 mg/kg once followed by 15 mg/kg per day in 2 divided doses for 10 days (Borio et al., 2002; CIDRAP, 2003).

Prevention

Except for yellow fever, none of the viral hemorrhagic fevers have an available vaccine. The risk of contracting naturally occurring viral hemorrhagic fevers can be reduced by avoiding areas of suspected or confirmed outbreaks. Those traveling in African forests should avoid contact with ill people, and stay away from nonhuman primates and their carcasses (Issacson, 2001). Mosquito precautions such as DEET, permethrin-impregnated clothing, bed nets, and staying in screened buildings during times of mosquito activity can be helpful in preventing yellow fever, Rift Valley fever, and dengue. Travelers, especially hikers and backpackers, can prevent Crimean-Congo hemorrhagic fever by using tick precautions such as permethrin-impregnated long-sleeved shirts, long pants tucked into socks, and regular tick inspections. People in rural and wilderness areas can reduce the risk of rodent-borne infections such as Lassa fever and hantavirus hemorrhagic fever and renal syndrome by avoiding rodents, sleeping on cots or ground covers, camping away from potential rodent dwellings, keeping food in rodent-proof containers, and not disturbing areas with rodent excreta.

— When health care workers are faced with a patient with possible viral hemorrhagic fever, it is essential to prevent secondary cases of nosocomial transmission by meticulously practicing blood and body fluid precautions: Use masks, eye protection, gloves, gowns, and boots. These precautions should also be observed around medical equipment, laboratory equipment, tissue samples, and cadavers. Airborne precautions, including negative-pressure rooms if available, are also recommended even though airborne transmission of viral hemorrhagic fevers is rare.

— Postexposure prophylaxis is not available except for Lassa fever, for which CDC guidelines recommend ribavirin for high-risk contacts. For viral hemorrhagic fevers in a potential biological weapons attack, exposed persons should be monitored closely and if fever greater than 101° F develops within 21 days of a high-risk exposure, empiric ribavirin should be started as described earlier in the Treatment section, and discontinued if the agent is found not to be an arenavirus or bunyavirus (Borio et al., 2002; CDC, 2002; Issacson, 2001; Tolan & Whitner, 2003).

Reporting

The CDC considers hemorrhagic fevers to be nationally notifiable diseases. The WHO considers hemorrhagic fevers important diseases in public health (Class 2A). See Appendix C for details and for upcoming changes in WHO reporting.

References

Borio, L., Inglesby, T., Peters, C.J., Schmaljohn, A.L., Hughes, J.M., et al. (2002). Hemorrhagic fever viruses as biological weapons, medical and public health management. *Journal of the American Medical Association, 287*, 2391-2405.

Center for Infectious Disease Research and Policy. (2003). Viral hemorrhagic fever (VHF): Current, comprehensive information on pathogenesis, microbiology, epidemiology, diagnosis, treatment, and prophylaxis. Retrieved November 16, 2003, from *www.cidrap.umn.edu/index.html*

Centers for Disease Control and Prevention. (2000). Biological and chemical terrorism: Strategic plan for preparedness and response. *MMWR: Morbidity and Mortality Weekly Report, 49*(RR-4), 1-14.

Centers for Disease Control and Prevention. (2002). Viral hemorrhagic fevers. Retrieved November 15, 2003, from *www.cdc.gov/ncidod/dvrd/spb/mnpages/dispages/vhf.htm*

Centers for Disease Control and Prevention. (2003a). Lassa fever. Retrieved November 15, 2003, from *www.cdc.gov/ncidod/dvrd/spb/mnpages/dispages/lassaf.htm*

Centers for Disease Control and Prevention. (2003b). Rift Valley fever. Retrieved November 15, 2003, from *www.cdc.gov/ncidod/dvrd/spb/mnpages/dispages/rvf.htm*

Cieslak, T.J., & Eitzen, E.M. (2000). Bioterrorism: Agents of concern. *Journal of Public Health Management Practice, 6,* 19-29.

Issacson, M. (2001). Viral hemorrhagic fever hazards for travelers in Africa. *Clinical Infectious Diseases, 33*, 1707-1712.

Tolan, R.W., & Whitner, M.L. (2003). Viral hemorrhagic fevers. Retrieved November 9, 2003, from *www.emedicine.com/PED/topic2406.htm*

Varkey, P., Poland, G.A., Cockerill, F.R., Smith, T.F., & Hagen, P.T. (2002). Confronting bioterrorism: Physicians on the front line. *Mayo Clinic Proceedings, 77*, 661-672.

Wells, R.M., Estani, S.S., Yadon, Z.E., Enria, D., Padula, D., et al. (1997). An unusual hantavirus outbreak in Argentina: Person-to-person transmission? *Emerging Infectious Diseases, 3*, 171-74.

40

HEPATITIS A

Geographic Distribution

Hepatitis A virus (HAV) is endemic throughout the world, with higher prevalence in areas with poorer sanitation. In some developing countries, nearly all preschool children are seropositive for HAV (Chin, 2000; Feinstone & Gust, 2000).

Agent and Vector

HAV is a member of the Picornaviridae family of RNA viruses. It is hardy, able to survive in dried stool for 4 weeks, in a live oyster for 5 days, and at 85° C for 1 min (Marsano, 2003). The virus is spread predominantly through the fecal-oral route and infects only humans. HAV may also be acquired through sexual contact, particularly among men who have sex with men, or by exchange of blood and body fluids, as occurs with needle sharing between intravenous drug users. The virus replicates in hepatocytes but is noncytopathic; the hepatocellular damage and symptoms of HAV disease are a result of the host's immune response. For 80% of children younger than age 2, HAV infection is asymptomatic. The older the patient, the more likely it is that illness and complications will occur. Consequently, in developing countries where almost all children are exposed at a young age, illness from HAV is mostly in travelers and expatriates from industrialized countries. As sanitary conditions improve in a country, the average age of infection increases, with a corresponding rise in the incidence of clinical disease (Feinstone & Gust, 2000).

Incubation

The incubation is usually between 2 and 4 weeks, but can be up to 6 weeks. Infected individuals may excrete HAV in their feces for 1 to 2 weeks before the onset of illness, and for more than a week afterward (Koff, 1998).

Clinical Findings and Treatment

Signs and Symptoms

Most symptomatic patients have some combination of fever, fatigue, anorexia, and nausea. Vomiting, weight loss, diarrhea, cough, and arthralgias may also be present. Symptoms usually last less than 8 weeks, though some with cholestatic hepatitis may have jaundice over 10 weeks, and up to 10% of patients may have relapsing hepatitis. In addition to jaundice, physical examination may reveal hepatosplenomegaly, sometimes with right upper quadrant tenderness, and spider nevi on the trunk, which disappear with recovery. About two-thirds of patients recover within 2 months, and almost all recover by 6 months (Feinstone & Gust, 2000; Marsano, 2003).

Complications

Cholestatic hepatitis with prolonged jaundice, fever, and pruritus may occur, usually with a favorable outcome. Relapsing disease with acute elevations of liver enzymes has also been observed. The most serious complication is fulminant hepatic failure, with hepatic encephalopathy and coagulopathy. Though this rarely occurs in HAV infection, in one U.S. study HAV accounted for 8% of cases of fulminant hepatic failure. Liver failure does occur in children, but is most common in adults (Feinstone & Gust, 2000; Zuckerman & Zuckerman, 2003).

Common Laboratory Findings

— Elevated aminotransferases up to 500 to 5000 units/L may be seen, as well as hyperbilirubinemia up to 12 to 29 mg/dL (Koff, 1998).

Diagnosis

— Detection of immunoglobulin M (IgM) anti-HAV is diagnostic of acute HAV infection. IgM antibody usually disappears by 3 to 6 months. IgG anti-HAV may occur with IgM in the early stages of infection, and it can persist for decades. When detected without IgM anti-HAV, IgG anti-HAV signifies past infection (or immunization) and resistance to reinfection (Koff, 1998).

Differential Diagnosis

— Before laboratory results are available, acute HAV is difficult to distinguish from other causes of viral hepatitis such as hepatitis B virus, hepatitis C virus, hepatitis D virus, and Epstein-Barr virus. Symptoms of acute viral hepatitis may also be similar to typhoid, malaria, viral hemorrhagic fever, leptospirosis, and amebic liver abscess. In HIV-infected patients, fungal or mycobacterial hepatitis should be considered. Autoimmune hepatitis, alcohol cirrhosis, toxic exposures, and metabolic diseases such as Wilson's disease are some of the noninfectious entities that should also be considered (Feinstone & Gust, 2000; Zuckerman & Zuckerman, 2003).

Treatment

— Treatment for HAV is supportive. Hospitalization may be required for those with dehydration and those with evidence of severe liver disease. Corticosteroids and nonsteroidal antiinflammatory drugs should not be used and alcohol should be avoided during the acute phase; otherwise, no dietary restrictions are necessary (Koff, 1998; Zuckerman & Zuckerman, 2003).

Prevention

- Improved sanitation and hygiene are the most effective means of controlling HAV. Hand washing is essential for food handlers and health care and child care workers. Travelers to developing countries should avoid untreated water, uncooked vegetables, and uncooked shellfish.
- Immunization with two doses of inactivated hepatitis A vaccine 6 to 12 months apart is safe and effective, providing at least 10 years of protection. Preexposure prophylaxis with hepatitis A vaccine should be given to anyone older than age 2 who is at increased risk for HAV, including travelers, military personnel, members of communities with higher rates of infection, men who have sex with men, intravenous drug users, and persons with occupational risk for exposure such as workers in institutions for people with developmental disabilities.
- Passive immunization with pooled immune globulin (IG) may be used for children younger than age 2 who are too young for the vaccine and who will be traveling to an endemic area. Because immunization requires around 2 weeks to achieve protective antibody levels, IG may also be useful for older patients who need protection against HAV before 2 weeks have elapsed. A dose of 0.02 mL/kg provides protection for up to 3 months, and 0.06 mL/kg is effective for up to 6 months. IG is also recommended as postexposure prophylaxis for unimmunized persons who have been exposed to HAV within 14 days (American Academy of Pediatrics, 2003; Chin, 2000; Feinstone & Gust, 2000). For more details on postexposure and preexposure prophylaxis, please see the American Academy of Pediatrics *Red Book* (2003).

Reporting

- The U.S. Centers for Disease Control and Prevention considers hepatitis A to be a nationally notifiable disease. The World Health Organization (WHO) considers it a Class 2A disease. See Appendix C for details and for upcoming changes in WHO reporting.

References

American Academy of Pediatrics. (2003). *2003 Red Book: Report of the Committee on Infectious Diseases* (26th ed.). Washington, DC: Author.

Chin, J. (Ed.). (2000). *Control of communicable diseases manual* (17th ed., pp. 238-242). Washington, DC: American Public Health Association.

Feinstone, S.M., & Gust, I.D. (2000). Hepatitis A. In G. Mandell, J. Bennett, & R. Dolin (Eds.), *Principles and practice of infectious diseases* (5th ed., pp 1920-1940). New York: Churchill Livingstone.

Koff, R.S. (1998). Hepatitis A. *Lancet, 35*, 1643-49.

Marsano, L.S. (2003). Hepatitis. *Primary Care, 30*, 81-107.

Zuckerman, J.N., & Zuckerman, A.J. (2003). Viral hepatitis. In G.C. Cook & A.I. Zumla (Eds.), *Manson's tropical diseases* (21st ed., pp. 707-723). Philadelphia: W.B. Saunders Company.

41

HEPATITIS B

Geographic Distribution

― Hepatitis B virus (HBV) is present throughout the world with especially high prevalence in Asia, Africa, southern Europe, and Latin America, where more than half of the population is infected at some time in their lives and 2% to 20% are chronic carriers. In most of the developed world the prevalence of chronic HBV infection is less than 1% (Alter, 2003; Kao & Chen, 2002).

Agent and Vector

― HBV is a member of the hepadnavirus family, which includes DNA viruses that cause hepatitis in birds and mammals. The virus particle consists of a sphere with a core surrounding the viral DNA. HBV is spread through blood and body fluids, but is capable of surviving long periods of time outside the host in ambient conditions. In areas of the world with high endemicity, transmission is usually either through vertical transmission from mother to neonate or horizontal transmission from person to person (Lee, 1997). The precise mechanism of horizontal transmission is not completely understood, because it often occurs among household contacts of chronically infected persons without a history of sexual contact or exposure to blood or serum-derived body fluids. In contrast, HBV infections in developed countries are usually the result of sexual activity, injection drug use, or occupational exposure (e.g., health care workers).

― HBV itself is typically not cytopathic; rather, it is the host's immune response to the virus that causes liver disease. The stages of infection are monitored through the detection of viral antigens and antibodies to different parts of the virus, as well as the measurement of liver enzymes (aminotransferases), which are elevated by hepatocellular damage. In the asymptomatic first stage, hepatitis B e-antigen (HBeAg) and hepatitis B surface antigen (HBsAg) are detectable as the virus replicates but liver enzymes are normal. Antibodies to hepatitis B core antigen (anti-HBc) also develop and remain detectable thereafter. As the host immune response develops and attacks virus-containing hepatocytes, liver enzymes increase and the patient develops symptoms. This acute second stage lasts 3 to 4 weeks, but in some patients with chronic HBV the second stage can last more than 10 years, leading to cirrhosis. In the third stage, active viral replication ends, liver enzymes normalize, and antibodies develop to HBeAg as the e-antigen itself ceases to be detectable but HBsAg remains present. Most patients then enter a fourth stage in which they are unlikely to become reinfected or have a reactivated infection; concurrently they become negative for HBsAg but positive for antibodies to HBsAg. The younger the age of infection, the less likely this fourth stage of infection is to occur: 95% of infected neonates become chronic carriers, compared to 30% of children under 6 years old and 3% to 5% of adults (Alter, 2003; Lee, 1997; Zuckerman & Zuckerman, 2003).

Incubation

The incubation period (the time from infection to the development of disease) of HBV is long, ranging from 45 to 160 days. For persons who are infected as neonates, the incubation period may last decades (Alter, 2003; Lee, 1997).

Clinical Findings and Treatment

Signs and Symptoms

Acute hepatitis B may be preceded by a prodrome of arthralgias, arthritis, and a transient rash. Low-grade fever with malaise, anorexia, nausea and vomiting, and myalgias then develop. Mild to moderate right upper quadrant and epigastric pain may also be present. Jaundice, if it occurs, presents 10 to 12 days after the onset of symptoms. On physical exam, patients may have mildly tender hepatomegaly, with splenomegaly in 5% to 15% of patients. Dermatologic findings include palmar erythema and spider angiomata, which disappear after a few weeks. Mental status changes, edema, asterixis, and abnormal bleeding may be signs of liver failure (Alter, 2003; Lee, 1997; Marsano, 2003; Zuckerman & Zuckerman, 2003).

Complications

In approximately 1% of patients, acute HBV infection develops into fulminant hepatitis B with liver failure, coagulopathy, encephalopathy, and cerebral edema. Approximately 25% of patients with chronic hepatitis will develop cirrhosis; of these, approximately 20% will develop hepatocellular carcinoma, which usually occurs 25 to 30 years after infection. Serum sickness, polyarteritis nodosa, and glomerulonephritis are some of the rare extrahepatic manifestations of HBV infection. Coinfection with hepatitis D virus (HDV) may also occur, presenting as a diphasic elevation of liver enzymes or bilirubin (Lee, 1997; Lok, 2002; Marsano, 2003).

Common Laboratory Findings

Elevated liver enzymes with ALT higher than AST may be seen in the range of 1000 to 2000 international units/L. Mild leukopenia with lymphocytosis is common. Laboratory signs of severe injury include bilirubin greater than 17.6 mg/dL and elongated prothrombin time. In chronic HBV infection, ALT is elevated for more than 6 months (Marsano, 2003; Zuckerman & Zuckerman, 2003).

Diagnosis

The diagnosis of HBV infection is usually made by the detection of HBV antigens or antibodies. In the acute stage these include HBsAg and greatly elevated immunoglobulin M (IgM) anti-HBc. Chronic HBV infection is marked by the presence of HBsAg (1) for more than 6 months, (2) with negative IgM anti-HBc with positive total anti-HBc, or (3) with evidence of chronic liver disease without another explanation. Confirmation is by measurement of HBV-DNA levels in serum. Negative HBsAg with positive hepatitis B surface antibody indicates either past exposure or past immunization. Occult HBV infection without detectable HBsAg is rare but often is associated with hepatitis C infection (Kao & Chen, 2002; Marsano, 2003; Zuckerman & Zuckerman, 2003).

Differential Diagnosis

Other causes of viral hepatitis include hepatitis A virus, hepatitis C virus, hepatitis D virus, and Epstein-Barr virus. Symptoms of acute HBV infection may also overlap with typhoid, malaria, viral hemorrhagic fever, leptospirosis, and amebic liver abscess. In HIV-infected patients, fungal or mycobacterial hepatitis should be considered. Other noninfectious etiologies to keep in mind include autoimmune hepatitis, metabolic diseases (e.g., Wilson's disease), alcohol cirrhosis, and toxins (e.g., acetaminophen overdose).

Treatment

The treatment of acute HBV infection is supportive. Chronic infection may be treated with alpha-interferon or lamivudine. A 3- to 6-month course of alpha-interferon is associated with a response rate of 30% to 40%. Lamivudine is well tolerated and less expensive than alpha-interferon, but long-term treatment is associated with drug-resistant mutants (Lok, 2002; Zuckerman & Zuckerman, 2003).

Prevention

— Hepatitis can be spread through contact with body fluids, including saliva, semen, vaginal fluids, breast milk, and others. Hepatitis B is also spread intrafamilially by unknown means. Thus universal precautions are essential in contact with infected patients. Education of at-risk people and communities, for example, sexually promiscuous individuals, intravenous drug users, and health care providers, is essential. Overall, the risk of hepatitis B infection can be reduced by using condoms, avoiding intravenous drug use, and practicing universal blood and body fluid precautions.

— Screening of at-risk groups, especially childbearing women is important. See the earlier Geographic Distribution section for populations at risk because of country of origin.

— The cornerstone of primary HBV prevention is universal vaccination with recombinant HBsAg. Immunization of infants and children with the three-dose series is 90% to 95% effective. Universal childhood HBV immunization is practiced in the United States, but the cost of the vaccine has slowed its implementation in developing countries where the burden of disease is much greater. All pregnant women should be screened for HBV infection, and when an infant is delivered to a mother who is known to be positive for HBsAg, the baby should be given hepatitis B hyperimmune globulin and the first dose of HBV vaccine within the first 12 hours after birth.

— HBV immunization should also be considered for travelers of all ages going to highly endemic areas, especially if they are staying for a prolonged period (more than 6 months), may have exposure to blood or body fluids (e.g., health care workers), or may have sexual contact with residents of these areas.

Secondary HBV prevention is also important to reduce the risk of cirrhosis and hepatocellular carcinoma in high-risk populations. All immigrants, refugees, and international adoptees should be screened for HBV with HBsAg, anti-HBs, and anti-HBc. Those found not to have evidence of past infection should be vaccinated, while those who have chronic infection should be referred for treatment. Some experts also recommend that clinicians screen chronic HBV carriers older than age 12 for hepatocellular carcinoma by obtaining alpha-fetoprotein levels every 6 months and right upper quadrant ultrasounds every 6 to 12 months (American Academy of Pediatrics, 2003; Kao & Chen, 2002; Marsano, 2003; Stauffer, Kamat, & Walker, 2002). For more details on HBV immunization, see the American Academy of Pediatrics *Red Book* (2003).

Reporting

The U.S. Centers for Disease Control and Prevention considers hepatitis B to be a nationally notifiable disease. The World Health Organization (WHO) considers it a Class 2A disease. See Appendix C for details and for upcoming changes in WHO reporting.

References

American Academy of Pediatrics. (2003). *2003 Red Book: Report of the Committee on Infectious Diseases* (26th ed.). Washington, DC: Author.

Alter, M.J. (2003). Epidemiology of hepatitis B in Europe and worldwide. *Journal of Hepatology, 39*(S1), 64-69.

Kao, J.H., & Chen, D.S. (2002). Global control of hepatitis B virus infection. *Lancet Infectious Disease, 2*, 395-403.

Lee, W.M. (1997). Hepatitis B virus infection. *New England Journal of Medicine, 337*, 1733-45.

Lok, A.S. (2002). Chronic hepatitis B. *New England Journal of Medicine, 346*, 1682-1683.

Marsano, L.S. (2003). Hepatitis. *Primary Care, 30*, 81-107.

Stauffer, W.M., Kamat, D., & Walker, P.F. (2002). Screening of international immigrants, refugees, and adoptees. *Primary Care, 29*, 879-905.

Zuckerman, J.N., & Zuckerman, A.J. (2003). Viral hepatitis. In G.C. Cook & A.I. Zumla (Eds.), *Manson's tropical diseases* (21st ed., pp. 707-723). Philadelphia: W.B. Saunders Company.

HEPATITIS, NON-A AND NON-B

Geographic Distribution

Hepatitis caused by viruses other than the hepatitis A virus (HAV) or hepatitis B virus (HBV) occurs worldwide. Enterically transmitted hepatitis E is more common in developing countries with poor sanitation. Hepatitis C has higher prevalence rates in Italy, Spain, central Europe, Japan, and parts of the Middle East. The geography of hepatitis D follows that of hepatitis B infection (Zuckerman & Zuckerman, 2003).

Agent and Vector

In addition to the most common pathogens, hepatitis A and B, the following viruses can also cause hepatitis (Marsano, 2003; Zuckerman & Zuckerman, 2003):

- Hepatitis C virus (HCV) is a member of the Flavivirus family of RNA viruses transmitted through intravenous drug use, transfusion of contaminated blood, and vertically from mother to infant. Most acute infections are asymptomatic, but fulminant hepatitis can occur, and a significant proportion develop chronic infection (defined as hepatitis lasting 6 months or more), of which 30% will have severe progression to cirrhosis.
- Hepatitis D virus (HDV) requires the presence of hepatitis B virus infection for replication and can increase the severity of acute HBV infections.
- Hepatitis E virus (HEV) is an enterically transmitted pathogen that affects older children and young adults.
- Epstein-Barr virus (EBV) is the causative agent of infectious mononucleosis and Burkitt's lymphoma, the most common childhood cancer in parts of equatorial Africa and Papua New Guinea.

- Cytomegalovirus (CMV or human herpesvirus type 5) can cause illness in infants and immunocompromised patients but usually is asymptomatic; more than 80% of healthy adults are seropositive for CMV.

Incubation

Hepatitis C virus has an incubation of 2 to 26 weeks, but usually is about 7 to 8 weeks. Hepatitis E virus has an incubation of 2 to 10 weeks. Epstein-Barr virus has an incubation of 30 to 50 days. CMV incubation is unknown for horizontal transmission, but it can occur 3 to 12 weeks following blood transfusion (Chin, 2000; Zuckerman & Zuckerman, 2003).

Clinical Findings and Treatment

Signs and Symptoms

Acute hepatitis commonly causes fatigue, anorexia, arthralgias, abdominal pain, and nausea and vomiting. Jaundice, fever, and rashes may also occur but are rare in HCV infection. Physical examination may reveal right upper quadrant tenderness (Marsano, 2003).

Complications

Fulminant hepatitis is the most feared complication, but fortunately is rare. See the hepatitis B chapter for more details.

Common Laboratory Findings

Laboratory findings in viral hepatitis include elevations of AST and ALT, the degree of which reflects the rate of hepatocellular damage. Values of more than 10,000 international units/mL are more consistent with toxic or ischemic injury; viral hepatitis typically causes elevations in the range of 1500 to 3000 international units/mL. Bilirubin and alkaline phosphatase may also be increased.

Marked lymphocytosis with atypical lymphocytes suggests Epstein-Barr virus, though atypical lymphocytes may also occur with other causes of viral hepatitis (Marsano, 2003).

Diagnosis

The diagnosis of hepatitis due to viral causes other than HAV or HBV is as follows (Marsano, 2003; Zuckerman & Zuckerman, 2003):

- *HCV.* Positive serology, which may not occur until 6 weeks after exposure; or detection of HCV RNA. For the diagnosis of chronic HCV, a patient must have detectable HCV RNA in addition to any of the following: (1) elevation of ALT for 6 months, (2) positive anti-HCV serology for 6 months, (3) HCV-RNA positivity for 6 months, or (4) liver biopsy consistent with chronic hepatitis.
- *HDV.* Positive immunoglobulin M (IgM) anti-HBc plus a positive IgM anti-HDV, followed by a positive IgG anti-HDV a few weeks later.
- *HEV.* Positive IgM anti-HEV, which usually is present at the peak of aminotransferase levels.
- *EBV.* Positive IgM to viral capsid antigen; heterophile antibodies are present in 85% of acute EBV infections.
- *CMV.* Viral culture, acute and convalescent serologies 2 weeks apart, or CMV antigen detection.

Differential Diagnosis

The differential diagnosis of viral hepatitis includes bacterial infections, fungal infections, malaria, immune disorders, metabolic disorders, and toxic injury.

Treatment

Treatment is supportive for most causes of viral hepatitis. HDV and HCV are treated with alpha-interferon (Zuckerman & Zuckerman, 2003).

Prevention

No vaccine exists for any of the causes of viral hepatitis except for HAV and HBV. Immunization against HBV is protective against HDV. The risk for HCV can be reduced by avoiding contaminated needles and by using condoms. Donor blood should also be screened for HCV. Sanitation and hygiene are keys to controlling HEV infection. Immune globulin has not proven effective for HCV or HEV prophylaxis. CMV transmission may be reduced by careful attention to hand washing, particularly by those who care for infants (Chin, 2000; Zuckerman & Zuckerman, 2003).

Reporting

The U.S. Centers for Disease Control and Prevention considers viral forms of hepatitis to be nationally notifiable diseases. The World Health Organization (WHO) considers them Class 2A diseases. See Appendix C for details and for upcoming changes in WHO reporting.

References

Chin, J. (Ed.). (2000). *Control of communicable diseases manual* (17th ed.). Washington, DC: American Public Health Association.

Marsano, L.S. (2003). Hepatitis. *Primary Care*, *30*(1), 81-107.

Zuckerman, J.N. & , Zuckerman, A.J. (2003). Viral Hepatitis. In G.C. Cook & A.I. Zumla (Eds.), *Manson's tropical diseases* (21st ed., pp. 707-723). Philadelphia: W.B. Saunders Company.

43

HISTOPLASMOSIS

Geographic Distribution

Histoplasmosis has a worldwide distribution. Endemic areas include the United States, West Indies, Central and South America, Africa, India, and the Far East. The areas with the highest incidence of new infections include the United States (Ohio and Mississippi River valleys) and Central and South America (Hay, 2003).

Agent and Vector

Histoplasma capsulatum is a thermally dimorphic fungus that can be found in soil or areas with large numbers of birds or bats. Histoplasmosis is acquired by the respiratory route when contaminated soil, bird excrement, or bat guano is disturbed and the spores are aerosolized. Cases of histoplasmosis were sporadic in the past, occurring mostly in high-risk populations such as farmers or cave explorers; however, the AIDS epidemic has seen an increased number of symptomatic cases in patients with decreased cell-mediated immunity (Hay, 2003; Navarro, Walsh, & Hay, 2000).

Incubation

Local pulmonary infection occurs when the spores are inhaled. Hematogenous spread ensues within 2 weeks of infection, before specific immunity has developed. In immunocompetent patients, cellular immunity then develops after 2 to 3 weeks and the infection is controlled. In immunocompromised patients, the infection may continue to progress (Wheat & Kauffman, 2003).

Clinical Findings and Treatment

Signs and Symptoms

- Most people who become infected with histoplasmosis remain asymptomatic, and the possibility for acquiring a symptomatic infection is determined largely by the magnitude of exposure and the immune status of the patient. The acute pulmonary form may develop 10 to 14 days after exposure and often consists of fever, dry cough, chest pain, joint pain, fatigue, and occasionally erythema multiforme. Chest X-rays may demonstrate patchy focal infiltrates and hilar enlargement. Patients infected with this type of histoplasmosis normally recover with only supportive care; however, chronic, progressive, or disseminated disease may develop.

- Chronic pulmonary histoplasmosis characteristically occurs in people who have underlying emphysema or lung disease. Patients develop recurrent pneumonia with night sweats, fatigue, productive cough, weight loss, hemoptysis, and chest radiographs with fibrous apical pulmonary infiltrates and cavitation.

- Disseminated infection most commonly occurs in immunocompromised patients, and HIV infection is a major risk factor. A more chronic progressive disseminated form, which may be present for years after exposure, can occur in older adults. Manifestations of disseminated disease can include fever, weight loss, hepatosplenomegaly, lymphadenopathy, pneumonia, subacute or chronic meningitis, stroke syndromes, encephalitis, adrenal insufficiency, endocarditis, and disseminated intravascular coagulation. Multiple skin lesions may be seen, including papules, pustules, ulcers, and nodules, and are most often seen in immunocompromised patients. Mucosal lesions, including ulcers, plaques, masses, and nodules, can occur anywhere along the gastrointestinal tract.

African histoplasmosis, caused by *H. capsulatum* var.
duboisii, occurs only in Central and West Africa. The
infection is not common, and the environmental source
of the fungus is not known. Patients present with chronic
ulcers, subcutaneous nodules, and osteolytic bone lesions
(Al-Abdely & Graybill, 1999; Hay, 2003; Saccente,
McDonnell, Baddour, Mathis, & Bradsher, 2003;
Wheat & Kauffman, 2003).

Complications

Enlarged mediastinal lymph nodes in patients with acute
pulmonary histoplasmosis can rarely lead to a pericarditis
or partial obstruction of the airway, pulmonary vessels,
or esophagus. Fibrosing mediastinitis, which is a fibrotic
response to a previous pulmonary histoplasmosis
infection, can also cause obstruction of mediastinal
structures; in rare cases it involves the recurrent laryngeal
nerve, thoracic duct, or right atrium, causing right heart
failure and respiratory insufficiency. Chronic pulmonary
histoplasmosis can be complicated by bronchopleural
fistulae, pneumothoraces, and concurrent bacterial
infections. Severe pulmonary disease, which may be
secondary to heavy exposure, can lead to pneumonia,
acute respiratory distress syndrome, and respiratory failure
(Al-Abdely & Graybill, 1999; Wheat & Kauffman, 2003).

Common Laboratory Findings

Disseminated disease may lead to anemia, leukopenia,
thrombocytopenia, and elevated liver enzymes. With
adrenal involvement, patients may develop hyponatremia
and hyperkalemia (Wheat & Kauffman, 2003).

Diagnosis

Histoplasmosis can be cultured from sputum in patients
with chronic pulmonary disease and from the blood,
bone marrow, lung, liver, or urine in patients with
disseminated disease. Cultures require several weeks to

grow and are held for up to 6 weeks before they are reported as negative. Histopathologic examination of silver-stained tissue biopsies has a high sensitivity, but not specificity, for histoplasmosis. Detection of the polysaccharide antigen in the urine, blood, cerebrospinal fluid, or bronchoalveolar lavage fluid can allow for rapid diagnosis of disseminated or acute pulmonary disease; however, this is only available in reference laboratories. Serologic studies, including the complement fixation and immunodiffusion tests, can also help lead to the diagnosis; however, their usefulness may be limited by the time period between infection and production of antibodies, availability of the tests, low antibody titers in immunosuppressed patients, cross-reaction of antibodies from other fungal infections, and previous histoplasmosis infection (Al-Abdely & Graybill, 1999; Wheat & Kauffman, 2003).

Differential Diagnosis

Chronic pulmonary histoplasmosis must be differentiated from primary lung carcinoma, sarcoidosis, and other cavitary lung diseases, such as tuberculosis and aspergillosis. Bacterial pulmonary infections, which are common to patients with emphysema, may be the cause of recurrent symptoms, rather than recurrent or progressive histoplasmosis. The persistent fever and hepatosplenomegaly associated with disseminated histoplasmosis may be confused with other chronic infections, such as malaria and typhoid fever. Skin lesions may resemble other systemic fungal infections, varicella, herpes, leishmaniasis, or molluscum contagiosum (Navarro et al., 2000; Wheat & Kauffman, 2003).

Treatment

Primary pulmonary histoplasmosis is usually self-limited but, if symptoms persist more than 1 month, patients can be treated with ketoconazole 400 mg/day or itraconazole 200 mg/day for 6 to 12 weeks.

— Severe primary pulmonary disease should be treated with amphotericin B (1 mg/kg) and prednisone (40 to 60 mg/day) for 2 weeks followed by itraconazole for 12 weeks. Children who are hypoxemic or need ventilation support should be given amphotericin B desoxycholate (0.7 mg/kg/24 hours IV) or lipid-complex amphotericin B (3 to 5 mg/kg/24 hours IV) until improved and then given itraconazole (3 to 5 mg/kg/24 hours PO once daily) for at least 12 weeks.

— Chronic pulmonary histoplasmosis can be treated with itraconazole (400 mg/day) or ketoconazole (400 mg/day) for 12 to 24 months, or amphotericin B (total dose of 35 mg/kg). Children should be treated with amphotericin B as previously mentioned and then a 12- to 24-month course of itraconazole.

— The less severe cases of disseminated histoplasmosis may be treated with itraconazole (400 mg/day) for 6 to 18 months; severe cases should be treated with amphotericin B (1 mg/kg/day) followed by itraconazole (400 mg/day) for 6 to 18 months. In AIDS patients, once the disseminated infection is treated with amphotericin B, itraconazole should be given for life (Al-Abdely & Graybill, 1999; Aronoff, 2004; Wheat & Kauffman, 2003).

Prevention

— There is currently no vaccine for histoplasmosis. AIDS patients with CD4 counts of less than 150 who are living in endemic areas or with a history of previous infection should be given prophylaxis with itraconazole 200 mg daily (Al-Abdely & Graybill, 1999).

Reporting

— The U.S. Centers for Disease Control and Prevention does not consider histoplasmosis to be a nationally notifiable disease. The World Health Organization (WHO) considers it a Class 3B disease. See Appendix C for details and for upcoming changes in WHO reporting.

References

Al-Abdely, H., & Graybill, J.R. (1999). Histoplasmosis, blastomycosis, coccidioidomycosis, and cryptococcosis. In R.L. Guerrant, D.H. Walker, & P.F. Weller (Eds.), *Tropical infectious diseases: Principles, pathogens, and practice* (pp. 626-636). New York: Churchill Livingstone.

Aronoff, S.C. (2004). Histoplasmosis (*Histoplasma capsulatum*). In R.E. Behrman, R.M. Kliegman, & H.B. Jenson (Eds.), *Nelson textbook of pediatrics* (17th ed., pp. 1018-1020). Philadelphia: W.B. Saunders Company.

Hay, R.J. (2003). Fungal infections. In G.C. Cook & A.I. Zumla (Eds.), *Manson's tropical diseases* (21st ed., pp. 1186-1187). Philadelphia: W.B. Saunders Company.

Navarro, E.E., Walsh, T.J., & Hay, R.J. (2000). Histoplasmosis. In G. Strickland (Ed.), *Hunter's tropical medicine and emerging infectious diseases* (8th ed., pp. 548-552). Philadelphia: W.B. Saunders Company.

Saccente, M., McDonnell, R.W., Baddour, L.M., Mathis, M.J., & Bradsher, R.W. (2003). Cerebral histoplasmosis in the azole era: Report of four cases and review. *Southern Medical Journal, 96*, 410-416.

Wheat, L.J., & Kauffman, C.A. (2003). Histoplasmosis. *Infectious Disease Clinics of North America, 17*, 1-19.

44

Hookworm

Geographic Distribution

Hookworm is present in all tropical and subtropical areas of the world. Worldwide, about 1.2 billion people are infected and, in some areas, the prevalence is more than 50%. The two parasites that cause human hookworm disease, *Ancylostoma duodenale* and *Necator americanus,* have different geographic distributions: *A. duodenale* is more common in southern Europe, the north coast of Africa, northern India, northern China, and Japan, while *N. Americanus* predominates in western, central, and southern Africa, southern Asia, the Pacific islands, and the Caribbean (Chin, 2000; Gilles, 2003; Hotez et al., 2003; Sinuon, Anantaphruti, & Socheat, 2003; Verle et al., 2003).

Agent and Vector

Hookworms include the intestinal parasites *Ancylostoma duodenale, Necator americana,* and *Uncinaria stenocephala.* Only *A. duodenale* and *N. americanus* cause disease in man; *U. stenocephala* affects canines. Adult male *A. duodenale* worms measure 8 to 11 mm while females measure 10 to 13 mm; male *N. americanus* worms are 7 to 9 mm and females 9 to 11 mm. Hookworm filariform larvae are transmitted from soil through the skin. Three days after penetrating the skin and entering the circulation, the larvae reach the lungs where they break into the alveoli and migrate up the trachea, down the esophagus, and into the stomach and small intestine. During the migration they molt and, once attached to the mucosa of the small intestine, they mature into adults. Bleeding from the attachment site leaks into the lumen of the intestine at an estimated rate of

0.03 mL/day for *N. americanus* and 0.15 mL/day for
A. duodenale. After 3 to 5 weeks, the adult females produce
thousands of eggs each day that are shed in the stool to
continue the life cycle. Adult worms can live in the
intestine for up to 9 years, though most are shed after
1 to 2 years. *A. duodenale* differs from *N. americanus*
in that the larvae can also infect through ingestion
(Centers for Disease Control and Prevention [CDC],
1999; Gilles, 2003).

Incubation

The incubation period is 2 to 8 weeks or sometimes
longer (CDC, 1999).

Clinical Findings and Treatment

Signs and Symptoms

Symptoms are more likely to occur in infected travelers
and expatriates than indigenous people living in endemic
areas, most of whom are asymptomatic. Entry points are
sometimes pruritic with a rash that may become
secondarily infected. Respiratory symptoms occur in a
minority of patients when larvae migrate through the
lungs. Chronic infection causes iron-deficiency anemia
and hypoalbuminemia secondary to ongoing blood loss.
Fatigue is common in persons with light parasite loads,
while heavier loads lead to apathy, anorexia or increased
appetite, weight loss, shortness of breath, abdominal
discomfort, nausea and vomiting, diarrhea, and/or
constipation. On examination, patients may have pallor,
a flow murmur, and generalized edema (CDC, 1999;
Gilles, 2003; Sinuon et al., 2003).

Complications

High-output heart failure may occur in patients with
severe anemia. Chronic anemia in children can lead to
stunting and developmental delay. Massive

gastrointestinal bleeding has been observed in infants (Gilles, 2003).

Common Laboratory Findings

Chronic blood loss causes anemia with decreased serum iron and increased total iron-binding capacity. Occult blood can be detected in stool. Eosinophilia (up to 7% to 14% of white blood cells) may be seen, particularly in the acute pulmonary stage (Gilles, 2003).

Diagnosis

Hookworm should be suspected in all patients with iron-deficiency anemia and a history of travel or residence in an endemic area. The diagnosis is made by identifying eggs in a wet-mount of formalin-fixed stool sediment (CDC, 1999).

Differential Diagnosis

Light infections in travelers may cause eosinophilia and symptoms similar to other helminth infections such as schistosomiasis and strongyloidiasis. Because asymptomatic infection is prevalent among people living in endemic areas, the presence of hookworm does not necessarily mean that the infection is causing the presenting illness. Abdominal pain can resemble that of duodenal ulcers or pancreatitis. Edema from hypoproteinemia must be differentiated from nephrotic syndrome and kwashiorkor (Gilles, 2003).

Treatment

Treatment of the anemia with ferrous sulfate or ferrous gluconate should be the first priority, and can usually be done concurrently with antiparasitic therapy. Antiparasitic therapy is often only temporarily successful and yearly retreatment is standard in some locales. In children, even light asymptomatic infections with mild anemia should be treated. Both adults and children may be treated with a single dose of albendazole 400 mg PO. Mebendazole at a dose of 100 mg bid for 3 days or 500 mg once may also be used. Pyrantel pamoate 11 mg/kg (maximum 1 g) per day for 3 days is another option. None of these medications is safe in pregnancy, and safety data for mebendazole and albendazole in children younger than age 1 are lacking. There is evidence that hookworm infection results in host anergy and immune hyporesponsiveness, thus contributing to very high rates of reinfection after treatment with antihelmintic drugs (Gilles, 2003; Hotez et al., 2003; Medical Letter, 2002).

Prevention

The risk of infection can be reduced by wearing shoes, washing hands, drinking only filtered or treated water, and eating properly cooked food. At the community level, improved sanitation and disposal of human feces are the keys to control. Latrines may be helpful for control in areas without running water. Health education to improve hygiene practices is also important. Progress is being made toward a recombinant hookworm vaccine, though success is unlikely in the immediate future (Chin, 2000; Gilles, 2003; Hotez et al., 2003).

Reporting

The CDC does not consider hookworm to be a nationally notifiable disease. The World Health Organization (WHO) considers it a Class 5 disease. See Appendix C for details and for upcoming changes in WHO reporting.

References

Centers for Disease Control and Prevention. (1999). Hookworm. Retrieved December 18, 2003, from *www.cdc.gov/ncidod/dpd/parasites/hookworm/factsht_hookworm.htm*

Chin, J. (Ed.). (2000). *Control of communicable diseases manual* (17th ed., pp. 265-268). Washington, DC: American Public Health Association.

Gilles, H.M. (2003). Hookworm. In G.C. Cook & A.I. Zumla (Eds.), *Manson's tropical diseases* (21st ed., pp. 1539-1544). Philadelphia: W.B. Saunders Company.

Hotez, P.J., Zhan, B., Bethony, J.M., Loukas, A., Williamson, A., et al. (2003). Progress in the development of a recombinant vaccine for human hookworm disease: The Human Hookworm Vaccine Initiative. *International Journal of Parasitology, 33,* 1245-1258.

Medical Letter. (2002). Drugs for parasitic infections. Retrieved October 30, 2003, from *www.medletter.com/freedocs/parasitic.pdf*

Sinuon, M., Anantaphruti, M.T., & Socheat, D. (2003). Intestinal helminthic infections in schoolchildren in Cambodia. *Southeast Asian Journal of Tropical Medicine and Public Health, 34,* 254-258.

Verle, P., Kongs, A., De, N.V., Thieu, N.Q., Depraetere, K., et al. (2003). Prevalence of intestinal parasitic infections in northern Vietnam. *Tropical Medicine & International Health, 8,* 961-964.

HYMENOLEPIASIS

Geographic Distribution

Hymenolepiasis, an intestinal infection with small cestodes (tapeworms), occurs primarily in warm, dry areas of the Americas, Australia, the Mediterranean countries, the Middle East, and India. In some populations (such as slum-dwellers in India), prevalence rates approach 10% (Chin, 2000; Mirdha & Samantray, 2002).

Agent and Vector

Hymenolepis nana (the dwarf tapeworm) is the only human cestode without an obligatory intermediate host; that is, the worm's life cycle is completed without any species other than humans. *H. nana* is also known as *Vampirolepis nana*. The adult *H. nana* is 25 to 30 mm in length and is comprised of around 200 or fewer proglottids (segments). It is often spread by direct fecal-oral transmission of eggs, such as occurs among small children or institutionalized, mentally impaired adults; or less commonly through ingestion of eggs in contaminated food or water. Other means of transmission include ingestion of infected insects such as fleas on pet rodents. Autoinfection can also occur, which amplifies the infection. Humans may also be infected with *H. diminuta*, a rodent cestode.

The ingested egg is passed to the small intestine where the oncosphere (embryo) is released and penetrates the intestinal mucosa. Once there, it encysts within a villus and grows to the larval stage. The larva reenters the intestinal lumen and reattaches to the intestinal wall where it matures and begins to lay eggs (Baily, 2003; Chin, 2000; Peters & Pasvol, 2002).

Incubation

Onset of symptoms after infection varies, probably according to parasite load. In some cases there are mild or no symptoms. The development of the adult worm takes 2 weeks (Chin, 2000).

Clinical Findings and Treatment

Signs and Symptoms

Symptoms primarily result from mucosal damage. Light or moderate infections may be asymptomatic or there may be only vague abdominal discomfort. The most common manifestations are diffuse, persistent abdominal pain and anorexia. Loose bowel movements or diarrhea with mucus may also occur, as may headache, dizziness, sleep disturbances, and irritability (Baily, 2003; Schantz, Tanowitz, & Wittner, 2000).

Complications

Complications are rare. Children with heavy parasite loads may have behavior problems that respond to antiparasitic treatment. Seizures have also been reported (Schantz et al., 2000).

Common Laboratory Findings

Moderate eosinophilia is common (Schantz et al., 2000).

Diagnosis

Diagnosis is through microscopic identification of eggs in feces (Chin, 2000).

Differential Diagnosis

The differential diagnosis would include other causes of chronic diffuse abdominal pain.

Treatment

Treatment for adults and children is with praziquantel 25 mg/kg once (Medical Letter, 2002).

Prevention

Prevention includes all basic fecal-oral disease measures (Chin, 2000), including the following:

- Provide clean toilet facilities.
- Practice hand washing after defecation or exposure to feces.
- Protect food and water from fecal (human and rodent) contamination.
- Eliminate rodents, including pet rodents, from the home environment.
- Educate the public on personal hygiene measures to prevent this and other fecal-oral illnesses.

Reporting

The U.S. Centers for Disease Control and Prevention does not consider hymenolepiasis to be a nationally notifiable disease. The World Health Organization (WHO) considers it a Class 5 disease. See Appendix C for details and for upcoming changes in WHO reporting.

References

Baily, G.G. (2003). Other cestode infections: Intestinal cestodes, cysticercosis, other larval cestode infections. In G.C. Cook & A.I. Zumla (Eds.), *Manson's tropical diseases* (21st ed., pp. 1583-1597). Philadelphia: W.B. Saunders Company.

Chin, J. (Ed.). (2000). *Control of communicable diseases manual* (17th ed., pp. 268-270). Washington, DC: American Public Health Association.

Medical Letter. (2002). Drugs for parasitic infections. Author. Retrieved November 1, 2003, from *www.medletter.com/freedocs/parasitic.pdf*

Mirdha, B.R., & Samantray, J.C. (2002). *Hymenolepis nana*: A common cause of paediatric diarrhoea in urban slum dwellers in India. *Journal of Tropical Pediatrics, 48*, 331-334.

Peters, W., & Pasvol, G. (2002). *Tropical medicine and parasitology* (5th ed.). Philadelphia: Mosby.

Schantz, P.M., Tanowitz, H.B., & Wittner, M. (2000). Tapeworm infections. In G.T. Strickland (Ed.), *Hunter's tropical medicine and emerging infectious diseases* (8th ed., pp. 854-862). Philadelphia: W.B. Saunders Company.

46 LASSA FEVER

Geographic Distribution

— Lassa fever is endemic in West Africa, including Guinea, Liberia, Sierra Leone, and some areas of Nigeria. There is also serologic evidence of human infection in other African countries (Chin, 2000).

Agent and Vector

— The Lassa virus is a member of the Arenaviridae family of RNA viruses. It is a zoonosis carried by several species of the multimammate rat *Mastomys* and is transmitted to humans via ingestion or inhalation of food, dust, and other materials contaminated with rat excreta. The virus can also be spread from human to human via body fluids, including the aerosol route (Box 46-1).

Incubation

— The incubation period for Lassa fever is 1 to 3 weeks (Chin, 2000).

Clinical Findings and Treatment

Signs and Symptoms

— The presentation of Lassa fever is variable with 80% of patients having mild or no symptoms and 20% suffering severe multiorgan disease. Common early symptoms are gradual onset of fever, malaise, headache, and abdominal pain. A severe exudative pharyngitis may also be present. Other symptoms are conjunctivitis, facial swelling, nonproductive cough, retrosternal pain, nausea, vomiting, diarrhea, back pain, and myalgia. Tachypnea, tachycardia, and hypotension may be seen. Neurologic involvement may also occur, including hearing loss, tremors, and encephalitis. Hemorrhagic manifestations (seen in about 17% of patients) may include mucosal bleeding and, less frequently, conjunctival, gastrointestinal, or vaginal bleeding (Borio et al., 2002; Center for Infectious Disease Research and Policy [CIDRAP], 2003; Chin, 2000).

Complications

In addition to hemorrhagic manifestations, severe infections produce pleural and pericardial effusions and shock with end-organ failure. Among hospitalized patients, case fatality rates are around 15% to 25% (CIDRAP, 2003). Case fatality rates are particularly high for pregnant women in their third trimester, and fetal loss rates are around 95% (Centers for Disease Control and Prevention [CDC], 2003). Some degree of hearing loss, sometimes permanent, occurs in about a third of patients and is independent of the severity of illness. Transient alopecia during recovery has been observed.

Common Laboratory Findings

Leukopenia is occasionally seen, but usually white blood cell counts are normal or moderately increased (CIDRAP, 2003). Thrombocytopenia if present is mild, though platelet function may be decreased. Elevated liver enzymes, proteinuria, and increased hematocrit may occur.

Diagnosis

Clinical diagnosis is difficult because of the nonspecificity of symptoms. The illness should be suspected in patients with the preceding signs and symptoms and a history of travel in an endemic area, or history of exposure to known cases. The Working Group on Civilian Biodefense adapted the following criteria from World Health Organization (WHO) surveillance standards for hemorrhagic fever to identify a suspected index case of viral hemorrhagic fever (Borio et al., 2002):

- Acute onset of temperature above 101° F for less than 3 weeks duration

BIOTERRORISM CONSIDERATIONS
BOX 46–1

The viral hemorrhagic fevers (see separate chapter for an overview) are considered by the Centers for Disease Control and Prevention to be Category A biological warfare agents, thus posing a risk to national security because they "can be easily disseminated or transmitted from person to person; cause high mortality, with potential for major public health impact; might cause public panic and social disruption; and require special action for public health preparedness" (CDC, 2000, p. 5). "All are potentially infectious by the aerosol route and most are stable as respirable aerosols" (Cieslak & Eitzen, 2000, p. 28).

Lassa fever virus has been weaponized by the former Soviet Union, Russia, and the United States prior to 1969. The Working Group on Civilian Biodefense determined that Lassa fever poses a serious threat as a biological weapon. The absence of vaccines and specific treatments for viral hemorrhagic fevers such as Lassa fever make their medical and public health management very challenging in a mass casualty situation (Borio et al., 2002).

- Severe illness, no predisposing factors for hemorrhagic manifestations
- No established alternative diagnosis
- At least two of the following hemorrhagic symptoms: hemorrhagic or purple rash, epistaxis, hematemesis, hemoptysis, blood in stools, or other hemorrhagic symptom.

Laboratory diagnosis is by indirect fluorescent antibody tests or enzyme-linked immunosorbent assay (ELISA) detection of immunoglobulin M (IgM) (present during the acute phase of illness) or acute and convalescent IgG antibody titers. Antigen-capture ELISA has also been helpful for early detection of Lassa fever. The virus can also be isolated by culture from pleural fluid, throat swabs, urine, placental fluid, and, in patients with encephalitis, cerebrospinal fluid. Reverse transcriptase-polymerase chain reaction is possible but usually limited to research settings (CIDRAP, 2003).

Differential Diagnosis

Mild cases are similar to common self-limited viral syndromes. For patients with severe symptoms, consider also typhoid fever, typhus, leptospirosis, rickettsial spotted fever, malaria, and meningococcemia. Other conditions include hemolytic uremic syndrome, thrombotic thrombocytopenic purpura, idiopathic thrombocytopenic purpura, and acute leukemia.

Treatment

In more severe infections, give supportive care similar to that for other viral hemorrhagic fevers: Avoid intramuscular injections, minimize invasive procedures such as vascular catheters, use acetaminophen instead of nonsteroidal antiinflammatory drugs for fever and comfort, and do not give anticoagulants. Maintain fluid and electrolyte balance, and consider early transfer to an intensive care unit for hemodynamic monitoring and vasopressor support. Mechanical ventilation and dialysis may also be needed.

Ribavirin has been effective in some cases of Lassa fever, so some experts recommend that it be started immediately in suspected cases pending diagnostic confirmation, and discontinued if the infection is determined not to be an arenavirus or bunyavirus. Ribavirin is given as a slow initial intravenous loading dose of 30 mg/kg (maximum 2 g) followed by 16 mg/kg (maximum 1 g) every 6 hours for 4 days, and then by 8 mg/kg (maximum 500 mg) every 8 hours for 6 days. In a mass casualty setting, it may be given orally with a loading dose of 2000 mg, followed by 600 mg twice a day for 10 days; for patients weighing less than 75 kg, the dose is 1200 mg followed by 400 mg in the morning and 600 mg in the evening for 10 days. Pregnant women are given the adult dosage. Children are given 30 mg/kg once followed by 15 mg/kg per day in two divided doses for 10 days (Borio et al., 2002).

Prevention

People in endemic areas can reduce the risk of Lassa fever by avoiding rodents, sleeping on cots or ground covers, camping away from potential rodent dwellings, keeping food in rodent-proof containers, and not disturbing areas with rodent excreta. For confirmed or suspected cases the following measures (CDC, 2003; Chin, 2000) should be taken:

- Immediate strict barrier isolation is essential. Strict isolation extends to the patient's body fluids and excreta.
- Keep laboratory tests to a minimum and make laboratory staff aware of risks and ensure that they follow isolation procedures for specimens. Conduct testing in a high containment area; if such an area is not available, use gloves, mask, and a biological safety cabinet. Serum may be disinfected by heating at 140° F or 60° C for 1 hour.
- Place patients in isolation units or, at a minimum, private rooms away from traffic patterns. A negative-pressure room and respiratory protection are preferred.
- Disinfect or incinerate body fluids, excreta, and all objects with which the patient has had contact. Effective disinfectants include 0.5% sodium hypochlorite or 0.5% phenol with detergent. Equipment and other materials with which the patient has had contact may be autoclaved or boiled to disinfect.
- Male patients should abstain from sexual contact for 3 months or until semen is free from virus.

- Upon death, immediately seal deceased patients in a casket or other container and cremate or bury immediately.
- Conduct surveillance of close contacts in the 3 weeks after the onset of illness, monitoring for fever at least twice a day.

Provide community education on prevention and safety measures.

Reporting

The CDC considers hemorrhagic fevers to be nationally notifiable diseases. The WHO considers hemorrhagic fevers important diseases in public health (Class 2A). See Appendix C for details and for upcoming changes in WHO reporting.

References

Borio, L., Inglesby, T., Peters, C.J., Schmaljohn, A.L., Hughes, J.M., et al. (2002). Hemorrhagic fever viruses as biological weapons, medical and public health management. *Journal of the American Medical Association, 287*, 2391-2405.

Center for Infectious Disease Research and Policy. (2003). Viral hemorrhagic fever (VHF): Current, comprehensive information on pathogenesis, microbiology, epidemiology, diagnosis, treatment, and prophylaxis. Retrieved November 16, 2003, from *www.cidrap.umn.edu/cidrap/content/bt/vhf/biofacts/vhffactsheet.html*

Centers for Disease Control and Prevention. (2000). Biological and chemical terrorism: Strategic plan for preparedness and response. *Morbidity and Mortality Weekly Report, 49(RR-4)*, 1-14.

Centers for Disease Control and Prevention. (2003). Lassa fever. Retrieved November 16, 2003, from *www.cdc.gov/ncidod/dvrd/spb/mnpages/dispages/lassaf.htm*

Chin, J. (Ed.) (2000). *Control of communicable diseases manual* (17th ed., pp. 278-281). Washington, DC: American Public Health Association.

Cieslak, T.J., & Eitzen, E.M. (2000). Bioterrorism: Agents of concern. *Journal of Public Health Management Practice, 6*, 19-29.

47

LEISHMANIASIS

Espundia (mucocutaneous leishmaniasis), Kala-azar (visceral leishmaniasis)

Geographic Distribution

Leishmaniasis is widely distributed throughout the world and is present in 88 countries on four continents. The most heavily affected areas include East and North Africa, the Middle East, Southern Europe, Central, South, and East Asia, South America, and Southern Mexico. The majority of visceral leishmaniasis is found in Bangladesh, India, Nepal, Sudan, and Brazil (Dedet & Pratlong, 2003).

Agent and Vector

The protozoal parasite species *Leishmania* is transmitted through the bite of female phlebotomine sandflies, causing three forms of disease (Dedet & Pratlong, 2003; Magill, 2000; Peters & Pasvol, 2002):

- Visceral leishmaniasis, or kala-azar, is caused primarily by *L. donovani* (in Bangladesh, China, India, Nepal, Pakistan), *L. chagasi* (in South and Central America), and *L. infantum* (in the Mediterranean, Central Asia, China, and the Middle East). The reservoirs for these organisms include humans in *L. donovani* and primarily dogs and foxes in *L. chagasi* and *L. infantum*.
- Cutaneous leishmaniasis is usually divided into (1) Old World leishmaniasis caused primarily by *L. tropica* (in the Middle East, Mediterranean, and southwest Asia), *L. major* (in central and southwest Asia, the Middle East, and sub-Saharan Africa), and *L. aethiopica* (in Ethiopia and Kenya); and

(2) New World leishmaniasis caused primarily by
L. mexicana (in Central America, Texas, and Mexico)
or *L. braziliensis* (in South America). Diffuse cutaneous
leishmaniasis is caused primarily by *L. aethiopica* or
L. mexicana. The reservoirs for these organisms
include humans and dogs in *L. tropica*, rodents in
L. major, *L. mexicana*, and *L. braziliensis*, and the
hyrax in *L. aethiopica*.

• Mucocutaneous leishmaniasis (espundia) is a
complication of cutaneous leishmaniasis caused
primarily by *L. braziliensis*.

Altogether, about 20 leishmanial species are transmitted
by approximately 30 species of sandflies. Cases of
congenital transmission as well as transmission by blood
transfusion and sexual contact have been reported.

Incubation

The incubation period is usually 2 to 6 months, but can
range from days to years. Relapse may occur in as many
as 10 years after the first episode. Local trauma
sometimes activates latent infection in cutaneous
leishmaniasis (Dedet & Pratlong, 2003).

Clinical Findings and Treatment: Visceral Leishmaniasis

Signs and Symptoms

The cardinal signs of visceral leishmaniasis include fever,
anemia, weight loss, muscle wasting, and splenomegaly,
an early sign that is almost always present. A cutaneous
nodule may or may not appear at the site of the bite
within several days of inoculation. If present, the nodule
remains, but in most cases, no other symptoms are
present for at least several months. Patients raised in
endemic areas may remain asymptomatic, have
subclinical disease, or experience a gradual onset of
systemic symptoms with a fever that often rises and falls

two to three times per day, lasting for weeks, and
sometimes becoming low grade. For those not from
endemic areas, the onset of symptoms is often more
acute, with a fever that appears suddenly and lasts several
days. Other systemic symptoms are fatigue, weight loss,
dizziness, cough, and diarrhea. Visceral manifestations
include a sometimes markedly enlarged, firm, nontender
spleen; hepatomegaly is less frequent and not as
pronounced. Patients may also have generalized
lymphadenopathy. Dermatologic signs include pallor,
gray hyperpigmentation of the skin (especially in India),
and polymorphic, diffuse, warty, nonulcerated papules
and plaques (most commonly in Africa). As the disease
progresses over months or years, patients in the late
stages may develop hemorrhagic symptoms, jaundice,
ascites, and cachexia (Dedet & Pratlong, 2003;
Magill, 2000).

Complications

Without specific antimicrobial therapy, visceral
leishmaniasis is almost universally fatal, from progressive
wasting, bleeding or secondary infections (e.g., measles,
bacterial pneumonia, tuberculosis, diarrhea).
Post–kala-azar cutaneous leishmaniasis may occur up to
10 years after successful treatment of visceral leishmaniasis
(Figure 47-1). Lesions can resemble lepromatous leprosy
and include hypopigmented macules, papules, and
nodules that are initially located on the face and
subsequently spread to rest of the body. Leishmaniasis
may occur as an opportunistic infection in
immunocompromised patients and often has an
atypical presentation (Dedet & Pratlong, 2003).

Common Laboratory Findings

Laboratory findings include pancytopenia,
hypergammaglobulinemia, and occasional liver enzyme
elevation. Both erythrocyte sedimentation rate and

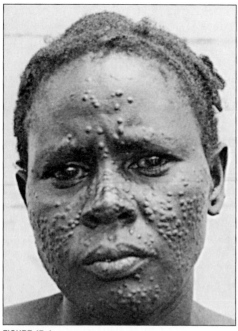

FIGURE 47–1

Nodular lesions of post–kala-azar dermal leishmaniasis. (*Source:* From Strickland, G.T. [2000]. *Hunter's tropical medicine and emerging infectious diseases* [8th ed., p. 675]. Philadelphia: W.B. Saunders Company.)

C-reactive protein may be elevated (Pearson, Jeronimo, & de Queiroz Sousa, 1999).

Diagnosis

Clinical presentation, in addition to living in or visiting an endemic area, leads to suspicion of leishmaniasis. The organism may be found in bone marrow, splenic aspirate (most sensitive), blood, and nasopharyngeal secretions. If parasites are present in sufficient concentration, light microscopy of Giemsa-stained slides reveals amastigotes, which are the tissue form of the parasite. Leishmania can be grown on Novy, MacNeal, Nicolle (NMN) medium, but cultures may take days to weeks to show a positive result. Direct agglutination and enzyme-linked immunosorbent assay (ELISA) are positive early. The intradermal leishmanin skin test, mostly useful in epidemiologic studies, turns positive weeks to months after active disease (Pearson et al., 1999).

Differential Diagnosis

The differential diagnosis of visceral leishmaniasis includes brucellosis, leprosy, schistosomiasis, trypanosomiasis (African), enteric fevers, malaria, histoplasmosis, lymphoma, leukemia, sarcoidosis, hepatic cirrhosis, tuberculosis, and bacterial endocarditis (Magill, 2000).

Treatment

Supportive care includes good nutrition and identification and treatment of secondary infections. Specific treatment has traditionally been unsatisfactory because of drug toxicity, poor response, multiple disease syndromes, and other factors including the emergence of antimony-resistant strains. Treatment is the same for adults and children. Orally administered miltefosine (100 mg/day or 2.5 mg/kg/day) for 4 weeks has recently shown great promise (cure rate of 95% at 6 months post-treatment) in the treatment of Indian visceral leishmaniasis. The treatment of choice at present is sodium stibogluconate, a pentavalent antimony compound (20 mg/kg/day IM or IV once daily) for 28 days, or 40 days if the disease is slow to respond or was contracted in India. Sodium stibogluconate is not FDA-approved and must be obtained from the U.S. Centers for Disease Control and Prevention (CDC).

Side effects of sodium stibogluconate include nausea, anorexia, malaise, headaches, lethargy, changes in liver function, elevations in serum lipase and amylase, electrocardiographic changes, musculoskeletal symptoms, thrombocytopenia, and anemia. Amphotericin B can be given as a second-line treatment (total IV dose of 6 to 20 mg/kg over 20 doses) as well as liposomal amphotericin B (3.0 mg/kg IV day 1, day 5, day 10). Other medications include IM pentamidine (2 to 4 mg/kg/day three times per week for 24 injections) or IM aminosidine (15 mg/kg/day for 30 days). Second-line medications (except for miltefosine) are sometimes given in combination with antimony compounds (Magill, 2000; Medical Letter, 2002; Melby, 2004).

Clinical Findings and Treatment: Cutaneous Leishmaniasis

Signs and Symptoms

The primary cutaneous lesion that develops at the site of inoculation starts as an erythematous papule and enlarges over several weeks. Mature lesions are typically painless, measure up to 10 cm in diameter, and are single or multiple, depending on the number of infecting bites. The most common lesion is the ulcerative type, which has an indurated border and a central crater (Figure 47-2). This is known as the "wet" lesion and is caused by *L. major* (oriental sore), *L. mexicana* (chiclero's ulcer), *L. peruviana* (uta), and *L. braziliensis*. The "dry" lesion is caused by *L. tropica* and is described as a papule or nodule with superficial scale. Low-grade fever, regional lymphadenopathy, lymphangitis, lesion pruritus, or pain may be present. In many cases, healing is spontaneous within months or years of onset. In other cases, however, the disease is progressive with visceral manifestations or spreading skin lesions (Dedet & Pratlong, 2003; Peters & Pasvol, 2002).

Complications

Diffuse cutaneous leishmaniasis is characterized by nonulcerating nodules and patches over the entire body,

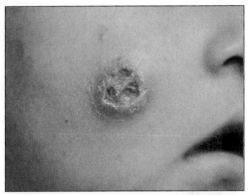

FIGURE 47–2

Ulcerated lesion in cutaneous leishmaniasis. (*Source:* From Bolognia, J.L., Jorizzo, J.L., & Rapini, R.P. [Eds.]. [2003]. *Dermatology* [p. 1298]. Philadelphia: Mosby.)

resembling lepromatous leprosy, and is usually associated with *L. mexicana* or *L. aethiopica* infection. Diffuse cutaneous leishmaniasis tends to be resistant to treatment. Leishmaniasis recidivans, due to *L. tropica* or *L. braziliensis*, is the recurrent, chronic form of leishmaniasis and usually presents as a continuously enlarging plaque on the face with central scarring. Cutaneous leishmaniasis may occur as an opportunistic infection in immunocompromised persons (Dedet & Pratlong, 2003; Peters & Pasvol, 2002). Mucocutaneous leishmaniasis is a sequela of New World cutaneous leishmaniasis and results from direct extension, hematogenous spread, or lymphatic metastasis to the nasal or oral mucosa. In most cases, naso-oropharyngeal symptoms appear several years after resolution of the primary lesion(s), but may also appear while the primary lesions are still present or decades later. Mucosal involvement usually starts in the nasal mucosa, and patients experience nasal congestion and/or epistaxis. The initial lesion is most often located in the anterior cartilaginous septum and leads to granulomatous destruction and perforation (Figure 47-3). The nose then appears flattened and the nasal tip is weighed down, leading to the classic "tapir nose." Other sites that may be affected at later stages include the buccal mucosa, palate, interior lips, and the larynx, which can cause death from airway obstruction. Mucocutaneous leishmaniasis can respond to treatment, but even when it is successful disfiguring facial scars may remain (Dedet & Pratlong, 2003; Peters & Pasvol, 2002).

Common Laboratory Findings

There are no specific laboratory findings characteristic of primary cutaneous leishmaniasis.

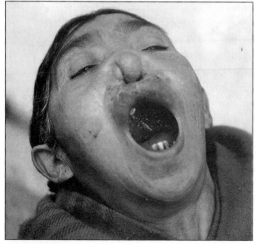

FIGURE 47–3

Partial destruction of nose, lip, and palate in mucocutaneous leishmaniasis. (*Source:* From Bolognia, J.L., Jorizzo, J.L., & Rapini, R.P. [Eds.]. [2003]. *Dermatology* [p. 1298]. Philadelphia: Mosby.)

Diagnosis

The clinical presentation and geographic risk lead to suspicion of leishmaniasis. The organism is present in histopathologic studies of slit skin smears or in cultures of ulcer aspirate, though neither technique is highly reliable. The leishmanin skin test is positive only after active disease (Dedet & Pratlong, 2003).

Differential Diagnosis

Numerous primary and secondary skin diseases, such as other tropical ulcers, impetigo, infected insect bites, leprosy, lupus vulgaris, tertiary syphilis, yaws, blastomycosis, and skin cancer, can mimic cutaneous leishmaniasis. For mucocutaneous leishmaniasis the differential diagnosis includes paracoccidioidomycosis, Wegener's granulomatosis, lymphoma, histoplasmosis, yaws, gummatous syphilis, tuberculosis, and nasopharyngeal carcinoma.

Treatment

Cutaneous leishmaniasis generally heals spontaneously in 6 to 12 months in immunocompetent patients. Treatment needs to be provided to immunocompromised patients, those at risk for mucosal leishmaniasis, patients with severe or obstructive lesions, and patients with metastatic skin lesions. First-line treatment is IM or IV sodium stibogluconate (20 mg/kg/day) for 20 days (adults and children). Alternative treatments include ketoconazole (400 to 600 mg/day) for 4 to 8 weeks, which is most effective against infection with *L. major* and *L. mexicana.* Topical treatment with 15% paromomycin and 12% methylbenzethonium has been used for Old World cutaneous leishmaniasis (Medical Letter, 2002; Melby, 2004; Pearson et al., 1999).

Prevention

The prevention of leishmaniasis (Chin, 2000; Darmstadt & Sidbury, 2004; Lane, 2003) includes the following:

- Control sandflies with residual-action insecticides; and eliminate or spray open trash heaps, stone walls, rodent holes, and other animal shelters. See Appendix D.
- Avoid exposure to sandflies during biting hours (usually sundown to sun-up and usually outdoors) in endemic areas. Use DEET-formulated insect repellant, and treat clothing with permethrin. Note, however, that some experts (Darmstadt & Sidbury, 2004) state that neither DEET nor permethrin is effective against sandflies.
- Avoid locating habitations in areas of heavy infestation. If such locations are unavoidable, practice increased vigilance and other prevention measures. In the New World, areas of infestation tend to be in forested areas, while in the Old World such areas tend to be dry and semiarid.
- Fine-mesh screens in homes are helpful, but are a luxury (as is insect repellent) in many of the endemic areas. Sandfly bed nets have very fine mesh and but are hot in tropical climates. Permethrin-impregnated mosquito nets offer some protection and are more comfortable to sleep under.
- Systematic case identification and prompt treatment help prevent complications and disability.
- Community education regarding these measures should be ongoing.

Reporting

The CDC does not consider leishmaniasis to be a nationally notifiable disease. The World Health Organization (WHO) considers it a Class 5 (no official report justified) disease. See Appendix C for details and for upcoming changes in WHO reporting.

References

Chin, J. (Ed.). (2000). *Control of communicable diseases manual* (17th ed., pp. 284-289). Washington, DC: American Public Health Association.

Darmstadt, G.L., & Sidbury, R. (2004). The skin. In R.E. Behrman, R.M. Kliegman, & H.B. Jenson (Eds.), *Nelson textbook of pediatrics* (17th ed., pp. 2153-2250). Philadelphia: W.B. Saunders Company.

Dedet, J.P., & Pratlong, F. (2003). Leishmaniasis. In G.C. Cook & A.I. Zumla (Eds.), *Manson's tropical diseases* (21st ed., pp. 1139-1161). Philadelphia: W.B. Saunders Company.

Lane, R.P. (2003). Family: Psychodidae; subfamily: Phlebotominae. In G.C. Cook & A.I. Zumla (Eds.), *Manson's tropical diseases* (21st ed., pp. 1733-1741). Philadelphia: W.B. Saunders Company.

Magill, A.J. (2000). Leishmaniasis. In G. Strickland (Ed.), *Hunter's tropical medicine and emerging infectious diseases* (8th ed., pp. 665-687). Philadelphia: W.B. Saunders Company.

Medical Letter. (2002). Drugs for parasitic infections. Retrieved October 8, 2003, from *www.medletter.com/freedocs/parasitic.pdf*

Melby, P.C. (2004). Leishmaniasis (Leishmania). In R.E. Behrman, R.M. Kliegman, & H.B. Jenson (Eds.), *Nelson textbook of pediatrics* (17th ed., pp. 1130-1133). Philadelphia: W.B. Saunders Company.

Pearson, R.D., Jeronimo, S.M, & de Queiroz Sousa, A. (1999). Leishmaniasis. In R.L. Guerrant, D.H. Walker, & P.F. Weller (Eds.), *Tropical infectious diseases: Principles, pathogens, and practice* (pp. 797-813). New York: Churchill Livingstone.

Peters, W., & Pasvol, G. (2002). *Tropical medicine & parasitology*. London: Mosby.

LEPROSY

Hansen's disease

Geographic Distribution

Approximately 2 to 3 million people worldwide are currently affected by active leprosy infection or postinfective sequelae. The most highly endemic areas include Africa, Asia, South America, and the Pacific. There are thousands of cases in the United States, with most occurring in immigrants; however, indigenous leprosy still exists in Texas, Louisiana, and Hawaii (Leprosy Group, World Health Organization [WHO], 2003; Meyers, 2000).

Agent and Vector

The method of transmission of the acid-fast bacilli that causes leprosy, *Mycobacterium leprae,* is not entirely known. Transmission is most likely via the respiratory route; however, other routes, such as via breaks in skin, have not been entirely dismissed. *M. leprae* has also been discovered in many animal reservoirs, such as armadillos, African chimpanzees, and monkeys, and this raises the possibility of a zoonotic source of infection (Leprosy Group, WHO, 2003; Meyers, 2000).

Incubation

The incubation period is usually 3 to 5 years but can range from a few weeks to more than 30 years (Leprosy Group, WHO, 2003).

Clinical Findings and Treatment

Signs and Symptoms

The type of leprosy acquired depends primarily on the immunologic response of the patient. Clinical and histopathologic features of leprosy exist on a spectrum, with lepromatous leprosy (Figure 48-1) at one end and tuberculoid leprosy at the other. Patients with characteristics of both types are classified as having borderline lepromatous, mid-borderline (Figure 48-2), or borderline tuberculoid leprosy. Those with vaguely defined (often early) lesions are classified as indeterminate. Initial and early skin lesions may be poorly defined anesthetic patches that are either hypopigmented or erythematous.

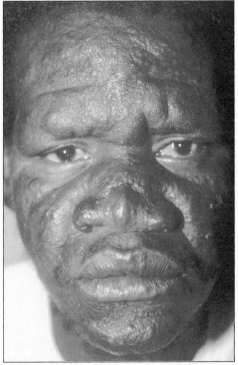

FIGURE 48–1

Lepromatous leprosy. (*Source:* From Bolognia, J.L., Jorizzo, J.L., & Rapini, R.P. [Eds.]. [2003]. *Dermatology* [p. 1149]. Philadelphia: Mosby.)

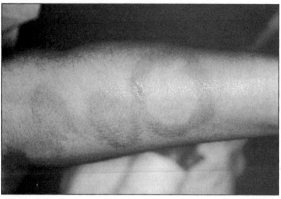

FIGURE 48–2

Borderline leprosy. (*Source:* From Bolognia, J.L., Jorizzo, J.L., & Rapini, R.P. [Eds.]. [2003]. *Dermatology* [p. 1148]. Philadelphia: Mosby.)

Most initial infections involve few symptoms and spontaneous recovery is common; however, a minority of patients develop clinical disease.

Lepromatous leprosy is a progressive process that occurs in persons with decreased cell-mediated immunity and often evolves from indeterminate or borderline leprosy. Bacilli are found in a variety of sites, including skin, nasal mucosa, nerves, lymph, liver, muscles, eyes, testes, and bone marrow. Early infection may demonstrate hypopigmented or slightly erythematous macules and patches, which eventually cover most of the body. If the infection is not treated at this stage, diffuse indurated plaques and nodules may develop. Cooler areas on the body are the most heavily affected, and these include the ears, face, extremities, and buttocks. Extensive induration and development of nodules on the face often leads to the characteristic "leonine facies." Loss of eyebrows, diminished body hair, thickened nerves, and sensory loss may also accompany this later stage of the disease. The nasal mucosa may become thickened and swollen, which can lead to ulceration and destruction. Nerve damage proceeds slowly, as opposed to the tuberculoid type. Later complications include symmetrical damage to facial, ulnar, median, lateral popliteal, and other nerves, resulting in decreased sensory and motor function; iritis, keratitis, and/or corneal damage; destructive bone lesions of the hands and feet; testicular atrophy and gynecomastia; and glomerulonephritis. Individuals from Central America or Mexico may present with a form of lepromatous leprosy known as Lucio leprosy. Infiltration of the skin is diffuse and is accompanied by an obstructive vasculitis (Lucio's phenomenon), which presents as infarcts and ulceration of the skin.

Tuberculoid leprosy is less malignant than lepromatous leprosy, and there is minimal to no deficiency in cell-mediated immunity. Skin lesions are anesthetic and include well-demarcated macules and plaques that range from less than 1 cm to large enough to cover entire body regions. The lesions are never diffuse and usually involve only one or a few areas. Tuberculoid leprosy lesions may heal spontaneously or continue to enlarge, leaving variously pigmented areas. Asymmetric peripheral nerve involvement is common and leads to gradual loss of sensation, especially in the hands, feet, and face. Nerve damage may eventually be accompanied by diminished ability to sweat in the affected area and loss of hair. Cutaneous nerves may be enlarged or tender.

Borderline leprosy is an unstable form of the disease that may have features of both lepromatous leprosy and tuberculoid leprosy, and can evolve into either form. Nerve damage tends to occur early and sensory (pain or anesthesia) or motor changes may be the presenting problem. Skin lesions can have characteristics of both tuberculoid leprosy and lepromatous leprosy. Lesions of borderline tuberculoid leprosy may resemble those of tuberculoid leprosy morphologically, but they are more numerous and less well defined. Skin lesions may also appear as annular plaques, small nodules, or bands.

Indeterminate leprosy is manifested by one or several poorly defined macules that may heal spontaneously, remain stable, or progress to the forms just described (Leprosy Group, WHO, 2003; Meyers, 1999, 2000; Sarkar, Kaur, Das, & Sharma, 1999).

Complications

Erythema nodosum leprosum is an antigen-antibody complex reaction, usually to therapy, which occurs in many patients with lepromatous and borderline lepromatous leprosy. Symptoms may occur before or during treatment and include acute onset of tender erythematous nodules, fever, iritis, and synovitis. Glomerulonephritis and secondary amyloidosis may also occur as part of erythema nodosum leprosum. Persons at greatest risk for erythema nodosum leprosum include those with lepromatous leprosy, skin infiltration or bacterial index > 4+ (10 to 100 bacilli per high power field), age younger than 40 years, and a previous episode of erythema nodosum leprosum. Reversal reactions, which are most frequent in borderline leprosy, are also a consequence of therapy. Reversal reactions can cause rapid irreversible nerve damage and must be quickly managed. Other features include swelling and increasing erythema of existing lesions, neuritis, and a transition of lesions to the tuberculoid type. Persons with the Lucio form of lepromatous leprosy are prone to developing septicemia, which may lead to death. Renal failure and hepatomegaly may result from secondary amyloidosis in long-standing disease. Advanced leprosy with disability and disfigurement is less common worldwide than in previous years and is essentially nonexistent in the Western world (Meyers, 1999, 2000).

Common Laboratory Findings

There are no common laboratory findings.

Diagnosis

Advanced lesions may be accurately diagnosed on
physical examination. The presence of hypoesthetic skin
lesions, enlarged cutaneous nerves, and acid-fast bacilli
on histopathologic exam allows for a definitive diagnosis.
Pathologists familiar with the histopathology of leprosy
are able to provide a diagnosis based on biopsies of
involved skin or nerves. Skin biopsies should be taken
from the edge of the lesion and extend down to
subcutaneous fat. Skin smears taken from the periphery
of multiple lesions, stained with Ziehl-Neelson, and
analyzed by experienced personnel can also lead to the
diagnosis. A negative skin smear does not rule out
leprosy because the test has a low sensitivity (but high
specificity). Serologic tests are available, and lepromatous
patients are usually positive; however, those with
tuberculoid leprosy and borderline tuberculoid leprosy
are more likely to be negative (Meyers, 1999;
Ustianowski & Lockwood, 2003).

Differential Diagnosis

The differential diagnosis of cutaneous leprosy, which
depends highly on the stage of the disease, includes
superficial fungal infections, postinflammatory pigment
changes, eczema, pellagra, syphilis, mycosis fungoides,
filariasis, granuloma annulare, leishmaniasis, lymphoma,
neurofibromatosis, lupus erythematosus, lupus vulgaris,
psoriasis, pityriasis rosea, yaws, and sarcoidosis. The
differential for peripheral nerve involvement includes
carpal tunnel syndrome, syringomyelia, lead toxicity,
diabetic neuropathy, primary amyloidosis, and familial
hypertrophic neuropathy (Leprosy Group, WHO, 2003;
Meyers, 1999).

Treatment

— Because of the development of dapsone resistance,
combination therapy is the currently accepted standard
for all types of leprosy. The length of treatment depends
on whether the patient has paucibacillary leprosy or
multibacillary leprosy.

— Multibacillary patients have more than three lesions or
have acid-fast bacilli positive skin smears at more than
one site, and include patients with borderline or
lepromatous leprosy. Patients with multibacillary leprosy
should be treated with a multiple-drug regimen such as
dapsone (100 mg daily for adults, 50 mg daily for
children ages 10 to 14), clofazimine (300 mg once a
month supervised and 50 mg daily self-administered,
150 mg once a month and 50 mg every other day for
children ages 10 to 14), and rifampin (600 mg once a
month supervised, 450 mg for children ages 10 to 14)
for at least 12 months.

— Paucibacillary patients have three or fewer lesions
without erythema or induration and no neuritis, and
include mostly patients with indeterminate or
tuberculous leprosy. These patients may be treated with
dapsone and rifampin (at the dosages just mentioned)
for 6 months.

— Minocycline, ofloxacin, and clarithromycin are
second-line drugs that can be used in patients who
cannot take rifampin because of liver disease or side
effects, clofazimine because of skin discoloration, or
dapsone because of toxicity. Clinical trials comparing
single-dose rifampin, ofloxacin, and minocycline to the
standard 6-month regimen for paucibacillary leprosy
patients have found the single-dose regimen to be
only a little less effective than standard treatment.

— Erythema nodosum leprosum and reversal reactions are
treated with prednisolone (1 mg/kg/day in children to a
maximum of 40 to 60 mg/day for adults) for several days

until improvement is seen and then tapered over several weeks. Erythema nodosum leprosum may also be treated with thalidomide (150 to 200 mg bid) for several days and then tapered over several weeks. Chronic erythema nodosum leprosum can be treated with thalidomide as well but can be tapered to a maintenance dose (50 to 100 mg at bedtime). Thalidomide is absolutely contraindicated in pregnancy (Leprosy Group, WHO, 2003; Rosenblatt, 1999; Ustianowski & Lockwood, 2003).

Prevention

Early detection and treatment is the best method of control and prevention. The efficacy of drug prophylaxis in close contacts has not been clearly demonstrated, and the use of rifampicin, ofloxacin, and minocycline is being investigated. The development of a vaccine is currently under way (Meyers, 2000; Ustianowski & Lockwood, 2003).

Reporting

The U.S. Centers for Disease Control and Prevention considers leprosy to be a nationally notifiable disease. In some cases leprosy excludes a person from immigrating to the United States. The WHO considers leprosy a disease important in public health (Class 2B). See Appendix C for details and for upcoming changes in WHO reporting.

References

Leprosy Group, WHO. (2003). Leprosy. In G.C. Cook & A.I. Zumla (Eds.), *Manson's tropical diseases* (21st ed., pp. 1065-1084). Philadelphia: W.B. Saunders Company.

Manandhar, R., LeMaster, J.W., & Roche, P.W. (1999). Risk factors for erythema nodosum leprosum. *International Journal of Leprosy and Other Mycobacterial Diseases, 67,* 270-278.

Meyers, W.M. (1999). Leprosy. In R.L. Guerrant, D.H. Walker, & P.F. Weller (Eds.), *Tropical infectious diseases: Principles, pathogens, and practice* (pp. 474-485). New York: Churchill Livingstone.

Meyers, W.M. (2000). Leprosy. In G.T. Strickland (Ed.), *Hunter's tropical medicine* (8th ed., pp. 513-523). Philadelphia: W.B. Saunders Company.

Rosenblatt, J.E. (1999). Antiparasitic agents. *Mayo Clinic Proceedings, 74*, 1161-1175.

Sarkar, R., Kaur, I., Das, A., & Sharma, V.K. (1999). Macular lesions in leprosy: A clinical, bacteriological, and histopathological study. *Journal of Dermatology, 26*, 569-576.

Ustianowski, A.P., & Lockwood, D.N. (2003). Leprosy: Current diagnostic and treatment approaches. *Current Opinions in Infectious Disease, 16*, 421-427.

LEPTOSPIROSIS

Canicola disease, Fort Bragg fever, Japanese autumnal fever, swineherd's disease, Weil's disease

Geographic Distribution

Leptospirosis has a worldwide distribution, with the highest prevalence in Latin America and Southeast Asia (Watt, 2000).

Agent and Vector

Leptospira interrogans is a motile spirochete that has more than 200 serovars. Different serovars seem to have a predilection for different hosts and geographical distribution. Infection by one serovar does not confer immunity to attacks by other serovars. The three most common serovars that cause leptospirosis are *Leptospira icterohaemorrhagiae* (carried by rats and causing the most severe form of leptospirosis), *L. canicola* (carried by dogs), and *L. pomona* (carried by cattle and swine). Infection is acquired via ingestion of food contaminated by infected urine or through contact of skin (especially abrasions) or mucous membranes with contaminated water, soil, or vegetation. High-risk occupations in endemic areas include sugar, rice, and rubber plantation workers, fish and poultry processors, butchers, and sewer workers. Other environments ideal for disease transmission are common in Asia: flooded rice fields, jungle swamps, and large cities with extensive rat populations that flood during rainy seasons (Chin, 2000; Scott & Coleman, 2003; Watt, 2000).

Incubation

‾ The incubation period is 2 to 26 days with an average of 7 to 12 days (Shieh, Edwards, Spiegal, & Zaki, 1999).

Clinical Findings and Treatment

Signs and Symptoms

‾ The degree of illness in leptospirosis varies from asymptomatic to severe or fatal. The most common forms are (1) anicteric and (2) icteric, or Weil's syndrome. Anicteric leptospirosis is the more common and milder form and often is biphasic. The first phase is characterized most frequently by sudden onset of high fever with chills, headache, cough, chest pain, abdominal pain, nausea, vomiting, and myalgias which often involve the muscles of the calves, abdomen, and paraspinal regions. Conjunctival suffusion is the most characteristic sign during this phase and is defined by a bulbar conjunctival redness that decreases in intensity toward the cornea and is not associated with pus or serous secretion (Figure 49-1). This sign is typically seen 2 to 3 days after the onset of fever. Other signs include lymphadenopathy, pharyngeal injection, hepatomegaly, and/or splenomegaly. A rash may be present that varies in clinical presentation from pretibial erythema nodosum-like lesions in Fort Bragg fever to transient urticaria, erythematous macules or papules, or purpura.

‾ In some cases, the illness resolves after about 1 week with no further manifestations. In other cases, the illness recurs in its second (immune) phase within 2 to 3 days. Second phase symptoms are more varied than in the first phase, but the hallmark is aseptic meningitis. The second phase usually lasts for several days, but it may persist for weeks. The fever tends to be milder, and gastrointestinal symptoms and myalgias are less severe. Uveitis is a late manifestation of leptospirosis and is usually seen after 4 to 8 months.

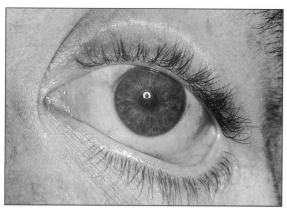

FIGURE 49–1

Subconjunctival hemorrhage in leptospirosis. (*Source:* From Peters, W., & Pasvol, G. [2002]. *Tropical medicine and parasitology* [5th ed., p. 172]. Chicago: Mosby.)

Icteric leptospirosis is the more severe form, with first and second phases that are less distinct. These patients develop persistent high fever, with subsequent deterioration and development of jaundice, hepatic dysfunction, myocarditis, decreased renal function, pulmonary complications, and hemorrhagic manifestations. Renal failure due to acute tubular necrosis may occur in the second week of illness but does not usually require dialysis. Early recognition of renal failure is critical to patient survival, and complete anuria is a poor prognostic sign. Pulmonary involvement may be characterized by infiltrates, cough, dyspnea, hemoptysis, and/or chest pain. Decreased hepatic function and jaundice are common, but hepatic failure is seldom a cause of death. On the other hand, jaundice is a poor prognostic sign as almost all deaths occur in jaundiced patients. Hemorrhagic manifestations include epistaxis, bleeding gums, purpura, petechiae, and, less frequently, gastrointestinal, pulmonary, and subarachnoid hemorrhage. (Chin, 2000; Jacobs, 1999; Scott & Coleman, 2003; Shieh et al., 1999; Speelman, 1998; Watt, 2000).

Complications

— In addition to the complications mentioned earlier, leptospirosis can be associated with acute respiratory distress syndrome, cerebral arteritis, pancreatitis, and disturbances in vision. Death is usually caused by renal failure, myocarditis, adrenal failure, hemorrhage, or cerebral artery thrombosis (Scott & Coleman, 2003).

Common Laboratory Findings

— Common laboratory findings in anicteric leptospirosis include low, normal, or elevated white blood cell count with neutrophilia, elevated erythrocyte sedimentation rate, elevated creatine phosphokinase and aldolase, anemia, proteinuria, pyuria, and hematuria. Lumbar puncture during the second phase may reveal changes consistent with aseptic meningitis, including normal glucose, normal to mildly elevated protein, early predominance of neutrophils, and late (after 7 days) predominance of lymphocytes.

— Laboratory findings in icteric leptospirosis are nonspecific but may include leukocytosis with neutrophilia, anemia, thrombocytopenia, elevated bilirubin and liver transaminases (up to three times the upper limit of normal), elevated erythrocyte sedimentation rate, elevated creatine phosphokinase, bilirubin and urobilinogen in the urine, proteinuria, pyuria, hematuria, and a rise in prothrombin time (Jacobs, 1999; Scott & Coleman, 2003; Speelman, 1998; Watt, 2000).

Diagnosis

— The diagnosis should be considered in patients with a flu-like illness with severe myalgias and conjunctival suffusion, particularly if the illness is biphasic with jaundice or aseptic meningitis, or if there is occupational or other exposure to contaminated water or infected urine. The Centers for Disease Control and Prevention (CDC) laboratory criteria for the diagnosis of leptospirosis are (1) isolation of leptospires from a clinical specimen, or (2) fourfold or greater increase in agglutination titer between acute and convalescent phases with serum specimens taken at least 2 weeks apart, or (3) demonstration of leptospires in a specimen with immunohistochemistry or immunofluorescence. Leptospires can be isolated from blood and cerebrospinal fluid during the first 10 days of the illness, but they may be found in the urine from the second week to several months after beginning of the illness. Isolation of the organisms requires special media, such as Fletcher's or EMJH semisolid media. Other tests include enzyme-linked immunosorbent assay (ELISA), complement fixation test, and polymerase chain reaction (PCR) assays (Shieh et al., 1999; Watt, 2000).

Differential Diagnosis

For anicteric leptospirosis, the principal differential diagnosis includes aseptic meningitis related to other entities, fever of unknown origin, influenza, appendicitis, and gastroenteritis. For icteric leptospirosis, the principal differential diagnosis includes viral hepatitis, malaria, typhoid fever, scrub typhus, dengue fever, and hantavirus infection (Watt, 2000).

Treatment

Leptospirosis responds best to treatment if started early in the illness; hence, treatment should be started as soon as the diagnosis is suspected. Anicteric or mild leptospirosis is treated with doxycycline 100 mg PO bid for 7 days or ampicillin 500 to 750 mg PO qid or amoxicillin 500 mg PO qid. Icteric or anicteric (moderate to severe) leptospirosis is treated with IV penicillin G 1.5 million units qid or IV ampicillin 1 g qid or IV amoxicillin 1 g qid or IV erythromycin 500 mg qid. The recommended treatment for children is with penicillin G 6 to 8 million units/m²/24 hours divided q4h IV for 7 days. Tetracycline 10 to 20 mg/kg/24 hours divided qid PO or IV for 7 days is the alternative for children older than 8 years. During therapy the release of toxic products from killed spirochetes can cause Jarisch-Herxheimer reactions characterized by fever, hypotension, rigors, headache, and myalgias. The reaction occurs usually within 24 hours of the start of therapy and subsides approximately 24 hours later. Therapy is continued unless symptoms are severe. Supportive care for leptospirosis includes careful attention to fluid and electrolyte balance, dialysis if necessary for renal failure, and transfusions as needed for severe anemia (Azimi, 2004; Chin, 2000; Sehgal, Sugunan, Murhekar, Sharma, & Vijayachari, 2000; Speelman, 1998).

Prevention

Prophylaxis with doxycycline 200 mg/week may be effective in preventing infection in those who may be at high risk for a short period of time. Vaccines have been developed against regional serovars and are used in domestic animals; however, despite occasional use in high-risk populations, their efficacy has not been conclusively demonstrated in humans. Moreover, vaccination of animals prevents illness, but not necessarily infection and infectiousness. Other preventive measures (Chin, 2000; Scott & Coleman, 2003; Watt, 2000) include the following:

- Avoid contact with contaminated water.
- Provide protective clothing for workers in high-risk agricultural, animal or meat production, or sewer-related occupations.

- Eliminate rodents in habitations and agricultural areas as much as is practical. Elimination of rubbish helps reduce the rodent population.
- Burn off cane fields before harvest, which markedly decreases sharp leaves and thus inoculation, but does not affect the canes themselves.

Readers will note that these measures are not always practical, for example, rice farmers are unlikely to wear boots and other protective clothing. Nevertheless, the disease can be reduced by instituting at least some or even partial measures and ongoing community education.

Reporting

The CDC does not consider leptospirosis to be a nationally notifiable disease. The World Health Organization (WHO) considers leptospirosis a disease important in public health (Class 2B). See Appendix C for details and for upcoming changes in WHO reporting.

References

Azimi, P. (2004). Leptospira. In R.E. Behrman, R.M. Kliegman, & H.B. Jenson (Eds.), *Nelson textbook of pediatrics* (17th ed., pp. 983-985). Philadelphia: W.B. Saunders Company.

Chin, J. (Ed.) (2000). *Control of communicable diseases manual* (17th ed., pp. 293-296). Washington, DC: American Public Health Association.

Jacobs, R.A. (1999). Infectious diseases: Spirochetal. In L.M. Tierney, S.J. McPhee, & M.A. Papadakis (Eds.), *Current medical diagnosis & treatment* (14th ed., pp.1332-1352). Stamford, CT: Appleton & Lange.

Scott, G., & Coleman, T.J. (2003). Leptospirosis. In G.C. Cook & A.I. Zumla (Eds.), *Manson's tropical diseases* (21st ed., pp. 1165-1171). Philadelphia: W.B. Saunders Company.

Sehgal, S.C., Sugunan, A.P., Murhekar, M.V., Sharma, S., & Vijayachari, P. (2000). Randomized controlled trial of doxycycline prophylaxis against leptospirosis in an endemic area. *International Journal of Antimicrobial Agents, 13*, 249-255.

Shieh, W-J., Edwards, C., Spiegal, R., & Zaki, S.R. (1999). Leptospirosis. In R.L. Guerrant, D.H. Walker, & P.F. Weller (Eds.), *Tropical infectious diseases: Principles, pathogens, and practice* (pp. 626-636). New York: Churchill Livingstone.

Speelman, P. (1998). Leptospirosis. In A.S. Fauci, E. Braunwald, K.J. Isselbacher, J.D. Wilson, J.B. Martin, et al. (Eds.), *Harrison's principles of internal medicine* (14th ed., pp. 1036-1038). New York: McGraw-Hill.

Watt, G. (2000). Leptospirosis. In G.T. Strickland (Ed.), *Hunter's tropical medicine* (8th ed., pp. 452-458). Philadelphia: W.B. Saunders Company.

50

LICE, HEAD

Geographic Distribution

— Head lice infestations occur throughout the world and can affect people of any age, race, or socioeconomic background. Head lice are more common in children, especially girls and those with long hair (Meinking, Burkhart, & Burkhart, 2003; Roberts, 2002; Wendel & Rompalo, 2002).

Agent and Vector

— Human head lice is caused by an infestation of the scalp with *Pediculus humanus capitis*, and transmission occurs by direct head-to-head contact or direct transfer with fomites. The adult louse is approximately 2 to 3 mm long and usually lives and lays eggs close to the scalp, except in warm climates. The female louse lives approximately 2 to 4 weeks and lays 50 to 150 eggs during her lifetime. The nits (eggs) are cemented to the hair, attached at an acute angle, and hatch within 1 week. Lice usually only survive a few hours off the host (Ko & Elston, 2004).

Incubation

— Incubation for lice may be anywhere from days to months. With the initial infection, symptoms may not develop for weeks; however, symptoms in subsequent infections may occur within 1 to 2 days since the individual has been sensitized (Meinking et al., 2003).

Clinical Findings and Treatment

Signs and Symptoms

— The clinical findings of head lice are confined to the scalp, neck, and area around the hair line. Patients often

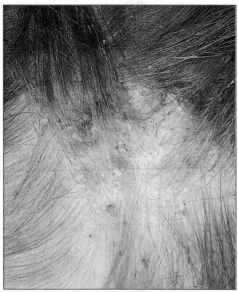

FIGURE 50–1

Pediculosis capitis. (*Source:* From Habif, T.P. [1996]. *Clinical dermatology* [4th ed., p. 507]. Chicago: Mosby.)

develop intense pruritus, excoriations, erythema, and/or scaling of the scalp and posterior neck (Figure 50-1). Other common manifestations include bite reactions (erythematous papules or wheals) on the surrounding skin, cervical lymphadenopathy, and conjunctivitis. Nits are seen attached to the hairs and may remain visible after infection is controlled, moving away from the scalp with the growth of the hair (Ko & Elston, 2004; Meinking et al., 2003; Roberts, 2002).

Complications

Complications of head lice include bacterial superinfection, fevers, or hypersensitivity reactions, which may mimic a viral exanthem, eczema, or urticaria

(Ko & Elston, 2004; Meinking et al., 2003; Wendel & Rompalo, 2002).

Common Laboratory Findings

— There are no common laboratory findings associated with head lice.

Diagnosis

— The diagnosis of head lice can be made when crawling lice are identified on head hair or are combed from the scalp. Louse combs can be a helpful tool in identifying lice, especially since lice crawl quickly and avoid light. Nits alone do not signify active infection; however, the likelihood is greater when they are very close to the scalp (Ko & Elston, 2004).

Differential Diagnosis

— Many entities resemble the nits found in head lice, including hair casts (pseudonits), debris from hairspray, flakes of seborrheic dermatitis, and psocids, which are louse-like insects that rarely cause infestations of the human scalp. Hair casts are formed by incomplete shedding of a portion of the hair shaft, thus creating a freely movable ring of keratin around the hair. This allows distinction from nits, which are firmly attached to one side of the hair. The superficial fungi that cause black and white piedra, *Piedraia hortae* and *Trichosporon beigelii*, can mimic head lice since they form concretions along the hair shaft (Ko & Elston, 2004).

Treatment

— Head lice can be treated with several topical therapies, including permethrin, lindane, malathion, and pyrethrins. All of these treatments are used by applying the medication to the dry scalp for 5 to 10 min (except for malathion, which is applied for 8 to 12 hours), rinsing the area, and repeating the treatment in 1 week.

Nits can be removed by combing through the hair with a fine-toothed comb. Resistance to permethrin is growing, and malathion treatment is indicated for treatment failure or resistant cases. Ivermectin (200 mcg/kg PO, repeated in 10 days) may also be an effective treatment (Jones & English, 2003; Ko & Elston, 2004; Nash, 2003; Orion, Matz, Ruocco, & Wolf, 2002; Roberts, 2002; Yoon et al., 2003).

Prevention

To avoid reinfection with lice, bed linens, towels, and clothing need to be washed during the treatment. Family members need not be treated except in cases of persistent mass infestations. The primary means of preventing lice is avoiding close contact with those who are infested (Elston, 2002; Wendel & Rompalo, 2002).

Reporting

The U.S. Centers for Disease Control and Prevention does not consider head lice to be a nationally notifiable disease. The World Health Organization (WHO) classifies head lice as a Class 5 disease. See Appendix C for details and for upcoming changes in WHO reporting.

References

Elston, D.M. (2002). Controversies concerning the treatment of lice and scabies. *Journal of the American Academy of Dermatology, 46,* 794-796.

Jones, K.N., & English, J.C., III. (2003). Review of common therapeutic options in the United States for the treatment of pediculosis capitis. *Clinical Infectious Diseases, 36,* 1355-1361.

Ko, C.J., & Elston, D.M. (2004). Pediculosis. *Journal of the American Academy of Dermatology, 50,* 1-12.

Meinking, T.L., Burkhart, C.N., & Burkhart, C.G. (2003). Infestations. In J.L. Bolognia, J.L. Jorizzo, & R.P. Rapini (Eds.), *Dermatology* (pp. 1321-1349). Philadelphia: Mosby.

Nash B. (2003). Treating head lice. *British Medical Journal, 326,* 1256-1257.

Orion, E., Matz, H., Ruocco, V., & Wolf, R. (2002). Parasitic skin infestations II, scabies, pediculosis, spider bites: Unapproved treatments. *Clinics in Dermatology, 20,* 618-625.

Roberts, R.J. (2002). Clinical practice. Head lice. *New England Journal of Medicine, 346,* 1645-1650.

Wendel, K., & Rompalo, A. (2002). Scabies and pediculosis pubis: An update of treatment regimens and general review. *Clinical Infectious Diseases, 35* (Suppl 2), S146-151.

Yoon, K.S., Gao, J.R., Lee, S.H., Clark, J.M., Brown, L., & Taplin, D. (2003). Permethrin-resistant human head lice, *Pediculus capitis,* and their treatment. *Archives of Dermatology, 139,* 994-1000.

51

LYME DISEASE

Lyme borreliosis

Geographic Distribution

Lyme disease is found in the United States, Canada, Europe, the Balkans, and from the Balkan sea heading east through Russia and continuing to the Pacific coast of Asia in the region of China and Korea (Dennis & Strickland, 2000).

Agent and Vector

Lyme disease is caused by the spirochete *Borrelia burgdorferi*, which is usually transmitted to humans by the *Ixodes scapularis* (hard) tick. The tick acquires the bacteria by feeding on infected hosts, usually deer and rodents, and then passing the infection on to humans through its saliva. The risk of transmitting the bacteria becomes significant after the tick has been attached for at least 48 hours. Such long attachment times are not uncommon because *Ixodes* ticks require hours to fully implant and days to become fully engorged (Blume, Levine, & Heymann, 2003).

Incubation

The incubation period is usually 1 week, but the primary rash associated with Lyme disease (erythema chronicum migrans) may not appear for up to 4 months (Singh-Behl, La Rosa, & Tomecki, 2003).

Clinical Findings and Treatment

Signs and Symptoms

The clinical presentation and characteristics of the infection can be divided into three categories: early localized infection, early disseminated infection, and late infection.

— Erythema chronicum migrans is the most prominent feature of early localized infection and can be described as a slowly expanding annular erythematous plaque, which can also be vesicular, edematous, or crusted (Figures 51-1A and B). Erythema chronicum migrans is present in approximately three-quarters of symptomatic patients and may be present along with fever, fatigue, anorexia, myalgias, arthralgias, and regional lymphadenopathy.

— Early disseminated infection may occur weeks after the initial localized infection. Patients may experience severe malaise, fatigue, and migratory joint and muscle pain. Multiple secondary lesions of erythema chronicum migrans occur in the minority of patients, and borrelial lymphocytomas, which appear as blue-red nodules or plaques on the earlobes of children or nipples of adults, may be seen in this stage. The most common neurologic feature is a cranial neuropathy (usually cranial nerve VII), which presents as unilateral or bilateral facial paralysis. Other neurologic signs and symptoms may include aseptic meningitis, motor or sensory radiculoneuritis, or encephalopathy. A rare manifestation of this stage of disease is atrioventricular block.

— Late disease can occur weeks to months after an untreated infection. The most common symptom in this stage is intermittent arthritis of one or more large weight-bearing joints. Acrodermatitis chronica atrophicans is a late skin manifestation that is biphasic in nature and presents as erythematous plaques and nodules on the distal extremities. Eventually, after weeks to years, these areas become atrophic and fibrous. Other possible manifestations at this stage include chronic encephalopathy, encephalomyelitis, paresthesias, and keratitis (Blume, Levine, & Heymann, 2003; Dennis & Strickland, 2000; Singh-Behl et al., 2003).

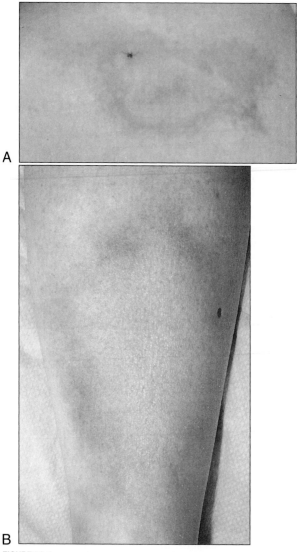

FIGURE 51–1

Erythema chronicum migrans. (*Source:* **A,** Courtesy of the University of Texas Southwestern Department of Dermatology. **B,** From Habif, T.P. [1996]. *Clinical dermatology* [3rd ed., p. 466]. Chicago: Mosby.)

Complications

— Early disseminated and late disease are complications of untreated or misdiagnosed early localized Lyme disease. Persistent symptoms after adequate treatment can sometimes occur and may be due to residual tissue inflammation, permanent tissue damage, postinfectious autoimmune response, residual infection, or misdiagnosis. Arthritis and neurologic symptoms, such as encephalopathy, are the most likely to be persistent. Potentially serious cardiac complications include ventricular conduction defects, atrioventricular block, and myopericarditis. (Dennis & Strickland, 2000; Singh-Behl et al., 2003).

Common Laboratory Findings

— None.

Diagnosis

— Diagnosis can be made clinically through the presence of erythema chronicum migrans in a patient from an endemic area, especially if they give the history of a recent tick bite. Serologic testing can be done when the diagnosis is not definitive and involves using enzyme-linked immunosorbent assay (ELISA) or Western blot to determine the presence of immunoglobulin M (IgM) and IgG antibodies to *B. burgdorferi*. IgM titers typically peak 3 to 6 weeks after the onset of illness but can be detected after 2 weeks; IgG titers are usually evident after 6 weeks. The sensitivity of serologic testing increases with the development of disseminated or late disease. The organism may also be isolated from the culture of a skin biopsy taken from an erythema chronicum migrans lesion. Polymerase chain reaction has been developed for the detection of *B. burgdorferi*, but the sensitivity is less than that of skin biopsy culture and the test is not easily obtained (Dennis & Strickland, 2000).

Differential Diagnosis

The initial febrile illness may be confused with influenza, infectious mononucleosis, Rocky Mountain spotted fever, babesiosis, or ehrlichiosis. The rash of erythema chronicum migrans may also resemble cellulitis or allergic contact dermatitis. Cranial nerve palsies can develop secondary to other viral illnesses, Bell's palsy, or may be idiopathic. Other causes of encephalopathy that may mimic the symptoms of Lyme disease include viral illnesses, multiple sclerosis, and amyotrophic lateral sclerosis. The severe myalgias, arthralgias, and fatigue that come with later disease may be similar to connective tissue diseases, such as systemic lupus erythematosus, dermatomyositis, or rheumatoid arthritis (Dennis & Strickland, 2000).

Treatment

Early disease in adults should be treated with doxycycline 100 mg bid for 2 to 3 weeks. An alternate regimen for children or pregnant women consists of amoxicillin 500 mg tid or 25 to 50 mg/kg/day divided tid for 2 to 3 weeks. Children may also be given cefuroxime 30 mg/kg/day in two divided doses or erythromycin 30 mg/kg/day in three divided doses, both for 2 to 3 weeks. Patients with severe neurologic, cardiac, or joint disease can be treated with intravenous ceftriaxone 2 g/day or penicillin G 20 to 24 million units/day for 2 to 4 weeks (Shapiro, 2004; Singh-Behl et al., 2003).

Prevention

Vaccinations for Lyme disease are available for dogs, and the outer-surface protein A (OspA) Lyme disease vaccine has been shown to be safe in humans. Other preventive measures (Nadelman et al., 2001; Shapiro, 2004; Singh-Behl et al., 2003) include the following:
- Avoid tick-infested areas.

- Wear protective permethrin-treated clothing and use insect repellent (DEET) on exposed skin when in potentially tick-infested areas. It is easier to see ticks on light-colored clothing.
- After leaving tick-infested areas, check the entire body, including creases, for ticks and remove them. Removal of a feeding tick is accomplished by using blunt-tipped forceps to grasp the tick as close to the skin as possible, then lifting away from the skin with steady, straight traction; take care not to leave the head embedded in the skin. Wash hands after touching ticks, and thoroughly wash the attachment site with antiseptic solution.
- Environmental control can be accomplished by removing wood piles and clearing trees in residential areas.
- In persons older than 8 years, a single 200-mg dose of doxycycline given within 72 hours after an *Ixodes* tick bite may prevent Lyme disease.

- Provide ongoing community education in endemic areas on the preceding points.

Reporting

- The U.S. Centers for Disease Control and Prevention considers Lyme disease to be a nationally notifiable disease. The World Health Organization (WHO) considers it a Class 3B disease. See Appendix C for details and for upcoming changes in WHO reporting.

References

Blume, J.E., Levine, E.G., & Heymann, W.R. (2003). Bacterial diseases. In Bolognia, J.L., Jorizzo, J.L., & Rapini, R.P. (Eds.), *Dermatology* (pp. 1138-1140). Philadelphia: Mosby.

Dennis, D.T., & Strickland, G.T. (2000). Lyme disease. In G.T. Strickland (Ed.), *Hunter's tropical medicine* (8th ed., pp. 458-465). Philadelphia: W.B. Saunders Company.

Nadelman, R.B., Nowakowski, J., Fish, D., Falco, R.C., Freeman, K., et al. (2001). Prophylaxis with single-dose doxycycline for the prevention of Lyme disease after an *Ixodes scapularis* tick bite. *New England Journal of Medicine, 345,* 79-84.

Shapiro, E.D. (2004). Lyme disease (*Borrelia burgdorferi*). In R.E. Behrman, R.M. Kliegman, & H.B. Jenson (Eds.), *Nelson textbook of pediatrics* (17th ed., pp. 986-990). Philadelphia: W.B. Saunders Company.

Singh-Behl, D., La Rosa, S.P., & Tomecki, K.J. (2003). Tick-borne infections. *Dermatology Clinics, 21,* 237-239.

Malaria

Geographic Distribution

Malaria is endemic in tropical Africa, Asia, South and Central Americas, East China, and the Middle East (Figure 52-1) at altitudes below 3000 meters. Cases in developed countries are among travelers to endemic areas, except for rare cases of "airport malaria" contracted from mosquitoes arriving on international flights from endemic areas (Nation's Health, 2000). Worldwide there are approximately 515 million cases and 2 million deaths each year from malaria, with increasing morbidity and mortality since the 1960s (Centers for Disease Control and Prevention [CDC], 2003; Gubler, 1998; Snow et al., 2005; White, 2003).

Agent and Vector

The obligate intracellular protozoa *Plasmodium falciparum* (Figure 52-2), *P. vivax*, *P. ovale*, and *P. malariae* are transmitted by female *Anopheles* mosquitoes. Transmission may also occur via parenteral injection or congenitally. The effects of malaria infection are caused by the destruction of red blood cells (RBCs), the release of parasites and RBC material into the circulation, the host inflammatory reaction to these events, and, in the case of *P. falciparum* (the most virulent form), microcirculatory obstruction (White, 2003). The cycle begins when sporozoites from the mosquito's salivary ducts enter the circulation and invade the liver, where they multiply asexually. At the end of the incubation period, the hepatocytes rupture to release merozoites into the bloodstream. The merozoites rapidly enter RBCs, where they grow into schizonts that eventually lyse the RBCs to release more merozoites into the circulation.

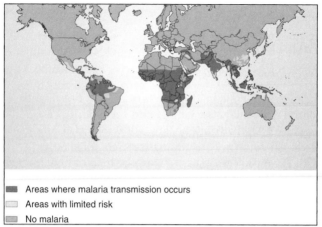

Areas where malaria transmission occurs
Areas with limited risk
No malaria

FIGURE 52–1

Global distribution of malaria (*Source:* From Wongsrichanalai, C., Pickard, A.L., Wernsdorfer, W.H., & Meshnick, S.R. (2002). Epidemiology of drug-resistant malaria. *Lancet Infectious Disease, 2,* 209-218.)

In *P. falciparum* infections, erythrocytes containing merozoites adhere to the vascular endothelium, causing microcirculatory obstruction and organ damage. After a series of asexual reproductive cycles, some of the malaria parasites develop into sexual forms (gametocytes) that infect biting anopheline mosquitoes during their blood meals. Inside the mosquito, the male and female forms fuse and produce more sporozoites to continue the life cycle (Chin, 2000; Taylor & Strickland, 2000).

Incubation

The incubation period is usually 1 to 4 weeks, but sometimes it is more than a year. *P. vivax* and *P. ovale* may remain dormant in the liver and cause relapses, which may occur as many as 10 years after first episode. Neither *P. falciparum* nor *P. malariae* has a dormant stage (Chin, 2000; Taylor & Strickland, 2000).

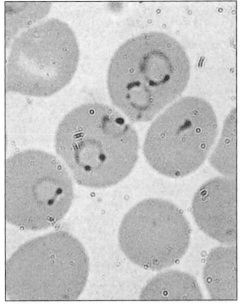

FIGURE 52–2

Plasmodium falciparum. (*Source:* From Peters, W., & Pasvol, G. [2002]. *Tropical medicine and parasitology* [5th ed., p. 26]. Chicago: Mosby.)

Clinical Findings and Treatment

Signs and Symptoms

Malaria is usually characterized by sudden onset of high fever, sweating, chills, uncontrollable shaking, headache, and splenomegaly. Fever tends to wax and wane in 48- to 72-hour cycles, although cycles may be irregular, especially with infection by *P. falciparum.* Onset may also be insidious, with low-grade fever, headache, dyspnea, abdominal pain, nausea, diarrhea, myalgias, and splenomegaly. Less severe illness may be seen in patients who have partial immunity from prior exposure to the disease. In endemic areas, childhood malaria is an important cause of as fever without a source (CDC, 2003; Taylor & Strickland, 2000; White, 2003).

Complications

P. falciparum causes death in as many as 25% of untreated cases. Life-threatening cerebral malaria, which is more common in children and nonimmune patients, is characterized by gradual onset of severe headache, drowsiness, delirium, and coma. Seizures may also occur and are most common in children. Other complications include splenic rupture, hypoglycemia, renal failure (especially among adults), severe anemia, pulmonary edema, and/or algid malaria (cold skin, profuse diarrhea, and profound weakness). Secondary infections such as pneumonia, sepsis, and urinary tract infections in patients with indwelling catheters may also occur.

"Blackwater fever" refers to a complication of chronic *P. falciparum* infection and is characterized by jaundice, hemoglobinuria, acute renal failure, and bloody dark red or black urine.

In children, respiratory distress with metabolic acidosis, pulmonary edema, shock, abnormal bleeding, anuria, hypothermia, and/or deep coma are danger signs and indicate a high risk of dying. Danger signs for adults include respiratory distress, pulmonary edema, anuria, shock, and hypothermia. Other signs of poor prognosis for adults include impaired consciousness, multiple seizures, and abnormal bleeding (CDC, 2003; White, 2003).

Common Laboratory Findings

Anemia, leukopenia, and thrombocytopenia are common. Hyponatremia and hypoglycemia may occur in patients with *P. falciparum* infection. Renal involvement can cause elevated serum creatinine as well as proteinuria and hemoglobinuria. Other laboratory findings indicative of severe illness include hyperparasitemia (>100,000/µL), acidosis (primarily lactic acidosis, but sometimes ketoacidosis in children), hyperbilirubine-mia, elevated liver enzymes, elevated creatine phosphoki-nase, and prolonged PT and PTT (White, 2003).

Diagnosis

— A history of geographic exposure combined with the findings of recurring fever, chills, anemia, and splenomegaly lead to suspicion of malaria. A febrile patient who has recently been in a malaria-endemic area should be considered to have malaria until proven otherwise. Though microscopy usually establishes the diagnosis, a negative blood smear does not exclude malaria. Clinicians should therefore consider repeating the test every 12 to 24 hours in a febrile patient with possible malaria until a definitive diagnosis is made or the fever has resolved. If neither rapid tests nor microscopic interpretation are immediately available, obtain blood smear and start presumptive treatment. Do not allow delays in slide interpretation to delay treatment (CDC, 2003; McLellan, 2002; White, 2003).
— Microscopic examination of Giemsa-stained thick smears (best for detection of organisms) and thin smears (best for identification of species) of blood are the standard for diagnosis. However, this technique requires specific expertise, and other commercially available techniques may yield more accurate (albeit more expensive) tests in laboratories with less malaria experience, especially where malaria is imported. Sensitive alternatives to microscopy (CDC, 2003; Hanscheid, 1999) include the following:
  • Fluorescent microscopy after centrifugation (QBC)
  • Dipstick antigen detection of HRP2 and pLDH (Parasight-F, ICT Malaria Pf, OptiMAL)
  • Polymerase chain reaction assays

Differential Diagnosis

— The differential diagnosis of malaria includes influenza, visceral leishmaniasis, leptospirosis, relapsing fever, typhoid fever, dengue fever, brucellosis, trypanosomiasis, gastroenteritis, urinary tract infection, amebic liver abscess, hepatitis, tuberculosis, and other causes of fever, splenomegaly, hepatomegaly, and anemia. Bacterial meningitis may cause symptoms similar to cerebral malaria.

Treatment

Treatment depends on the organism, immune status of the patient, and severity of the attack (Table 52-1). Start treatment promptly, especially if exposure to *P. falciparum* is a possibility. Because the initial clinical presentation can be deceiving, pregnant women and children with malaria and all patients with *P. falciparum* should be admitted to the hospital regardless of the severity of their symptoms (Medical Letter, 2004).

Oral chloroquine is a mainstay of treatment except for infection with chloroquine-resistant *P. falciparum*. *P. falciparum* presents the greatest challenge because of the rapidity of onset and severity of attacks as well as the existence of multiple-drug–resistant (MDR) strains. Combination drug treatment is commonly used, for example, mefloquine combined with artesunate for MDR strains.

Response to treatment (White, 2003) is classified as the following:

- *Early treatment failure.* The development of severe malaria or danger signs (see earlier Complications and Common Laboratory Findings sections) during the first 3 days of treatment, axillary temperature 37.5° C or above, and parasitemia.
- *Late treatment failure.* The development of severe malaria or danger signs and axillary temperature 37.5° C or above during days 4 to 14 of treatment.
- *Adequate clinical response.* Measured during "the 14-day test" starting when treatment starts. An adequate clinical response occurs either when there is no early

TABLE 52-1 Treatment of Malaria Specific to Parasite

Infection	Adults	Children	Comments
All malaria except when caused by chloroquine-resistant *P. falciparum* or chloroquine-resistant *P. vivax*	Chloroquine phosphate 1 g (600 mg base) PO; then 500 mg (300 mg base) 6 hours later; then 500 mg (300 mg base) 24 and 48 hours later OR	Chloroquine phosphate 10 mg base/kg (maximum 600 mg base) PO,;then 5 mg base/kg 6 hours later, then 5 mg base/kg 24 and 48 hours later	*P. falciparum* in the Dominican Republic, Haiti, Central America west of the Panama Canal, Egypt, and some countries in the Middle East is still sensitive to chloroquine
	Hydroxychloroquine sulfate: 400 mg hydroxychloroquine is equivalent to 500 mg chloroquine phosphate OR		
	Quinine dihydrochloride 20 mg/kg loading dose IV in 5% dextrose over 4 hours, followed by 10 mg/kg over 2-4 hours q8h (maximum 1800 mg/day) until PO treatment started OR	Same as adult dose	Side effects include cinchonism (tinnitus, high-tone hearing impairment, dysphoria, and nausea and vomiting), hypoglycemia, and (rarely) cardiac conduction disorders

continued

Table 52-1 continued

Infection	Adults	Children	Comments
P. falciparum or chloroquine-resistant *P. vivax* —cont'd	Quinidine gluconate 10 mg/kg loading dose (maximum 600 mg) in NS IV over 1-2 hours, followed by continuous IV infusion 0.02 mg/kg/min until PO treatment is started **Alternative** Artemether 3.2 mg/kg IM; then 1.6 mg/kg daily for 5-7 days IM	Same as adult dose Same as adult dose	More toxic than quinine and seldom used. Decrease or omit loading dose for patients who have received quinine or mefloquine. If >48 hours IV treatment is needed, decrease quinine or quinidine dose by 30% to 50%. Continuous ECG, blood pressure, and glucose monitoring are recommended, especially in young children and pregnant women Not available in the United States
Chloroquine-resistant *P. falciparum*	Quinine sulfate 650 mg PO tid for 3 days except in Southeast Asia where quinine is taken for 7 days + doxycycline 100 mg PO bid for 7 days OR	Quinine sulfate 25 mg/kg/day PO in 3 doses for 3 days except in Southeast Asia where quinine is taken for 7 days + doxycycline 2 mg/kg/day PO for 7 days OR	Chloroquine-resistant *P. falciparum* occurs in all endemic areas except Central America west of the Panama Canal, Mexico, Haiti, the Dominican Republic, and much of the Middle East (resistance is found in Yemen, Oman, Saudi Arabia, and Iran)

Quinine + tetracycline 250 mg PO qid for 7 days OR	Quinine + tetracycline 6.25 mg/kg PO qid for 7 days OR	Tetracycline and doxycycline may cause tooth discoloration for children 8 years old
Quinine + pyrimethamine-sulfadoxine (Fansidar = 25 mg pyrimethamine and 500 mg sulfadoxine) 3 tablets PO at once on last day of quinine OR	Quinine + pyrimethamine-sulfadoxine <1 year, 1/4 tablet PO; 1-3 years, 1/2 tablet PO; 4-8 years, 1 tablet PO; 9-14, years, 2 tablets PO at once on the last day of quinine OR	Resistance to pyrimethamine-sulfadoxine reported from SE Asia, Amazon basin, sub-Saharan Africa, Bangladesh, Oceania
Quinine + clindamycin 900 mg PO tid for 5 days OR	Quinine + clindamycin 20-40 mg/kg/day PO in 3 doses for 5 days OR	Clindamycin is used in pregnancy Take within 45 minutes of eating to decrease stomach upset
Atovaquone/proguanil 2 adult tablets (atovaquone 250 mg/proguanil 100 mg) PO bid for 3 days	Atovaquone/proguanil: 11-20 kg, 1 adult tablet PO qd × 3 days; 21-30 kg 2 adult tablets/day PO for 3 days;	Significant side effects common; not for use in pregnancy; not given with quinine, quinidine, or halofantrine; caution when giving

continued

Table 52–1 continued

Infection	Adults	Children	Comments
Chloroquine resistant *P. falciparum*—cont'd		31–40 kg, 3 adult tablets PO for 3 days; >40 kg, 2 adult tablets PO bid for 3 days (pediatric tablets contain atovaquone 62.5 mg/proguanil 25 mg)	quinine, quinidine, or halofantrine to patients who have taken mefloquine for prophylaxis
	Alternatives Mefloquine 750 mg PO followed by 500 mg in 12 hours	Mefloquine 15 mg/kg PO followed by 10 mg/kg in 8–12 hours (not FDA approved). On the Thailand-Burma and Cambodian borders, 25 mg/kg	May cause arrhythmias, heart monitoring recommended; do not give to patients with conduction defects or seizure disorder; safety during pregnancy not established; do not take 1 hour before or 2 hours after eating
	OR	OR	
	Halofantrine 500 mg PO q6h for 3 doses; repeat in 1 week	Halofantrine <40 kg give 8 mg/kg PO q6h for 3 doses; repeat in 1 week	Prolongs QTc interval; do not give to patients with conduction disorders or ventricualr dysrhythmias; interaction with mefloquine may lead to fatal prolongation of QTc interval; do not give to pregnant or lactating women
	OR		

Chloroquine-resistant *P. vivax*	Artesunate 4 mg/kg/day PO for 3 days + mefloquine 750 mg PO followed by 500 mg in 12 hours	Same as adult dose; may be given PO or PR + mefloquine 15 mg/kg PO followed by 10 mg/kg in 12 hours (not FDA approved)	Common in Papua New Guinea and Indonesia; resistance also occurs in Burma, India, Thailand, Vanuatu, Guyana, Brazil, Columbia, and Peru
	Quinine sulfate 650 mg PO tid for 3 days except in Southeast Asia where quinine is taken for 7 days + doxycycline 100 mg PO bid for 7 days OR Mefloquine 750 mg PO followed by 500 mg in 12 hours *Alternatives* Halofantrine 500 mg PO q 6h × 3 doses; repeat in 1 week	Quinine sulfate 25 mg/kg/day PO in 3 doses for 3 days except in Southeast Asia where quinine is taken for 7 days + doxycycline 2 mg/kg/day PO for 7 days OR Mefloquine 15 mg/kg PO followed by 10 mg/kg in 8-12 hours Halofantrine <40 kg give 8 mg/kg PO q6h for 3 doses; repeat in 1 week	See previous comments on prolongation of QTc

continued

Table 52–1 continued

Infection	Adults	Children	Comments
Chloroquine-resistant *P. vivax*—cont'd	OR Chloroquine 25 mg base/kg PO in 3 doses over 48 hours + primaquine 2.5 mg base/kg in 3 doses over 48 hours		Primaquine may cause hemolytic anemia and is contraindicated in patients deficient in glucose-6-phosphate dehydrogenase (G-6-PD); screen prior to treatment; not for use during pregnancy
Prevention of relapse with *P. vivax* or *P. ovale* only	Primaquine phosphate 26.3 mg (15 mg base)/day for 14 days or 79 mg (45 mg base)/week for 8 weeks (see comments)	Primaquine phosphate 0.3 mg base/kg/day for 14 days	See warnings above Relapse may occur – treat with 2nd 14-day course of 30 mg base/day; in Somalia and SE Asia, first course is with 30 mg base/day
Presumptive treatment	Atovaquone/proguanil 2 adult tablets bid PO × 3 days	Atovaquone/proguanil	Take with food

	11-20 kg, 1 tablet daily for 3 days; 21-30 kg, 2 tablets daily for 3 days; 31-40 kg, 3 tablets daily for 3 days; >40 kg, same as adults	
OR	OR	
Pyrimethamine-sulfadoxine (Fansidar) take single dose (3 tablets) for treatment of febrile illness when medical care unavailable	Pyrimethane-sulfadoxine <1 yr, ¼ tablet; 1-3 years, ½ tablet; 4-8 years, 1 tablet; 9-14 years, 2 tablets	Resistance to pyrimethamine-sulfadoxine reported from SE Asia, Amazon basin, sub-Saharan Africa, Bangladesh, Oceania

Sources: Gomez, Jurado, & Cambon, 2003; Medical Letter, 2004; Rosenblatt, 1999; White, 2003.

or late treatment failure and there is an absence of parasitemia regardless of temperature or there is an axillary temperature of 37.5° C or less. However, White (2003) notes that "at low levels of resistance nearly all recrudescences occur *after* 14 days" (p. 1263).

— Supportive care includes careful attention to fluid and electrolyte balance, blood transfusion for severe anemia, frequent blood glucose monitoring with immediate correction of hypoglycemia, and empiric antibiotics to cover secondary infections.

— Readers are referred to the World Health Organization (WHO) or the CDC for updates on outbreaks, geographic risks, treatment, and prevention.

Prevention

— The search for a vaccine for malaria has been challenging. One promising vaccine called RTS,S has shown 71% efficacy in clinical trials, but protection drops off after 2 months. Other candidate vaccines in development include DNA vaccines and vaccines aimed at blocking the mosquito stage of the malaria life cycle (Whitty, Rowland, Sanderson, & Mutabingwa, 2002).

— Preventive measures in endemic areas (Chin, 2000; Koren, Matsui, & Bailey, 2003; White, 2003) include the following:

  • Kill adult mosquitoes by spraying inside and outside human habitations and surrounding areas with residual insecticides. The goal is to kill as many female mosquitoes as possible, thus decreasing the likelihood of disease transmission.
  See Appendix D.
  • Kill larvae and eliminate breeding areas as much as possible. Elimination of breeding areas includes draining standing water such as swamps, emptying open water-filled containers and used tires, and

reducing the number of plants that hold standing water, for example, bromeliads.

— Personal protection includes the following:

- Close off living and working quarters with door and window screens.
- Use a residual insecticide inside homes and work areas. See Appendix D.
- Use insecticide-impregnated mosquito netting over beds. Nets must be retreated with insecticide annually. See Appendix D.
- Stay inside as much as possible during hours when mosquitoes are biting, which, in the case of *Anopheles* mosquitoes is from dusk to dawn.
- Use DEET repellant on exposed skin and wear permethrin-treated clothing when outside during biting hours. DEET may be used to protect pregnant and lactating women traveling to endemic areas (CDC, 2003). Formulations with concentrations of 30% or less can be used safely in children and infants older than 2 months (American Academy of Pediatrics, 2003). Long-acting repellents in which DEET is bound in a polymer have the advantages of longer duration and decreased systemic absorption.
- Take chemoprophylaxis when traveling to endemic areas, especially if doing relief work or visiting rural or less developed settings (Table 52-2). Persons with seizure disorders or neuropsychiatric disorders should not take mefloquine for prophylaxis. Primaquine should not be given to individuals with glucose-6-phosphate dehydrogenase deficiency. Patients taking doxycycline should be cautioned about photosensitivity reactions.

— Provide ongoing community education regarding the preceding measures.

TABLE 52-2 Chemoprophylaxis of Malaria Specific to Parasite

Area	Adults	Children	Comments
Chloroquine-sensitive areas	Chloroquine phosphate 500 mg (300 mg base) weekly starting 1-2 weeks before travel to endemic areas and continuing for 4 weeks after leaving	Chloroquine phosphate 5 mg/kg base weekly up to adult dose and according to adult schedule	Take on a full stomach; may worsen psoriasis
Chloroquine-resistant areas	Mefloquine 250 mg 1 × week beginning 1-2 weeks before travel and continuing for 4 weeks after leaving OR Doxycycline 100 mg daily starting 1-2 days before travel and continuing 4 weeks after leaving area	Mefloquine <15 kg, 5 mg/kg; 15-19 kg, ¼ tablet; 20-30 kg, ½ tablet; 31-45 kg, ¾ tablet; >45 kg, 1 tablet 1 × week according to adult schedule OR Doxycycline 2 mg/kg/d up to 100 mg/day according to adult schedule	Contraindicated for patients with depression or major psychiatric disorder, seizures, (except simple febrile seizure), cardiac conduction abnormalities Doxycycline contraindicated in pregnancy and children younger than age 8; take with food; counsel patients on photosensitivity

	OR	OR	
	Atovaquone/proguanil 250 mg/100 mg (adult tablet) daily starting 1-2 days before travel and continuing 1 week after leaving area	Atovaquone/proguanil 11-20 kg, ¼ tablet; 21-30 kg, ½ tablet; 31-40 kg, ¾ tablet; >40 kg, 1 tablet daily according to adult schedule	Do not give to pregnant women, children under 11 kg, patients with severe renal impairment
	OR	OR	
	Primaquine 30 mg base daily starting 1 day before travel and continuing 1 week after leaving area	Primaquine 0.5 mg/kg daily starting 1 day before travel and continuing 1 week after leaving area	Primaquine may cause hemolytic anemia and is contraindicated in patients deficient in glucose-6-phosphate dehydrogenase; screen before treatment; not for use during pregnancy or lactation unless infant has a normal G6PD level

Sources: Medical Letter, 2002; Rosenblatt, 1999; White, 2003.

Reporting

The CDC considers malaria to be a nationally notifiable disease. The WHO classifies it as a disease important in public health (Class 1A in nonendemic areas; 3C in endemic areas). See Appendix C for details and for upcoming changes in WHO reporting.

References

American Academy of Pediatrics. (2003). Follow safety precautions when using DEET on children. Retrieved December 7, 2003, from *www.aap.org/family/wnv-jun03.htm*

Centers for Disease Control and Prevention. (2003). Malaria. Retrieved November 3, 2003, from *www.cdc.gov/travel/diseases/malaria/index.htm*

Chin, J. (Ed.). (2000). *Control of communicable diseases manual* (17th ed., pp. 310-313). Washington, DC: American Public Health Association.

Gomez, L-E.A., Jurado, M.H., & Cambon, N. (2003). Randomised efficacy and safety study of two 3-day artesunate rectal capsule/mefloquine regimens versus artesunate alone for uncomplicated malaria in Ecuadorian children. *Acta Tropical, 89,* 47-53.

Gubler, D.J. (1998). Resurgent vector-borne diseases as a global health problem. *Emerging Infectious Diseases, 4.* Retrieved November 10, 2003, from *www.cdc.gov/ncidod/eid/vol4no3/gubler.htm*

Hanscheid, T. (1999). Diagnosis of malaria: A review of alternatives to conventional microscopy. *Clinical Laboratory Haematology, 21,* 235-245.

Koren, G., Matsui, D., & Bailey, B. (2003). DEET-based insect repellents: Safety implications for children and pregnant and lactating women. *Canadian Medical Association Journal.* Retrieved November 27, 2003, from *www.cmaj.ca/pdfs/deet-koren.pdf*

McLellan, S.L. (2002). Evaluation of fever in the returned traveler. *Primary Care, 29,* 47-69.

Medical Letter. (2004). Drugs for parasitic infections. *The Medical Letter,* August 2004., Retrieved March 23, 2005, from *www.medletter.com/freedocs/parasitic.pdf*

Nation's Health. (2000). World health leaders fear spread of "airport malaria." *Nation's Health,* October 2000, p. 14.

Rosenblatt, J.E. (1999). Antiparasitic agents. *Mayo Clinic Proceedings, 74,* 1161-1175.

Snow, R.W., Guerra, C.A., Noor, A.M., Myint, H.Y., & Hay, S.I. (2005). The global distribution of clinical episodes of *Plasmodium falciparum* malaria. *Nature, 434,* 214-217.

Taylor, T.E., & Strickland, G.T. (2000). Malaria. In G.T. Strickland (Ed.), *Hunter's tropical medicine and emerging infectious diseases* (8th ed., pp. 614-643). Philadelphia: W.B. Saunders Company.

White, N.J. (2003). Malaria. In G.C. Cook & A.I. Zumla (Eds.), *Manson's tropical diseases* (21st ed., pp. 1205-1295). Philadelphia: W.B. Saunders Company.

Whitty, C.J., Rowland, M., Sanderson, F., & Mutabingwa, T.K. (2002). Malaria. *British Medical Journal, 325,* 1221-1224.

Wongsrichanalai, C., Pickard, A.L., Wernsdorfer, W.H., & Meshnick, S.R. (2002). Epidemiology of drug-resistant malaria. *Lancet Infectious Disease, 2,* 209-218.

53

MEASLES
Hard measles, red measles, morbilli, Rubeola

Geographic Distribution

Each year approximately 800,000 people die from measles—nearly all in developing nations. Measles is endemic worldwide with epidemics occurring primarily in developing nations with inadequate vaccination coverage. Measles is also one of the leading causes of mortality in complex humanitarian emergencies such as refugee camps (Medicin sans Frontieres [MSF USA], 2003; Sphere, 2000). In temperate climates measles tends to occur in late winter and early spring, whereas in tropical climates the disease occurs primarily in the dry season (Aaby et al., 2003; Chin, 2000; Horm, Dumas, Svay, Feldon, & Reynes, 2003; Shetty & Shetty, 2003).

Agent and Vector

The measles virus is a member of the genus *Morbillivirus*, family Paramyxoviridae. Humans are the only natural host for wild measles virus, and children are most affected. Measles is spread by contact with respiratory secretions of infected persons (either airborne or direct contact), especially during the prodromal catarrhal stage of illness. Infection begins in the nasopharynx and spreads to the reticuloendothelial system and epithelial cells. After the necrosis of reticuloendothelial cells affected by the initial viremia, a second wave of viremia occurs. Measles virus then spreads to involve the entire respiratory mucosa. Measles virus infection also involves the skin, conjunctivae, mouth, larynx, and gastrointestinal tract, and causes depression of cellular immunity as well. When the characteristic rash occurs, antibody to measles virus becomes detectable and the patient is no longer infectious. Though the virus is quite labile and sensitive to strong light and drying, measles is one of the most highly contagious diseases with about 90% of household contacts of index cases becoming infected (CDC, 2003; Cook & Zumla, 2003; Gershon, 2000; Maldonado, 2004).

Incubation

The incubation period is 10 to 12 days, but 7 to 18 days may elapse from exposure to onset of fever (Chin, 2000).

Clinical Findings and Treatment

Signs and Symptoms

Measles is manifested first by the gradual onset of 3 to 5 days of prodromal symptoms of low-grade to moderate fever, conjunctivitis, coryza, cough, and malaise. Two to 3 days after the onset of symptoms, the pathognomonic sign of measles, Koplik spots, appear on the buccal mucosa (Figure 53-1). Koplik spots are small red spots likened to grains of sand in size, with bluish-white centers that persist for only about 12 to 18 hours and may not be noticed except on careful exam.

On about the third day of illness, a characteristic maculopapular exanthem (red in light-skinned persons, deep red to purple in dark-skinned persons) appears on the face and neck, and during the next 3 to 4 days generalizes to the entire body (Figure 53-2). The exanthem is only slightly pruritic. It is during the first several days of the rash that fever is highest and patients feel the worst. The severity of the rash correlates to the severity of the illness: A widespread confluent rash indicates severe illness. As the rash clears in the same order that it developed about 5 days later, desquamation and a brownish discoloration occur and then clear after another 7 to 10 days.

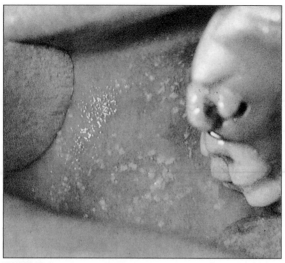

FIGURE 53–1

Koplik spots. (*Source:* From Peters, W., & Pasvol, G. [2002]. *Tropical medicine and parasitology* [5th ed., p. 276]. Chicago: Mosby.)

Brief generalized convulsions with complete recovery may occur during the febrile phase.

— A hemorrhagic and severe form of measles ("black measles") sometimes occurs, with purpura and bleeding from mouth, nose, and bowel.

— An atypical form of measles occurs in persons who were vaccinated with killed virus (versus the currently used live virus) between 1963 and 1967 in the United States. Atypical measles is characterized by headache, abdominal pain, vomiting, myalgia, cough, congestion, pneumonia, and pleural effusion. The rash of atypical measles is a maculopapular exanthem that begins on the palms, wrists, soles, and ankles and progresses centripetally, becoming vesicular and later purpuric or hemorrhagic.

— Among adults, clinical features are similar to the typical course described. Liver involvement is relatively

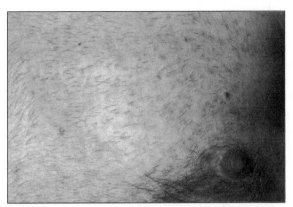

FIGURE 53–2
Measles. (*Source:* Courtesy of the University of Texas Southwestern Department of Dermatology.)

common, with abdominal pain, sometimes jaundice, and elevated aspartate aminotransferase (AST) levels (CDC, 2003; Cook & Zumla, 2003; Gershon, 2000; Maldonado, 2004).

Complications

- The case fatality rate for measles ranges from 1 to 3 per 1000 in developed nations to 100 per 1000 in rural undeveloped areas. The risk of death increases with malnutrition, age younger than 5 years, and preexisting immune deficiency, such as leukemia or HIV.
- Death is often from one of the two most common complications of measles: pneumonia or acute encephalitis (Gershon, 2000). Pneumonia may be caused by direct viral invasion of the respiratory tree, or from bacterial superinfection facilitated by viral damage to local defenses as well as immune system depression. Acute measles encephalitis occurs in approximately 1 in 1000 cases, and presents as a return of fever during the convalescent phase with headache, irritability, seizures,

and alterations in consciousness. Chronic measles encephalitis, called subacute sclerosing panencephalitis (SSPE), may become apparent 5 to 10 years after the initial measles virus infection and is characterized by behavior changes, deterioration in cognitive abilities, and seizures. A high proportion of acute and chronic encephalitis survivors have neurologic sequelae.

— Other complications of measles infection include otitis media, conjunctivitis with corneal perforation and blindness (associated with vitamin A deficiency), cancrum oris (gangrene of the lips and cheeks, also known as noma), laryngotracheobronchitis, exacerbation of tuberculosis, and diarrhea.

— Measle in pregnancy is not associated with congenital anomalies as is rubella (German measles). However, spontaneous abortion and premature delivery may occur. Pregnant women with measles tend to be very sick (Cook & Zumla, 2003; Gershon, 2000; Maldonado, 2004).

Common Laboratory Findings

— Leukopenia may be seen (Gershon, 2000).

Diagnosis

— Diagnosis is usually based on the characteristic clinical picture. Infection may be serologically confirmed by the presence of immunoglobulin M (IgM) measles antibodies, or by a fourfold or greater rise in measles antibody titers in acute and convalescent sera. Measles virus can also be detected by immunofluorescent detection of measles virus antigen in infected tissues, by reverse transcriptase-polymerase chain reaction (RT-PCR), or by viral culture of urine, blood, or nasopharyngeal secretions.

Differential Diagnosis

— The differential diagnosis includes rubella, roseola infantum (human herpesvirus type 6), echovirus infection, coxsackievirus infection, adenovirus infection, tick-borne and louse-borne typhus, meningococcemia, scarlet fever, infectious mononucleosis, Kawasaki disease, and serum sickness.

Treatment

There is no specific treatment for measles. Supportive measures include management of fever, oral pain, and hydration. Oral vitamin A for 2 days at a dose of 200,000 international units for children age 1 and older (100,000 international units for children ages 6 months to 1 year) should be given to children in developing countries to prevent blindness and decrease mortality. In developed countries, vitamin A should be considered for children ages 6 months to 2 years hospitalized for measles or its complications, or children older than 6 months with immune deficiency, malnutrition, clinically evident vitamin A deficiency, or recent immigration from an area with a high measles mortality rate. Children with ocular manifestations of vitamin A deficiency should receive another dose 4 weeks later (American Academy of Pediatrics [AAP], 2003).

Prevention

In the United States, the first dose of measles, mumps, and rubella (MMR) vaccine is given at 12 to 15 months when maternal antibody levels have waned. MMR induces antibody formation to all three viruses in at least 95% of recipients. The second dose is typically given at ages 4 to 6 but may be given earlier as long as it is separated from the first dose by at least 28 days. In travelers to high-risk areas, the monovalent measles vaccine may be given as early as 6 months but should be followed by the routine two-dose MMR series beginning at 12 to 15 months. Children living in developing countries are given measles vaccine beginning at age 9 months.

— Measles immunization and vitamin A supplementation should be one of the top priorities during a refugee influx, even if no cases have been reported and the population is thought to be highly immunized (MSF-USA, 2003; Sphere Project, 2000). During the emergency phase, all children between ages 6 months and 12 to 15 years should be vaccinated. Infants age 6 months or younger born to immune mothers are protected by maternal antibody (Cook & Zumla, 2003; Maldonado, 2004). But because measles vaccine given at 9 months has only 85% efficacy, vaccine coverage has to be close to 100% in the target population to prevent an epidemic (MSF-USA, 2003). There may also be a nonspecific beneficial effect in vulnerable populations, because a reduction in mortality from diseases *other than measles* has been observed after measles vaccination, especially for girls (Aaby et al., 2003).

— Contraindications to the use of live-virus vaccine includes severe primary immune deficiency diseases (HIV is not an absolute contraindication), severe acute illness, anaphylactic reaction to a previous dose of measles vaccine or allergy to gelatin or neomycin, high-dose corticosteroids given for 14 days or more, and recent administration of immune globulin or blood products (AAP, 2003). Measles vaccine should not be given to pregnant women because of the theoretical risk of fetal infection, though no evidence substantiates this risk (AAP, 2003; Chin, 2000, p. 334). Egg allergy is no longer a contraindication (Box 53-1).

— Despite concerns arising in 2002 following a report from a small study that MMR vaccine might be a cause of autism, large population-based studies have failed to find evidence that the MMR vaccine is associated with autism (Jacobson, 2004; Offit & Coffin, 2003).

— Postexposure prophylaxis with immune globulin 0.25 mL/kg IM (0.5 mL/kg in immunocompromised patients, maximum 15 mL) can modify or prevent

---

A NOTE ON TUBERCULOSIS TESTING AND MEASLES BOX 53–1

Purified protein derivative (PPD) tuberculin testing has no effect on the response to the MMR vaccination. However, measles vaccine (and possibly mumps, rubella, and varicella vaccines) can suppress the response to PPD in a person infected with *Mycobacterium tuberculosis*.

To minimize the risk of a false-negative interpretation, PPD testing should be delayed for 4 to 6 weeks after MMR vaccination. If PPD testing is needed, it should be done before MMR vaccination. PPD may be applied at the same time as MMR is administered, because the mild immunosuppressive effect of the vaccine will not occur for several days after vaccination. MMR does not worsen tuberculosis disease (CDC, 2003).

---

measles when given within 6 days of exposure (AAP, 2003; CDC, 2003; Chin, 2000).

Reporting

The CDC considers measles to be a nationally notifiable disease. The World Health Organization (WHO) classifies measles as 2A. See Appendix C for details and for upcoming changes in WHO reporting.

References

Aaby, P., Garly, M-L., Balé, C., Martins, C., Jensen, H., et al. (2003). Survival of previously measles-vaccinated and measles unvaccinated children in an emergency situation: An unplanned study. *Pediatric Infectious Diseases, 22,* 798-805.

American Academy of Pediatrics. (2003). *2003 Red Book: Report of the Committee on Infectious Diseases* (26th ed.). Washington, DC: Author.

Centers for Disease Control and Prevention. (2003). Measles. Retrieved December 20, 2003, from *www.cdc.gov/travel/diseases/measles.htm*

Chin, J. (Ed.). (2000). *Control of communicable diseases manual* (17th ed., pp. 330-335). Washington, DC: American Public Health Association.

Cook, G.C., & Zumla, A. (2003). Cutaneous viral diseases. In G.C. Cook & A.I. Zumla (Eds.), *Manson's tropical diseases* (21st ed., pp. 841-859). Philadelphia: W.B. Saunders Company.

Gershon, A.A. (2000). Measles virus (rubeola). In G. Mandell, J. Bennett, & R. Dolin (Eds.), *Principles and practice of infectious diseases* (5th ed., pp. 1801-1809). New York: Churchill Livingstone.

Horm, S.V., Dumas, C., Svay, S., Feldon, K., & Reynes, J.M. (2003). Genetic characterization of wild-type measles viruses in Cambodia. *Virus Research, 97,* 31-37.

Jacobson, R.M. (2004). Association of autistic spectrum disorder and the measles, mumps, and rubella vaccine—A systematic review of current epidemiological evidence. *Child: Care, Health and Development, 30,* 91-92.

Maldonado, Y. (2004). Measles. In R.E. Behrman, R.M. Kliegman, & H.B. Jenson (Eds.), *Nelson textbook of pediatrics* (17th ed., pp. 1026-1032). Philadelphia: W.B. Saunders Company.

Medicin sans Frontieres. (2003). *Measles immunization.* Retrieved January 4, 2004, from *www.refugeecamp.org/learnmore/vaccination/measles_immunization.htm*

Offit, P.A., & Coffin, S.E. (2003). Communicating science to the public: MMR vaccine and autism. *Vaccine, 22,* 1-6.

Shetty, N., & Shetty, P.S. (2003). Epidemiology of disease in the tropics. In G.C. Cook & A.I. Zumla (Eds.), *Manson's tropical diseases* (21st ed., pp. 19-31). Philadelphia: W.B. Saunders Company.

Sphere Project. (2000). Humanitarian charter and minimum standards in disaster response. Retrieved January 3, 2004, from *www.sphereproject.org/handbook/*

MELIOIDOSIS
Whitmore's disease
Geographic Distribution

— Melioidosis is endemic in Southeast Asia (Vietnam, Cambodia, Laos, Thailand, and Malaysia). It was originally discovered in Burma (Myanmar), but no confirmed indigenous cases have been documented there since 1945 (White, 2003). Melioidosis is found to a lesser extent in Oceania (including northern Australia), Africa, India, and the Middle East. Isolated cases have occurred in the Western Hemisphere (Centers for Disease Control and Prevention [CDC], 2000a; Chin, 2000).

Agent and Vector

— Melioidosis is any infection caused by *Burkholderia pseudomallei* (formerly *Pseudomonas pseudomallei*), a gram-negative, oxidase-positive, motile bacillus. There remain questions about the exact mode of transmission, but inhalation of contaminated soil (dust) or water is the primary means of acquisition. Direct inoculation through breaks in the skin is another route. Infection is apparently not spread through ingestion. Most infections occur during the rainy season and most persons with infection have an underlying chronic illness such as diabetes, alcoholism, cystic fibrosis, or renal failure. Approximately 50% of adult patients with symptomatic melioidosis have poorly managed type 2 diabetes. Person-to-person transmission is rare (Box 54-1). Animals susceptible to melioidosis include most domesticated or farm animals, rodents, and birds (CDC, 2000a; Chin, 2000; Currie, 2003; Dance, 2003).

BIOTERRORISM CONSIDERATIONS   BOX 54–1

Burkholderia pseudomallei and the related *B. mallei* (glanders agent) are considered by the CDC to be Category B biological warfare agents. Category B agents are moderately easy to disseminate and cause moderate morbidity and low mortality. *B. pseudomallei* and *B. mallei* have the potential for production and dissemination in quantities sufficient to affect large populations (CDC, 2000b; Rotz, Khan, Lillibridge, Ostroff, & Hughes, 2002).

In endemic areas, up to 80% of the population older than 4 years of age has antibodies to the bacteria, implying that most infections are mild or asymptomatic. Antibodies are not protective, so people are still susceptible after exposure. Patients with symptomatic melioidosis most often present with pneumonia. Acute melioidosis pneumonia ranges from mild undifferentiated pneumonia to severe pneumonia with fulminant septic shock. Lung abscesses can also occur, with empyema sometimes resulting from abscess rupture into the pleural space. Melioidosis also frequently presents as bacteremia with no other focus. Focal suppuration (nodule, lymphangitis, lymphadenopathy) often results from inoculation through breaks in the skin. Inoculating skin injuries may also result in pneumonia. Abscesses may also appear on other organs, especially the liver, spleen, skeletal muscle, joints, and prostate. Direct inoculation of the eye results in rapid corneal ulceration. In children, especially in Thailand, melioidosis may also appear as a unique acute suppurative parotitis.

Incubation

The incubation period is variable, ranging from around 24 hours after aspiration of water in near drowning experiences to weeks. Reactivation occasionally occurs after many disease-free years (29 years documented), such as among former soldiers who served in Southeast Asia (Currie, 2003; Warawa & Woods, 2002).

Clinical Findings and Treatment

Signs and Symptoms

Melioidosis has a variable presentation and, consequently, is difficult to identify clinically. In most symptomatic cases, melioidosis presents with influenza-like symptoms of fever, chills, headache, arthralgia, and respiratory symptoms. Other signs include decreased consciousness, jaundice, and diarrhea. Skin abscesses have light green or brown odorless pus. Chronic pulmonary melioidosis is usually a slowly progressive condition characterized by fever, weight loss, productive cough, and sometimes hemoptysis. Chest X-ray almost always shows upper lobe infiltrates and/or cavitation. The illness may progress over months or follow a remitting and relapsing course over years (Currie, 2003; Dance, 2003; White, 2003).

Complications

Acute fulminant septicemic melioidosis pneumonia is most common among debilitated persons and those with chronic illnesses as previously mentioned. These patients present as toxic, with high fever and prostration. In most cases, chest X-rays show unilateral diffuse nodular infiltrates, which tend to coalesce, cavitate, and progress rapidly; in other cases chest X-ray shows discrete and progressive consolidation in one or more lobes, especially the upper lobes. Deterioration tends to be rapid with the development of widespread abscesses, metabolic acidosis, and hypotension. The mortality rate in Asia is about 50%, but is lower in Australia (Dance, 2003; White, 2003).

Common Laboratory Findings

— Laboratory findings in acute illness include anemia, leukocytosis with neutrophilia, coagulopathy, and evidence of renal and hepatic impairment (Dance, 2003).

Diagnosis

— Definitive diagnosis is by isolation of *B. pseudomallei*. Commercially available blood culture agar and Ashdown's selective medium are used to culture sputum, blood, throat swabs, ulcer swabs, and rectal swabs. Rapid diagnosis may be made with direct immunofluorescence microscopy of infected sputum, urine, or pus. Antigen- and DNA-detection techniques exist, but are not commercially available and their usefulness in endemic areas is limited because of high rates of background positivity (Currie, 2003; White, 2003).

Differential Diagnosis

— The differential diagnosis of acute septicemic melioidosis includes enteric fever or any of the numerous diseases that mimic enteric fever, such as bartonellosis, plague, leptospirosis, relapsing fever, hepatitis, dengue fever, and many others. Clinicians should also think of common causes of bacteremia and sepsis. For those with pulmonary disease, other causes of bacterial or viral pneumonia should be considered. Melioidosis is clinically and pathologically similar to glanders disease, but the ecology and epidemiology of melioidosis are different.
— Chronic melioidosis is often mistaken for tuberculosis. Geographic location and presence of risk factors are important considerations in diagnosing melioidosis (Currie, 2003; Pearson & Guerrant, 2000).

Treatment

— Treatment of melioidosis includes intravenous and oral
medications. For initial therapy, the treatment of choice
is IV ceftazidime 40 mg/kg q8h (120 mg/kg/24 hours)
for at least 10 days and until clear improvement is
documented and the patient is able to take oral
medications. Therapeutic response is slow, so although
new abscesses may develop or old abscesses grow in
the first week of therapy, premature switching of antibiotics should be avoided. Ceftazidime is safe for use in
neonates. Renal impairment requires dose adjustment.
Alternative intravenous treatment is with imipenem
20 mg/kg up to 1 g q8h (efficacy equal to ceftazidime);
or meropenem 20 mg/kg up to 1 g q8h; or amoxicillin-
clavulanate 27 mg/kg q4h (total 162 mg/kg day,
though intravenous form not commonly used in the
United States). Other third-generation cephalosporins
are not as effective as these. When possible, abscesses
should be incised and drained, especially in the case of
suppurative parotitis.

— A combination of oral medications (for eradication therapy)
is given for at least 3 months when intravenous
treatment is discontinued. Exceptions are children with
the singular syndrome of melioidosis acute suppurative
parotitis, which is treated with oral medications for 8 weeks
after discontinuation of intravenous therapy. In the past,
standard eradication therapy was with doxycycline
alone, but it is now recognized that the addition of
trimethoprim/sulfamethoxazole produces far better outcomes (Currie, 2003; White, 2003). Oral eradication
therapy includes a combination of chloramphenicol
40 mg/kg/day qid for the first 8 weeks; doxycycline
4 mg/kg/day bid; and trimethoprim/sulfamethoxazole
8 mg (of trimethoprim)/kg/day bid. Children younger
than age 8 and pregnant women are treated with
amoxicillin-clavulanate with 60 mg/kg/day of the

amoxicillin component and 15 mg/kg/day of clavulanic acid (White, 2003).

Prevention

Eradication of the disease from endemic areas is impossible because of the ubiquitous nature of the agent. Progress is being made toward developing a vaccine for melioidosis, but there is unlikely to be a vaccine available in the near future. Persons at risk because of chronic illness should thus avoid endemic areas or, if that is not possible, tightly manage high-risk conditions such as diabetes (Chin, 2000; Warawa & Woods, 2002).

Reporting

The CDC considers melioidosis to be a nationally notifiable disease. The World Health Organization (WHO) classifies melioidosis as 5. See Appendix C for details and for upcoming changes in WHO reporting.

References

Centers for Disease Control and Prevention. (2000a). Melioidosis. Retrieved November 7, 2003, from *www.cdc.gov/ncidod/dbmd/diseaseinfo/melioidosis_g.htm*

Centers for Disease Control and Prevention. (2000b). Biological and chemical terrorism: Strategic plan for preparedness and response. *Morbidity and Mortality Weekly Report, 49*(RR-4), 1-14.

Chin, J. (Ed.). (2000). *Control of communicable diseases manual* (17th ed., pp. 335-338). Washington, DC: American Public Health Association.

Currie, B.J. (2003). Melioidosis: An important cause of pneumonia in residents of and travelers returned from endemic regions. *The European Respiratory Journal, 22,* 542-550.

Dance, D. (2003). In G. Mandell, J. Bennett, & R. Dolin (Eds.), *Principles and practice of infectious diseases* (5th ed., pp. 1134-1136). New York: Churchill Livingstone.

Pearson, R.D., & Guerrant, R.L. (2000). Enteric fever and other causes of abdominal symptoms with fever. In G. Mandell, J. Bennett, & R. Dolin (Eds.),

Principles and practice of infectious diseases (5th ed., pp. 1137-1150). New York: Churchill Livingstone.

Rotz, L.D., Khan, A.S., Lillibridge, S.R., Ostroff, S.M., & Hughes. J.M. (2002). Public health assessment of potential biological terrorism agents. *Emerging Infectious Diseases, 8,* 225-230.

Warawa, J. & Woods, D.E. (2002). Melioidosis vaccines. *Expert Review of Vaccines, 1,* 477-482.

White, N.J. (2003). Melioidosis. *The Lancet, 361,* 1715-1722.

55

MENINGITIS, BACTERIAL

Note: Numerous diseases and pathogens cause neurologic manifestations and meningeal signs. See Appendix A, Identification and Diagnosis of Diseases by Presentation and Geographic Distribution, for a listing of such diseases and conditions. Because viral meningitis is well known, generally less severe, and resolves without specific treatment, and because bacterial meningitis can be a devastating disease, this chapter addresses only acute bacterial meningitis.

Geographic Distribution

Bacterial meningitis occurs worldwide. Most pathogens that cause bacterial meningitis are nonepidemic, with geographic differences in incidence depending mostly on the presence of routine childhood immunization and the level and accessibility of health care. An exception is *Neisseria meningitidis* group A, which is responsible for periodic epidemics in the expanding "meningococcal meningitis belt" of sub-Saharan Africa (Senegal, Gambia, Mali, Upper Volta, Ghana, Togo, Benin, Nigeria, Niger, Cameroon, Chad, Central African Republic, Sudan, southern Egypt, Democratic Republic of Congo, and Ethiopia), extending now to Tunisia, Algeria, Kenya, Tanzania, Uganda, and Rwanda (Figure 55-1) (Centers for Disease Control and Prevention [CDC], 2003a; Chin, 2000; Tan, 2003).

Meningococcal epidemics, which usually occur during the dry season, are reported in other African countries and to a lesser extent elsewhere in the world. Bacterial meningitis is one of 15 diseases covered by the World Health Organization's (WHO's) Communicable Disease Surveillance & Response program (Greenwood, 2000; Hart & Cuevas, 2003; WHO, 2003a, 2003b).

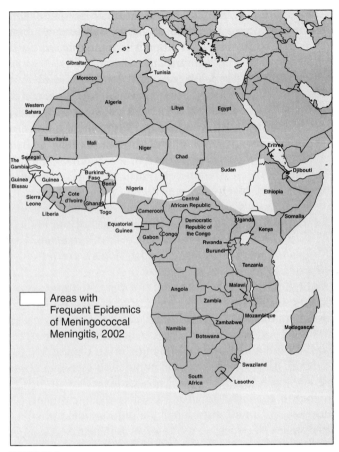

FIGURE 55–1

Areas with frequent epidemics of meningococcal meningitis, 2002
(*Source:* CDC, 2003a).

Agent and Vector

Many bacteria are capable of causing meningitis (infection of the meninges), but only three organisms are responsible for more than 90% of cases outside the neonatal period: *N. meningitidis* (meningococcus), which are nonmotile, gram-negative cocci; *Streptococcus pneumoniae* (pneumococcus), which appear as gram-positive cocci usually in pairs; and *Haemophilus influenzae* type b, a pleomorphic gram-negative coccobacillus (Hart & Cuevas, 2003). *H. influenzae* type b is a common cause only for children younger than age 5 in countries without routine childhood immunization against the bacteria, whereas pneumococcus is the most common cause among children in developed countries and older adults. Among neonates, who often acquire infection from the birth canal or maternal perineum, common agents are *Streptococcus agalactiae* (group B streptococcus) and *Escherichia coli*. Other neonatal pathogens include *N. meningitidis*, *H. influenzae* type b, *S. pneumoniae*, *Klebsiella* species, *Salmonella* species, *Staphylococcus aureus*, and *Listeria monocytogenes*.

Among non-neonates, infection is spread by droplet or saliva exchange from close contacts, often in crowded living conditions. Colonization usually occurs first in the nasopharynx, with many people becoming asymptomatic carriers and a minority developing clinical disease. Between 10% and 25% of the population carries *N. meningitidis* at any given time, with the rate probably higher in epidemic situations. Possible risk factors for developing clinical disease include immune deficiency, anatomic defects, sickle cell disease, asplenism, malnutrition, and damage to the local defenses of the nasopharynx such as occurs with upper respiratory tract infections.

The means by which the pathogens reach the brain after entering the circulation is incompletely understood. Once at the brain the bacteria localize in the pia and arachnoid maters and induce secretion of several chemical mediators, including tumor necrosis factor, interleukin, eicosanoids, and platelet activating factor. Meningococcal and *H. influenzae* type b bacteria also release endotoxins. These mediators potentiate inflammation and increase the permeability of the blood-brain barrier. As inflammation continues, cerebral vasculitis, thrombosis, and edema can occur, leading to increased intracranial pressure and ischemia.

Bacterial pathogens can cause meningitis with or without bacteremia, or bacteremia without meningitis. Bacteremia can lead to sepsis with shock, diffuse vasculitis, disseminated intravascular coagulopathy, multiple organ failure, and death or long-term disability (Greenwood, 2000; Hart & Cuevas, 2003; WHO, 2003a; Woods, 2004). Fulminant meningococcemia can rapidly progress from fever to shock and death in a matter of hours.

Incubation

The incubation period ranges from 2 to 3 days to several months (Hart & Cuevas, 2003).

Clinical Findings and Treatment

Signs and Symptoms

The various pathogens that cause bacterial meningitis produce many common signs and symptoms. In neonates the early signs are nonspecific and may resemble sepsis with a toxic or ill appearance, irritability, lethargy, poor feeding, and fever or hypothermia. Among infants with bacterial meningitis, less than 20% have bulging fontanel, less than 35% have opisthotonos, less than 25% have neck stiffness, and less than 15% have seizures.

In persons older than age 2, common symptoms of meningitis are high fever, headache, and stiff neck developing over several hours to several days and often preceded by signs and symptoms of an upper respiratory tract infection. Other signs and symptoms are nausea, vomiting, photophobia, delirium, headache, hyper- or hypotonia, hypotension, somnolence, and coma. Physical examination may show a positive Kernig's sign (pain when the knee is extended while the hip is in flexion) or Brudzinski's sign (flexion of the hips and knees when the neck is flexed). In patients with meningococcemia, a maculopapular rash may precede more serious illness, often evolving to petechiae and purpura particularly on the distal extremities.

Complications

Death may occur within a few hours of onset and is strongly associated with shock, coma, and seizures. Patients of any age may have seizures, especially those living in developing and tropical locales (Akpede, Akuhwa, Ogiji, & Ambe, 1999; CDC, 2003b; Greenwood, 2000; WHO, 2003a; Woods, 2004). The syndrome of inappropriate antidiuretic hormone secretion (SIADH) may complicate meningitis by causing hyponatremia and fluid overload. In up to 15% of meningitis survivors, persistent and sometimes global neurologic defects occur, including hearing loss, speech disorders, mental retardation, and paralysis. Loss of limbs from gangrene (especially in meningococcemia), suppurative arthritis, pneumonia, myocarditis, and purulent pericarditis may also be seen (Greenwood, 2000; WHO, 2003b).

Common Laboratory Findings

Common laboratory findings in blood include elevated WBC counts with an increased percentage of neutrophils, and thrombocytopenia. Blood culture is positive in approximately two-thirds of patients with *H. influenzae* meningitis and is negative in many patients with pneumococcal and meningococcal meningitis. Cerebrospinal fluid (CSF) is usually turbid (from large numbers of neutrophils) except in early infection, when it may be clear. CSF examination may reveal WBCs with predominantly neutrophils, high protein levels, and low glucose levels (Greenwood, 2000). In contrast, the CSF in viral (aseptic) meningitis has mostly lymphocytes as opposed to neutrophils, though early in the illness the proportion of neutrophils may be similar to that in bacterial meningitis. Table 55-1 summarizes the CSF findings in bacterial versus viral meningitis.

Diagnosis

In adults and older children, characteristic signs and symptoms may suggest the diagnosis of meningitis; in infants and the elderly, signs and symptoms are less definitive so a high degree of suspicion is required. Gram-stain of centrifuged CSF establishes a specific diagnosis in many cases; CSF culture confirms the species and identifies antimicrobial susceptibility to guide treatment (Greenwood, 2000; Hart & Cuevas, 2003).

TABLE 55–1

Cerebrospinal Fluid in Meningitis

CSF	Normal	Bacterial meningitis	Aseptic meningitis
Volume (ml)	40–120	-	-
Appearance	Clear	Turbid	Clear to opalescent
Pressure (mmH$_2$O)	<180–200	Raised	Normal
Protein (g/l)	0.15–0.4	0.5–6.0	0.5–1.0
Mononuclear cells (x10^6/l)	0–5	Can be raised	15–500
Neutrophils (x10^6/l)	0	100–6,000	<15
Glucose (mmol)	2.2–3.3	0–2.2	2.2–3.3

Source: Hart, C.A., & Cuevas, L.E. (2003). Bacterial meningitis. In G.C. Cook & A.I. Zumla (Eds.), *Manson's tropical diseases* (21st ed., pp. 981-994). Philadelphia: W.B. Saunders Company.

In patients with meningococcemia, Gram stain of a scraping from a petechial or purpural lesion may reveal the organism.

Differential Diagnosis

The differential diagnosis includes cerebral malaria, typhus, relapsing fever, Rocky Mountain spotted fever, ehrlichiosis, tuberculosis meningitis, cryptococcal infection, amebic meningoencephalitis, viral meningitis, and viral encephalitis (e.g., herpes simplex virus). Noninfectious etiologies to consider include the vasculitides and intracranial tumors.

Treatment

Early antibiotic therapy improves outcomes. Clinicians should admit patients with suspected meningitis to the hospital, obtain blood cultures, perform a lumbar puncture to obtain CSF for analysis and culture, and start empiric antibiotic therapy until the specific pathogen is identified. In developed countries, empiric therapy is usually with a third-generation cephalosporin such as ceftriaxone or cefotaxime, with ampicillin added for infants younger than 3 months old. In developing countries, where expensive cephalosporins are often not available, ampicillin and chloramphenicol are used together, with gentamicin substituted for chloramphenicol in infants younger than 3 months old (WHO, 1997). After identification and antibiotic sensitivities are obtained, treatment can be tailored to specific pathogens as follows, usually for a 10- to 14-day course with dosing as summarized in Table 55-2:

- *Neisseria meningitidis.* Penicillin G is the first-line antibiotic, but because of the possibility of penicillin-resistant strains, some recommend cefotaxime or ceftriaxone. Chloramphenicol may also be used when cephalosporins are not available.

TABLE 55-2

Dosing Guidelines for Antibiotics Used to Treat Meningitis

Antibiotic	Dose	Maximum daily dose
Penicillin G	300,000 units/kg/day divided q 4 to 6 hours	24 million units
Ceftriaxone	100 mg/kg/day divided q 12 hours	4 g
Cefotaxime	300 mg/kg/day divided q 8 hours	12 g
Ampicillin	400 mg/kg/day divided q 6 hours	10 g
Chloramphenicol	100 mg/kg/day divided q 6 hours	4 g
Vancomycin	60 mg/kg/day divided q 6 hours	4 g

Note: See Kumar (2003) for dosing adjustment for neonates.

- *Haemophilus influenzae* type b. Cefotaxime or ceftriaxone are most effective, because they will also cover beta-lactamase–producing strains. Chloramphenicol may also be used for sensitive strains when cephalosporins are not available. Ampicillin can be used for beta-lactamase negative strains. Neither ampicillin nor chloramphenicol eliminate nasopharyngeal carriage.
- *Streptococcus pneumoniae.* Penicillin G is the standard therapy for sensitive strains. Ceftriaxone or cefotaxime should be used for strains that are not penicillin sensitive, with vancomycin added for highly resistant strains. Chloramphenicol may be used when cephalosporins are not available.

There are some important considerations with respect to supportive therapy for bacterial meningitis. Careful attention to fluid and electrolyte balance is essential.

Fluid restriction was once routinely recommended for
children to reduce the risk of hyponatremia and fluid
overload from SIADH; however, because evidence to
support the practice is limited and small trials have
suggested better outcomes without fluid restriction,
additional studies are needed (WHO, 1997). Steroid
therapy with dexamethasone before antibiotic
administration has been shown in randomized clinical
trials to decrease neurologic sequelae such as hearing loss
in children with meningitis caused by *H. influenzae* or
S. pneumoniae. However, in developed countries the
incidence of *H. influenzae* type b has fallen dramatically
with the use of conjugate vaccine, and there are
unanswered questions regarding the use of steroids with
antibiotic-resistant *S. pneumoniae*.

Additional concerns surround the use of steroids for
meningitis in developing countries, where it is sometimes
difficult to differentiate bacterial meningitis from TB
meningitis or cerebral malaria at the time empiric
therapy begins. The patient should be monitored for
signs of increased intracranial pressure, which may be
treated by hyperosmolar agents such as mannitol or by
mechanical hyperventilation. Anticonvulsants may be used
to treat seizures, but clinicians using chloramphenicol
should note that phenobarbital and phenytoin may
increase the rate of conjugation, thereby decreasing blood
levels of the antibiotic (Akpede et al., 1999; Hart &
Cuevas, 2003; WHO, 2003a; Woods, 2004). Patients
with meningococcemia or sepsis often require intensive care
with mechanical ventilation, plasma, vasopressor support,
and inotropes. Steroids do not alter the course of sepsis.

Prevention

VACCINATION

Vaccines are available for the three major pathogens as
discussed next:

- *Neisseria meningitidis (meningococcal)*. A nonconjugate
  polysaccharide (A, C, Y, and Y135) is widely available

and recommended by the WHO for mass emergency immunizations at the start of epidemics, but is unreliable in children younger than age 2. It is recommended for people who are asplenic or who have complement deficiencies, and it should be offered to young adults living in dormitories as well as persons traveling to endemic or epidemic areas (American Academy of Pediatrics [AAP], 2003). Conjugate polysaccharide vaccines (against group C) are highly efficacious and available for infants and young children in the developed world (though not routinely in the United States), but are less available in the developing world. A new quadrivalent meningococcal conjugate vaccine (MCV4) is being incorporated into the routine childhood immunization schedule for young adolescents and teens in the United States (AAP, 2005).

- *Haemophilus influenzae* type b (Hib). Conjugate Hib vaccine is widely available, well tolerated, and more than 93% effective in clinical trials. It also eliminates carriage, thus providing herd immunity. The United States and other developing countries saw a dramatic decline in incidence after its incorporation into routine immunization for infants and children younger than age 5.
- *Streptococcus pneumoniae (pneumococcal).* Pneumococcal vaccine is available in two forms: a polysaccharide vaccine useful for adults who are elderly, chronically ill, with sickle cell disease, or asplenic; and a conjugate vaccine that has recently been incorporated into the routine childhood immunization schedule in the United States for infants and children younger than age 5.

CHEMOPROPHYLAXIS

Chemoprophylaxis should be provided for close household contacts, day care contacts, and any others who may have been exposed to secretions; it is not generally recommended for health care personnel unless they have had exposure to an infected person's oral secretions as might occur with mouth-to-mouth resuscitation. Chemoprophylaxis for individual pathogens is as follows:

- *Neisseria meningitidis (meningococcal).* Chemoprophylaxis is usually with rifampin 600 mg bid PO for 2 days for adults; 10 mg/kg bid PO for 2 days for children (maximum dose for children is 600 mg); and 5 mg/kg/dose for infants younger than 1 month old. However, because rifampin treatment may result in the selection of rifampin-resistant meningococci, alternatives should be considered such as ceftriaxone 250 mg IM in a single dose for persons older than age 12; 125 mg IM in a single dose for children younger than age 12; or ciprofloxacin 500 mg PO in a single dose for persons age 18 and older.
- *Haemophilus influenzae* type b. Chemoprophylaxis is with rifampin 20 mg/kg/day in a single dose for 4 days, to a maximum dose of 600 mg/day.
- *Streptococcus pneumoniae (pneumococcal).* There is no standard means of chemoprophylaxis for pneumococcal meningitis. However, patients with sickle cell anemia may reduce their risk of invasive pneumococcal disease with daily penicillin prophylaxis.

Other prevention measures include reduction of overcrowding in living quarters such as military barracks, ships, and schools, and education of the public on how to reduce exposure from direct contact or droplet infection. Early index case identification and subsequent chemoprophylactic measures for close contacts as discussed earlier are important (Chin, 2000; Hart & Cuevas, 2003; WHO, 2003a; Woods, 2004).

Reporting

The CDC considers bacterial meningitis to be a nationally notifiable disease. The WHO classifies bacterial meningitis as Class 2A. See Appendix C for details and for upcoming changes in WHO reporting.

References

Akpede, G.O., Akuhwa, R.T., Ogiji, E.O., & Ambe, J.P. (1999). Risk factors for an adverse outcome in bacterial meningitis in the tropics: A reappraisal with focus on the significance and risk of seizures. *Annals of Tropical Pediatrics, 19,* 151-159.

American Academy of Pediatrics. (2003). *2003 Red Book: Report of the Committee on Infectious Diseases* (26th ed.). Washington, DC: Author.

American Academy of Pediatrics. (2005). ACIP recommends meningococcal vaccine. Retrieved March 10, 2005, from *http://aapnews.aappublications.org/cgi/content/full/e2005163v1*

Centers for Disease Control and Prevention. (2003a). Areas with frequent epidemics of meningococcal meningitis, 2002. Retrieved July 5, 2004, from *www.cdc.gov/travel/diseases/maps/menin_map.htm*

Centers for Disease Control and Prevention. (2003b). Meningococcal disease. Retrieved September 8, 2003, from *www.cdc.gov/ncidod/dbmd/diseaseinfo/meningococcal_g.htm*

Chin, J. (Ed.). (2000). *Control of communicable diseases manual* (17th ed., pp. 340-348). Washington, DC: American Public Health Association.

Greenwood, B.M. (2000). Acute bacterial meningitis. In G.T. Strickland (Ed.), *Hunter's tropical medicine and emerging infectious diseases* (8th ed., pp. 372-379). Philadelphia: W.B. Saunders Company.

Hart, C.A., & Cuevas, L.E. (2003). Bacterial meningitis. In G.C. Cook & A.I. Zumla (Eds.), *Manson's tropical diseases* (21st ed., pp. 981-994). Philadelphia: W.B. Saunders Company.

Kumar, A. (2003). Meningitis, bacterial. *eMedicine Journal.* Retrieved January 2, 2004, from *http://author.emedicine.com/PED/topic198.htm*

Tan, T.Q. (2003). Chronic meningitis. *Seminars in Pediatric Infectious Diseases, 14,* 131-139.

Woods, C.R. (2004). *Neisseria meningitidis* (meningococcus). In R.E. Behrman, R.M. Kliegman, & H.B. Jenson (Eds.), *Nelson textbook of pediatrics* (17th ed., pp. 896-899). Philadelphia: W.B. Saunders Company.

World Health Organization. (1997). Antimicrobial and support therapy for bacterial meningitis in children. Retrieved December 23, 2003, from *www.who.int/child-adolescent-health/New_Publications/child_health/who_chd_98.6.htm*

World Health Organization. (2003a). Meningococcal meningitis. Retrieved November 22, 2003, from *www.who.int/mediacentre/factsheets/2003/fs141/en/*

World Health Organization. (2003b). Communicable disease surveillance & response (CSR). Retrieved November 20, 2003, from *www.who.int/csr/disease/en/*

MYCETOMA
Madura foot, maduromycosis
Geographic Distribution

— Mycetoma is generally found in tropical areas and is most commonly seen in Africa, India, Mexico, and Central and South America (Hay, 2000, 2003).

Agent and Vector

— Mycetoma can be caused either by true fungi or actinomycetes, which are filamentous bacteria. When maduromycosis is caused by fungi it is termed *eumycetoma,* and when it is caused by filamentous bacteria it is termed *actinomycetoma.*

— The most common causes of eumycetoma are *Madurella mycetomatis*, found in Africa and India, and *Madurella grisea*, found in Central and South America. Other less common causes of eumycetoma include *Leptosphaeria senegalensis, Exophiala jeanselmei, Aspergillus* species, *Acremonium* species, and *Fusarium* species.

— The most common causes of actinomycetoma include *Actinomadura madurae*, found mainly in Africa and the Middle East, and *Nocardia brasiliensis,* which is the main cause of maduromycosis in Central America. Other less common causes of actinomycetoma include *Streptomyces somaliensis* and *Actinomadura pelletieri.*

— The organisms tend to form aggregates (called *grains*) in the subcutaneous tissue, and infections are sometimes characterized by grain color. Only eumycetomas can create black grains, and the likely organisms include *M. mycetomatis, M. grisea, L. senegalensis*, and *E. jeanselmei. A. pelletieri* is the only organism that creates red grains. White or yellow grains are the most common, found in eumycetomas or actinomycetomas, and are caused by *Acremonium* spp., *Fusarium* spp., *N. brasiliensis*, *A. madurae,* and *S. somaliensis.*

Maduromycosis is usually seen in male agricultural workers. The organisms are present in the environment, and the infection may be introduced into the subcutaneous tissue through penetrating injury (Hay, 2003; Mahgoub, 1999; Queiroz-Telles, McGinnis, Salkin, & Graybill, 2003).

Incubation

The development of maduromycosis may occur rapidly, but it usually takes many years for the first sign of clinical disease to become apparent (Hay, 2003; Sobera & Elewski, 2003).

Clinical Findings and Treatment

Signs and Symptoms

The infection can occur at any site that is subject to trauma, including the feet, lower extremities, hands, trunk, and scalp. The infection usually begins with a painless papule or nodule, which then leads to tissue swelling and draining sinus tracts (Figures 56-1A and B) (Hay, 2003; Sobera & Elewski, 2003).

Complications

If not treated, the infection can spread to the deep tissue, including muscle and bone, or become extensive, with involvement of an entire limb. Eumycetomas tend to progress slowly, but actinomycetomas are more likely to progress rapidly and become extensive. Dissemination is rare. The infection may cause a loss of function, leading to the inability to work (Hay, 2000, 2003).

Common Laboratory Findings

There are no common laboratory findings.

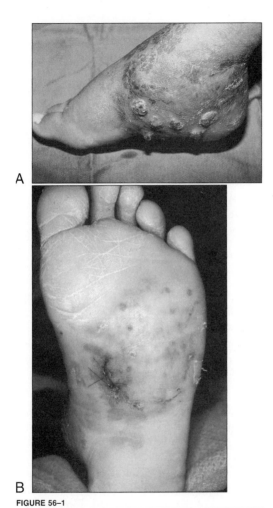

FIGURE 56–1

Madura foot. (*Source:* **A,** From Bolognia, J.L., Jorizzo, J.L., & Rapini, R.P. [Eds.] [2003]. *Dermatology* [p. 1188]. Philadelphia: Mosby. **B,** Courtesy of the University of Texas Southwestern Department of Dermatology.)

Diagnosis

A biopsy taken from the lesion can be examined by routine histology, and grains can be identified and characterized. Fungal grains give a coarse texture, measure 2 to 5 μm, and occasionally carry a black pigment. Bacterial grains have a finer texture, measure 1 μm or less, and are never black. Discharge from the sinus tracts can also be examined with direct microscopy, and characteristics of the grains and filaments can help identify the cause. Eumycotic filaments are typically broad, and actinomycotic filaments are thin. If the etiology is unclear, a culture of the exudate can be performed (Hay, 2000).

Differential Diagnosis

The differential diagnosis includes other causes of chronic osteomyelitis, botryomycosis, which is a deep chronic bacterial infection with sinus formation, and actinomycosis, which is an infection caused by *Actinomyces israelii* or *A. bovis* that occurs around areas where the bacteria is found, including the oral cavity, thorax, and abdomen (Hay, 2000, 2003).

Treatment

Actinomycetomas respond to medical treatment more often than eumycetomas. Actinomycetoma treatment consists of the combination of dapsone 100 mg PO twice daily for adults and streptomycin 1 g daily for at least 1 month. Trimethoprim-sulfamethoxazole (TMP-SMX) can be used instead of dapsone if needed. For children dapsone is given 1 to 1.5 mg/kg PO daily. The treatment is usually continued for approximately 9 months. Children may be given amikacin 7.5 mg/kg IV q12h for 3 weeks in addition to the dapsone or TMP-SMX. An alternative for adults is amikacin 500 mg IM q12h for 3 weeks in addition to the dapsone or TMP-SMX.

Ketoconazole, itraconazole, or griseofulvin can be tried in the treatment of eumycetomas; however, surgical excision is often the only chance for cure (Hay, 2000).

Prevention

In endemic areas, workers need to wear shoes and protective clothing. Education and early treatment are the best ways to prevent extensive infection and loss of function (Mahgoub, 1999).

Reporting

The U.S. Centers for Disease Control and Prevention does not consider mycetoma to be a nationally notifiable disease. The World Health Organization (WHO) considers mycetoma a Class 5 disease. See Appendix C for details and for upcoming changes in WHO reporting.

References

Hay, R.J. (2000). Subcutaneous mycoses: General principles. In G.T. Strickland (Ed.), *Hunter's tropical medicine* (8th ed., pp. 537-541). Philadelphia: W.B. Saunders Company.

Hay, R.J. (2003). Fungal infections. In G.C. Cook & A.I. Zumla (Eds.), *Manson's tropical diseases* (21st ed., pp. 1180-1182). Philadelphia: W.B. Saunders Company.

Mahgoub, E. (1999). Mycetoma. In R.L. Guerrant, D.H. Walker, & P.F. Weller (Eds.), *Tropical infectious diseases: Principles, pathogens, and practice* (pp. 616-620). New York: Churchill Livingstone.

Queiroz-Telles, F., McGinnis, M.R., Salkin, I., & Graybill, J.R. (2003). Subcutaneous mycoses. *Infectious Disease Clinics of North America, 17*(1), 59-85.

Sobera, J.O., & Elewski, B.E. (2003). Fungal diseases. In Bolognia, J.L., Jorizzo, J.L., & Rapini, R.P. (Eds.), *Dermatology* (pp. 1187-1188). Philadelphia: Mosby.

57

MYIASIS

Blowfly, fleshfly, human botfly infestation, tumbu fly

Geographic Distribution

— The geographic distribution of myiasis varies according to the type of fly causing the disease and the location of the infestation on the body. Cutaneous tissue myiasis can be caused by the Congo floor maggot (in tropical Africa), the tumbu fly (in sub-Saharan Africa and Southern Spain), and the human botfly (in Central and South America). Wound myiasis is found worldwide, but the dominant fly species varies with the location. Dermal myiasis is caused by the horse or cattle botfly, which is a common parasite found worldwide. Nasal myiasis is caused by many types of flies and is found primarily in Asia and less commonly in Africa (White, 2003; Wirtz & Azad, 2000).

Agent and Vector

— Cutaneous myiasis can be caused by the blood-sucking Congo floor maggot. The adult fly is named *Auchmeromyia luteola.* This fly lays its eggs in the crevices of mud floors of thatched huts, takes blood meals by attaching its mouth hooks into cutaneous blood vessels, and then retreats under sleeping mats or into the floor.

— Subcutaneous myiasis can be caused by the tumbu fly, *Cordylobia anthropophaga,* or the human botfly, *Dermatobia hominis.* The female tumbu fly lays eggs on clothing or in the sand. The hatched larvae can remain alive for 9 to 15 days without feeding, and they eventually attach to a living host, painlessly penetrate unbroken skin, and slowly mature within the subcutaneous tissue. The human botfly lays her eggs on day-flying mosquitoes or muscoid flies. The eggs are then deposited in the host's skin at the site of penetration when the mosquito or fly bites. Maturation of the larvae takes from 1 to 12 weeks, at which time the larvae drop to the ground to pupate in the soil.

–   Wound myiasis is caused by flies that lay their eggs in wounds or gangrenous tissues. *Wohlfahrtia magnifica* is the predominant source of infection in southern Europe, Russia, Africa, and the Middle East. *Chrysomyia bezziana* is the most common cause of wound myiasis in Asia and sub-Saharan Africa. In the Americas, *Cochliomyia hominivorax* is the primary culprit.

–   Dermal myiasis, or creeping eruption, is caused by the horse botfly, *Gasterophilus* species, or the cattle botfly, *Hypoderma* species. The larvae penetrate the skin but cannot develop in the human host, creating a wandering burrow in the epidermis.

–   Nasal myiasis is most commonly caused by the Old World screw fly, *C. bezziana*; however, other causes include the sheep nasal botfly, *Oestrus ovis*, and the Russian gadfly, *Rhinoestrus purpureus*. The flies lay eggs in the nasal cavity and burrow into nearby tissue, including cartilage and bone.

–   Other types of myiasis include ocular myiasis (caused by *Oestrus*, *Wohlfahrtia*, *Gasterophilus*, *Rhinoestrus*, and *Hypoderma* species), myiasis of the anus and vagina (caused by *Wohlfahrtia* species), urogenital myiasis (caused by *Psychoda*, *Musca*, *Calliphora*, and *Sarcophaga* species), and intestinal myiasis (caused by *Musca*, *Fannia*, *Chrysomyia*, *Calliphora*, *Sarcophaga*, and *Lucilia* species) (Meinking, Burkhart, & Burkhart, 2003; White, 2003; Wirtz & Azad, 2000).

Incubation

— The time that larvae spend developing in human tissue ranges from days to weeks, depending on the type of fly.

Clinical Findings and Treatment

Signs and Symptoms

— Cutaneous myiasis, caused by the blood-sucking Congo floor maggot, leads to painless bites on the skin and relatively little blood loss. The only symptoms present may be itching and redness in the area of the bite.

— Subcutaneous myiasis, also known as furuncular myiasis, causes boil-like skin lesions. The lesions caused by the tumbu fly are usually on the trunk, thighs, and buttocks; however, the human botfly most commonly affects exposed areas, including the scalp, face, arms, and legs. A small erythematous pruritic papule develops within 1 day of penetration and slowly grows to a nodule 1 to 3 cm in diameter. The larvae or larval feces may be seen extruding from the apex of the nodule. The lesions are often itchy, painful, crusted, and occasionally purulent.

— In wound myiasis, larvae may sometimes be seen within the wound. Occasionally they burrow to nearby tissue, creating erythematous subcutaneous nodules.

— Dermal myiasis caused by *Gasterophilus* larvae has an erythematous wandering tract that resembles cutaneous larva migrans. The *Hypoderma* species are able to penetrate deeper into subcutaneous tissue and may also form subcutaneous nodules. The predominant symptom is itching.

— Initial symptoms of nasal myiasis include sneezing, pain, and nasal obstruction, which may progress to edema and purulent discharge (Meinking et al., 2003; White, 2003; Wirtz & Azad, 2000).

Complilcations

— Some larvae can migrate into the eye from nearby cutaneous lesions; however, certain species specifically involve the ocular structures. The *Oestrus* species and *Wohlfahrtia* species lay eggs on the external surface of the eye, causing conjunctival irritation known as external ophthalmomyiasis. Other species are capable of causing internal ophthalmomyiasis, leading to blindness and loss of the eye.

— The maggots of *Hypoderma ovis* have been reported to invade the central nervous system. In nasal myiasis, the larvae may migrate through the nasal bones into the brain, leading to meningitis and death. Larvae may also invade the ear canal, leading to pain, deafness, and tinnitus.

— Other structures that may be invaded by the larvae include the vagina, anus, bladder, and intestinal tract. This may lead to symptoms such as abdominal pain, vomiting, diarrhea, dysuria, and cutaneous erosions around the genitals and anus (White, 2003).

Common Laboratory Findings

— There are no laboratory findings commonly associated with myiasis.

Diagnosis

— The diagnosis of subcutaneous myiasis can be made by identifying the respiratory spiracles of the larvae or fecal exudates at the apex of the furuncular skin lesion. If these are not seen, petroleum jelly can be applied on the surface of the lesion and the presence of bubbles or emergence of the larvae is pathognomonic.

— Dermal myiasis needs to be differentiated from other causes of creeping eruptions. The *Gasterophilus* larvae can be identified by applying mineral oil to the skin lesion and visualizing the larvae with black transverse spines.

Nasal myiasis can be diagnosed by visualizing and extracting the larvae with the aid of a nasal speculum. Any extracted larvae, whether from the nose, eye, gastrointestinal tract, bladder, or genitals, can be preserved in alcohol and sent to a laboratory for identification (White, 2003).

Differential Diagnosis

The differential diagnosis for subcutaneous myiasis includes furunculosis, cellulitis, onchocerciasis, leishmaniasis, infected epidermal inclusion cysts, tungiasis, other arthropod bites, and lymphadenopathy. Dermal myiasis resembles other creeping eruptions, such as cutaneous larva migrans caused by *Ancylostoma*, *Strongyloides*, *Gnathostoma*, or *Fasciola* (Meinking et al., 2003; White, 2003).

Treatment

Subcutaneous myiasis can be treated in many ways. The larvae can be surgically removed; however, if they are forcibly extracted or parts of the larvae are left behind, then a foreign body reaction can occur. Substances, such as petrolatum, oil, or paraffin, can be applied to the surface of the skin lesion in order to suffocate or extrude the larvae (Figure 57-1). The base of the furuncular lesion can also be injected with lidocaine, which causes tissue swelling and forces the larvae to the surface. Dermal myiasis can be excised or removed with a needle. Wound myiasis is treated with debridement and irrigation or surgical removal.

Treatment of myiasis involving other organs also involves manual extraction or surgical removal of the larvae. Widespread cutaneous or body cavity myiasis can be treated with a one-time dose of oral ivermectin (total of 300 μg/kg); however, it often takes weeks for the larvae to be sloughed. Once this occurs, the erythema and inflammation will slowly resolve (Meinking et al., 2003;

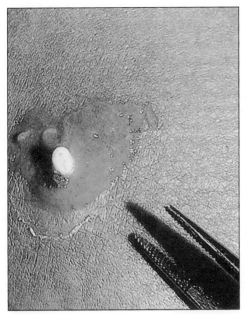

FIGURE 57–1

Removing a larva after covering it with oil to block the respiratory spiracles. (*Source:* From Peters, W., & Pasvol, G. [2002]. *Tropical medicine and parasitology* [5th ed., p. 271]. Chicago: Mosby.)

Ribeiro, Pereira, & Alves, 2001; White, 2003; Wirtz & Azad, 2000).

Prevention

Prevention is best accomplished by limiting contact with areas or conditions where fly eggs are laid. Other measures (Meinking et al., 2003; White, 2003) include the following:

- Avoid lying on the ground, especially sandy areas contaminated with urine or feces.
- Hang newly washed clothes to dry indoors with the windows closed, or hang newly washed clothes to dry in bright sunlight rather than shade (because eggs are

laid only in shaded areas). Do not lay clothes on the ground to dry.

- Use window screens and avoid sleeping on dirt floors.
- Iron both sides of all clothing and towels.
- Reduce the host population (dogs and brown rats) and transmitting mosquito or fly populations as much as possible.
- Keep wounds scrupulously clean.
- Use DEET insect repellant when in infested areas.
- Widespread sterilization of male insects or extermination may help control the fly population.

Community education in endemic areas should be ongoing.

Reporting

The U.S. Centers for Disease Control and Prevention does not consider myiasis to be a nationally notifiable disease. The World Health Organization (WHO) considers myiasis a Class 5 disease. See Appendix C for details and for upcoming changes in WHO reporting.

References

Meinking, T.L., Burkhart, C.N., & Burkhart, C.G. (2003). Infestations. In J.L. Bolognia, J.L. Jorizzo, & R.P. Rapini (Eds.), *Dermatology* (pp. 1321-1349). Philadelphia: Mosby.

Ribeiro, F., Pereira, C., & Alves, A. (2001). Treatment of human cavitary myiasis with oral ivermectin. *Revista Brasileira de Otorrinolaringologia, 67,* 755-761.

White, G.B. (2003). Ectoparasites: Leeches and leech infestation, myiasis, jigger fleas, scabies, louse infestation. In G.C. Cook & A.I. Zumla (Eds.), *Manson's tropical diseases* (21st ed., pp. 1599-1609). Philadelphia: W.B. Saunders Company.

Wirtz, R.A., & Azad, A.F. (2000). Injurious arthropods. In G. Strickland (Ed.), *Hunter's tropical medicine and emerging infectious diseases* (8th ed., pp. 910-925). Philadelphia: W.B. Saunders Company.

58

PARACOCCIDIOIDOMYCOSIS
Brazilian blastomycosis, South American blastomycosis

Geographic Distribution

‒ Paracoccidioidomycosis is found in the tropical areas of Central and South America, with Brazil, Colombia, and Venezuela being the areas of highest endemicity (Graybill & Al-Abdely, 1999).

Agent and Vector

‒ Paracoccidioidomycosis is caused by *Paracoccidioides brasiliensis,* a dimorphic fungus. The organism is found in the soil of endemic regions with abundant vegetation, rivers, and rainfall, and infection is most common among young male rural agricultural workers. Infection is likely caused by inhalation of aerosolized conidia (asexual fungal spores), leading to pulmonary disease and occasionally dissemination. Primary infection of the skin and mucous membranes occurs rarely (Graybill & Al-Abdely, 1999; Negroni, 2000; Sobera & Elewski, 2003).

Incubation

‒ The period between exposure to the organism and clinical disease may be many years (Graybill & Al-Abdely, 1999).

Clinical Findings and Treatment

Signs and Symptoms

‒ Paracoccidioidomycosis infection is often asymptomatic or very mild, and primary pulmonary infections are usually overlooked since they may mimic common bacterial or viral respiratory infections. People living in endemic areas frequently have positive skin tests to paracoccidioidomycosis without a known history of prior infection.

— The two main forms of symptomatic disease are the acute juvenile type and the chronic adult type. The acute juvenile type makes up a small percentage of paracoccidioidomycosis infections and manifests as rapid disseminated disease with involvement of the spleen, liver, lymph nodes, lungs, bone marrow, and mucocutaneous surfaces. Patients may present with fever, anorexia, weight loss, diarrhea, pneumonia, lymphadenopathy, hepatosplenomegaly, mucosal and skin ulcerations, subcutaneous abscesses, and/or acneiform papules of the skin.

— The chronic adult form progresses over months to years and accounts for the majority of symptomatic paracoccidioidomycosis infections. The lungs are sometimes the only site of infection, and progressive pulmonary disease is characteristic. Symptoms may include cough, sputum production, weight loss, exertional dyspnea, and fever. A chest X-ray may show bilateral symmetric parahilar infiltrates and small nodules. Although lung disease is common, the majority of patients with the chronic adult form present with involvement of multiple sites, including the skin, mucous membranes, lungs, lymph nodes, adrenal glands, liver, spleen, and central nervous system (CNS). Mucocutaneous lesions are often ulcerative, destructive, or verrucous, and they are commonly found on the face, oral mucosa, or nasal mucosa (Figure 58-1). The lips and gingiva may have a firm violaceous edema, which makes eating painful. Lymphangitic spread commonly results in cervical lymphadenopathy, which may be firm, suppurative, or necrotic. (Graybill & Al-Abdely, 1999; Negroni, 2000; Sobera & Elewski, 2003).

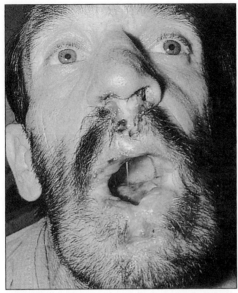

FIGURE 58–1

Mucocutaneous lesions in paracoccidioidomycosis. (*Source:* From Peters, W., & Pasvol, G. [2002]. *Tropical medicine and parasitology* [5th ed., p. 259]. Chicago: Mosby.)

Complications

Laryngeal attacks can occur in the chronic adult form and may be associated with dysphonia, dysphagia, and dyspnea. When the lesions of the chronic adult form heal, the resulting dense fibrosis may cause chronic dyspnea, dysphonia, microstomia, glottic or tracheal stenosis, cor pulmonale, or adrenal insufficiency. Paracoccidioidomycosis infections may occur as an AIDS-associated opportunistic infection and are usually aggressive with common involvement of the meninges. CNS involvement may result in posterior fossa abscesses or meningoencephalitis (Graybill & Al-Abdely, 1999; Negroni, 2000).

Common Laboratory Findings

The acute juvenile form may present with anemia, leuko-cytosis with eosinophilia, and elevated bilirubin levels (Negroni, 2000).

Diagnosis

The diagnosis can be established based on history of exposure, physical examination, and the demonstration of typical large narrow-based budding yeast cells from tissue. The characteristic budding yeast can be found in tissue sections of involved organs, especially skin, and bronchoalveolar lavage fluid or sputum. In tissue sections, periodic acid-Schiff stains can be used to more easily visualize the yeast. Potassium hydroxide prepara-tions or methenamine silver stains of sputum samples may be used to demonstrate the yeast forms. Culture of sputum, bronchoalveolar lavage fluid, or other infected tissue may be performed on Sabouraud agar at room temperature. Specific antibodies can be demonstrated using complement fixation or enzyme-linked immunosorbent assays (ELISA). The paracoccidioidin skin test has little value in the diagnosis because it does not confirm active disease, and false-positive reactions may occur in patients with infections with other fungi (Graybill & Al-Abdely, 1999; Negroni, 2000; Vega-Lopez & Chopra, 2003).

Differential Diagnosis

The acute juvenile form may clinically resemble severe tuberculosis, leukemia, or lymphoma. The endemic areas of paracoccidioidomycosis infection overlap with those of histoplasmosis. The pulmonary and disseminated forms of these diseases are very similar, making these entities difficult to distinguish. The differential diagnosis of the skin lesions may include leishmaniasis, syphilis, Wegener's granulomatosis, and natural killer (NK) cell lymphoma (Graybill & Al-Abdely, 1999; Negroni, 2000; Sobera & Elewski, 2003).

Treatment

Sulfadiazine (6 g/day) and trimethoprim-sulfamethoxazole (TMP-SMX) DS, (160/800 mg q12h) can be used to treat paracoccidioidomycosis, and the combination is frequently used for recently diagnosed patients with no previous therapy, patients with chronic focal disease, for maintenance therapy after treatment with amphotericin B, or as prophylaxis in AIDS patients. Treatment must continue for 2 to 3 years when using these medications due to the high relapse rate. Ketoconazole (200 mg/day for 12 months) or itraconazole (100 mg/day for 6 months) can also be used and seem to have a higher response rate and lower relapse rate than sulfonamides. For severe disease, amphotericin B (0.7 to 0.8 mg/kg/day to a total maximum dose of 35 mg/kg) can be used initially (Graybill & Al-Abdely, 1999; Negroni, 2000).

Prevention

No control measures or vaccinations have been developed to prevent paracoccidioidomycosis infection in endemic areas (Negroni, 2000).

Reporting

The U.S. Centers for Disease Control and Prevention does not consider paracoccidioidomycosis to be a nationally notifiable disease. The World Health Organization (WHO) considers it a Class 5 disease. See Appendix C for details and for upcoming changes in WHO reporting.

References

Graybill, J.R., & Al-Abdely, H. (1999). Paracoccidioidomycosis. In R.L. Guerrant, D.H. Walker, & P.F. Weller (Eds.), *Tropical infectious diseases: Principles, pathogens, and practice* (pp. 637-640). New York: Churchill Livingstone.

Negroni, R. (2000). Paracoccidioidomycosis. In G.T. Strickland (Ed.), *Hunter's tropical medicine and emerging infectious diseases* (8th ed., pp. 559-561). Philadelphia: W.B. Saunders Company.

Sobera, J.O., & Elewski, B.E. (2003). Fungal diseases. In J.L. Bolognia, J.L. Jorizzo, & R.P. Rapini (Eds.), *Dermatology* (pp. 1193-1194). Philadelphia: Mosby.

Vega-Lopez, F., & Chopra, S. (2003). Dermatologic problems. In G.C. Cook & A.I. Zumla (Eds.), *Manson's tropical diseases* (21st ed., pp. 380-381). Philadelphia: W.B. Saunders Company.

59

Parastrongyliasis, Abdominal

Formerly angiostrongyliasis

Geographic Distribution

— Abdominal parastrongyliasis occurs in Central and South America, especially in Costa Rica (Chin, 2000).

Agent and Vector

— *Parastrongylus costaricensis* is a small (33 mm in length) filiform nematode of rodents, especially the cotton rat. The mature worms live in and lay eggs in the mesenteric arteries of the cecal area. The eggs are carried into the intestinal wall, where they hatch and migrate as first-stage larvae through the wall and into the lumen and are excreted. Feces are a food source for the intermediate host, usually slugs. In the intermediate host, the larvae mature to the infective third stage. When rodents eat the slugs with larvae, they are infected or reinfected. Humans are infected when infected slugs (or their mucus, as may be found on poorly washed vegetables) are ingested. The larvae penetrate the gut wall, where they mature in lymph nodes and vessels, and then migrate to the mesenteric arterioles of the ileocecal region of the gastrointestinal tract where eggs are laid. In rodents, this reinitiates the life cycle, but in humans, the eggs and larvae die, causing eosinophilic granuloma masses ("Morera's disease"). Another pathogenic mechanism is the thrombosis of mesenteric arteries, with resultant necrosis of tissue (Chin, 2000; Morera, 2000; Peters & Pasvol, 2002).

Incubation

— The incubation period is approximately 24 days (Morera, 2000).

Clinical Findings and Treatment

Signs and Symptoms

— Abdominal parastrongyliasis is most commonly found in children and is often mistaken for acute abdomen or appendicitis when the worms are in the ileocecal area. Signs and symptoms include abdominal pain and tenderness in the right iliac fossa and right flank; in about 50% of cases, a tumor-like mass may be felt in the lower right quadrant on palpation. Fever, anorexia, nausea and vomiting, constipation, abdominal rigidity, and pain on rectal examination are common. Less common are complaints of upper right quadrant pain, with hepatomegaly and tenderness to palpation (Morera, 2000; Peters & Pasvol, 2002).

Complications

— The testicles may be affected, causing acute pain and redness, with the testicles later becoming purple and necrotic (Morera, 2000).

Common Laboratory Findings

— Leukocytosis and eosinophilia are common.

Diagnosis

— Diagnosis is based on endemicity and clinical features. It is complicated by the lack of excreted larvae in feces. Because of similarity to appendicitis (or testicular torsion), diagnosis is often at surgery (Morera, 2000; Peters & Pasvol, 2002).

Differential Diagnosis

— The differential diagnosis includes appendicitis, malignancy, and (with testicular involvement) testicular torsion (Morera, 2000; Peters & Pasvol, 2002).

Treatment

Because abdominal parastrongyliasis is self-limiting, treatment is usually supportive, with surgery sometimes required with heavy loads. Antihelminthics such as diethylcarbamazine or thiabendazole have been used, but efficacy in humans has not been demonstrated; in rats, these drugs disrupt the parasites and cause erratic migration and worsened lesions (Morera, 2000; Nash, 2000).

Prevention

Prevention of abdominal parastrongyliasis caused by *P. costaricensis* (Chin, 2000; Zanini & Graeff-Teixeira, 2001) is aided by the following:

- Control rodents by coordinated and simultaneous campaigns to rat-proof buildings, store food in secure areas, bury or burn garbage, rid community of uncontrolled rubbish accumulations, and poison rodents. Rodent control is the most important means of prevention.
- Avoid consumption of raw or undercooked mollusks (snails, prawns, shrimp, crabs) and fish. These foods may be safely eaten after boiling for 3 to 5 min or freezing at $-15°$ C ($5°$ F) for 12 hours.
- Avoid consumption of raw vegetables, especially leafy greens, in endemic areas, because even thorough cleaning of vegetables is not effective unless done with 1.5% bleach solution for 15 min.
- Control mollusks and land planarians (worms).

Community education regarding the above measures is important.

Reporting

The U.S. Centers for Disease Control and Prevention does not classify abdominal parastrongyliasis as a nationally notifiable disease. The World Health

Organization (WHO) considers it to be a Class 5 disease. See Appendix C for details and for upcoming changes in WHO reporting.

References

Chin, J. (Ed.). (2000). *Control of communicable diseases manual* (17th ed., pp. 15-17). Washington, DC: American Public Health Association.

Morera, P. (2000). Abdominal angiostrongyliasis. In G.T. Strickland (Ed.), *Hunter's tropical medicine and emerging infectious diseases* (8th ed., pp. 795-797). Philadelphia: W.B. Saunders Company.

Nash, T.E. (2000). Visceral larva migrans and other unusual helminthic infections. In G. Mandell, J. Bennett, & R. Dolin (Eds.), *Principles and practice of infectious diseases* (5th ed., pp. 2965-2970). New York: Churchill Livingstone.

Peters, W., & Pasvol, G. (2002). *Tropical medicine and parasitology* [5th ed.]. Chicago: Mosby.

Zanini, G.M., & Graeff-Teixeira, C. (2001). Inactivation of infective larvae of *Angiostrongylus costaricensis* with short time incubations in 1.5% bleach solution, vinegar, or saturated cooking salt solution. *Acta Tropica, 78,* 17-21.

Parastrongyliasis Meningitis

Eosinophilic meningoencephalitis, formerly angiostrongyliasis

Geographic Distribution

Parastrongyliasis meningitis occurs in the Caribbean Islands, Southeast Asia, Pacific Islands, and Taiwan (Chin, 2000; Nash, 2000).

Agent and Vector

Parastrongylus cantonensis is a nematode also known as the rat lung worm. The mature worms live in the pulmonary arteries of rodents. Eggs are laid in the arteries and first-stage larvae migrate to the alimentary tract and are excreted in the rodent feces. The feces are then eaten by snails, slugs, freshwater shrimp, or other mollusks (notably, the giant African land snail); these animals become the intermediate hosts in which the larvae further mature. When infected mollusks (or their mucus left on poorly washed vegetables) are ingested, the infective third-stage larvae migrate to the brain to mature into young adults. In rats, the life cycle continues with migration through the subarachnoid space and on to the pulmonary arteries. In humans, the worms seldom survive past the central nervous system (CNS) (Bunnag, 2000; Peters & Pasvol, 2002).

Incubation

The incubation period ranges from 1 to 45 days, and is most commonly 13 to 16 days (Hughes & Biggs, 2002; Nash, 2000).

Clinical Findings and Treatment

Signs and Symptoms

Depending on larval loads, eosinophilic meningoencephalitis from parastrongylus infection ranges from benign and subclinical to severe and fatal. In general, patients are not as ill as those with bacterial meningitis. Soon after ingesting the larvae there may be symptoms of nausea, vomiting, and abdominal discomfort. After the parasites have reached the CNS, the chief complaint is usually severe bitemporal or occipital headache of insidious or sudden onset. Other signs and symptoms include stiff neck, low-grade fever, paresthesias of trunk and extremities, and unilateral facial paralysis. Cranial nerve involvement is most commonly optic (II), abducens (VI), or facial (VII). Young adult worms are rarely found in the optic chambers. The disease is usually self-limiting with severe symptoms lasting a few days and the illness resolving in 2 to 8 weeks (Bunnag, 2000; Hughes & Biggs, 2002; Nash, 2000).

Complications

Retinal hemorrhage and detachment, coma, and death are uncommon complications (Bunnag, 2000).

Common Laboratory Findings

Common laboratory findings include elevation of the initial cerebrospinal fluid (CSF) pressure above 200 mm water and up to 500 mm. The CSF is opalescent or turbid but not purulent, has elevated protein, and contains between 500 and 2,00 leukocytes/mm^3, usually with a high percentage of eosinophils. Peripheral eosinophilia (15% to 50%) lasts about 3 months (Bunnag, 2000).

Diagnosis

Diagnosis is on the basis of characteristic clinical and laboratory findings (especially of the CSF), combined with a history of travel to or residence in endemic areas and consumption of undercooked foods such as freshwater shrimp or contaminated salad greens. Rarely, larvae may be found in the CSF. A definitive diagnosis may be made by serologic examination of paired specimens using a specific adult worm antigen or (on autopsy) by recovery of *P. cantonensis* larvae from the CNS or ocular chambers (Bunnag, 2000; Peters & Pasvol, 2002).

Differential Diagnosis

The syndrome of eosinophilic meningoencephalitis may occur with cysticercosis, paragonimiasis, toxocariasis, schistosomiasis, and *Gnathostoma spinigerum* infections. The differential diagnosis also includes other illnesses with meningeal signs and symptoms such as bacterial and viral meningitis (see Appendix A on presenting symptoms).

Treatment

Treatment is supportive, and includes corticosteroids, repeated lumbar punctures to relieve intracranial pressure, and analgesics. Anthelminthics are not used because of danger of eliciting a host inflammatory reaction to dead worms in the CNS (Bunnag, 2000).

Prevention

Prevention of parastrongyliasis meningitis (Bunnag, 2000; Chin, 2000; Zanini & Graeff-Teixeira, 2001) includes the following:

- Control rodents by coordinated and simultaneous campaigns to rat-proof buildings, store food in secure areas, bury or burn garbage, rid community of uncontrolled rubbish accumulations, and poison rodents. Rodent control is the most important means of prevention.

- Avoid consumption of raw or undercooked mollusks (snails, prawns, shrimp, crabs) and fish. These foods may be safely eaten after boiling for 3 to 5 min or freezing at $-15°$ C ($5°$ F) for 12 hours.
- Avoid consumption of raw vegetables, especially leafy greens, in endemic areas, because even thorough cleaning of vegetables is not completely effective unless done with 1.5% bleach solution for 15 min.
- Control mollusks and land planarians (worms).

Community education regarding the preceding measures is important.

Reporting

The U.S. Centers for Disease Control and Prevention does not classify parastrongyliasis meningitis as a nationally notifiable disease. The World Health Organization (WHO) considers it to be a Class 5 disease. See Appendix C for details and for upcoming changes in WHO reporting.

References

Bunnag, T. (2000). Angiostrongylus meningitis. In G.T. Strickland (Ed.), *Hunter's tropical medicine and emerging infectious diseases* (8th ed., pp. 793-797). Philadelphia: W.B. Saunders Company.

Chin, J. (Ed.). (2000). *Control of communicable diseases manual* (17th ed., pp. 15-17). Washington, DC: American Public Health Association.

Hughes, A.J., & Biggs, B.A. (2002). Parasitic worms of the central nervous system: An Australian perspective. *Internal Medicine Journal, 32,* 541-553.

Nash, T.E. (2000). Visceral larva migrans and other unusual helminthic infections. In G. Mandell, J. Bennett, & R. Dolin (Eds.), *Principles and practice of infectious diseases* (5th ed., pp. 2965-2970). New York: Churchill Livingstone.

Peters, W., & Pasvol, G. (2002). *Tropical medicine and parasitology* (5th ed.). Chicago: Mosby.

Zanini, G.M., & Graeff-Teixeira, C. (2001). Inactivation of infective larvae of *Angiostrongylus costaricensis* with short time incubations in 1.5% bleach solution, vinegar or saturated cooking salt solution. *Acta Tropica, 78,* 17-21.

61

PEMPHIGUS, ENDEMIC FOLIACEUS
Fogo selvagem (wild fire), Brazilian pemphigus foliaceus
Geographic Distribution

― Pemphigus foliaceus is endemic to Brazil and certain areas of Colombia, Bolivia, Paraguay, and Argentina (Vega-Lopez & Chopra, 2003).

Agent and Vector

― Endemic pemphigus foliaceus is clinically and histologically identical to the sporadic form of pemphigus foliaceus; however, unlike the sporadic form, cases are clustered in rural endemic regions and occur with high frequency in children and young adults. Most affected people live near rivers and within flying range of the black flies (*Simulium pruinosum*) that may be the vectors of this disease.

― The clinical findings associated with all forms of pemphigus foliaceus are caused by autoantibodies directed against desmoglein-1, a desmosome-associated glycoprotein in the skin. There is a high prevalence of these autoantibodies among asymptomatic people living in the endemic areas of pemphigus foliaceus, and disease onset is thought to be preceded by a sustained antibody response. The production of these autoantibodies is likely initiated by an environmental factor, such as exposure to *S. pruinosum;* however, people with certain human leukocyte antigen (HLA) classes may have a higher predisposition to developing clinical disease (Amagai, 2003; Chiossi & Roselino, 2001; Hans-Filho et al., 1999; Nisihara et al., 2003; Warren et al., 2000).

Incubation

- The incubation period is unknown, given that the environmental exposure or cause of the disease is not entirely clear.

Clinical Findings and Treatment

Signs and Symptoms

- The primary lesions of pemphigus foliaceus are superficial blisters; however, these rupture easily and typically present as erythematous, crusted, scaly erosions (Figure 61-1). The lesions favor a seborrheic distribution, including the scalp, face, and upper trunk, and mucosal involvement is very rare. Some patients complain of burning or pain at the site of the lesions (hence the name of the illness).

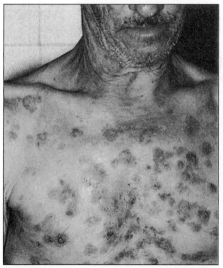

FIGURE 61-1

Man with "fogo selvagem." (*Source:* From Peters, W., & Pasvol, G. [2002]. *Tropical medicine and parasitology* [5th ed., p. 312]. Chicago: Mosby.)

Pemphigus foliaceus has several forms, such as the classic localized form, classic generalized form, probable localized form, pemphigus foliaceus under treatment, and cured pemphigus foliaceus. The localized form often presents as erosions in focal areas of the face and trunk; however, some patients may only have erythematous, violaceous, or hyperpigmented papules and plaques. These localized lesions may remain unchanged for months to years, undergo spontaneous regression, or progress to the generalized form.

The generalized form has three presentations, including a bullous-exfoliative, exfoliative erythroderma, and generalized keratotic and nodular form. The bullous-exfoliative form is acute, aggressive, and may present with widespread bullae, fever, arthralgias, and malaise. The primary lesions in the exfoliative erythroderma form are widespread crusted erosions. The generalized keratotic form presents as widespread keratotic plaques and nodules, especially in the seborrheic and acral areas.

The probable localized form may show clinical and histologic evidence of pemphigus foliaceus but the immunofluorescent studies are negative. Once the autoantibodies are detected, these patients may be reclassified as the classic localized form. Occasionally patients who are either being treated or undergoing remission will develop a hyperpigmentation syndrome, and the pigmentation may be diffuse or confined to areas with previous lesions. Patients are considered cured when they show no clinical or immunologic evidence of pemphigus foliaceus for at least 5 years (Amagai, 2003; Hans-Filho et al., 1999; Vega-Lopez & Chopra, 2003).

Complications

Patients with the bullous-exfoliative type of the generalized form are susceptible to life-threatening severe infections with herpes simplex virus. Patients with the exfoliative erythroderma type of the generalized form are susceptible to superinfection with dermatophytes, scabies, and warts. Delay in diagnosis in early childhood can lead to azoospermia and dwarfism. Forty percent of patients who do not receive treatment will die within 2 years (Hans-Filho et al., 1999; Vega-Lopez & Chopra, 2003).

Common Laboratory Findings

There are no common laboratory findings.

Diagnosis

The history and physical examination of a patient living in an endemic area may suggest the diagnosis of pemphigus foliaceus. The clinical, histologic, and immunologic features of endemic pemphigus foliaceus are identical to sporadic pemphigus foliaceus, and only the history can help differentiate these two entities. A skin biopsy of an early blister will reveal acantholysis, or separation of the epidermis, in or adjacent to the granular layer; however, this can also be present in pemphigus vulgaris, staphylococcal scalded skin syndrome, or bullous impetigo. Demonstration of autoantibodies against the cell surface of keratinocytes through direct immunofluorescence of perilesional normal skin or indirect immunofluorescence of the patients' sera to normal human skin or guinea pig esophagus will help establish the diagnosis; however, pemphigus vulgaris and foliaceus will often have indistinguishable staining patterns. To differentiate these, specific autoantibodies against desmoglein-1 can be identified using immunoprecipitation, immunoblotting, or enzyme-linked immunosorbent assay (ELISA) (Amagai, 2003).

Differential Diagnosis

When few crusted lesions are present, fogo selvagem is often mistaken for impetigo. The localized form of pemphigus foliaceus may be confused with discoid lupus erythematosus (DLE), given the involvement of sun-exposed areas on the face and trunk; however, pemphigus foliaceus lacks many features of DLE, such as follicular involvement, epidermal atrophy, and hypopigmentation. In the generalized form of exfoliative erythroderma, other causes of erythroderma should be ruled out, including atopic dermatitis, psoriasis, drug reactions, and dermatophyte infection. Endemic pemphigus foliaceus can be differentiated from the sporadic form of pemphigus foliaceus by the history of exposure to an endemic area and from pemphigus vulgaris by the lack of mucosal involvement (Amagai, 2003; Hans-Filho et al., 1999)

Treatment

When disease is localized, superpotent topical steroids may be sufficient for treatment. In the case of widespread active lesions, systemic steroids are the treatment of choice (1.0 mg/kg/day initially), and they are slowly tapered according to the disease response. Pulse methylprednisolone may be given at a dose of 1 g/day over 2 to 3 hours for 3 to 5 consecutive days. Other immunosuppressants that may be used as steroid sparing agents to control disease include azathioprine 2 to 4 mg/kg/day, cyclophosphamide 1 to 3 mg/kg/day, mycophenolate mofetil 2 to 3 g/day, or cyclosporine 5 mg/kg/day. Before receiving immunosuppressants, patients should first be evaluated for concurrent infection, such as tuberculosis. During therapy, many of the medications mentioned require monthly clinical and laboratory monitoring for possible pancytopenia, liver toxicity, renal toxicity, and carcinogenesis (Amagai, 2003; Vega-Lopez & Chopra, 2003).

Prevention

Prevention is difficult because the exact cause is not known and the prevalence of disease is so high in endemic areas.

Reporting

The U.S. Centers for Disease Control and Prevention does not classify pemphigus foliaceus as a nationally notifiable disease. The World Health Organization (WHO) considers it as a Class 5 disease. See Appendix C for details and for upcoming changes in WHO reporting.

References

Amagai, M. (2003). Pemphigus. In J.L. Bolognia, J.L. Jorizzo, & R.P. Rapini (Eds.), *Dermatology* (pp. 449-460). Philadelphia: Mosby.

Chiossi, M.P., & Roselino, A.M. (2001). Endemic pemphigus foliaceus ("Fogo selvagem"): A series from the Northeastern region of the State of Sao Paulo, Brazil, 1973-1998. *Revista do Instituto de Medicina Tropical de Sao Paulo, 43,* 59-62.

Hans-Filho, G., Aoki, V., Rivitti, E., Eaton, D.P., Lin, M.S., & Diaz, L.A. (1999). Endemic pemphigus foliaceus (fogo selvagem)—1998. The Cooperative Group on Fogo Selvagem Research. *Clinics in Dermatology, 17,* 225-235.

Nisihara, R.M., et al. (2003). Prevalence of autoantibodies in patients with endemic pemphigus foliaceus (fogo selvagem). *Archives of Dermatological Research, 295,* 133-137.

Vega-Lopez, F., & Chopra, S. (2003). Dermatologic problems. In G.C. Cook & A.I. Zumla (Eds.), *Manson's tropical diseases* (21st ed., pp. 395-396). Philadelphia: W.B. Saunders Company.

Warren, S.J., et al. (2000). The prevalence of antibodies against desmoglein 1 in endemic pemphigus foliaceus in Brazil. Cooperative Group on Fogo Selvagem Research. *New England Journal of Medicine, 343,* 23-30.

PERTUSSIS

Whooping cough

Geographic Distribution

— Pertussis is endemic worldwide, with epidemics occurring in limited geographic areas in 3- to 5-year cycles (Centers for Disease Control and Prevention [CDC], 2002).

Agent and Vector

— Most cases of pertussis are caused by *Bordetella pertussis*, a small gram-negative coccobacilli spread by airborne droplets from the respiratory mucous membranes of infected persons. Pertussis is highly contagious with as many as 90% of susceptible household contacts developing the illness after exposure to an index case. *B. parapertussis* also causes pertussis, especially in Europe and Russia. *B. pertussis* and *B. parapertussis* infect only humans and primates, although the related *B. bronchiseptica* commonly infects animals and, occasionally, immunocompromised humans. *B. pertussis* produces several biologically active substances, most notably pertussis toxin (PT), that account for local and systemic manifestations of the disease (CDC, 2002; Long, 2004).

Incubation

— The incubation period is 3 to 12 days and up to 20 days (Chin, 2000; Long, 2004).

Clinical Findings and Treatment

Signs and Symptoms

— In most cases, pertussis is a three-stage disease with severe cough and relatively mild systemic symptoms lasting approximately 6 weeks. Fever is either low grade or absent.

— The catarrhal or prodromal stage lasts 1 to 2 weeks and is marked by the gradual onset of rhinorrhea, sneezing, and cough similar to the common cold. Toward the end of the catarrhal stage, the cough becomes increasingly severe and secretions thicken.

— The paroxysmal stage is characterized by episodes of severe and often protracted paroxysmal coughing, which for some *but not all* patients ends with a loud inspiration or "whoop." There may be 2 to 50 coughing episodes per day, with 10 to 30 coughs in each episode. Paroxysms of coughing are exhausting and sometimes followed by vomiting of swallowed secretions. The paroxysmal stage usually lasts 3 to 4 weeks but ranges from a few days to several months. Paroxysms are worrisome if they are associated with:

- Cyanosis
- Oxygen desaturation or tachycardia that does not resolve within 30 sec after the end of the paroxysm
- Bradycardia (less than 60 beats per minute in infants)
- Duration longer than 60 sec
- Weak or absent self-rescue breaths
- Unresponsiveness at the end of the paroxysm.

— Even infants with potentially fatal illness may appear well between paroxysms.

— The convalescent stage is characterized by a gradual shift from paroxysmal coughing to a chronic cough. In most cases, the cough decreases in frequency and severity over 3 to 4 weeks but may last longer in some cases. Among infants, however, cough and whoop may increase during convalescence (Bass & Vincent, 2000; Bortolussi, Miller, Ledwith, & Halperin, 1995; Tozzi, Ravà, Ciofi degli Atti, Salmaso, and the Progetto Pertosse Working Group, 2003).

— Because the vaccine is not 100% effective, persons who are immunized against pertussis are still potentially susceptible, but the course is shorter and less severe than among those who are not immunized. Note that in infants and young adults the usual stages and manifestations are often absent or atypical. For example, infants may be toxic with apnea and cyanosis more prominent than cough, and the whoop may not be present. In older children and adults, the whoop may not be present and the illness may present as simply a prolonged cough with post-tussive vomiting.

Complications

The most common complication is pneumonia, either from a secondary bacterial infection or aspiration, characterized by fever, tachypnea, or respiratory distress between paroxysms. Other secondary infections include otitis media and sinusitis. Atelectasis shifting to several different areas of the lung is sometimes followed by bronchiectasis. Severe coughing may result in seizures (from hypoxemia), intracranial hemorrhage, subconjunctival hemorrhage, retinal hemorrhage, pneumothorax and subcutaneous emphysema, umbilical and inguinal hernia, and laceration of frenulum. Encephalopathy may be secondary to hypoxia, intracranial hemorrhage, or pertussis toxin. Poor feeding and vomiting may lead to significant weight loss. Pertussis early in life may lead to abnormal pulmonary function into adulthood. Death is most common among infants younger than age 6 months and is often related to pneumonia (Long, 2004; Luo, Brabin, & Bunn, 2003).

Common Laboratory Findings

Common laboratory findings include leukocytosis with absolute lymphocytosis consisting of normal small cells rather than large and atypical lymphocytes. Increased neutrophils suggest either a secondary infection or an alternate diagnosis. Extreme leukocytosis and thrombocytosis (platelet count of several hundred thousand) are associated with a poor prognosis. Chest X-rays usually have only mild abnormalities with perihilar infiltrates and atelectasis.

Diagnosis

Because laboratory diagnosis is imperfect, the diagnosis is often made clinically. A commonly accepted case definition is an acute cough illness lasting at least 2 weeks with either paroxysms of coughing, inspiratory whoop, or post-tussive vomiting without other apparent cause.

B. pertussis can be cultured on special media by obtaining nasopharyngeal secretions by aspiration or with a Dacron or calcium alginate swab. Direct testing of nasopharyngeal secretions by direct fluorescent antibody has low sensitivity and requires an experienced laboratory. Polymerase chain reaction is very sensitive, but not universally available. In unimmunized patients these tests are usually positive during the catarrhal and paroxysmal stages, but in partially or completely immunized individuals the tests are less sensitive during the paroxysmal stage. Serologic testing is sensitive, but not widely available (Long, 2004; Preziosi & Halloran, 2003).

Differential Diagnosis

The differential diagnosis for pertussis includes pneumonia (mycoplasma, chlamydia, and other bacteria), viral infections such as adenovirus or respiratory syncytial virus, tuberculosis, and cystic fibrosis.

Treatment

Infants younger than 3 months old, or any patient with concerning paroxysms, should be hospitalized for supportive care such as monitoring for episodes of apnea, oxygen, and suctioning. Mist by tent is useful when secretions are tenacious and airways are highly reactive. Patients with severe disease may require hospitalization in the intensive care unit for intubation, paralysis, and ventilation.

Antibiotic therapy can modify the course of illness only when started in the catarrhal stage. Afterward, the role of antibiotic therapy is to reduce the spread of the disease. Infected individuals should be considered contagious for 5 days after antibiotic therapy begins. The standard treatment is erythromycin estolate, 40 to 50 mg/kg/day (maximum 2 g/day) PO divided qid for 14 days. However, in infants younger than 6 weeks, erythromycin increases the risk of infantile hypertrophic pyloric stenosis by 7- to 10-fold. Azithromycin, which is as effective and better tolerated than erythromycin, may also be used at a dose of 10 mg/kg/day on day 1 followed by 5 mg/kg/day on days 2 through 5 as a single dose. Clarithromycin is also as effective as erythromycin and is given at 15 to 20 mg/kg/day (maximum 1 g) PO divided bid for 7 days. (Bass & Vincent, 2000; Langley, Halperin, Boucher, & Smith, 2004; Long, 2004).

Prevention

Pertussis can be prevented to a large extent by immunization with a five-dose series starting at 6 to 8 weeks of age through age 6 years. Acellular DTaP vaccine, consisting of multiple diphtheria and tetanus toxoids combined with acellular pertussis, has fewer and less severe adverse reactions than the older whole-cell DTP vaccine. Only DTaP is used in the United States, though DTP is still used in many countries. Local reactions are more likely and more severe with each successive dose. Contraindications to additional doses of vaccine are either an immediate anaphylactic reaction or encephalopathy within 7 days of immunization. Precautions that are not absolute contraindications include a seizure within 3 days of immunization, or any of the following within 48 hours of immunization: persistent or unusually severe screaming lasting more

than 3 hours, collapse or shock-like state, or unexplained
fever higher than 40.5° C (104.8° F).

For postexposure prophylaxis, family members and close
contacts of index cases should be given a 14-day
chemoprophylactic course of erythromycin as discussed
in the Treatment section. Health care workers should
practice droplet precautions in addition to standard
precautions. In an outbreak, chemoprophylaxis should be
considered for exposed health care personnel, especially
for those who develop cough (American Academy of
Pediatrics, 2003; Bortolussi et al., 1995; Chin, 2000;
Long, 2004).

Reporting

The CDC considers pertussis to be a nationally notifiable
disease. The World Health Organization (WHO)
considers it as a Class 2B disease. See Appendix C
for details and for upcoming changes in WHO reporting.

References

American Academy of Pediatrics. (2003). *Red Book: 2003 Report of the
Committee on Infectious Diseases* (26th ed. pp. 472-486). Chicago: Author.

Bass, J.W. & Vincent, J.M. (2000). Pertussis. In G.T. Strickland (Ed.),
Hunter's tropical medicine and emerging infectious diseases (8th ed.,
pp. 310-313). Philadelphia: W.B. Saunders Company.

Bortolussi, R., Miller, B., Ledwith, M., & Halperin, S. (1995). Clinical course
of pertussis in immunized children. *The Pediatric Infectious Diseases Journal,
14,* 870-874.

Centers for Disease Control and Prevention. (2002). Pertussis. Retrieved
December 10, 2003, from *www.cdc.gov/ncidod/dbmd/diseaseinfo/pertussis_t.htm*

Chin, J. (Ed.). (2000). *Control of communicable diseases manual* (17th ed.,
pp. 375-379). Washington, DC: American Public Health Association.

Langley, J.M., Halperin, S.A., Boucher, F.D., Smith, B., & Pediatric
Investigators Collaborative Network on Infections in Canada (PICNIC).
(2004). Azithromycin is as effective as and better tolerated than erythromycin
estolate for the treatment of pertussis. *Pediatrics, 114,* 96-91.

Long, S.S. (2004). Pertussis (*Bordetella pertussis* and *B. parapertussis*). In
R.E. Behrman, R.M. Kliegman, & H.B. Jenson (Eds.), *Nelson textbook of
pediatrics* (17th ed., pp. 908-912). Philadelphia: W.B. Saunders Company.

Luo, C., Brabin, B.J., & Bunn, J. (2003). Paediatrics in the tropics. In
G.C. Cook & A.I. Zumla (Eds.), *Manson's tropical diseases* (21st ed.,
pp. 467-483). Philadelphia: W.B. Saunders Company.

Preziosi, M.P., & Halloran, M.E. (2003). Effects of pertussis vaccination on
disease: Vaccine efficacy in reducing clinical severity. *Clinical Infectious
Diseases, 15,* 772-779.

Tozzi, A.E., Ravà, L., Ciofi degli Atti, M.L., Salmaso, S. & Progetto Pertosse
Working Group. (2003). Clinical presentation of pertussis in unvaccinated and
vaccinated children in the first six years of life. *Pediatrics, 112,* 1069-1075.

Pinta

Azul, carate, Mal de pinto

Geographic Distribution

— Pinta is found primarily in rural areas of southern Mexico and northern South America (Kapembwa, 2003).

Agent and Vector

— Pinta is caused by *Treponema pallidum* spp. *carateum,* an organism that is microscopically and serologically identical to the organism that causes venereal syphilis, *Treponema pallidum* spp. *pallidum.* Pinta is a nonvenereal skin disease, and the mode of transmission is unknown; however, direct prolonged skin-to-skin contact is thought to play a role. Primary infection is most common in children and young adults, but skin lesions may last for many years and result in chronic changes when untreated (Antal, Lukehart, & Meheus, 2002; Blume, Levine, & Heymann, 2003; Hook III, 1999; Perine & Bell, 2000).

Incubation

— Primary lesions of pinta occur 1 week to several months after inoculation (Blume et al., 2003)

Clinical Findings and Treatment

Signs and Symptoms

— In the early stage of infection, the primary lesion occurs at the site of inoculation, which is usually an exposed area such as the face, arms, or legs. The initial lesion may consist of minute macules or papules with an erythematous halo, a single small erythematous papule, or a scaly plaque with surrounding satellite lesions. After several months, the primary lesions enlarge to form irregular, scaly, erythematous plaques (up to 10 cm in diameter) with an infiltrative border and pale center. After months to years, secondary lesions, known as *pintids,* appear as small scaly papules that enlarge and coalesce to form psoriasiform plaques. During this stage, patients may develop regional lymphadenopathy, but there is no evidence that the infection causes other systemic involvement. The primary and secondary lesions may then merge and often undergo color changes from red to blue, brown, gray, or black. In the tertiary stage of infection, patients develop hypopigmented to depigmented atrophic or hyperkeratotic plaques (Figure 63-1). At this stage, patients are no longer considered infectious (Antal et al., 2002; Blume et al., 2003; Kapembwa, 2003; Perine & Bell, 2000).

Complications

The main complication is leukoderma, which is often considered a social stigmata in areas where the disease occurs (Kapembwa, 2003).

Common Laboratory Findings

There are no common laboratory findings.

Diagnosis

The history and characteristic physical examination may help make the diagnosis, especially if the patient lives in an endemic area. Dark-field microscopy of scrapings taken from the border of primary or secondary lesions allows visualization of the organism. A skin biopsy taken from primary or secondary lesions may demonstrate treponemes when stained with silver stain. Venereal Disease Research Laboratory tests are positive in the majority of patients during secondary and tertiary infections (Blume et al., 2003; Perine & Bell 2000).

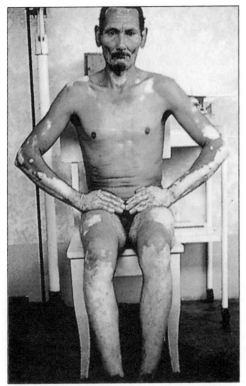

FIGURE 63–1

Depigmented lesions of pinta. (*Source:* From Peters, W., & Pasvol, G. [2002]. *Tropical medicine and parasitology* [5th ed., p. 253]. Chicago: Mosby.)

Differential Diagnosis

— Secondary skin lesions of pinta may resemble leprosy, psoriasis, lichen planus, eczema, or tinea corporis. The depigmented tertiary lesions can mimic vitiligo (Blume et al., 2003; Perine & Bell, 2000).

Treatment

— A single IM dose of benzathine penicillin G is the recommended treatment. Dosages include 0.6 million units for children younger than age 6, 1.2 million units for children ages 6 to 15, and 2.4 million units for persons older than age 15. When treatment is administered in the early stages of disease, cutaneous lesions resolve; however, the chronic lesions of tertiary pinta often will not respond to therapy (Kapembwa, 2003).

Prevention

The prevalence of pinta has drastically decreased due to treatment campaigns and improved standards of living. Control programs have recommended treatment of entire communities if active infection is apparent in more than 10% of the population; treatment of patients, their contacts, and all children in communities where active infection occurs in 5% to 10% of the population; and treatment of the patients and close contacts in communities where less than 5% of the population is affected. Health education and screening of schoolchildren may also help control the spread of pinta. Barriers to effective treatment and prevention include the fact that health care providers in endemic areas have to deal with many other overwhelming health needs, limited resources make this disease a low priority, the economic impact is not felt since the disease occurs mainly in young people, and the most commonly affected are remote poor populations (Antal et al., 2002; Kapembwa, 2003).

Reporting

The U.S. Centers for Disease Control and Prevention does not classify pinta as a nationally notifiable disease. The World Health Organization (WHO) considers it to be a Class 2B disease. See Appendix C for details and for upcoming changes in WHO reporting.

References

Antal, G.M., Lukehart, S.A., & Meheus, A.Z. (2002). The endemic treponematoses. *Microbes and Infection, 4,* 83-94.

Blume, J.E., Levine, E.G., & Heymann, W.R. (2003). Bacterial diseases. In Bolognia, J.L., Jorizzo, J.L., & Rapini, R.P. (Eds.), *Dermatology* (p. 1141). Philadelphia: Mosby.

Hook III, E.W. (1999). Treponemal infections. In R.L. Guerrant, D.H. Walker, & P.F. Weller (Eds.), *Tropical infectious diseases: Principles, pathogens, and practice* (pp. 527-534). New York: Churchill Livingstone.

Kapembwa, M. (2003). Endemic treponematoses. In G.C. Cook & A.I. Zumla (Eds.), *Manson's tropical diseases* (21st ed., pp. 1149-1151). Philadelphia: W.B. Saunders Company.

Perine, P.L., & Bell, T.A. (2000). Syphilis and the endemic treponematoses. In G.T. Strickland (Ed.), *Hunter's tropical medicine and emerging infectious diseases* (8th ed., pp. 354-364). Philadelphia: W.B. Saunders Company.

64

PLAGUE

Geographic Distribution

- Plague is widely distributed throughout the world, affecting more than 200 species of wild rodents in central, eastern, and southern Africa, South America, the western part of North America, and areas of Asia. In the past decade, more than 75% of plague cases and deaths have been reported from Africa (World Health Organization [WHO], 2002).

Agent and Vector

- Plague is a zoonosis caused by *Yersinia pestis*, a nonmotile microaerophilic bacillus (sometimes coccobacillus) of the family *Enterobacteriaceae*. It is spread among its wild rodent reservoir through fleas, which sporadically transmit *Y. pestis* to rats and humans (Figure 64-1). The three common forms of plague are bubonic (the most common form), pneumonic (the most rapid and most deadly), and septicemic.
- Bubonic plague occurs when the bacteria are transmitted either by the bite of an infected flea or by direct inoculation, as might occur from handling an infected animal carcass. The organisms migrate to regional lymph nodes where they multiply, resulting in swollen, painful, erythematous lymph nodes called buboes.
- Pneumonic plague occurs when the bacteria infect the lungs, either as a result of hematogenous spread from a primary infection, or by inhaling infected droplets from a person with pneumonic plague (Box 64-1).
- Septicemic plague may be secondary to hematogenous spread from a buboe, or primary when septicemia occurs

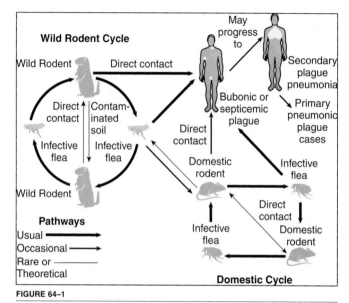

FIGURE 64–1

Life cycle of plague. (*Source:* From Strickland, G.T. [2000]. *Hunter's tropical medicine and emerging infectious diseases* [8th ed., p. 404]. Philadelphia: W.B. Saunders Company.)

without buboes (Center for Infectious Disease Research and Policy [CIDRAP], 2005; WHO, 2002).

Throughout history, plague has caused approximately 200 million deaths in pandemics in various parts of the world. Its effects are ingrained in the common nursery rhyme:

Ring around the rosy	(rose-colored purpuric lesions)
Pocket full of posies	(flowers carried to prevent the disease and cover the stench)
Ashes, ashes	(death, or in an alternate version, "A'choo, a'choo" referring to sneezing in pneumonic plague)
We all fall down.	(dead)

Incubation

— Patients develop symptoms of bubonic plague 2 to
8 days after the bite of an infected flea. Aerosolized
Y. pestis causes pneumonic plague 1 to 6 days
(usually 2 to 4 days) after exposure (Inglesby
et al., 2000).

Clinical Findings and Treatment

Signs and Symptoms

— Naturally occurring bubonic plague is manifested by
the abrupt onset of high fever, severe headache, severe
myalgias, prostration, and, in some cases, delirium. An
ulcer may develop at the inoculation site. Lymphadenitis
is followed by painful, nonfluctuant bubo(es) occurring
most often in the groin, axilla, and neck. Buboes rarely
develop fluctuance and suppuration. Bacteremia and
sepsis ensue and can rapidly lead to disseminated
intravascular coagulation (DIC), shock, coma, and death.
— Patients with pneumonic plague develop an acute
fulminant pneumonia with high fever, malaise,
dyspnea, and cough that sometimes produces watery
blood-tinged sputum or, less commonly, purulent
sputum. Gastrointestinal symptoms can include
abdominal pain, nausea, vomiting, and diarrhea.
Buboes seldom appear after exposure to aerosolized
plague. Sepsis can develop rapidly, with progression
to cyanosis, shock, and respiratory failure. Common
radiographic findings are bilateral alveolar infiltrates
and consolidation.
— Septicemic plague is characterized by rapid decline,
DIC, coma, and multiple-organ-system failure.
Cutaneous manifestations include purpura and large
ecchymoses. Necrosis of the digits and nose may
also occur in the later stages (CIDRAP, 2005;
Heddurshetti, Pumpradit, & Lutwick, 2001;
Inglesby et al., 2000; McGovern, Christopher, &
Eitzen, 1999).

BIOTERRORISM CONSIDERATIONS BOX 64-1

Plague is considered by the Centers for Disease Control and Prevention to be a Category A critical biological agent. Category A agents have the greatest potential for mass casualties and a moderate to high potential for large-scale dissemination. Japan reportedly used plague as a weapon during World War II by dropping infected fleas over parts of China. During the postwar period both the United States and the Soviet Union developed the ability to aerosolize plague directly. In a biowarfare attack, inhaled organisms would cause primary pneumonic plague, with significant numbers of septicemic cases. Secondary pneumonic cases would continue to spread the disease after the initial attack. The bacillus may remain viable for as long as an hour, for a distance of up to 10 km (Chin, 2000; Heddurshetti et al., 2001; Inglesby et al., 2000; Rotz et al., 2002).

Complications

Rare manifestations include plague pharyngitis, which is associated with cervical lymphadenopathy, and plague meningitis, which is manifested by fever and meningismus. When the diagnosis of pneumonic plague is made more than 24 hours after the onset of symptoms, death is likely (Inglesby et al., 2000).

Common Laboratory Findings

Plague causes leukocytosis with toxic granulation and other nonspecific findings seen with sepsis from other causes.

Diagnosis

Gram-negative bacilli or coccobacilli and bipolar "safety-pin" staining organisms may be detected in sputum, peripheral blood, or buboe aspirate. Diagnosis is confirmed by culture, antigen detection, IgM immunoenzyme, immunostaining, or polymerase chain reaction. These tests are only available at some state health departments, military

facilities, and the Centers for Disease Control and
Prevention (CDC) (CIDRAP, 2003; Inglesby et al., 2000).

Differential Diagnosis

A single case of pneumonic plague would resemble a
severe case of common bacterial pneumonia. The sudden
appearance of large numbers of otherwise healthy
patients with severe pneumonia and sepsis should raise
suspicion for either plague or anthrax; hemoptysis
increases the likelihood of plague. Specific differential
diagnosis considerations include the following (CIDRAP,
2003; Heddurshetti et al., 2001; Inglesby et al., 2000):

- *Pneumonic plague.* Inhalational anthrax, tularemia,
  community-acquired pneumonia, viral pneumonia,
  Q fever.
- *Bubonic plague.* Streptococcal or staphylococcal
  adenitis, tularemia, cat scratch fever, mycobacterial
  infection, lymphogranuloma venereum, chancroid,
  primary genital herpes, primary or secondary
  syphilis, strangulated inguinal hernia.
- *Septicemic plague.* Meningococcemia, septicemia
  from other gram-negative bacteria.

Treatment

Treatment must begin within 24 hours of the onset of
symptoms to alter the outcome. Because of the lack of
experience in treating plague in humans, some of the
therapies discussed here have not been adequately
studied and are not approved by the Food and Drug
Administration. The following are the recommendations
of the Working Group on Civilian Biodefense, which
have been confirmed by CIDRAP (CIDRAP, 2003;
Inglesby et al., 2000).

CONTAINED CASUALTIES

Treat for 10 days as follows:

- Adults may be treated with streptomycin 1 g IM
  twice daily or gentamicin 5 mg/kg IM or

IV once daily or 2 mg/kg loading dose followed by 1.7 mg/kg IM or IV three times daily (gentamicin is the choice for pregnant women). Alternatives are doxycycline 100 mg IV twice daily or doxycycline 200 mg IV once daily or ciprofloxacin 400 mg IV twice daily or chloramphenicol 25 mg/kg IV four times daily.

- Children may be treated with streptomycin 15 mg/kg IM twice daily (maximum daily dose 2 g) or gentamicin 2.5 mg/kg IM or IV three times daily. Alternatives include doxycycline: If the patient weighs 45 kg or more, give adult dose. If less than 45 kg, give 2.2 mg/kg IV twice daily (maximum 200 mg/24 hours) or ciprofloxacin 15 mg/kg IV twice daily or chloramphenicol (if older than 2 years) 25 mg/kg IV four times daily. Doxycycline may cause tooth discoloration in children younger than 8 years.

MASS CASUALTIES AND POSTEXPOSURE PROPHYLAXIS

Begin treatment without waiting for laboratory confirmation, and treat for 10 days; postexposure prophylaxis requires only 7 days:

- Adults may be treated with ciprofloxacin 500 mg PO twice daily or doxycycline 100 mg twice daily. An alternative for adults is chloramphenicol 25 mg/kg PO four times daily.
- Children may be treated with doxycycline (the preferred choice). If the child weighs 45 kg or more, give adult dose. If less than 45 kg, give 2.2 mg/kg (maximum 200 mg/24 hours) PO twice daily or, for older children, ciprofloxacin 20 mg/kg (up to adult dose) PO twice daily. An alternative for children older than age 2 is chloramphenicol 25 mg/kg PO four times daily.

Prevention

There is no vaccine for plague. Patients should be isolated until 48 hours of antibiotic treatment and there is improvement. Unnecessary contact with others should be avoided. Close contacts should receive prophylactic treatment. Isolation of close contacts who refuse prophylaxis is not recommended; but such persons should be closely monitored for fever or cough for the first 7 days after exposure and treatment started if either occurs. Patients and others in contact with patients should wear disposable surgical masks. Rooms of patients with pneumonic plague should be terminally cleaned and contaminated linens disinfected according to hospital protocol. Plague aerosol is infectious for only an hour after release, hence later environmental decontamination of areas exposed to aerosolized plague is not necessary (Chin, 2000; Inglesby et al., 2000). Other preventive measures include the following:

- Control fleas by using insecticides, especially when instituting a rodent control program. See Appendix D on vector control.
- Control rodents by coordinated and simultaneous campaigns to rat-proof buildings, store food in secure areas, bury or burn garbage, rid community of uncontrolled rubbish accumulations, and poison rodents. Rodent control is the most important means of prevention. See Appendix D on vector control.

Community education regarding the above measures is important.

Reporting

The CDC considers plague to be a nationally notifiable disease. Plague is one of three diseases that the WHO requires its member states to report (Class 1). See Appendix C for details and for upcoming changes in WHO reporting.

References

Center for Infectious Disease Research and Policy. (2005). Plague: Current, comprehensive information on pathogenesis, microbiology, epidemiology, diagnosis, and treatment. Retrieved April 4, 2005, from *www.cidrap.umn.edu/cidrap/content/bt/plague/index.html*

Chin, J. (Ed.). (2000). *Control of communicable diseases manual* (17th ed., pp. 381-387). Washington, DC: American Public Health Association.

Heddurshetti, R., Pumpradit, W., & Lutwick, L.I. (2001). Pulmonary manifestations of bioterrorism. *Current Infectious Disease Reports, 3,* 249-257.

Inglesby, T.V., et al. (2000). Plague as a biological weapon: Medical and public health management. *JAMA, 283,* 2281-2290.

McGovern, T.W., Christopher, G.W., & Eitzen, E.M. (1999). Cutaneous manifestations of biological warfare and related threat agents. *Archives of Dermatology, 135,* 1417-1418.

Rotz, L.D, Khan, A.S., Lillibridge, S.R., Ostroff, S.M., & Hughes. J.M. (2002). Public health assessment of potential biological terrorism agents. *Emerging Infectious Diseases, 8,* 225-230.

World Health Organization. (2002). Plague. Retrieved February 24, 2004, from *www.who.int/csr/disease/plague/en/*

POLIOMYELITIS

Geographic Distribution

— Poliomyelitis was found worldwide until widespread immunization was instituted in the 1950s, culminating in the Global Polio Eradication Initiative beginning in 1988. The last case in the Western Hemisphere was in 1991. Today, three countries (Nigeria, Pakistan, and India) account for 98% of new cases and there are only three other countries (Afghanistan, Egypt, and Niger) where wild polio virus is endemic (Aylward, Acharya, England, Agocs, & Linkins, 2003; Centers for Disease Control and Prevention [CDC], 2003; World Health Organization [WHO], 2002a).

Agent and Vector

— Poliomyelitis is caused by the three serotypes of poliovirus, genus *Enterovirus*, in the family *Picornaviridae*. Almost 90% of the time the disease is from infection with wild poliovirus, but live attenuated oral polio vaccine can cause vaccine-associated paralytic polio (VAPP) either in vaccine recipients or their close contacts, especially if immune compromised.

— Humans are the only known reservoir for poliovirus. Transmission is usually by the fecal-oral route, but it can also occur through pharyngeal secretions. Ingested viruses replicate in the pharynx, gastrointestinal tract, and local lymphatics, with primary viremia occurring 2 to 3 days after infection. The virus seeds to multiple sites, including the reticuloendothelial system, fat, and muscle. Most infections are asymptomatic and are contained after this "minor viremia." But in some patients, viral replication in the reticuloendothelial system gives way to a "major viremia" in which infection spreads to the central nervous system (CNS), probably along peripheral nerves. The virus causes cell death in multiple sites in the CNS, most commonly motor neurons in the spinal cord and the medulla oblongata, resulting in muscle weakness, paralysis, hyperesthesia, and myalgia (CDC, 2003; Simoes, 2004).

Incubation

The incubation period ranges from 3 to 35 days and is usually 6 to 20 days (CDC, 2003).

Clinical Findings and Treatment

Signs and Symptoms

Poliovirus infections are classified by the severity of clinical presentation as follows:

- *Inapparent* or *asymptomatic* infection occurs in 90% to 95% of all poliovirus infections. Despite the absence of symptoms, infected persons shed virus in their stool and thus may transmit the disease to others.
- *Abortive poliomyelitis* accounts for 4% to 8% of poliovirus infections. Abortive poliomyelitis resembles mild, nonspecific upper respiratory virus infections with 2 to 3 days of fever, malaise, headache, sore throat, anorexia, nausea, and, less commonly, myalgia and vomiting. There is no evidence of neurologic involvement and no long-term complications.
- *Nonparalytic aseptic meningitis* or *nonparalytic poliomyelitis* occurs in 1% to 2% of poliovirus infections. The nonparalytic form is preceded by a prodromal illness similar to but more intense than abortive poliomyelitis, followed (sometimes after a short symptom-free period) by pain and stiffness of posterior neck, trunk, and extremities, manifested on physical exam by positive Kernig and Brudzinski signs. Symptoms last 2 to 10 days, and recovery is complete.

- *Paralytic poliomyelitis* occurs in about 0.1% of persons with poliomyelitis infection.

There are three paralytic syndromes: spinal paralytic poliomyelitis, bulbar poliomyelitis, and polioencephalitis.

- *Spinal paralytic poliomyelitis* is the most common paralytic syndrome. Presentation varies, but often there is first severe headache, fever, and muscle pain. Then after about a day, acute flaccid paralysis or paresis, most often involving one leg or one arm. Intramuscular injection or injury to an extremity in the 2 to 4 weeks prior to illness increases the risk that the extremity will be affected.

- *Bulbar poliomyelitis* primarily involves cranial nerves and medullary centers; when the spinal nerves are also involved, it is called bulbospinal poliomyelitis. The lesions cause symptoms corresponding to their location, such as dysphagia, aspiration, inability to cough, and cardiovascular and respiratory irregularities. In bulbospinal polio, the trunk and muscles of the thorax and abdomen may be involved, resulting in quadriplegia, respiratory insufficiency and the need for ongoing ventilatory support.

- *Polioencephalitis* is the rarest form and involves higher centers of the brain, thus producing alterations in consciousness and other neurologic symptoms such as seizures, coma, spastic paralysis, and respiratory insufficiency.

Polio is a disease whose manifestations occur on a continuum; consequently, a patient's presentation may not be as clearly defined as the clinical syndromes presented here (CDC, 2003; Simoes, 2004; WHO, 2002a).

Complications

Paralytic poliomyelitis is, in itself, a complication. Those who need ongoing artificial ventilation live an enormously restricted life and suffer numerous medical complications such as pneumonia. In developing nations, the resources necessary to sustain life may simply not be available. Intestinal erosion, acute gastric dilatation, hypertension, seizures, cardiac irregularities, pulmonary edema, and hypercalcemia are other complications of paralytic poliomyelitis. Post-polio syndrome (PPS) occurs in about 40% of persons who have full or partial recovery from paralytic polio. PPS appears 15 to 40 years after the original illness and is usually manifested by slowly progressive muscle weakness, myalgia, and arthralgia, and less commonly by muscle atrophy, dysphagia, dyspnea, sleep disorders, and cold intolerance (WHO, 2001).

Common Laboratory Findings

The cerebrospinal fluid (CSF) findings are similar to aseptic meningitis caused by other enteroviruses: a moderately elevated white blood cell count (primarily lymphocytes or sometimes neutrophils early in the infection) and mildly elevated protein. Peripheral blood may show leukocytosis or leukopenia (CDC, 2003; Solomon & Willison, 2003)

Diagnosis

The diagnosis of poliomyelitis is confirmed by isolation of poliovirus from stool or from throat secretions. Virus can be detected in the feces for several weeks. Oligonucleotide mapping or genomic sequencing can determine if the virus is wild or vaccine type (CDC, 2003). Isolation of the virus from CSF is uncommon, but important when investigating a potential case of VAPP. Infection can also be diagnosed by paired acute and convalescent sera, but this cannot distinguish wild from vaccine viruses.

Differential Diagnosis

The differential diagnosis for acute flaccid paralysis includes Guillain-Barré syndrome, transverse myelitis, traumatic neuritis secondary to sciatic nerve injury, toxic and infectious neuropathies (especially West Nile virus and enterovirus 71), tick paralysis, myasthenia gravis, porphyria, botulism, insecticide poisoning, polymyositis, trichinosis, and periodic paralysis (Chin, 2000; Solomon & Willison, 2003). Sensory changes are unusual in polio and should prompt consideration of other etiologies.

Treatment

— Treatment is supportive in all types of poliomyelitis and prevention of immobility-related disability and/or complications is a priority from the beginning of treatment. In the acute phase, patients should be hospitalized and placed on bed rest, because physical activity can increase the risk and distribution of paralysis.

Prevention

— Vaccination is the key to preventing the spread of poliovirus. The WHO and partner organizations used a fourfold strategy in the Global Polio Eradication Initiative: (1) routine immunizations, (2) national immunization days, (3) acute flaccid paralysis surveillance, and (4) mopping up immunization. Improved sanitation and sewage treatment have also played an important role in polio control.

— Two types of polio vaccine are in use worldwide: inactivated polio vaccine (IPV) and live attenuated oral polio vaccine (OPV). Both are given in a four-dose series during infancy and childhood. OPV is available in less developed nations, whereas in developed nations where cases of VAPP outnumber cases caused by wild poliovirus, the more expensive IPV is used. Because of the risk of VAPP, it is hoped that IPV will replace OPV worldwide. Nonimmunized adults should receive three doses of IPV. Adults who have completed the primary immunization and are at increased risk of exposure to wild-type poliovirus (e.g., through travel to an endemic country) should receive a single dose of IPV (American Academy of Pediatrics, 2003; Chin, 2000; WHO, 2002b).

Reporting

The CDC considers poliomyelitis to be a nationally notifiable disease. The WHO considers poliomyelitis to be a Class 1A disease. See Appendix C for details and for upcoming changes in WHO reporting.

References

American Academy of Pediatrics. (2003). *2003 Red Book: Report of the Committee on Infectious Diseases* (26th ed.). Washington, DC: Author.

Aylward, R.B., Acharya, A., England, S., Agocs, M., & Linkins, J. (2003). Global health goals: Lessons from the worldwide effort to eradicate poliomyelitis. *Lancet, 362,* 909-914.

Centers for Disease Control and Prevention. (2003). Poliomyelitis. Retrieved December 1, 2003, from *www.cdc.gov/nip/publications/pink/polio-sm.pdf*

Chin, J. (Ed.). (2000). *Control of communicable diseases manual* (17th ed., pp. 393-405). Washington, DC: American Public Health Association.

Simoes, E.A. (2004). Polioviruses. In R.E. Behrman, R.M. Kliegman, & H.B. Jenson (Eds.), *Nelson textbook of pediatrics* (17th ed., pp. 1036-1042). Philadelphia: W.B. Saunders Company.

Solomon, T., & Willison, H. (2003). Infectious causes of acute flaccid paralysis. *Current Opinion in Infectious Diseases, 16,* 375-381.

World Health Organization. (2001). Post-polio syndrome. Retrieved November 20, 2003, from *www.who.int/vaccines-polio/all/background/files/PostPolioSyndrom.pdf*

World Health Organization. (2002a). Global polio status 2002. Retrieved December 2, 2003, from *www.polioeradication.org/*

World Health Organization. (2002b). Global polio progress 2002. Retrieved December 2, 2003, from *www.who.int/vaccines-polio/all/news/files/pdf/PolioProgressReport2002.pdf*

66

Psittacosis
Ornithosis, parrot fever
Geographic Distribution

Psittacosis occurs worldwide and is strongly linked to contact with psittacine birds such as parrots, parakeets, cockatiels, and canaries (Chin, 2000).

Agent and Vector

Psittacosis is a zoonosis caused by *Chlamydia psittaci*, an obligate intracellular parasitic bacterium (Box 66-1). Though psittacine birds are the most common source, humans may also contract the illness from infected turkeys, squabs, ducks, or other birds that may or may not appear ill. Imported birds, especially those imported illegally, tend to be strongly associated with psittacosis. Humans usually acquire the illness by inhalation of dried feces or dust from feathers, but may also be infected from kissing birds or being bitten or pecked. Other animals such as cattle, horses, dogs, and cats may also contract and spread psittacosis. In up to 20% of confirmed cases, there is no known contact with birds.

Infection occurs when the bacteria are in the form of metabolically inactive elementary bodies. The elementary bodies are inhaled, phagocytosed, and then become metabolically active and grow as reticulate bodies. Infected macrophages carry the organisms to the reticuloendothelial system where replication occurs. From there, bacteremia begins and spreads the organism to target organs (Centers for Disease Control and Prevention [CDC], 2002; Elliot, 2001; Gregory & Schaffner, 1997; Ward, 2000).

BIOTERRORISM CONSIDERATIONS   BOX 66–1

Chlamydia psittaci is considered by the CDC to be
a Category B biological warfare agent. Category B agents
are moderately easy to disseminate and cause moderate
morbidity and low mortality. *C. psittaci* has the potential
for production and dissemination in quantities sufficient to
affect large populations. The biological warfare route of
infection is most likely aerosol. Treatment of mass casualties would be doxycycline or erythromycin as discussed in
the Treatment section (CDC, 2000; Rotz, Khan, Lillibridge,
Ostroff, & Hughes, 2002).

Incubation

The incubation period is 1 to 3 weeks (CDC, 2002).

Clinical Findings and Treatment

Signs and Symptoms

Onset is most often rapid, but it may be insidious. The
clinical presentation of psittacosis is varied, usually
including fever, chills, malaise, headache, upper or
lower respiratory symptoms, dry cough (sometimes
with scant purulent or blood-tinged sputum), backache,
hepatosplenomegaly, and myalgia. Relative bradycardia
for the degree of fever is common. Atypical pneumonia
is the most frequently seen manifestation with a history
of several days of fever and cough, as well as heard on
auscultation of the chest. Splenomegaly in a patient with
atypical pneumonia should raise suspicion for psittacosis
(Elliot, 2001; Gregory & Schaffner, 1997; Ward, 2000).

Complications

Encephalitis, endocarditis, myocarditis, and
thrombophlebitis occasionally occur. Older persons
may have severe respiratory symptoms (Chin, 2000).

Common Laboratory Findings

White blood cell count is normal or decreased with a left shift. Increased C-reactive protein and erythrocyte sedimentation rate are common. The most frequent radiologic finding is consolidation of a single lower lobe (Elliot, 2001; Ward, 2000).

Diagnosis

Atypical pneumonia and a history of contact with birds is sufficient for a presumptive diagnosis. The most common test for psittacosis is serologic testing by complement fixation of acute and convalescent specimens obtained 2 to 3 weeks apart. Cultures are very infectious and should be done only in appropriately equipped laboratories. Polymerase chain reaction (PCR) is available, but only in specialized laboratories (CDC, 2002; Elliot, 2001; Ward, 2000).

Differential Diagnosis

The differential diagnosis includes other atypical pneumonias (such as legionellosis, *C. pneumoniae, Mycoplasma pneumoniae*), acute viral pneumonia, viral pneumonitis, and Q fever. Other considerations include typhoid fever, brucellosis, rheumatic fever, tularemia, influenza, and HIV infection (Ward, 2000).

Treatment

Clinical response to antibiotics is usually seen within 1 to 3 days, but therapy should be given for 10 to 14 days beyond defervescence to decrease the chance of relapse. Doxycycline 100 mg PO bid is the treatment of choice. For children who weigh less than 45 kg, doxycycline may be given at a dose of 5 mg/kg/day divided bid up to a maximum of 100 mg PO bid. Children who weigh more than 45 kg are given the adult dose. Erythromycin is less effective than doxycycline for severe infection but is an option for those who are allergic to doxycycline, children younger than 8 years old, and pregnant women. For adults, erythromycin (as ethylsuccinate) may be given at 1.6 to 4 g/day PO in three or four divided doses (maximum 4 g). For children, erythromycin (as ethylsuccinate) may be given at 50 mg/kg/day PO in three or four divided doses (maximum 2 g/day). There is insufficient data concerning the use of newer macrolides such as clarithromycin and azithromycin (Elliot, 2001; Ward, 2000).

Prevention

Preventive measures include avoiding sick birds and imported birds from unregulated sources such as flea markets. Persons who work in pet shops, markets, processing plants, and other places of frequent contact should be educated about psittacosis and early identification of the illness. Infected birds should be treated with tetracyclines or destroyed, and their cages cleaned and disinfected (Chin, 2000).

Reporting

The CDC considers psittacosis to be a nationally notifiable disease. The World Health Organization (WHO) considers psittacosis to be a Class 2A disease. See Appendix C for details and for upcoming changes in WHO reporting.

References

Centers for Disease Control and Prevention. (2000). Biological and chemical terrorism: Strategic plan for preparedness and response. *Morbidity and Mortality Weekly Report*, *49*(RR-4), 1-14.

Centers for Disease Control and Prevention. (2002). Psittacosis. Retrieved December 23, 2003, from *www.cdc.gov/ncidod/dbmd/diseaseinfo/psittacosis_t.htm*

Chin, J. (Ed.). (2000). *Control of communicable diseases manual* (17th ed., pp. 405-407). Washington, DC: American Public Health Association.

Elliot, J.H. (2001). Psittacosis. *Australian Family Physician, 30,* 739-741.

Gregory, D.W., & Schaffner, W. (1997). Psittacosis. *Seminars in Respiratory Infections, 12,* 7-11.

Rotz, L.D., Khan, A.S., Lillibridge, S.R., Ostroff, S.M., & Hughes, J.M. (2002). Public health assessment of potential biological terrorism agents. *Emerging Infectious Diseases, 8,* 225-230.

Ward, B.J. (2000). Psittacosis. In G.T. Strickland (Ed.), *Hunter's tropical medicine and emerging infectious diseases* (8th ed., pp. 308-310). Philadelphia: W.B. Saunders Company.

67

Q FEVER
Query fever
Geographic Distribution

Q fever is endemic in every country in the world except New Zealand. Its incidence is especially high where humans are in close contact with sheep and cattle; exposure is often occupational. Most identified cases occur in Canada, the United Kingdom, France, and Australia, but the incidence of Q fever is significantly underestimated (Chin, 2000; de Alarcón et al., 2003).

Agent and Vector

Q fever is a zoonosis caused by *Coxiella burnetii,* an obligate intracellular coccobacillus of the *Rickettsiaceae* family that infects mammals, birds, and arthropods. Although *Coxiella* is classified as gram negative, the stain can be gram variable. The organism is very hardy and resistant to heat, drying, and many disinfectants. Transmission among its reservoir hosts (including sheep, goats, and cattle) is through tick bites. Transmission to humans, however, is usually from exposure to the urine, feces, placenta, and amniotic fluids of infected animals. Contaminated dust and hay are also relatively common sources of human infection. Infection from ingesting contaminated milk is rare, as is human-to-human transmission (Box 67-1) (Centers for Disease Control and Prevention [CDC], 2003; de Alarcón et al., 2003; Madariaga, Rezai, Trenholme, & Weinstein, 2003).

Incubation

The incubation period is 2 to 4 weeks (CDC, 2003).

BIOTERRORISM CONSIDERATIONS

BOX 67-1

Coxiella burnetii is considered by the CDC to be a Category B biological warfare agent. Category B agents are moderately easy to disseminate and cause moderate morbidity and low mortality. *C. burnetii* is stable in aerosol and has a very low respiratory infective dose, so the biological warfare route of infection with Q fever would most likely be aerosol. Treatment of mass casualties would be with doxycycline or, alternatively, erythromycin or trimethoprim-sulfamethoxazole. Priority would be given to pregnant women, immunosuppressed persons, and persons with valvular heart disease (CDC, 2000, 2003; Madariaga et al., 2003; Rotz, Khan, Lillibridge, Ostroff, & Hughes, 2002).

Clinical Findings and Treatment

Signs and Symptoms

- About 50% of people infected with *C. burnetii* have no symptoms. Naturally occurring Q fever is usually a self-limiting illness with a highly variable presentation ranging from asymptomatic to pneumonia and hepatitis. In addition, there are differences in presentation according to geographic distribution, with the illness presenting more often as pneumonia in some regions (such as the Basque region of Spain), and as hepatitis and fever in others (such as Southern Spain).
- Most symptomatic cases present with acute onset of high fever (up to 104° to 105° F), chills, sweats, malaise, confusion, severe headache, sore throat, nonproductive cough, chest pain, nausea, vomiting, diarrhea, abdominal pain, and myalgia. The fever usually lasts 1 to 2 weeks. Persistent weight loss sometimes occurs.
- Thirty percent to 50% of patients with symptomatic infection develop pneumonia. The most common signs

and symptoms of Q fever pneumonia include fever, anorexia, very severe headache, cough, chills, and pleuritic chest pain in addition to the manifestations described earlier.

— Hepatitis sometimes occurs with Q fever and may or may not be symptomatic. Patients with even mildly elevated liver enzymes may have focal hepatocellular necrosis. Liver granulomata are present in more severe cases.

— Most patients with Q fever recover with no disability or long-term sequelae after several months of illness (CDC, 2003; de Alarcón et al., 2003; Madariaga et al., 2003; Marrie, 2003).

Complications

— Complications of Q fever include osteomyelitis, hepatitis, endocarditis, chronic Q fever, and Q fever fatigue syndrome. Miscarriage is a complication of infection in the first trimester and prematurity is a common complication of infection in the second trimester. Low birth weight and neonatal death may also occur.

— Chronic Q fever occurs from 1 to 20 years after the initial acute infection and persists for more than 6 months. Risk factors for chronic Q fever include immunosuppression, pregnancy, and preexisting valvular heart disease. Endocarditis is a very serious complication of the chronic form of Q fever and, rarely, of acute Q fever. Others at risk for chronic Q fever include persons with organ transplants, cancer, and chronic renal disease. Up to 65% of persons with chronic Q fever may die of the disease.

— Q fever fatigue syndrome (QFFS) occurs as a sequelae of acute infection in about 20% of patients. Symptoms of QFFS include fatigue, headaches, blurred vision, sweats, lymphadenopathy, myalgia, muscle fasciculations, and arthralgias (CDC, 2003; Hatchette, Hayes, Merry, Schlech, & Marrie, 2003).

Common Laboratory Findings

— In acute Q fever, the white blood cell count is usually normal, although in some cases it is slightly elevated. The erythrocyte sedimentation rate is usually raised, and liver enzymes may be mildly elevated. Hyponatremia occurs in about 25% of patients. Transient thrombocytopenia in the acute phase and thrombocytosis in the recovery phase are common.

— Radiologic features include lower lobe (especially left) involvement (about 37%), air bronchograms (about 26%), pleural effusions (about 10%), and bilateral opacities (about 8%).

— In chronic Q fever, laboratory findings include anemia, increased sedimentation rate, thrombocytopenia, increased liver enzymes, elevated creatinine, and microscopic hematuria (Kagawa, Wehner, & Mohindra, 2003; Madariaga et al., 2003; Marrie, 2003).

Diagnosis

— Diagnosis on the basis of signs and symptoms is difficult because of the nonspecific presentation of Q fever. A history of contact with animal reservoirs raises suspicion. The very high infectivity of *C. burnetii* makes culture unacceptably hazardous in most laboratory settings, hence diagnosis is usually by serology. Indirect immunofluorescence assay is the most commonly used method and becomes positive from 7 to 15 days after the onset of symptoms. Other assays include microagglutination, enzyme-linked immunosorbent assay (ELISA), and complement fixation testing (CDC, 2003; Kagawa et al., 2003).

Differential Diagnosis

— The differential diagnosis of an isolated acute infection includes other atypical pneumonias, typhoid, toxoplasmosis, Epstein-Barr, HIV, cytomegalovirus, psittacosis, viral hepatitis, miliary tuberculosis, and syphilis. With mass casualties, the differential diagnosis would include influenza, anthrax, plague, and tularemia (Cowan, 2003; Madariaga et al., 2003).

Treatment

- In all cases, treatment is most effective if begun within 3 days of onset of illness. For adults, acute Q fever is treated with doxycycline 100 mg PO bid for 14 to 21 days. Alternatives include erythromycin 500 mg PO qid for 14 to 21 days or clarithromycin 500 mg PO bid for 14 days. Note that in some cases erythromycin has failed in severe disease. Marrie (2003) suggests combining rifampin with macrolide (or fluoroquinolone) treatment. Children may be treated with erythromycin (e.g., as ethylsuccinate) 50 mg/kg/day PO in three or four divided doses or clarithromycin 7.5 mg/kg PO bid.
- Chronic Q fever requires long-term treatment, and the recommended treatment for Q fever endocarditis is longer than for any other bacterial disease. Treatment regimens for chronic Q fever and endocarditis include doxycycline (as given earlier) in combination with a quinolone, such as ciprofloxacin 500 mg PO bid for at least 4 years, or doxycycline in combination with hydroxychloroquine for 1.5 to 3 years. Long-term hydroxychloroquine use has significant risk and requires close monitoring and routine eye exams. To assess the response and duration of treatment, serologic testing is recommended once monthly for the first 6 months and then every 3 months. Surgery to remove damaged valves is required in some cases of Q fever endocarditis but there is a risk of reinfection of the prosthetic valve.
- In mass casualty situations, acute Q fever can be treated with doxycycline, erythromycin, clarithromycin, or a fluoroquinolone as discussed earlier (CDC, 2003; Kagawa et al., 2003; Madariaga et al., 2003; Raoult et al., 1999).

Prevention

Prevention measures should be directed primarily at persons in contact with reservoir animals and nearby environs and to persons at risk for chronic Q fever (see earlier section). Specific measures include the following:

- Educate high-risk individuals on the sources, risks, and manifestations of infection.
- Avoid raw milk products.
- Quarantine imported reservoir animals.
- Maintain holding facilities for sheep away from populated areas.
- Routinely test reservoir animals for antibodies to *C. burnetii*.
- Appropriately dispose of placenta and other birth products at facilities housing cattle, sheep, and goats.
- Vaccinate (where possible) people engaged in research with pregnant sheep or live *C. burnetii*. Vaccine is available in Australia, but not the United States. Previous exposure to *C. burnetii* is a contraindication because of the potential for severe local reactions (CDC, 2003; Chin, 2000).

Reporting

The CDC classifies Q fever as a nationally notifiable disease. The World Health Organization (WHO) considers it to be a Class 3B disease. See Appendix C for details and for upcoming changes in WHO reporting.

References

Centers for Disease Control and Prevention. (2000). Biological and chemical terrorism: Strategic plan for preparedness and response. *Morbidity and Mortality Weekly Report, 49*(RR-4), 1-14.

Centers for Disease Control and Prevention. (2003). Q fever. Retrieved December 22, 2003, from */www.cdc.gov/ncidod/dvrd/qfever/index.htm*

Chin, J. (Ed.). (2000). *Control of communicable diseases manual* (17th ed., pp. 407-411). Washington, DC: American Public Health Association.

Cowan, G.O. (2003). Rickettsial infections. In G.C. Cook & A.I. Zumla (Eds.), *Manson's tropical diseases* (21st ed., pp. 891-906). Philadelphia: W.B. Saunders Company.

de Alarcón, A., et al. (2003). Q fever: Epidemiology, clinical features and prognosis. A study from 1983 to 1999 in the south of Spain. *Journal of Infection, 47,* 110-116.

Hatchette, T.F., Hayes, M., Merry, H., Schlech, W.F., & Marrie, T.J. (2003). The effect of *C. burnetii* infection on the quality of life of patients following an outbreak of Q fever. *Epidemiology and Infection, 130,* 491-495.

Kagawa, F.T., Wehner, J.H., & Mohindra, V. (2003). Q fever as a biological weapon. *Seminars in Respiratory Infections, 18,* 183-195.

Madariaga, M.G., Rezai, K., Trenholme, G.M., & Weinstein, R.A. (2003). Q fever: A biological weapon in your backyard. *Lancet Infectious Diseases, 3,* 709-721.

Marrie, T.J. (2003). *Coxiella burnetii* pneumonia. *European Respiratory Journal, 21,* 713-719.

Raoult, D., Houpikian, P., Tissot Dupont, H., Riss, J.M., Arditi-Djiane, J., & Brouqui, P. (1999). Treatment of Q fever endocarditis: Comparison of 2 regimens containing doxycycline and ofloxacin or hydroxychloroquine. *Archives of Internal Medicine, 159,* 167-173.

Rotz, L.D, Khan, A.S., Lillibridge, S.R., Ostroff, S.M., & Hughes. J.M. (2002). Public health assessment of potential biological terrorism agents. *Emerging Infectious Diseases, 8,* 225-230.

RELAPSING FEVER

Recurrent fever, spirillum fever, tick fever, tick bite fever

Geographic Distribution

— Louse-borne (or epidemic) relapsing fever occurs in areas of South America, Europe, Africa (especially Ethiopia and Sudan), and Asia. Tick-borne (or endemic) relapsing fever occurs in parts of all the Americas, southern Europe, throughout Africa except the Sahara and rain forest belt, and in most of Asia (Butler, 2000).

Agent and Vector

— The causative agents for relapsing fever are blood spirochetes of the *Borrelia* species.

— Louse-borne relapsing fever is caused by *B. recurrentis,* which is carried by the human body louse, *Pediculus humanus.* Humans are the only known natural reservoir. Because the spirochetes are not carried in the salivary glands of the louse, infection occurs not with bites, but when an infective louse is crushed, thus releasing spirochetes to enter the skin through louse bite sites or scratched skin. *Borrelia* species invade systemic and lymphatic circulation and multiply in the blood. Symptoms begin when concentrations reach 10^6 to 10^8/mL of blood. Spirochetes are pyrogenic. Although there is no extravascular replication, sequestration of platelets and disseminated intravascular coagulation occur, resulting in petechiae and hemorrhage. In most cases, relapsing fever is self-limited with immunity developed to the same serotype of *Borrelia.* Lice tend to leave excessively warm environments, such as the body of a person with high fever. This may help spread infection from sick to well people.

— Tick-borne relapsing fever is caused by different species of *Borrelia* carried by fast-feeding argasid (soft-bodied) ticks (genus *Ornithodoros*). The primary reservoirs are rodents and, to a lesser extent, birds, reptiles, and amphibians. Humans are accidental hosts, with infection acquired by a bite from an infected tick. Unlike the lengthy time required for Lyme disease transmission from the slow-feeding ixodid tick, relapsing fever is transmitted within minutes of an *Ornithodoros* tick bite. Pathogenesis is as described earlier under louse-borne relapsing fever, except that illness tends to be less severe (Butler, 2000; Cook, 2003; Schwan & Piesman, 2002).

Incubation

— The incubation period ranges from 2 to 15 days (Chin, 2000; Cook, 2003).

Clinical Findings and Treatment

Signs and Symptoms

— Louse-borne relapsing fever tends to be more severe than tick-borne. Other differences between the two forms include potential for more relapses with tick-borne, shorter episodes with tick-borne, and fewer neurologic sequelae with tick-borne. Mortality may reach 40% in untreated patients during louse-borne epidemics.

— Relapsing fever is characterized by abrupt onset of fever, chills, fatigue, and headache, all of which tend to worsen over the first days of illness. Other common, but not universal, manifestations include confusion, dizziness, dry cough, dyspnea, dysphagia, nausea and vomiting, hepatosplenomegaly, jaundice, chest and back pain, myalgia, and arthralgia. Skin manifestations include a petechial rash on flanks, shoulders, and into mucous membranes (with conjunctival suffusion and/or epistaxis) and/or (during the first episode only) an erythematous papular rash on the upper body. The first episode may last 5 to 7 days with sudden defervescence. Most patients experience relapse in 5 to 9 days, with the second episode less severe than the first. A third episode occurs in less than half of patients and a fourth rarely occurs (Butler, 2000; Cook, 2003; Peters & Pasvol, 2002).

Complications

— Complications include pneumonia, nephritis, parotitis, arthritis, neuropathy (especially of cranial nerves), ophthalmitis and iritis, meningoencephalitis, meningitis, and induction of labor in pregnant women. Causes of death include liver failure, cerebral hemorrhage, and cardiac arrhythmia secondary to myocarditis.

— Treatment may be complicated by the Jarisch-Herxheimer reaction, characterized by restlessness and rigors lasting 10 to 30 min with increased temperature, tachycardia, tachypnea, and hypertension. As the rigors pass there is flushing, sweating, and decreased blood pressure, followed by relief from symptoms. The entire episode may last 24 to 48 hours (Butler, 2000; Cook, 2003; Shapiro, 2004).

Common Laboratory Findings

— Common laboratory findings include abnormal liver function tests, anemia, leukocytosis, elevated cerebrospinal fluid pressure with lymphocytic pleocytosis and sometimes *Borrelia* species present in cerebrospinal fluid. Albuminuria and microscopic hematuria are common (Butler, 2000; Cook, 2003).

Diagnosis

— Peripheral blood during a febrile stage shows *Borrelia* species in thin or thick film with Wright's or Giemsa stain (Chin, 2000; Cook, 2003).

Differential Diagnosis

— The differential diagnosis includes louse-borne versus tick-borne relapsing fever, rat-bite fever, influenza, yellow fever, viral hepatitis, leptospirosis, malaria, typhoid fever, louse-borne typhus, and trench fever.

Treatment

— Treatment for adults with louse- or tick-borne relapsing fever is tetracycline 500 mg PO qid for 7 to 10 days with or without procaine penicillin G 400,000 to 600,000 units IM once or twice at a 12-hour interval. Erythromycin (as ethylsuccinate) may be given in place of tetracycline at 500 mg PO qid for 7 days. Note that in Ethiopia, a single 500-mg dose of tetracycline or erythromycin has been effective in adults.

— Children under 9 years old may be treated with erythromycin (as ethylsuccinate) 30 to 50 mg/kg/day (maximum 100 mg/kg/day) in three or four evenly divided doses for 7 to 10 days. Penicillin may be given at a dose of 30,000 units/kg/day in 3 to 6 divided doses. Chloramphenicol is also effective.

— There are differences of opinion about the efficacy of nonsteroidal antiinflammatory drugs in ameliorating Jarisch-Herxheimer reaction, with some authors recommending them (e.g., Shapiro, 2004) and others seeing them as not useful (e.g., Azimi, 2004). In either case, reassurance, intravenous fluids as necessary, and support are indicated (Azimi, 2004; Butler, 2000; Cook, 2003; Shapiro, 2004).

Prevention

— Prevention of louse- and tick-borne relapsing fever is accomplished by avoidance of vector-infected areas, using permethrin-impregnated bed netting and protective clothing, and applying insect repellent

containing *N,N*-diethylmetatoluamide (DEET) to
exposed skin. DEET may be used to protect pregnant
and lactating women traveling to endemic areas.
Formulations with concentrations of 30% or less can be
used safely in children and infants older than 2 months.
DEET repellants are effective against ticks for 3 to
8 hours, depending on the strength of the formulation
(American Academy of Pediatrics, 2003; Centers for
Disease Control and Prevention [CDC], 2003;
U.S. Environmental Protection Agency, 2003).

LOUSE-BORNE RELAPSING FEVER

Individual prevention in non-mass situations includes
washing clothing according to guidelines given next.
Discarding or treating infested clothing (see next
paragraph) and bathing in hot water is sufficient to rid
a person of body lice because the lice live in the clothing
as opposed to on the body.

In mass population situations where conditions favor
lice infestation, such as refugee crises, Chin (2000)
recommends that residual insecticide powders be applied
to the clothes and bodies of persons at risk; for instance,
10% DDT insufflating powder for clothing and 1%
malathion or 0.5% permethrin under clothing (Butler,
2000). The U.S. military guidelines for prevention of
louse-borne diseases include (1) treatment of persons
infected with the disease(s), (2) bathing infested persons,
and (3) laundering all clothing with regimes lethal to
lice and eggs. For example, immersion for 15 min in
water heated to 140° F (60° C) kills all life stages of lice.
Alternatively, exposing clothing for 15 min to circulating
air at a temperature of 140° F (60° C) kills all stages of
lice (Armed Forces Pest Management Board, 2002;
Butler, 2000; Chin, 2000).

TICK-BORNE RELAPSING FEVER

As noted earlier, soft ticks of the Argasidae family are
fast feeding with infection occurring within a minute of

the bite. Prevention (Butler, 2000; Chin, 2000; Cook, 2003) includes the following:

- Use DEET insect repellent on skin and permethrin-impregnated protective clothing when in endemic areas.
- Avoid rodent-infested buildings, earthen-floored structures, and mud houses, especially ones in which migrant workers have slept. Also avoid old campsites in endemic areas.
- Do not sleep on the floor or on the ground.
- Environmental control can be accomplished by controlling rodents and other carriers, removing wood piles, and clearing trees in residential areas.
- Install concrete floors and impervious walls (rather than mud or thatch) in new structures in endemic areas.

Provide community education on the preceding guidelines.

Reporting

The CDC does not consider relapsing fevers to be nationally notifiable diseases. The World Health Organization (WHO) considers them to be Class 4 diseases. See Appendix C for details and for upcoming changes in WHO reporting.

References

American Academy of Pediatrics. (2003). Follow safety precautions when using DEET on children. Retrieved December 7, 2003, from *www.aap.org/family/wnv-jun03.htm*

Armed Forces Pest Management Board. (2002). Delousing procedures for the control of louse-borne disease during contingency. Retrieved December 26, 2003, from *www.afpmb.org/pubs/tims/TG6/TG6.pdf*

Azimi, P. (2004). Relapsing fever (*Borrelia*). In R.E. Behrman, R.M. Kliegman, & H.B. Jenson (Eds.), *Nelson textbook of pediatrics* (17th ed., pp. 985-986). Philadelphia: W.B. Saunders Company.

Butler, T. (2000). Relapsing fever. In G.T. Strickland (Ed.), *Hunter's tropical medicine and emerging infectious diseases* (8th ed., pp. 448-452). Philadelphia: W.B. Saunders Company.

Centers for Disease Control and Prevention. (2003). Malaria. Retrieved November 3, 2003, from *www.cdc.gov/travel/diseases/malaria/index.htm*

Chin, J. (Ed.). (2000). *Control of communicable diseases manual* (17th ed., pp. 541-548). Washington, DC: American Public Health Association.

Cook, G.C. (2003). Other spirochaetal diseases (excluding *Treponema* spp. and *Leptospira* spp.). In G.C. Cook & A.I. Zumla (Eds.), *Manson's tropical diseases* (21st ed., pp. 1153-1164). Philadelphia: W.B. Saunders Company.

Peters, W., & Pasvol, G. (2002). *Tropical medicine and parasitology* (5th ed.). Chicago: Mosby.

Schwan, T.G., & Piesman, J. (2002). Vector interactions and molecular adaptations of Lyme disease and relapsing fever spirochetes associated with transmission by ticks. *Emerging Infectious Diseases, 8,* 115-121.

Shapiro, E.D. (2004). Lyme disease (*Borrelia burgdorferi*). In R.E. Behrman, R.M. Kliegman, & H.B. Jenson (Eds.), *Nelson textbook of pediatrics* (17th ed., pp. 986-990). Philadelphia: W.B. Saunders Company.

U.S. Environmental Protection Agency. (2003). Reregistration of the insect repellant DEET. Retrieved December 26, 2003, from *www.epa.gov/pesticides/factsheets/chemicals/deet.htm*

69

SCABIES

Geographic Distribution

Scabies is found throughout the world and can affect people of any age, race, or socioeconomic background. The highest incidence of scabies is in overcrowded conditions, urban areas, and tropical countries. Crusted scabies can be found in those with decreased sensation or compromised immune systems, including the elderly or patients with a history of an organ transplant, HIV, HTLV-1, or malignancy. Scabies epidemics have been reported in hospitals and nursing homes (Meinking, Burkhart, & Burkhart, 2003; Wendel & Rompalo, 2002).

Agent and Vector

Scabies is caused by the human mite, *Sarcoptes scabiei* var. *hominis*, and is transmitted primarily by close physical contact. These mites are usually too small to be seen by the naked eye; however, they can often be scraped or curetted from superficial skin burrows and seen under the microscope (Figure 69-1). The burrowing female mite lives approximately 30 to 60 days in the stratum corneum of the skin and lays 60 to 90 eggs, which mature within 10 days. Most people with scabies infections have less than 100 mites; however, those with crusted scabies may contain thousands to millions of mites. Mites cannot usually live longer than 3 days without a host, except in the case of crusted scabies, where they can live up to a week by feeding on the shed stratum corneum (Meinking et al., 2003; Wendel & Rompalo, 2002).

Incubation

Incubation for scabies may be anywhere from days to months. With the initial infection, symptoms may not

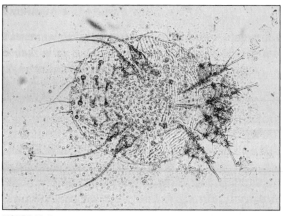

FIGURE 69–1

Sarcoptes scabiei seen at 40× magnification. (*Source:* From Habif, T.P. [1996]. *Clinical dermatology* [3rd ed., p. 498]. Chicago: Mosby.)

develop for weeks; however, symptoms with subsequent infections may occur within 1 to 2 days since the person has been sensitized (Meinking et al., 2003).

Clinical Findings and Treatment

Signs and Symptoms

Scabies most commonly manifests with pruritus, which may be more severe at night, skin lesions, and often a history of pruritus in close contacts or family members. Skin manifestations may include erythematous papules, excoriations, blisters, eczematous plaques, nodules, or characteristic 2- to 10-mm, thin, elevated, superficial tracts, known as *burrows* (Figure 69-2). Occasionally patients will develop lymphadenopathy. Typical sites of involvement are the interdigital spaces, wrists, axillae, waist, feet, ankles, buttocks, nipples, and genitals. In the elderly, infants, and immunocompromised persons, lesions can occur anywhere on the body. Crusted scabies may present with diffuse crusted, hyperkeratotic or

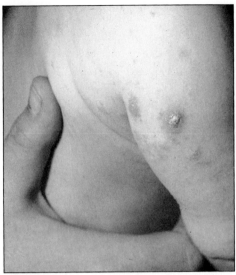

FIGURE 69–2

The effects of scabies. (*Source:* Courtesy of the University of Texas Southwestern Department of Dermatology.)

psoriasiform plaques and dystrophic nails (Meinking et al., 2003; Wendel & Rompalo, 2002).

Complications

Complications of scabies include bacterial superinfection, fevers, or hypersensitivity reactions, which may mimic a viral exanthem, eczema, or urticaria. The extensive lesions that may develop in crusted scabies can cause pain on movement, skin fissuring, and loss of skin integrity. Leukocytoclastic vasculitis is a rare complication of scabies (Meinking et al., 2003; Wendel & Rompalo, 2002).

Common Laboratory Findings

Scabies occasionally has associated eosinophilia.

Diagnosis

The diagnosis of scabies is made by demonstration of the mite, eggs, or feces (scybala) on microscopic examination. A specimen can be collected by using a curette or scalpel to scrape the stratum corneum of the burrows or papules onto a glass slide. The mites can also be visualized within the stratum corneum on skin biopsy; however, this test is invasive, takes longer to receive results, and is lower yield than vigorous scraping of suspicious lesions. Demonstration of the mite is sometimes difficult, and the presence of characteristic skin lesions, intense pruritus, and similar symptoms in close contacts is often enough evidence to treat for scabies (Meinking et al., 2003; Wendel & Rompalo, 2002).

Differential Diagnosis

Scabies is the only disease where burrows can be identified. If no burrows are seen, scabies can be confused with atopic dermatitis, impetigo, other insect bites, or any entity where pruritus is the primary complaint (Meinking et al., 2003).

Treatment

Scabies can be treated with topical or oral medications. Lindane is the traditional topical treatment and is used by applying the lotion to the whole body from the neck down and then rinsing in 8 to 14 hours. This should be repeated in 1 week. Adults are typically not affected on the head and neck; however, infants commonly have the infestation on the scalp and need to be treated in this area as well, with caution. Lindane has a risk of central nervous system toxicity, including nausea, vomiting, and seizures, but is usually a result of overuse, misuse, or application to skin with an extremely compromised barrier. Lindane is not recommended for children younger than age 2, pregnant women, or those with extremely damaged skin.

Resistance to lindane is increasing, and permethrin is the preferred topical treatment. Permethrin is used in the same manner as lindane; however, the risk of toxicity is much lower. The major side effect is allergic or irritant contact dermatitis. Other topical treatments include precipitate sulfur (5% to 10%) in petrolatum (which is approved for use in infants and pregnant or breast-feeding women), benzyl benzoate, and crotamiton. Resistance to topical treatment is becoming a problem in some areas, and rotational therapy (alternating permethrin and lindane treatment for several nights) may help to combat this dilemma.

Ivermectin is an extremely successful and safe oral medication used in treating scabies. The medication is given as 200 mcg/kg and is repeated in 1 week. Ivermectin should be avoided in pregnant or breast-feeding women and anyone who weighs less than 15 kg (Elston, 2002; Meinking et al., 2003; Orion, Matz, Ruocco, & Wolf, 2002; Wendel & Rompalo, 2002).

Prevention

To avoid reinfection with scabies, close contacts and family members need to be treated, and bed linens, towels, and clothing need to be washed during treatment. This is generally not required for lice except in cases of persistent mass infestations. The major means of prevention is the avoidance of close contact or shared bedding with others who have these infestations (Elston, 2002; Wendel & Rompalo, 2002).

Reporting

The U.S. Centers for Disease Control and Prevention does not consider scabies a nationally notifiable disease. The World Health Organization (WHO) classifies scabies as a Class 5 disease. See Appendix C for details and for upcoming changes in WHO reporting.

References

Elston, D.M. (2002). Controversies concerning the treatment of lice and scabies. *Journal of the American Academy of Dermatology, 46,* 794-796.

Meinking, T.L., Burkhart, C.N., & Burkhart, C.G. (2003). Infestations. In J.L. Bolognia, J.L. Jorizzo, & R.P. Rapini (Eds.), *Dermatology* (pp. 1321-1349). Philadelphia: Mosby.

Orion, E., Matz, H., Ruocco, V., & Wolf, R. (2002). Parasitic skin infestations II, scabies, pediculosis, spider bites: Unapproved treatments. *Clinics in Dermatology, 20,* 618-625.

Wendel, K., & Rompalo, A. (2002). Scabies and pediculosis pubis: An update of treatment regimens and general review. *Clinical Infectious Diseases, 35*(Suppl 2), S146-S151.

SCHISTOSOMIASIS
Bilharzia, bilharziasis
Geographic Distribution

Schistosomiasis is found throughout the world, especially in the Middle East, the Mediterranean, Brazil, Venezuela, China, the Philippines, Indonesia, and Africa. Four important species of *Schistosoma* cause human disease, and each has a particular geographic distribution:

- *S. japonicum* is found in Central and Eastern China, the Philippines, Indonesia, and nearby islands.
- *S. mansoni* is found in Africa, the Arabian peninsula, the eastern Mediterranean, the Caribbean, and South America.
- *S. haematobium* is found in sub-Saharan Africa, the Middle East, the eastern Mediterranean, and Southwest Asia.
- *S. mekongi* is found in Southeast Asia (Davis, 2003; King & Mahmoud, 1999; Strickland & Ramirez, 2000).

Agent and Vector

Schistosomiasis is caused by *Schistosoma,* which are blood flukes (trematodes) carried by freshwater snails (the intermediate host). Infected humans (the definitive host, though some schistosomes also infect birds and other mammals) pass eggs via stool or urine into the water where the parasites grow inside the snails. The parasite then leaves the snail in the form of cercaria (a worm-like early developmental form of a trematode) and directly penetrates the skin of persons working (e.g., planting rice), bathing, or swimming in the water. The worms migrate in host vessels and eventually arrive in the intrahepatic vasculature, where maturation and mating take place. Mating adults can then migrate to the venous plexus of the bladder and bowel, where they lay eggs that are eventually shed into the environment by the host to continue the cycle (Figure 70-1).

Incubation

Symptoms of acute schistosomiasis begins 5 to 7 weeks after initial infection, corresponding to the start of schistosome egg production (Strickland & Ramirez, 2000).

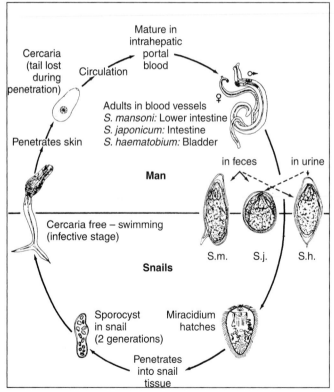

FIGURE 70–1

Life cycle of schistosomes in human infection. (*Source:* From Strickland, G.T. [2000]. *Hunter's tropical medicine and emerging infectious diseases* [8th ed., p. 808]. Philadelphia: W.B. Saunders Company.)

Clinical Findings and Treatment

Signs and Symptoms

- There are several syndromes, not all of which occur in every infected person. The manifestation of the chronic stage varies according to species. *S. japonicum*, *S. mansoni*, and *S. mekongi* primarily affect the liver and gastrointestinal tract, whereas *S. haematobium* primarily affects the urinary tract.

- Cercarial dermatitis (swimmer's itch) is a rash that may appear within 24 hours of exposure to cercaria-containing water. This results from incomplete, or abortive, skin penetration by the cercariae and manifests differently depending on whether the person has been previously sensitized. Nonsensitized people may develop a few macules that disappear within 12 hours and may not be noticed. Sensitized persons usually develop a more fulminant response with erythema, papules, vesicles, and pruritus that may last more than 1 week.

- Acute schistosomiasis, or Katayama fever, occurs as a primary infection approximately 5 to 7 weeks after exposure to a heavy cercarial load. Acute schistosomiasis is most common with *S. japonicum* and *S. mansoni* infection, and symptoms may include fever, sweats, chills, headache, urticaria (Figure 70-2), diarrhea, and cough. Physical examination may reveal hepatosplenomegaly and lymphadenopathy. Symptoms tend to gradually diminish over several weeks; however, overwhelming infection may result in death.

- Chronic hepatosplenic schistosomiasis is a consequence of prolonged infection with *S. mansoni* or *S. japonicum*, in which eggs retained in the liver provoke a delayed hypersensitivity granulomatous reaction. Patients usually present at least 6 months after the initial infection with lethargy, mucoid diarrhea, abdominal pain, and hepatomegaly. Granuloma formation and liver fibrosis

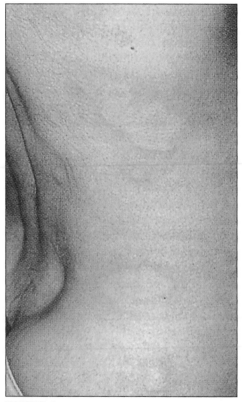

FIGURE 70–2

Urticaria in Katayama fever. (*Source:* From Peters, W., & Pasvol, G. [2002]. *Tropical medicine and parasitology* [5th ed., p. 140]. Chicago: Mosby.)

may lead to portal hypertension, splenomegaly, esophageal or gastric varices, and ascites.

— Intestinal schistosomiasis can also occur in chronic infection with *S. mansoni* or *S. japonicum.* The entire intestinal tract may be affected with granulomatous disease, but the large intestine is more frequently and severely involved. With mild disease, patients may present with fatigue, mucoid or hemorrhagic diarrhea, cramping, abdominal tenderness, and hyperactive bowel sounds. Patients rarely have both severe intestinal and hepatosplenic involvement. Severe intestinal involvement, or intestinal granulomatosis, is most common with *S. mansoni* infections in the Middle East, where patients manifest with severe mucohemorrhagic diarrhea, anemia, weight loss, abdominal tenderness, and occasionally large bowel obstruction.

Genitourinary schistosomiasis is associated with chronic *S. haematobium* infection. Granulomas in the bladder mucosa result from masses of eggs laid repeatedly by female worms residing in the bladder. Most infections are mild or asymptomatic. Hematuria, urinary frequency, and dysuria are common in the acute and chronic stages. Chronic infection may lead to obstructive uropathy, chronic bacteriuria, or bladder calcification. Obstructive uropathy develops when granulomas block ureteral orifices, leading to possible urethral dilation, hydronephrosis, uremia, and renal failure. Pyelonephritis can develop due to obstruction and may lead to septicemia, which is a common cause of death in urinary schistosomiasis. Salmonella infection concurrent with schistosomiasis is common and is resistant to treatment unless the schistosomiasis is also treated. In endemic areas, chronic genitourinary schistosomiasis is suspected to be the main factor behind increased rates of bladder cancer, which presents with gross hematuria, weight loss, and lymphadenopathy (Davis, 2003; King & Mahmoud, 1999; Strickland & Ramirez, 2000).

Complications

Intestinal granulomatosis can lead to focal intussusception, rectal prolapse, anorectal fistulas, or perirectal abscess formation. The portal hypertension that develops with hepatosplenic disease may lead to massive ascites, hemolytic anemia, or fatal hemorrhage due to large rupture of large varices. Nephrotic syndrome, manifesting as edema, hypoalbuminemia, proteinuria, and hyperlipidemia, occasionally occurs with *S. mansoni* infections. Larval pneumonitis can develop days to weeks after a heavy cercarial exposure; manifests as fever, cough, wheezing, and eosinophilia; and resolves within several weeks. Cor pulmonale may occur in *S. mansoni* hepatosplenic disease, and patients present with dyspnea on exertion, cough, right ventricular hypertrophy, and pulmonary hypertension. Cerebral schistosomiasis most commonly occurs with *S. japonicum* infections and presents with focal or generalized seizures (Strickland & Ramirez, 2000).

Common Laboratory Findings

Eosinophilia is seen in most cases of acute schistosomiasis. Anemia, hypoalbuminemia, and hypergammaglobulinemia are common findings in all types of schistosomiasis. Albuminuria and red cells in the urine are commonly found with *S. haematobium* infection (Strickland & Ramirez, 2000).

Diagnosis

Diagnosis is usually established by eggs in the feces, as in *S. japonicum* and *S. mansoni,* or in urine sediment, as in *S. haematobium.* Biopsy of infected tissue, such as the intestine, liver, or bladder, may also show eggs; however, it is often difficult to distinguish current versus past infection. On the other hand, ova loads are not always sufficient for diagnosis, especially in long-standing chronic illness. Identification of species-specific antischistosomal antibodies can be accomplished using techniques such as Western blot or enzyme-linked immunosorbent assay (ELISA). These are also not specific for active disease, and people living in endemic areas may have elevated antibody titers for long periods of time. Antigen detection assays are increasingly being used since the development of assays that detect antigens known as the circulating anodic antigen and cathodic antigen. "Fetal head" bladder calcification is a specific sign that may be seen in X-rays of patients with chronic *S. haematobium* infection. Ultrasound examinations may be useful and can reveal a thickened bladder wall, hydronephrosis, calcification, ureteral dilation, thickened portal tracts and portal veins, and esophageal varices. Colonoscopy and cystoscopy allow for biopsies to be taken in order to identify granulomatous disease or eggs in the tissue (Davis, 2003; King & Mahmoud, 1999; Strickland & Ramirez, 2000).

Differential Diagnosis

The differential diagnosis for acute schistosomiasis includes any prolonged febrile illness, including typhoid fever, brucellosis, malaria, and leptospirosis. Strongyloidosis and trichinosis cause fever with eosinophilia, which makes them more difficult to distinguish from schistosomiasis. Genitourinary schistosomiasis may be confused with other causes of hematuria, including malignancy, nephritic syndromes, and bacterial infection. Intestinal schistosomiasis may be confused with other infectious causes of diarrhea, peptic ulcer disease, pancreatitis, or appendicitis. The differential diagnosis for hepatosplenic schistosomiasis includes visceral leishmaniasis, myeloproliferative diseases, hemoglobinopathies, and viral hepatitis (Davis, 2003).

Treatment

Praziquantel is the primary treatment for susceptible cases of schistosomiasis. For *S. haematobium* and *S. mansoni* infections, the recommended single oral dose of praziquantel is 40 mg/kg. In patients with a high infectious load with *S. mansoni*, a total dose of 50 to 60 mg/kg may be needed and is given in two divided doses on a single day. *S. japonicum* should be treated with a single dose of 40 mg/kg. The oral dose recommended for *S. mekongi* is 60 mg/kg; however, repeated treatments are often required. Side effects of praziquantel are usually of short duration and include abdominal pain, nausea, and vomiting. *S. mansoni* may also be treated with oxamniquine in a single oral dose of 15 mg/kg (20 mg/kg for children), but a repeat dose may be required in 6 months for patients who are still excreting ova. *S. mansoni* infections in North and Eastern Africa are less susceptible and require doses up to 30 mg/kg. Drowsiness and dizziness are the most common side effects.

Systemic corticosteroids are sometimes required in severe disease, such as those manifesting with acute schistosomiasis, pneumonitis, or central nervous system symptoms (Davis, 2003; Richter, 2003; Strickland & Ramirez, 2000).

Prevention

There are many possible ways to attempt to prevent transmission of infection including reduction in snail vectors and habitats, sanitation to prevent contamination of water sources, improved accessibility of clean water sources, and the distribution of medications for either mass distribution in a population with high prevalence rates or cure of persons with high infectious loads. Elimination of schistosomiasis has been achieved in Japan and Venezuela through water sanitation projects. Vaccines are currently being developed, and Bilhvax is currently in phase II trials. Specific measures (Chin, 2000; Pearce, 2003; Strickland & Ramirez, 2000) to prevent or reduce the occurrence of schistosomiasis include the following:

- Provide sanitary facilities away from water that may contain the intermediate snail hosts. Because a number of animals are hosts in addition to humans, this may not eliminate transmission, but it may reduce transmission rates from some sources, for example, water where people regularly swim.

- Ensure that water for drinking, cooking, bathing, and washing clothes is free of mollusks. Effective water treatment includes the use of iodine or chlorine or water filters, including paper filters.
- Reduce mollusk habitats through removing vegetation or draining and filling mollusk habitats.
- Minimize exposure to contaminated water. Use of rubber boots is recommended. If exposed to contaminated water, immediately and vigorously rub dry with a towel and apply 70% alcohol to exposed skin to kill any remaining cercaria.
- Use molluscicides to treat water sources in high prevalence areas. Currently, the only molluscicide in broad use is niclosamide, which should be applied by a specialist.

Provide community education on these measures in endemic areas.

Reporting

The U.S. Centers for Disease Control and Prevention does not consider schistosomiasis to be a nationally notifiable disease. The World Health Organization (WHO) classifies schistosomiasis as a Class 3C disease. See Appendix C for details and for upcoming changes in WHO reporting.

References

Chin, J. (2000). Schistosomiasis. In J. Chin (Ed.), *Control of communicable diseases manual* (17th ed., pp. 447-450). Washington, DC: American Public Health Association.

Davis, A. (2003). Schistosomiasis. In G.C. Cook & A.I. Zumla (Eds.), *Manson's tropical diseases* (21st ed., pp. 1431-1469). Philadelphia: W.B. Saunders Company.

King, C.H., & Mahmoud, A.A.F. (1999). Schistosomiasis. In R.L. Guerrant, D.H. Walker, & P.F. Weller (Eds.), *Tropical infectious diseases: Principles, pathogens, and practice* (pp. 1031-1038). New York: Churchill Livingstone.

Pearce, E.J. (2003). Progress towards a vaccine for schistosomiasis. *Acta Tropica, 86,* 309-313.

Richter, J. (2003). The impact of chemotherapy on morbidity due to schistosomiasis. *Acta Tropica, 86,* 161-183.

Strickland, G.T., & Ramirez, B.L. (2000). Schistosomiasis. In G.T. Strickland (Ed.), *Hunter's tropical medicine and emerging infectious diseases* (8th ed., pp. 804-832). Philadelphia: W. B. Saunders Company.

71

SEVERE ACUTE RESPIRATORY SYNDROME

SARS

Geographic Distribution

— SARS first emerged in southern China in November 2002 and, by early 2003, expanded into a major global outbreak facilitated by international air travel. The pandemic caused more than 8000 cases including 774 deaths in more than two dozen countries before it was contained. Sporadic cases have since occurred in Asia (Centers for Disease Control and Prevention [CDC], 2004; Lingappa, McDonald, Simone, & Parashar, 2004).

Agent and Vector

— SARS is caused by SARS-CoV, a previously undescribed member of the coronavirus family of single-stranded RNA viruses. Other known coronaviruses in humans cause only the common cold. SARS-CoV is thought to have spread from mammals to humans in markets in southern China that specialize in selling live exotic game animals such as macaques, civets, ferrets, and raccoon dogs. The disease is highly transmissible through respiratory droplets and aerosol. The virus causes illness by inflicting diffuse alveolar damage and inflammation, pulmonary edema, and hyaline membrane formation, but in autopsy has also been isolated from bowel, lymph nodes, spleen, liver, and kidneys (Lingappa et al., 2004; Peiris, Yuen, Osterhaus, & Stohr, 2003).

Incubation

— The incubation period is 2 to 10 days, with a mean of 6 days (Peiris et al., 2003).

Clinical Findings and Treatment

Signs and Symptoms

SARS presents with nonspecific symptoms similar to
common respiratory illnesses: fever, cough, myalgias, and
malaise. Over time, shortness of breath and tachypnea
develop. Rhinorrhea and sore throat are uncommon.
Defervescence sometimes begins around the 10th day of
illness, but many patients will clinically worsen in the
second and third week. Diarrhea is more common in the
later stages. Common findings on physical examination
include tachycardia (46%), tachypnea (39%), and rales
(27%). Around 20% to 30% of patients will require
admission to an intensive care unit for mechanical
ventilation and other supportive measures. The overall
case fatality rate for SARS is around 10% (Peiris et al.,
2003; Wang & Chang, 2004; Wang et al., 2004).

Complications

Secondary infections and multisystem organ failure
are potential complications during hospitalization.
After discharge SARS-CoV survivors may suffer from
post-traumatic stress disorder, depression, and respiratory
impairment from residual pulmonary fibrosis (Peiris
et al., 2003).

Common Laboratory Findings

Lymphopenia, thrombocytopenia, and elevated liver
enzymes, lactate dehydrogenase, creatine phosphokinase,
and C-reactive protein have been observed. Plain chest
radiography often shows a "ground glass appearance"
with underlying consolidation (Peiris et al., 2003; Wang
et al., 2004).

Diagnosis

The challenge of SARS-CoV is that it requires a rapid
public health response for containment, yet has initial

symptoms that are indistinguishable from common community-acquired respiratory illnesses. Therefore, the diagnosis is usually made on the basis of clinical and epidemiologic findings.

— If at the time of presentation there are no reports of person-to-person SARS-CoV transmission anywhere in the world, the disease should be suspected in a hospitalized patient with radiographically confirmed pneumonia who within 10 days of the onset of symptoms:

- Has a history of recent travel to mainland China, Hong Kong, or Taiwan or close contact with ill persons with a history of recent travel to such areas, or
- Is employed in an occupation at particular risk for SARS-CoV exposure, such as a health care worker with direct patient contact or a worker in a laboratory that contains live SARS-CoV, or
- Is part of a cluster of cases of atypical pneumonia without an alternative diagnosis.

— If person-to-person transmission of SARS-CoV is occurring anywhere in the world, all patients with fever or lower respiratory tract symptoms should be screened for the preceding factors as well as the following additional risk factors:

- Close contact with someone suspected of having SARS-CoV disease, or
- History of foreign travel (or close contact with an ill person with a history of travel) to a location with documented or suspected SARS-CoV, or
- Exposure to a domestic location with documented or suspected SARS-CoV (including a laboratory that contains live SARS-CoV), or close contact with an ill person with such an exposure history.

— Reverse transcriptase-polymerase chain reaction (RT-PCR) testing for SARS-CoV may be done for patients who fit the clinical and epidemiologic profiles just described. Despite the high sensitivity and specificity of the test, the positive predictive value (the probability that a person with a positive test actually has the disease) is low in the absence of epidemiologic risk factors. Also, because the test is less sensitive in the early stages of illness, samples should be obtained from more than one body site (e.g. nasopharyngeal swab, throat swabs, sputum, serum, or stool), and over multiple times during the course of the illness. Antibody assays are also available but are valuable primarily for retrospective diagnosis, because they are most accurate when done more than 28 days following the onset of symptoms (CDC, 2004).

Differential Diagnosis

The differential diagnosis for SARS-CoV includes community-acquired pneumonias (particularly atypical pneumonias from *Mycoplasma, Chlamydia, Legionella*) and influenza. Co-infection with SARS-CoV and other respiratory pathogens is possible (Peiris et al., 2003).

Treatment

There are no specific therapies for SARS. Interferon alpha, corticosteroids, and ribavirin have been tried, but no randomized, placebo-controlled trials supporting their use have been conducted. Because it presents similarly to community-acquired pneumonias, patients are usually started on broad-spectrum antibiotics empirically until the diagnosis is made (Peiris et al., 2003).

Prevention

Current evidence suggests that persons with SARS become contagious at the onset of symptoms, and are most contagious during the second week of illness. A patient recovering from SARS should be considered contagious until 10 days have passed after the resolution of fever and respiratory symptoms.

Basic respiratory infection control measures are effective at preventing SARS. Patients presenting to a health care facility for evaluation for SARS should be quickly taken to separate area and given a face mask to wear. Staff involved in triaging and assessing the patient should also wear masks in addition to eye protection and should wash their hands before and after patient contact. Contaminated gloves should be disposed of, and stethoscopes and other equipment that can potentially spread infection should be cleaned with disinfectants. Public health authorities should be notified immediately of a patient suspected of having SARS.

Travelers should consult the CDC and World Health Organization (WHO) to learn of any current SARS outbreaks and travel restrictions. They should also be educated about the main symptoms of SARS (fever of more than 100.4° F, dry cough, shortness of breath or breathing difficulties) and be instructed to see a physician if they develop these symptoms within 10 days of visiting an area where local transmission of SARS has occurred (CDC, 2004; WHO, 2004).

Reporting

The CDC considers SARS to be a nationally notifiable disease. The WHO considers it a Class 1 disease. See Appendix C for details and for upcoming changes in WHO reporting.

References

Centers for Disease Control and Prevention. (2004). Severe Acute Respiratory Syndrome (SARS). Retrieved May 13, 2004, from *www.cdc.gov/ncidod/sars/index.htm*

Lingappa, J.R., McDonald, L.C., Simone, P., & Parashar, U.D. (2004). Wrestling SARS from uncertainty. *Emerging Infectious Diseases, 10,* 167-70.

Peiris, J.S., Yuen, K.Y., Osterhaus, A.D., & Stohr, K. (2003). The severe acute respiratory syndrome. *New England Journal of Medicine, 349,* 2431-41.

Wang, J.T., & Chang, S.C. (2004). Severe acute respiratory syndrome. *Current Opinion in Infectious Diseases, 17,* 143-48.

Wang, J.T., et al. (2004). Clinical manifestations, laboratory findings, and treatment outcomes of SARS patients. *Emerging Infectious Diseases, 10,* 818-824.

World Health Organization. (2004). Severe acute respiratory syndrome (SARS). Retrieved May 18, 2004, from *www.who.int/csr/sars/en/*

SMALLPOX

Variola

Geographic Distribution

Through the use of a massive vaccination campaign by the World Health Organization (WHO), smallpox was officially eradicated in 1977. Routine vaccinations for smallpox were stopped in the United States in 1972, leaving most young people today unprotected. The use of smallpox as a weapon of bioterrorism could therefore be devastating (Box 72-1). Although smallpox exists today only in small stockpiles in the United States and the former Soviet Union, this disease is still a potential global threat (Kiang & Krathwohl, 2003).

Agent and Vector

Smallpox is caused by the DNA virus, *Orthopoxvirus*. The organism is passed from human to human

---

BIOTERRORISM CONSIDERATIONS | BOX 72–1

Smallpox is considered by the Centers for Disease Control and Prevention (CDC) to be a Category A biological warfare agent. Category A agents are easily disseminated or transmitted, have high mortality rates and epidemic potential, and require special preparedness. Weaponized smallpox can be spread by aerosol and can be delivered directly (e.g., sprayed or released in enclosed spaces) or by bombs or missiles. The virus is stable and the infectious dose is small. The biological warfare route of infection is most likely aerosol. There is currently no proven treatment for this infection. See the Prevention section later in this chapter for specifics on the currently available vaccine (CDC, 2000; Johns Hopkins University, 2000).

predominantly by respiratory droplets and less so by direct contact with infected bodily fluids or scabbed cutaneous lesions. Because aerosolized virus can survive for many hours outside of the host, and only a small amount of virus is needed for infection, smallpox can potentially spread rapidly in unimmunized populations. The efficacy of transmission of smallpox from an infected person depends on several factors; however, the rate of transmission to unvaccinated contacts can be as high as 90%. Factors that increase infectiousness include high viral load in the oropharynx, severe disease, lack of previous vaccination, exposure to others during the first week of the rash, and frequent close face-to-face contact with those who are not immunized (Dacko, Hardick, & Yoshida, 2003; Kiang & Krathwohl, 2003).

Incubation

The incubation period is approximately 12 to 14 days after exposure (Dacko et al., 2003).

Clinical Findings and Treatment

Signs and Symptoms

Affected individuals first develop a prodrome consisting of sudden-onset high fever, chills, malaise, severe headache, backache, and occasionally vomiting, diarrhea, and delirium. Several days after the onset of symptoms, the fever drops and erythematous macules appear in the mouth and on the face, quickly spreading to involve the extremities and trunk (Figures 72-1 and 72-2). The rash evolves in a characteristic manner, with the macules becoming papules, then firm, often umbilicated, deep vesicles, and finally pustules after approximately 1 week. Lesions appear as a single crop, with all in the same stage of evolution at any particular time. Vesicles that develop in the oral mucosa easily rupture and allow for the release of large amounts of viral particles into the saliva and respiratory droplets. After 2 weeks, the vesicles and pustules scab over and eventually fall off, leaving depigmentation or pitted scars. Affected individuals remain contagious until the scabs are resolved. Although most patients have this characteristic presentation, there are several less common subtypes of smallpox. Variola minor is a less severe form with fewer systemic symptoms and may occur in patients with previous vaccination. Two forms of smallpox, flat and hemorrhagic, are uncommon, atypical in presentation, and nearly always fatal. Flat smallpox presents as slowly developing erythematous, velvety, rubbery nodules with little fluid inside. Hemorrhagic smallpox begins with dusky erythema and progresses to hemorrhage into the skin and mucous membranes (Dacko et al., 2003; Hull, Danila, & Ehresmann, 2003).

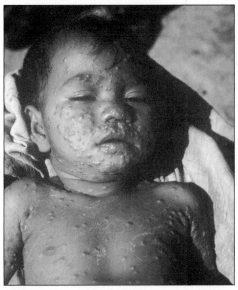

FIGURE 72–1

Smallpox. (*Source:* From Centers for Disease Control and Prevention, Health Image Library ID #3261.)

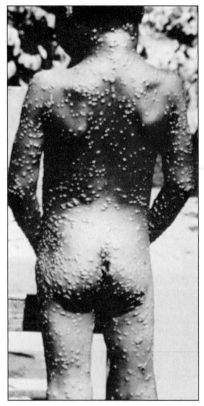

FIGURE 72–2

A monkeypox eruption (day 8) that resembles smallpox. (*Source:* From Strickland, G.T. [2000]. *Hunter's tropical medicine and emerging infectious diseases* [8th ed., p. 209]. Philadelphia: W.B. Saunders Company.)

Complications

Respiratory complications, including pneumonia and bronchitis, occur frequently. Bacterial superinfection, hemorrhage, arthritis, tubulointerstitial nephritis, and encephalitis are other possible complications. Ocular complications may include eyelid and conjunctival infection, corneal ulceration, keratitis, iritis, optic neuritis, and blindness. Case-fatality rates range from 20% to 50% in unvaccinated individuals, and death usually occurs during the second week of illness (Hull et al., 2003; Semba, 2003).

Common Laboratory Findings

Granulocytopenia, with an absolute increase in the number of lymphocytes, is generally present during the eruptive period, but this typically reverts to leukocytosis during the late pustular phase (Fenner, Henderson, Arita, Jezek, & Ladnyi, 1988).

Diagnosis

If a smallpox outbreak occurs, laboratory testing will be needed initially to confirm the clinical diagnosis. Definitive testing is currently only done by the CDC, and patients with a high risk of infection need to be reported immediately to the state health department. The CDC defines high-risk patients as those with a febrile prodrome and classic smallpox lesions which are all in the same stage of evolution. These people should be placed in contact and airborne isolation, and diagnostic tests immediately initiated. Possible specimens that may be obtained for testing include scrapings from the base of a vesicle or pustule, skin biopsies, throat swabs, and blood. To confirm the diagnosis in a high-risk patient, the samples obtained should be tested at the CDC or CDC-designated laboratory using the following available methods: electron microscopy, polymerase chain reaction (PCR) for variola, vaccinia, and orthopoxviruses, orthopox viral culture, serology, and other tests (i.e., direct fluorescent antibody, Tzanck preparation, PCR) to rule out varicella, herpes simplex, and other infections. For patients at low risk for smallpox, initial testing may be done at reference or local laboratories that are biosafety level 2 or higher (Besser, Crouch, & Sullivan, 2003; Hull et al., 2003).

Differential Diagnosis

Varicella is the primary disease that needs to be distinguished from smallpox. Characteristics of varicella that allow it to be differentiated from smallpox include the appearance of the lesions in crops, characteristic superficial vesicles surrounded by erythema, typically a less toxic picture (especially in children), and a centripetal distribution. Other diseases that may possibly resemble smallpox include herpes simplex virus, vaccinia vaccine reaction, molluscum contagiosum, monkeypox, secondary syphilis, scabies, and erythema multiforme (Besser et al., 2003; Hull et al., 2003).

Treatment

There is no specific treatment for smallpox. The most important measures for those affected include containment of the disease and supportive care consisting of nutrition, hydration, and treatment of secondary bacterial infections. Individuals who have been exposed to smallpox need to be vaccinated within 4 days of exposure, if vaccination is not contraindicated. Vaccinia immunoglobulin is available in limited quantities and may be used for severe cutaneous reactions to the immunization or for those who need protection but cannot be vaccinated due to their risk for complications. The antiviral drugs cidofovir and ribavirin have shown in vitro activity against smallpox and may prevent infection if taken 1 to 2 days after exposure (Dacko et al., 2003; Henderson, 1999; Hull et al., 2003).

Prevention

Three methods of prevention include isolation of infected individuals, vaccination of high-risk individuals, and chemoprophylaxis with agents such as cidofovir or ribavirin.

— The smallpox vaccine is made from vaccinia, which is a less virulent poxvirus with cross-protection to variola. Duration of immunity with the original vaccine varied from 3 to 10 years; however, even after immunity wanes, immunized individuals infected with smallpox may be less infectious and have a milder form of the disease. The current vaccine is a live attenuated vaccinia virus and, therefore, may have several adverse reactions that can be classified into three categories:

- Local reactions, including autoinoculation of other sites and vaccinia keratitis
- Widespread reactions, such as erythema multiforme and generalized vaccinia
- Systemic reactions, which are commonly mild and may include fever, chills, headache, and myalgias. Potentially fatal severe systemic reactions are rare, and include progressive vaccinia (vaccinia necrosum), eczema vaccinatum, encephalitis, congenital vaccinia, and myopericarditis

— Many individuals should not receive the vaccination because of a high risk of complications: pregnant women; patients with eczema or exfoliative dermatitis, hereditary immune deficiencies, history of organ transplantation, generalized malignancy, autoimmune diseases, or HIV infection; and those taking immunosuppressive medications. If these people are exposed to smallpox, the vaccine may be coadministered with vaccinia immunoglobulin. Household contacts of high-risk persons should also not be immunized. Recently, it has been recommended that patients with previous myocardial infarctions, heart failure, cardiomyopathy, and other heart conditions should not be vaccinated due to the possible association with cardiac events (Aragon, Ulrich, Fernyak,

& Rutherford, 2003; Bonilla-Guerrero & Poland, 2003; Dacko et al., 2003; Kiang & Krathwohl, 2003).

Reporting

An outbreak of smallpox would be an unparalleled public health disaster. The CDC considers smallpox to be a nationally notifiable disease. The WHO considers smallpox a Class 1 disease. See Appendix C for details and for upcoming changes in WHO reporting.

References

Aragon, T.J., Ulrich, S., Fernyak, S., & Rutherford, G.W. (2003). Risks of serious complications and death from smallpox vaccination: A systematic review of the United States experience, 1963-1968. *Biomed Central Public Health, 11.* Retrieved February 22, 2004, from *www.pubmedcentral.nih.gov/articlerender.fcgi?tool=pubmed&pubmedid= 12911836*

Besser, J.M., Crouch, N.A., & Sullivan, M. (2003). Laboratory diagnosis to differentiate smallpox, vaccinia, and other vesicular/pustular illnesses. *Journal of Laboratory and Clinical Medicine, 142,* 246-251.

Bonilla-Guerrero, R., & Poland, G.A. (2003). Smallpox vaccines: Current and future. *Journal of Laboratory and Clinical Medicine, 142,* 252-257.

Centers for Disease Control and Prevention. (2000). Biological and chemical terrorism: Strategic plan for preparedness and response. *MMWR: Morbidity and Mortality Weekly Report, 49*(RR-4), 1-14.

Dacko, A., Hardick, K., & Yoshida, T. (2003). Smallpox. *Cutis, 71,* 319-322.

Fenner, F., Henderson, D.A., Arita, I., Jezek, Z., & Ladnyi, I.D. (1988). *Smallpox and its eradication.* Geneva, Switzerland: World Health Organization. Retrieved February 29, 2004, from *www.who.int/emc/diseases/smallpox/Smallpoxeradication.html*

Henderson, D.A. (1999). Smallpox and monkeypox. In R.L. Guerrant, D.H. Walker, & P.F. Weller (Eds.), *Tropical infectious diseases: Principles, pathogens, and practice* (pp. 1095-1108). New York: Churchill Livingstone.

Hull, H.F., Danila, R., & Ehresmann, K. (2003). Smallpox and bioterrorism: public-health responses. *Journal of Laboratory and Clinical Medicine, 142,* 221-228.

Johns Hopkins University Center for Civilian Biodefense Studies. (2000). Retrieved September 24, 2001, from *www.hopkins-biodefense.org/*

Kiang, K.M., & Krathwohl, M.D. (2003). Rates and risks of transmission of smallpox and mechanisms of prevention. *Journal of Laboratory and Clinical Medicine, 142,* 229-238.

Semba, R.D. (2003). The ocular complications of smallpox and smallpox immunization. *Archives of Ophthalmology, 121,* 715-719.

73

Sporotrichosis

Geographic Distribution

Sporotrichosis is most commonly found in Mexico, Central and South America, Africa, and Japan. Occasionally cases are reported from the southern United States, the Far East, Australia, Guatemala, Peru, and South Africa (Hay, 2003).

Agent and Vector

Sporotrichosis is caused by the dimorphic mold *Sporothrix schenckii*, which grows on dead plant material in temperate and tropical environments. The organism most commonly causes infection through traumatic inoculation of the skin with contaminated environmental sources, such as thorns, barbs, sphagnum moss, or soil. The disease primarily affects individuals whose occupations require contact with plants and soils in endemic areas (Bustamante & Campos, 2001; Queiroz-Telles, McGinnis, Salkin, & Graybill, 2003).

Incubation

The incubation period usually ranges from 1 to 4 weeks (Hay, 2003).

Clinical Findings and Treatment

Signs and Symptoms

The most common manifestation of sporotrichosis infection is cutaneous involvement of an extremity, although any exposed area of skin has the potential for infection. The organism may gain entry into the skin through traumatic inoculation or contact with an abrasion. Cutaneous sporotrichosis initially manifests as a small, firm subcutaneous nodule at the site of inoculation that may subsequently ulcerate or form granulomatous lesions (Figures 73-1A and B). Lymphangitic spread often occurs and satellite nodules or ulcers become apparent along the course of local lymphatic vessels. Regional lymphadenopathy may also occur. Occasionally cutaneous disease remits spontaneously, but it often recurs or requires treatment. Although the skin is overwhelmingly the most common site of infection, other areas of involvement have been described.

Primary pulmonary infection can occur in endemic areas and is most often caused by inhalation of the organism.

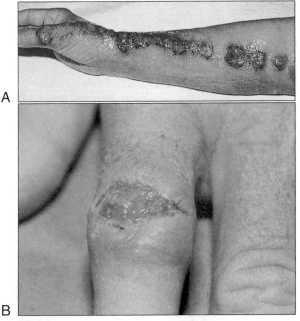

A

B

FIGURE 73–1

Sporotrichosis lesions. (*Source:* **A,** From Peters, W., & Pasvol, G. [2002]. *Tropical medicine and parasitology* [5th ed., p. 261]. Chicago: Mosby. **B,** Courtesy of the University of Texas Southwestern Department of Dermatology.)

The infection is usually asymptomatic but may cause a productive cough, dyspnea, or hemoptysis. Chronic cavitary disease and fibrosis can develop and, if untreated, may ultimately lead to progressive disease and death.

Disseminated sporotrichosis may develop in patients with underlying conditions, such as alcoholism, diabetes, HIV, or other types of immunosuppression, and is spread hematogenously from a cutaneous or pulmonary site of infection. These patients usually develop multiple widespread cutaneous nodules that may subsequently ulcerate. The infection can eventually involve the joints, bones, mucous membranes, and central nervous system, leading to meningitis, brain abscesses, and arthritis. Mortality in disseminated disease is high, especially if the patient has severe comorbid illnesses, has a delayed diagnosis, or is not treated in a timely manner (Hay, 2000, 2003; Hospenthal & Bennett, 1999; Queiroz-Telles et al., 2003).

Complications

Osteomyelitis can occur at a site of trauma or primary inoculation. Bursitis may occur under skin lesions, most often on the knees and elbows. Multiple joint effusions may be seen in immunosuppressed patients with widespread disease. Primary pulmonary sporotrichosis can lead to fibrosis of the lungs, and disseminated disease may result in chronic meningitis or debilitating arthritis (Queiroz-Telles et al., 2003).

Common Laboratory Findings

There are no common laboratory findings.

Diagnosis

The diagnosis may be suspected with the classic lymphangitic sporotrichosis presentation, especially when the history reveals potential exposure. Confirmation of the diagnosis can be achieved in several ways. *S. schenckii* can be cultured on Sabouraud's agar, and sample tissue should be obtained from the edge of skin lesions using a swab or biopsy. Growth can be detected on culture media after approximately 3 to 10 days. Direct examination of exudate or scrapings from a skin lesion is usually not helpful.

— Skin biopsies taken from the edge of a lesion may reveal a granulomatous reaction with neutrophils; however, few organisms are usually present which makes visualization of the fungus difficult without special stains, such as periodic acid-Schiff (PAS) and Giemsa. Occasionally the characteristic "asteroid body," which represents a central yeast structure with a radiating eosinophilic halo, can be seen in histologic sections. Immunohistochemical staining, although not widely available in endemic areas, can greatly enhance the sensitivity of tissue examination.

— The Sporotrichin skin test, which is an intradermal reaction to an agent prepared from *Sporothrix* antigens, can be useful in identifying those who have been exposed during outbreaks of the disease; however, many uninfected individuals in endemic areas will already have positive reactions. Although current serologic tests are not always reliable, they may be useful in diagnosing disseminated disease or chronic meningitis due to sporotrichosis. Enzyme-linked immunosorbent assays (ELISAs) and slide latex agglutination are the most useful serologic tests in these situations (Bustamante & Campos, 2001; Hays, 2000, 2003; Hospenthal & Bennett, 1999).

Differential Diagnosis

— The differential diagnosis of sporotrichoid nodules or ulcers with lymphatic spread includes infection with *Nocardia*, *Actinomyces*, nontuberculous mycobacteria, such as *M. marinum* and *M. fortuitum*, *Francisella tularensis*, *Staphylococcus aureus*, *Bartonella*, *Leishmania*, blastomycosis, histoplasmosis, and coccidioidomycosis. Other infections that may be confused with a solitary sporotrichoid nodule or ulcer may include paracoccidioidomycosis, blastomycosis, chromoblastomycosis, phaeohyphomycosis, tuberculosis, syphilis, or protozoa. Noninfectious entities that may mimic sporotrichosis include sarcoidosis and primary skin cancers (Queiroz-Telles et al., 2003).

Treatment

The primary treatment of cutaneous sporotrichosis consists of potassium iodide in saturated solution 1 mL tid with incremental increases to 4 to 6 mL tid after 1 month for 3 months, but treatment should be continued for at least 3 to 4 weeks after a clinical cure is achieved. Side effects include nausea, dry mouth, metallic taste, and swollen salivary glands. Alternative therapies include externally applied heat, liquid nitrogen, itraconazole 100 to 200 mg/day for 3 to 6 months, fluconazole 400 mg/day for 6 months, and terbinafine 250 mg/day for 3 to 6 months. HIV-infected patients should continue on long-term prophylactic treatment with itraconazole 200 mg bid.

Pulmonary disease is best treated with surgery, followed by amphotericin B 0.5 mg/kg/day to total of 1 to 2 g or itraconazole 200 mg bid, since it is often refractory to medical treatment alone. Osteoarticular disease is treated with itraconazole 300 mg bid for 6 to12 months followed by 200 mg bid. Disseminated disease is best treated with parenteral amphotericin B 0.5 mg/kg/day to a total of 1 to 2 g followed by itraconazole 200 mg bid or fluconazole 800 mg daily (Gilbert, Moellering, & Sande, 2002; Hays, 2000, 2003; Hospenthal & Bennett, 1999).

Prevention

Avoidance of traumatic inoculation by contaminated plant material is the best way to prevent infection. Individuals who work closely with plants in endemic areas should wear gloves and protective clothing. Fungicide treatment of high-risk wooded areas has been used during epidemics of disease (Hospenthal & Bennett, 1999).

Reporting

The U.S. Centers for Disease Control and Prevention does not consider sporotrichosis to be a nationally notifiable disease. The World Health Organization (WHO) classifies sporotrichosis as a Class 5 disease. See Appendix C for details and for upcoming changes in WHO reporting.

References

Bustamante, B., & Campos, P.E. (2001). Endemic sporotrichosis. *Current Opinion in Infectious Disease, 14,* 145-149.

Gilbert, D.N., Moellering Jr., R.C., & Sande, M.A. (Eds.) (2002). *The Sanford guide to antimicrobial therapy* (32nd ed.). Hyde Park, VT: Antimicrobial Therapy, Inc.

Hay, R.J. (2000). Sporotrichosis. In G.T. Strickland (Ed.), *Hunter's tropical medicine and emerging infectious diseases* (8th ed., pp. 541-542). Philadelphia: W.B. Saunders Company.

Hay, R.J. (2003). Fungal infections. In G.C. Cook & A.I. Zumla (Eds.), *Manson's tropical diseases* (21st ed., pp. 1184-1185). Philadelphia: W.B. Saunders Company.

Hospenthal, D.R., & Bennett, J.E. (1999). Entomophthoramycosis, lobomycosis, rhinosporidiosis, and sporotrichosis. In R.L. Guerrant, D.H. Walker, & P.F. Weller (Eds.), *Tropical infectious diseases: Principles, pathogens, and practice* (pp. 668-671). New York: Churchill Livingstone.

Queiroz-Telles, F., McGinnis, M.R., Salkin, I., & Graybill, J.R. (2003). Subcutaneous mycoses. *Infectious Disease Clinics of North America, 17,* 59-85.

STAPHYLOCOCCAL SKIN INFECTION
Pyoderma
Geographic Distribution

Staphylococcal skin infections are common worldwide, in both urban and rural settings, developed and underdeveloped countries, and in healthy and immunocompromised individuals.

Agent and Vector

Both *Staphylococcus aureus* and *S. epidermidis* are normally found on the skin; however, *S. aureus* is the more pathogenic. Infections occur when there is direct inoculation of the skin with the bacteria, which may arise secondary to minor trauma, insect bites, burns, surgery, superficial fungal infections, eczema, or other conditions that compromise the integrity of the skin. Once the bacteria gains access to the tissue, damage can be caused by proteases, coagulases, and, in the cases of staphylococcal scalded skin syndrome (SSSS) and staphylococcal toxic shock syndrome (Staph TSS), by exfoliative toxins (Vega-Lopez & Chopra, 2003).

Incubation

Incubation periods are variable, and there may be a long delay between colonization and clinical infection (Vega-Lopez & Chopra, 2003).

Clinical Findings and Treatment

Signs and Symptoms

Skin infection with *Staphylococcus* can manifest in many ways, including folliculitis, furuncles, carbuncles, abscesses, impetigo, cellulitis, botryomycosis, SSSS, and

Staph TSS. Each of these is discussed in separate paragraphs next.

— Folliculitis is most commonly caused by *S. aureus* and manifests as erythematous perifollicular pustules that are sometimes pruritic or painful. The head, neck, trunk, axilla, and buttocks are the areas most frequently involved. Occasionally the pustules rupture and only erythematous papules with collarettes of scale remain.

— A furuncle is a collection of pus around a hair follicle, a carbuncle is a collection of furuncles, and an abscess is a collection of pus that can occur anywhere and is not confined to a hair follicle. *S. aureus* is the most common organism that causes furuncles, and predisposing factors that lead to their development include nasal carriage of *S. aureus*, diabetes mellitus, poor hygiene, and immunodeficiency states. Other aerobic bacteria, anaerobic bacteria, and foreign body reactions may also cause furuncles. Furuncles and carbuncles develop most commonly on the face, neck, axilla, buttocks, thighs, and groin. Furuncles appear as firm, tender, erythematous nodules that enlarge and may drain purulent fluid. Carbuncles are similar in appearance, except they often extend deeper into the subcutaneous tissues and have multiple draining sinus tracts.

— Impetigo is a superficial skin infection that is common in children and is highly contagious. Conditions that predispose patients to impetigo include warm humid climates, poor hygiene, overcrowding, nasal carriage of *S. aureus*, and skin trauma. Nonbullous impetigo is the most common type and is caused by *S. aureus* in the majority of cases, with *Streptococcus pyogenes* accounting for a minority. Patients initially manifest with a small erythematous macule or papule, which eventually erodes and develops the characteristic honey-colored crust (Figure 74-1). The most likely affected sites include the face, especially the nose and mouth, and the

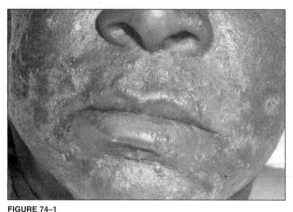

FIGURE 74–1

Impetigo. (*Source:* Courtesy of the University of Texas Southwestern Department of Dermatology.)

extremities. Lymphadenopathy may be present. Impetigo may also occur secondary to other skin conditions when the skin barrier is already compromised, such as scabies, eczema, and superficial fungal infections. Bullous impetigo is always caused by *S. aureus* and characteristically develops in neonates. Superficial vesicles and bullae develop on the face, trunk, buttocks, or extremities, which easily rupture and leave behind an erosion and collarette of scale. There is usually minimal to no erythema or crust, nor are systemic symptoms usually associated with bullous impetigo. Cellulitis is caused by *S. aureus* or *S. pyogenes* and usually develops secondary to skin trauma in immunocompetent individuals. Bacteria may also be introduced into the skin through hematogenous spread, causing cellulitis in immunocompromised patients. Other predisposing factors for cellulitis include diabetes mellitus, alcoholism, malignancy, peripheral vascular disease, and conditions of poor or damaged lymphatic drainage. Cellulitis is characterized by an ill-defined, erythematous, warm plaque, which may have bullae, pustules, or necrotic

areas in severe cases. Fever and chills may precede the
onset of skin findings, and the extremities are the most
commonly affected areas in adults.

— Botryomycosis is a rare type of a chronic granulomatous
bacterial skin infection that is most commonly caused by
S. aureus, but may also be due to *Pseudomonas*, *Proteus*,
or *Corynebacterium*. Affected individuals may present
with abscesses, nodules, ulcers, verrucous plaques,
and/or sinus tracts, which discharge granules made up
of bacterial aggregates. These lesions typically occur at
sites of trauma on the extremities in individuals with
defective cellular immunity.

— SSSS is caused by strains of *S. aureus* that produce
exfoliative toxins, ET-A and ET-B. These toxins are
renally excreted, thus SSSS occurs more often in young
children with immature kidneys and adults with renal
insufficiency. Patients initially present with fever,
malaise, and tender skin. Erythema of the skin begins
on the head and neck, rapidly spreads to the body,
develops widespread flaccid bullae, and slough in
flexural areas within 1 to 2 days. Patients continue
to desquamate and often develop perioral crusting,
fissuring, and facial edema. Skin re-epithelializes and
heals without scarring within a couple of weeks when
treated.

— Staph TSS is caused by strains of *S. aureus* that produce
the exfoliative toxin, toxic shock syndrome toxin-1
(TSST-1). Predisposing factors for the development of
Staph TSS include surgery, cutaneous *S. aureus* infection,
postpartum infection, deep abscesses, pneumonia, and
nasal picking. One to 2 weeks before development
of skin manifestations, patients develop fever, chills,
myalgias, and lethargy. The illness progressively worsens,
with the development of hypotension, tachycardia, and
skin involvement. Patients develop an erythematous
macular rash that spreads centripetally, erythema of the
mucous membranes, and edema and erythema of the

palms and soles, which desquamate within 1 to 3 days
(Blume, Levine, & Heymann, 2003; Hay, 2003; Kelly,
2003; Mahe, 2001; Stevens, 2000).

Complications

— Complications of Staph TSS include decreased renal
function, myalgias, paresthesias, arthralgias, and
gangrene. Untreated cases of Staph TSS can result in
death. Mortality rates for SSSS are low for children
but exceed 50% in adults and those with underlying
disease.
— Unsuccessfully treated lesions of botryomycosis may
extend into the underlying muscle or bone.
Visceral botryomycosis most often occurs in
immunocompromised patients and is sometimes
related to prior surgery (Blume et al., 2003).

Common Laboratory Findings

— There may be an increased leukocyte count and
a left shift, depending on the extent of the infection.
Inflammatory markers such as erythrocyte sedimentation
rate (ESR) and C-reactive protein may also be elevated.

Diagnosis

— The diagnosis of these entities is usually based on the
history, physical examination, and distribution of the
lesions; however, the specific causative organism can
only be identified by culturing the contents of intact
pustules or bullae, superficial crusts, or erosions. This
is particularly important in cases that are recurrent or
resistant to treatment. A needle aspiration or skin biopsy
can be taken from lesions of cellulitis in order to
determine the organism. This should especially be
considered in children or immunocompromised persons
who may not be infected with the usual bacteria.
Botryomycosis can be diagnosed by Gram staining or
culturing of crushed granules. A skin biopsy and

histologic examination of the lesion may also help to confirm the diagnosis.

In patients suspected of having SSSS, *S. aureus* may be cultured from the nares, conjunctiva, or established pyogenic skin infection; however, it will not be found in the new bullae or desquamating plaques. Blood cultures may be positive in adults but are usually negative in children. The diagnosis of SSSS can be confirmed with frozen sections of skin lesions, which reveals a cleavage plane within or just below the stratum granulosum, or enzyme-linked immunosorbent assay (ELISA) identification of the ET-A and ET-B toxins. Staph TSS is often a clinical diagnosis, and all cultures are usually negative (Blume et al., 2003).

Differential Diagnosis

The differential diagnosis of staphylococcal folliculitis includes folliculitis caused by other bacteria (*Pseudomonas*) or fungi (*Candida* or *Pityrosporum*), eosinophilic folliculitis, acne, rosacea, pseudofolliculitis barbae, and keratosis pilaris. Furunculosis may be confused with a ruptured cyst, hidradenitis suppurativa, or cystic acne. Impetigo is fairly characteristic clinically; however, the causative organism should be established with a culture. It is also necessary to determine if there is an underlying skin condition that predisposes the patient to impetigo, such as scabies or eczema.

The differential diagnosis of cellulitis includes superficial or deep-venous thrombosis, stasis dermatitis, and vasculitis. Cellulitis may be caused by a mixture of bacteria in the setting of diabetic ulcers, decubitus ulcers, and chronic venous insufficiency, and a culture needs to be done to determine to causative organism(s). Necrotizing fasciitis, which is caused by group A streptococcus or is sometimes polymicrobial, may resemble staphylococcal cellulitis but typically has severe pain with rapidly spreading edema and bulla, and signs of shock. Because necrotizing fasciitis progresses so rapidly and often requires surgical intervention, treatment must be started immediately.

— Botryomycosis may resemble mycetoma, actinomycosis, cutaneous tuberculosis, blastomycosis, chromoblastomycosis, and atypical mycobacterial infections.

— SSSS may be confused with Kawasaki disease, toxic shock syndrome (caused by *Streptococcus* or *Staphylococcus*), a viral exanthem, a drug reaction, or toxic epidermal necrolysis. The differential diagnosis for Staph TSS is similar (Blume et al., 2003).

Treatment

— Localized bacterial folliculitis or impetigo can be treated with antibacterial washes (chlorhexidine or triclosan) or antibacterial ointments (bacitracin or mupirocin) applied topically for 1 to 2 weeks. For widespread folliculitis or impetigo, oral antibiotics that cover *S. aureus* should be used. Some options include cephalexin 500 mg every 6 hours in adults and 25 to 50 mg/kg/day divided bid to qid in children for 7 to 10 days, or erythromycin 500 mg qid in adults and 10 mg/kg qid in children for 7 to 10 days.

— For small furuncles, warm compresses may help to promote maturation and resolution of the lesion. Oral antibiotics are not needed in this situation. Large furuncles, carbuncles, recurrent lesions, lesions with surrounding cellulitis, or those not responding to compresses may need surgical drainage or antibiotic treatment as listed earlier for impetigo.

— Mild cellulitis caused by *S. aureus* can be treated with the oral antibiotic regimen as above. Complicated or extensive cellulitis may need intravenous antibiotic therapy with nafcillin 1 to 2 g IV q4-6h in adults or 37 mg/kg q6h in children or cefazolin 1 to 2 g IV q8h in adults or 20 mg/kg q8h in children.

~ Botryomycosis is treated with surgical excision and debridement, because antibiotics are not usually successful.

~ SSSS is treated with intravenous antibiotics, such as those listed earlier for complicated cellulitis, for at least 1 week. Bland emollients may decrease the tenderness of the skin and help promote healing. Patients should also be treated with mupirocin ointment for possible nasal *S. aureus* carriage.

~ Staph TSS treatment requires hospitalization and supportive care, such as intravenous fluids and vasopressor medications. Patients should be treated with intravenous antibiotics, such as nafcillin 1 to 2 g IV q4-6h in adults or 37 mg/kg q6h in children or cefazolin 1 to 2 g IV q8h in adults or 20 mg/kg q8h in children. Affected individuals should also be treated with mupirocin ointment for possible nasal *S. aureus* carriage (Blume et al., 2003; Gilbert, Moellering, & Sande, 2002).

~ Methicillin-resistant *S. aureus* (MRSA) is an emerging pathogen that should be suspected in patients who do not respond to standard therapy. Infection with MRSA is confirmed by antibiotic sensitivity testing of isolates. Critically ill patients infected with MRSA should be treated with vancomycin 500 mg IV q6h for adults or 10 mg/kg/dose q6h for children; q12h for neonates less than 1 week old after an initial loading dose of 15 mg/kg; q8h for infants 1-4 weeks old. The evidence for ideal therapy of less serious infections is not clear. Some experts recommend sulfamethoxazole/ trimethoprim (TMP/SMX), 1 DS tablet PO bid for adults, 8 to 10 mg TMP/kg/day divided bid for children. Clindamycin, 300 to 450 mg PO tid in adults or 8 to 16 mg/kg/day divided tid in children, is often effective but may not work against erythromycin-resistant MRSA. Fluoroquinolones are another option, but there are concerns that their use could contribute to the development of further antibiotic resistance. Rifampin at a dose of 300 mg PO bid to tid in adults or 20 mg/kg/day divided bid in children is sometimes added to TMP/SMX or clindamycin to reduce the possibility of resistance. For abscesses, the most important treatment is incision and drainage. Mupirocin ointment (applied tid to qid) may be used on MRSA infected lesions in conjunction with oral antibiotics, as well as intranasally to eliminate carriage (Cohen & Grossman, 2004).

Prevention

Underlying skin conditions, such as eczema and scabies, should be treated in order to avoid superinfection with *S. aureus*. Good hygiene and hand washing are helpful, as is tight glucose control in diabetics. Treatment of *S. aureus* carriers with mupirocin ointment to the nares can prevent disease recurrence and passage of infection to others; however, recolonization is common.

Reporting

The U.S. Centers for Disease Control and Prevention does not consider *S. aureus* infection to be a nationally notifiable disease. The World Health Organization (WHO) considers *S. aureus* infection to be a Class 4 disease. See Appendix C for details and for upcoming changes in WHO reporting.

References

Blume, J.E., Levine, E.G., & Heymann, W.R. (2003). Bacterial diseases. In J.L. Bolognia, J.L. Jorizzo, & R.P. Rapini, (Eds.), *Dermatology* (pp. 1117-1144). Philadelphia: Mosby.

Cohen, P.R., & Grossman, M.E. (2004). Management of cutaneous lesions associated with an emerging epidemic: Community-acquired methicillin-resistant *Staphylococcus aureus* skin infections. *Journal of the American Academy of Dermatology, 51,* 132-135.

Gilbert, D.N., Moellering Jr., R.C., & Sande, M.A. (Eds.) (2002). *The Sanford guide to antimicrobial therapy* (32nd ed.). Hyde Park, VT: Antimicrobial Therapy, Inc.

Hay, R.J. (2003). Pyoderma and scabies: A benign association? *Current Opinion in Infectious Disease, 6,* 69-70.

Kelly, P. (2003). Folliculitis and the follicular occlusion tetrad. In J.L. Bolognia, J.L. Jorizzo, & R.P. Rapini, (Eds.), *Dermatology* (pp. 553-554). Philadelphia: Mosby.

Mahe, A. (2001). Bacterial skin infections in a tropical environment. *Current Opinion in Infectious Disease, 14,* 123-126.

Stevens, D.L. (2000). Streptococcal and staphylococcal infections. In G. Strickland (Ed.), *Hunter's tropical medicine and emerging infectious diseases* (8th ed., pp. 195-199). Philadelphia: W.B. Saunders Company.

Vega-Lopez, F., & Chopra, S. (2003). Dermatological problems. In G.C. Cook & A.I. Zumla (Eds.), *Manson's tropical diseases* (21st ed., pp. 364-366). Philadelphia: W.B. Saunders Company.

75

STRONGYLOIDIASIS

Larva currens

Geographic Distribution

Strongyloidiasis is found worldwide but favors tropical and subtropical areas. It is endemic in regions of Asia, Africa, Latin America, and the southern United States. In temperate climates, the infection can sometimes be a problem in prisons, psychiatric hospitals, or other crowded institutions. Severe or refractory cases of strongyloidiasis may be associated with human T-lymphotropic virus type 1 (HTLV-1) in areas where the infection is endemic (Gilles, 2003; Gilman, 2000; Terashima et al., 2002).

Agent and Vector

Strongyloidiasis is caused by infection with the threadworm *Strongyloides stercoralis*. Infection begins when the filiform larvae, which are found in fecally contaminated moist soil, penetrate the skin. The larvae then migrate through blood vessels into the lungs, where they enter alveoli and travel up the respiratory tree into the trachea and glottis. The larvae are then swallowed and complete their life cycle by maturing into adult worms in the small intestine. One month after the initial infection, the adult female worms lay eggs in the intestinal mucosa. The eggs hatch into noninfectious larvae, which either pass in the feces or mature into infectious filiform larvae in the intestines or perianal skin. These filiform larvae can cause internal autoinfection by penetrating the intestinal mucosa or perianal skin and proceeding through the blood vessels into the lungs, continuing the life cycle.

The noninfectious larvae that are passed in feces can complete their life cycle in the soil as well. There they transform into adult worms and lay eggs that hatch into noninfectious larva and eventually mature into the filiform infectious larvae.

Due to the balance between autoinfection and immunity, most affected people carry a small number of adult worms in the small intestine for many years even without further outside exposure. However, individuals who become immunocompromised secondary to medications or disease states can develop severe invasive disease. Decreased cellular immunity allows the rapid, uncontrolled conversion of noninfectious to infectious filiform larvae in the intestine, with subsequent widespread dissemination (Gilles, 2003; Gilman, 2000).

Incubation

The time period from exposure of an individual to the development of larvae in the feces is approximately 1 month, but the time to appearance of symptoms may be years (Gilles, 2003).

Clinical Findings and Treatment

Signs and Symptoms

Most affected people are asymptomatic or have mild nonspecific symptoms. As the number of worms in the intestine increases, symptoms may become more apparent. The initial infection is not usually recognized. The first sign may be a pruritic erythematous plaque or migrating linear urticaria (a.k.a. larva currens) at the site of larval penetration. As the larvae move to the lungs and glottis, a cough or sore throat may develop. Rarely, the migration of the larvae through the lungs is associated with Löffler's syndrome, characterized by cough, wheezing, transient pulmonary infiltrates, and eosinophilia. Once the larvae mature into adult worms in the intestine, abdominal fullness, pain, and diarrhea alternating with constipation may occur.

Chronic infection is characterized by intermittent gastrointestinal and cutaneous manifestations. Gastrointestinal signs and symptoms may include epigastric or right upper quadrant abdominal pain, abdominal fullness, nausea, diarrhea sometimes alternating with constipation, weight loss, and occasionally occult blood in the stool. Cutaneous manifestations include chronic recurrent urticaria and larva currens, which is a pruritic urticarial linear track under the skin caused by migrating larvae (Figure 75-1). This characteristically occurs in the perianal area secondary to autoinoculation by larvae in the feces. Disseminated infection may cause gastrointestinal or pulmonary disease. Gastrointestinal symptoms that can develop include malabsorption, severe diarrhea with electrolyte abnormalities, protein-losing enteropathy, hypoalbuminemia and generalized edema,

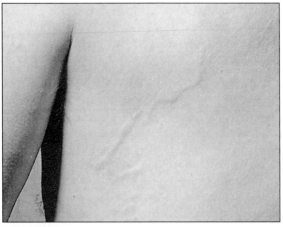

FIGURE 75-1

Migrating *Strongyloides* larvae. (*Source:* From Peters, W., & Pasvol, G. [2002]. *Tropical medicine and parasitology* [5th ed., p. 118]. Chicago: Mosby.)

ileus, and necrotic bowel. Lung manifestations can be severe and may consist of chronic diffuse bronchopneumonia, bronchospasm, intra-alveolar hemorrhage, cavitation, pleural effusions, pulmonary abscesses, and respiratory failure (Genta, 1999; Gilles, 2003; Gilman, 2000).

Complications

Most complications occur with severe infection. Mortality is high with disseminated disease, especially when patients develop bacterial sepsis with enteric organisms carried by migrating larvae from the bowel. Other complications include peritonitis, endocarditis, and neurologic manifestations, such as meningitis, seizures, confusion, and focal neurologic signs (Gilles, 2003; Gilman, 2000).

Common Laboratory Findings

During the initial infection, patients develop high leukocytosis with prominent eosinophilia. As the disease becomes chronic, eosinophils are only moderately elevated. The disappearance of eosinophilia in severe disseminated disease is a poor prognostic indicator (Gilles, 2003).

Diagnosis

Stool examination for larvae is the main diagnostic method; however, in mild or chronic infections, the parasite load may not be high enough to allow for fecal detection. To increase the sensitivity of stool examination, the test should be performed on multiple samples over the course of several days. A more sensitive test that allows detection of larvae is the duodenal aspirate, which is obtained using endoscopy. In disseminated infection, the larvae are more numerous and may be found in the feces, sputum, bronchoalveolar lavage, ascitic fluid, cerebrospinal fluid, or pleural fluid.

Culture can be performed on fecal specimens using damp charcoal or filter paper techniques; however, the preferred method is with nutrient agar plates into which the larvae burrow. Once they are cultured, the larvae need to be distinguished microscopically from hookworms and other possible infections. Many immunodiagnostic assays are sensitive for detecting the larvae, but they lack specificity. The antibody tests to *Strongyloides* cross-react with other filariae and helminth infections, thus limiting their usefulness. Currently, an enzyme-linked immunosorbent assay (ELISA) to detect genus-specific immunoglobulin E (IgE) in human strongyloidiasis is being developed that provides the specificity needed for an accurate diagnosis (Costa-Cruz et al., 2003; Genta, 1999; Gilles, 2003; Gilman, 2000; Siddiqui & Berk, 2001).

Differential Diagnosis

Symptoms of chronic gastrointestinal infection may mimic inflammatory bowel disease. Larva currens resembles the persistent linear tracks created by cutaneous larva migrans; however, larva currens moves rapidly and disappears within hours. Pulmonary manifestations of disseminated disease may be similar to tropical pulmonary eosinophilia, caused by *Wuchereria bancrofti* or *Brugia malayi*, or other migrating parasitic infections such as *Ascaris*, hookworm, or schistosomiasis (Genta, 1999; Gilles, 2003).

Treatment

Strongyloidiasis should be treated even in asymptomatic patients since there is potential for chronic symptomatic infection and severe disease. Ivermectin has been shown to be very effective, has few side effects, and may be given in a single dose of 200 µg/kg PO. Thiabendazole can also be used (25 mg/kg PO bid) for 2 to 3 days, then repeated in 2 weeks to ensure eradication. The side effects, which include nausea, vomiting, foul-smelling urine, unpleasant taste, and dizziness, may not be tolerated. Other possible treatments include albendazole and mebendazole (Gann, Neva, & Gam, 1994; Genta, 1999; Gilman, 2000).

Prevention

Prevention of infection with *S. stercoralis* (Gilles, 2003; Gilman, 2000) includes the following:
- Dispose of human feces in a sanitary manner. Ventilated improved pit latrines and double vault latrines are adequate and inexpensive.
- Wear shoes in endemic areas.
- Treat infected pets and domestic animals that come in contact with humans.
- Use caution when starting patients on immunosuppressive agents if they have chronic gastrointestinal symptoms and are from an endemic area. Patients with strongyloidiasis should be treated for the helminthic infection before immunosuppressive therapy to avoid development of a severe disseminated infection.

Community education on the preceding points is important.

Reporting

The U.S. Centers for Disease Control and Prevention does not consider strongyloidiasis to be a nationally notifiable disease. The World Health Organization (WHO) considers strongyloidiasis to be a Class 5 disease. See Appendix C for details and for upcoming changes in WHO reporting.

References

Costa-Cruz, J.M., Madalena, J., Silva, D.A., Sopelete, M.C., Campos, D.M., & Taketomi, E.A. (2003). Heterologous antigen extract in ELISA for the detection of human IgE anti-*Strongyloides stercoralis*. *Revista do Instituto de Medicina Tropical de Sao Paulo, 45,* 265-268.

Gann, P.H., Neva, F.A., & Gam, A.A. (1994). A randomized trial of single- and two-dose ivermectin versus thiabendazole for treatment of strongyloidiasis. *Journal of infectious disease, 169,* 1076-1079.

Genta, R.M. (1999). Strongyloides. In R.L. Guerrant, D.H. Walker, & P.F. Weller (Eds.), *Tropical infectious diseases: Principles, pathogens, and practice* (pp. 975-984). New York: Churchill Livingstone.

Gilles, H.M. (2003). Soil-transmitted helminths (geohelminths). In G.C. Cook & A.I. Zumla (Eds.), *Manson's tropical diseases* (21st ed., pp. 1545-1549). Philadelphia: W.B. Saunders Company.

Gilman, R.H. (2000). Intestinal nematodes that migrate through the skin and lung. In G. Strickland (Ed.), *Hunter's tropical medicine and emerging infectious diseases* (8th ed., pp. 736-740). Philadelphia: W.B. Saunders Company.

Siddiqui, A.A., & Berk, S.L. (2001). Diagnosis of *Strongyloides stercoralis* infection. *Clinical Infectious Disease, 33,* 1040-1047.

Terashima, A., Alvarez, H., Tello, R., Infante, R., Freedman, D.O., & Gotuzzo, E. (2002). Treatment failure in intestinal strongyloidiasis: An indicator of HTLV-I infection. *International Journal Infectious Disease, 6,* 28-30.

76

Syphilis
Lues, venereal syphilis
Geographic Distribution

— Venereal syphilis is present worldwide, but recently the largest increases have been in urban areas of developing countries in Africa and Asia. The worldwide incidence in industrialized countries has been steadily declining, except for a temporary increase in the infection rate in the southern United States in the early 1990s. Pandemics of HIV have also allowed for increased rates of infection in some areas, because transmission of these two diseases is synergistic (Perine & Bell, 2000; Stary, 2003).

Agent and Vector

— Venereal syphilis is caused by the spirochete *Treponema pallidum* spp. *pallidum* and is transmitted when the organism penetrates the skin or mucous membranes. This occurs when there is exposure to moist mucosal or cutaneous lesions during sexual contact. The treponemes are quickly disseminated throughout the body by way of blood vessels and lymphatics.

— Syphilis is the most common cause of genital ulcer disease in developing countries and most commonly occurs in sexually active people between the ages of 18 and 40. Risk factors include high-risk sexual behavior, multiple sexual partners, and other concurrent sexually transmitted diseases, including HIV. Syphilis can also be transmitted in utero, leading to congenital syphilis (Hook, 1999; Mabey & Richens, 2003; Stary, 2003).

Incubation

— Chancres develop 2 to 6 weeks after exposure (Stary, 2003).

Clinical Findings and Treatment

Signs and Symptoms

The chancre, which is the characteristic lesion of primary syphilis, begins as a small erythematous papule that erodes into a painless, shallow, indurated, clean ulceration (Figure 76-1). It is most commonly located on the penis in men and cervix or vulva in women; however, the chancre can occur anywhere on the body. Regional lymph nodes are often enlarged. Due to the painless nature of the chancre, this stage may not be noticed by the patient, especially when located on the cervix or in the rectum. The chancre heals spontaneously over several weeks, and patients often do not believe they require further treatment. When these individuals are not treated

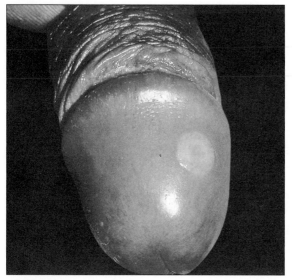

FIGURE 76-1

Primary syphilis. (*Source:* From Bolognia, J.L., Jorizzo, J.L., & Rapini, R.P. [Eds.]. [2003]. *Dermatology* [p. 1275]. Philadelphia: Mosby.)

at the primary stage, progression to secondary syphilis occurs 3 weeks to several months after the appearance of the chancre.

— With the dissemination of untreated primary syphilis, patients often develop a prodrome of fever, malaise, and headache, sometimes accompanied by weight loss, sore throat, iridocyclitis, periostitis, arthritis, meningitis, and mild hepatitis. The most common manifestation of secondary syphilis is a generalized, nonpruritic, papulosquamous rash; however, the eruption may also be macular, papular, follicular, annular, or pustular. Other possible clinical features of secondary syphilis include granulomatous nodules, papules with a collarette of scale on the palms and soles (Figure 76-2), soft moist papules in the genital area (condylomata lata) or oral mucosa (mucous patches), split papules in the commissures of the mouth, small shallow ulcers on the oral mucosa, and patchy "moth-eaten" nonscarring alopecia. Lesions of secondary syphilis typically resolve

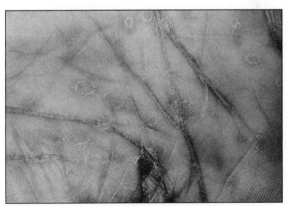

FIGURE 76–2

Secondary syphilis. (*Source:* From Bolognia, J.L., Jorizzo, J.L., & Rapini, R.P. [Eds.]. [2003]. *Dermatology* [p. 1277]. Philadelphia: Mosby.)

within several weeks; however, when untreated, patients may either relapse or enter a latent stage.

— Latent syphilis is an asymptomatic stage that can last many years. Early latent disease is the period within 1 year of initial infection, and secondary syphilis relapses often occur within this time frame. Late latent disease occurs after 1 year, and relapses are rare. Approximately one-third of patients with latent disease go on to develop lesions of tertiary syphilis.

— The most common manifestations of tertiary syphilis are gummas, which are destructive nodules or ulcerations that can develop in the skin, bones, and rarely the visceral organs. Neurosyphilis is often asymptomatic, but many patients manifest with chronic meningitis. More severe manifestations of neurosyphilis include endarteritis leading to focal neurologic deficits; generalized cerebral disease causing paresis, dementia, and seizures; tabes dorsalis leading to painless arthropathies (Charcot joints) and ulcers; and optic nerve atrophy. Cardiovascular syphilis affects the thoracic aorta and can result in aortic aneurysms, aortic valve disease, and narrowing of the coronary ostia.

— The risk for congenital syphilis is the greatest when the mother has primary or secondary syphilis and decreases with the duration of latent syphilis. Transplacental infection can occur as early as the ninth week and is fatal in almost half of the untreated cases. Early congenital syphilis, which is defined as symptoms within the first 3 months of life, can present with bullous or papulosquamous skin lesions (Figure 76-3), mucopurulent nasal discharge ("snuffles"), periorificial fissures, lymphadenitis, osteochondritis, anemia, hepatosplenomegaly, syphilitic pneumonitis, or congenital neurosyphilis. Late congenital syphilis presents later in childhood and manifestations include interstitial keratitis, neural deafness, and dental abnormalities (Mabey & Richens, 2003; Perine & Bell, 2000; Stary, 2003).

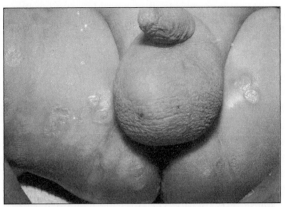

FIGURE 76–3

Congenital syphilis. (*Source:* Courtesy of the University of Texas Southwestern Department of Dermatology.)

Complications

Gumma formation of the bones may lead to periostitis, causing pain and limited range of motion. Gummas may also be very destructive by ulcerating through the hard palate, nasal septum, vertebral bodies, or other bones. In the heart, gummas can destroy myocardium, causing conduction abnormalities. Neurosyphilis is a complication of untreated syphilis, leading to great morbidity and mortality as noted earlier, and is more common in patients with concurrent HIV infection. Possible complications of cardiovascular syphilis include aortic valve insufficiency, myocardial infarction, aneurysm rupture, and death (Mabey & Richens, 2003; Perine & Bell, 2000; Stary, 2003).

Common Laboratory Findings

Nontreponemal tests, such as rapid plasma reagin (RPR) and Venereal Disease Research Laboratory (VDRL) tests, are positive in approximately 80% to 90% of primary syphilis cases, in all cases of secondary syphilis, and variably in latent and tertiary syphilis. Titers of these antibodies are useful in monitoring disease activity, and a fourfold decrease in the titer indicates successful treatment. Some limitations of these tests include false-positive results with endemic treponematoses or borreliosis, false-negative results, temporary negative results in HIV infection, and biologic false positives due to tissue damage in pregnancy, connective tissue diseases, malignancy, and infection.

Treponemal tests are more specific, remain positive indefinitely, and are used to confirm the diagnosis of syphilis. These tests include the microhemagglutination-*T. pallidum* test (MHA-TP) and fluorescent treponemal antibody assays (FTA-ABS). The specificity of these tests ranges from 70% to 100% in primary syphilis, 100% in secondary and latent syphilis, and slightly less than 100% in tertiary syphilis. The enzyme-linked immunosorbent assay (ELISA) technique for detection of *T. pallidum* antibodies allows for an accurate, reliable diagnosis of syphilis in all stages.

Other possible laboratory findings in primary, secondary, tertiary, and congenital syphilis include leukocytosis, elevated sedimentation rate, hypergammaglobulinemia, elevated rheumatoid factor, and cryoglobulinemia. Cerebrospinal fluid abnormalities can occur during any stage and may include mononuclear cell pleocytosis, reactive RPR, and increased protein (Castro, Prieto, Santo, Azevedo, & Exposto Fda, 2003; Mabey & Richens, 2003; Perine & Bell, 2000; Stary, 2003).

Diagnosis

The most specific method for diagnosing primary, secondary, and early congenital syphilis is the examination of fluid from a skin lesion or lymph node aspirate with dark-field microscopy. Using this method,

T. pallidum appears as a long, thin, coiled, light-colored thread on a dark background, which has characteristic episodic movements. Serologic tests, such as RPR, VDRL, MHA-TP, and FTA-ABS, can detect syphilis-associated antibodies with varying sensitivity and specificity, depending on the stage of disease, as described earlier. Biopsy of characteristic skin lesions in primary or secondary syphilis may reveal spirochetes when examined histologically with the Warthin-Starry stain. *T. pallidum* nucleic acid sequences can also be detected using polymerase chain reaction (PCR), but this is not routinely available (Perine & Bell, 2000; Stary, 2003).

Differential Diagnosis

The chancre of primary syphilis can resemble genital herpes, genital trauma, chancroid, and lymphogranuloma venereum. The differential diagnosis of secondary syphilis includes pityriasis rosea, guttate psoriasis, eczema, drug eruptions, folliculitis, and viral exanthems. Condyloma lata may be confused with genital warts or squamous cell carcinoma. The bullous lesions of congenital syphilis may resemble neonatal herpes infection, and hepatosplenomegaly in a newborn can be associated with several intrauterine infections, such as cytomegalovirus, toxoplasmosis, and rubella. The differential diagnosis of tertiary syphilis is very broad, depending on the presenting symptoms (Mabey & Richens, 2003; Stary, 2003).

Treatment

Adults with primary, secondary, or early latent syphilis should be treated with 2.4 million units of benzathine penicillin IM in a single dose. Children should be evaluated for potential abuse and treated with benzathine penicillin 50,000 units/kg up to 2.4 million units. Individuals allergic to penicillin can receive tetracycline

500 mg PO qid, erythromycin 500 mg PO qid, or
doxycycline 100 mg PO bid for 14 days. Late latent
and tertiary syphilis without central nervous system
(CNS) involvement is treated with 2.4 million units
of benzathine penicillin IM weekly for three doses.
Alternatively, patients may be treated with doxycycline
200 mg PO daily for 28 days. In cases of neurosyphilis,
aggressive treatment is needed with intravenous aqueous
penicillin G 2 to 4 million units q4h for 10 to 14 days.
Alternatively, patients may be given intramuscular
procaine penicillin 2.4 million units daily plus
probenecid 500 mg PO qid for 10 to 14 days.

During pregnancy, women should be treated with
2.4 million units of benzathine penicillin IM weekly
for three doses. If they are allergic to penicillin, they
should either undergo desensitization and be treated
with penicillin or use azithromycin 500 mg PO daily for
10 days as an alternative regimen. Patients with HIV
infection should also be treated with 2.4 million units
of benzathine penicillin IM weekly for three doses.
Patients should be warned of possible Jarisch-Herxheimer
reactions, which consist of fever, chills, and aggravation
of syphilitic lesions 6 to 12 hours after initial penicillin
treatment.

Congenital syphilis should be treated with either IM
benzathine penicillin 50,000 units/kg in a single dose
or IM procaine penicillin 50,000 units/kg daily for
10 to 14 days when there is no CNS involvement. If
there is CNS involvement, treatment in the newborn
period should consist of either intramuscular procaine
penicillin (dosed as above) or intravenous aqueous
penicillin G 50,000 units/kg q12h for 7 days, and then
50,000 units/kg q8h for another 3 to 7 days. When
possible, children allergic to penicillin should undergo
desensitization and then be treated with penicillin
(Perine & Bell, 2000; Stary, 2003).

Prevention

— Follow-up should consist of RPR or VDRL tests
at 1, 3, and 6 months after treatment of early syphilis
and then every 6 months for several years. Late syphilis
should be followed every couple of years. Following these
titers allows for evaluation of the response to treatment
and helps to prevent further spread of the disease.

— Sexual partners (within the past 3 months for primary
disease and 12 months for secondary disease) should be
tested for syphilis. The affected individual should also
be evaluated for other sexually transmitted diseases.
Screening pregnant women with serologic tests and
treatment of those affected may prevent many cases
of congenital syphilis. Health department notification
of new syphilis cases is required in many countries
(Perine & Bell, 2000).

Reporting

— The U.S. Centers for Disease Control and Prevention
considers syphilis to be a nationally notifiable disease.
The World Health Organization (WHO) considers
syphilis to be a Class 2A disease. See Appendix C for
details and for upcoming changes in WHO reporting.

References

Castro, R., Prieto, E.S., Santo, I., Azevedo, J., & Exposto Fda, L. (2003).
Evaluation of an enzyme immunoassay technique for detection of antibodies
against *Treponema pallidum*. *Journal of Clinical Microbiology, 41,* 250-253.

Hook, E.W. (1999). Treponemal infections. In R.L. Guerrant, D.H. Walker,
& P.F. Weller (Eds.), *Tropical infectious diseases: Principles, pathogens, and
practice* (pp. 527-534). New York: Churchill Livingstone.

Mabey, D., & Richens, J. (2003). Sexually transmitted infections (excluding
HIV). In G.C. Cook & A.I. Zumla (Eds.), *Manson's tropical diseases* (21st ed.,
pp. 445-448). Philadelphia: W.B. Saunders Company.

Perine, P.L., & Bell, T.A. (2000). Syphilis and the endemic treponematoses. In G. Strickland (Ed.), *Hunter's tropical medicine and emerging infectious diseases* (8th ed., pp. 354-363). Philadelphia: W.B. Saunders Company.

Stary, A. (2003). Sexually transmitted diseases. In J.L. Bolognia, J.L. Jorizzo, & R.P. Rapini, (Eds.), *Dermatology* (pp. 1271-1282). Philadelphia: Mosby.

Tapeworm

Geographic Distribution

- *Taenia solium*, the pork tapeworm, was once prevalent worldwide but is now found primarily in less developed areas of Central and South America, Asia, and non-Islamic areas of Africa. It is the most common etiology of acquired seizure disorder in the developing world, causing neurologic disease in more than 400,000 people in Latin America alone (Baily, 2003; Garcia et al., 2004).

- Other cestodes that are briefly discussed in this chapter include *Diphyllobothrium latum*, the fish tapeworm (Russia and Americas), *Taenia saginata*, the beef tapeworm (developing countries with poor sanitation and unregulated meat production), *Dipylidium caninum* (Europe, Latin America, east Asia, South Africa, North America), *Spirometra* (most common in east Asia), and *Taenia multiceps* (Africa and South America).

- Information on *Echinococcus* species and *Hymenolepis* species may be found in their specific chapters.

Agent and Vector

- Adult tapeworms of most species have a scolex or head with which the parasite attaches to the host. Some cestodes have sucking grooves or cups on their scolex, while others have sucking cups and hooklets. The distal portion of the scolex is called the neck, and it is from this area that the segments of the worm, called proglottids, are formed. As new segments are formed, the maturing proglottids are displaced distally. Mature or gravid proglottids are filled with eggs, thousands of which are released daily. Treatment of tapeworm infection is directed to the scolex because it is the means of reproduction and growth.

— *T. solium* is a small (2 to 7 mm in length) cestode that causes disease in pigs (intermediate hosts) and humans (definitive hosts). The two forms of *T. solium* infection are taeniasis and cysticercosis. Humans acquire taeniasis by ingesting undercooked (or "measly") pork containing larvae (cysticerci). In the intestinal lumen, larvae are activated by the digestive process, attach to the jejunal wall, and mature over 5 to 12 weeks. An adult *T. solium* worm lives for about 5 years, during which time countless eggs are released. Persons with taeniasis are at high risk of cysticercosis infection, most likely by autoinfection.

— Cysticercosis occurs *not* from eating infected pork but from ingesting food contaminated with human feces containing eggs or proglottids. Unlike taeniasis, where the larva attaches to the intestine, in cysticercosis the activated eggs develop into oncospheres that invade the intestinal wall and migrate to distal sites, especially subcutaneous tissue, muscle, eyes, and the central nervous system. There the oncospheres mature in about 2 months into cysticerci that can grow to more than 2 cm. The larger cysticerci tend to be in the central nervous system (CNS) where they can be asymptomatic for variable amounts of time, sometimes more than several years. Neurologic manifestations appear when the cysticerci begin to degenerate and a host inflammatory response occurs. Less frequently, neurologic symptoms result from mass effect or from blockage of cerebrospinal fluid (CSF) flow (Baily, 2003; Garcia, Gonzalez, Gilman, for The Cysticercosis Working Group in Peru, 2003a; Garcia, Gonzalez, Evans, Gilman, for The Cysticercosis Working Group in Peru, 2003b; Schantz, Tanowitz, & Wittner, 2000).

— Many other cestodes infect humans. *Echinococcus* and *Hymenolepis* are discussed in their own chapters. Some tapeworm species are of little clinical significance to humans, whereas others can cause devastating illness.

— *Diphyllobothrium latum* is acquired through ingesting infected fish. Infection is usually asymptomatic or characterized by vague complaints such as malaise and headache. Treatment is with praziquantel or niclosamide. Other *Diphyllobothrium* spp. cause human infection of small clinical significance.

— *Dipylidium caninum* is a common tapeworm of dogs that occasionally infects humans, especially children, through ingestion of infected fleas. It is usually asymptomatic and treatment is with praziquantel or niclosamide.

— *Spirometra* species are tapeworms of variable sizes (1 to 50 cm) that infect dogs and other carnivores, including snakes and amphibians. In humans, *Spirometra* species cause sparganosis. Human infection occurs through the ingestion of water contaminated with fleas containing the larval stage. Manifestations of sparganosis include inflamed subcutaneous swelling, often of the chest and legs and sometimes periorbital. Rarely the parasite enters the brain, with devastating consequences. Surgical excision is the only effective treatment.

— *Taenia multiceps* is a tapeworm of dogs (definitive host) and sheep (intermediate host) that causes coenurosis, a rare neurologic condition. Transmission is fecal-oral. Manifestations of coenurosis are the result of a space-occupying cyst/lesion and inflammation of the CNS and/or eye, and may include hydrocephalus, increased intracranial pressure, seizures, and blindness. Treatment may include surgery and/or praziquantel along with antiinflammatory drugs.

— *Taenia saginata* is the beef tapeworm. Its intermediate hosts are cattle, and humans are the only definitive host. Raw or undercooked beef is the usual means of transmission. Infection is generally asymptomatic, except for vague irritable bowel symptoms and distress related to feeling the very motile proglottids emerging from the anus. Treatment is with praziquantel or niclosamide (Baily, 2003; Centers for Disease Control and Prevention [CDC],

2002; Chin, 2000; Garcia et al., 2003a, 2004; *Medical Letter,* 2002; Peters & Pasvol, 2002).

Incubation

— The incubation period (from ingestion to eggs appearing in stool) for taeniasis is about 10 to 14 weeks. Cysticercosis develops in about 2 months, though symptoms may take years to develop (Baily, 2003; Chin, 2000).

Clinical Findings and Treatment

Signs and Symptoms

— Taeniasis is usually asymptomatic or causes mild gastrointestinal symptoms such as nausea and vague abdominal pain. Unlike infection with *T. saginata*, patients infected with *T. solium* seldom notice proglottids in stool because *T. solium* proglottids are smaller and less motile.

— Neurocysticercosis manifestations depend on the site, number, and size of lesions, as well as the degree of the host immune response. Seizures are the most common symptom and are followed in frequency by symptoms of intracranial hypertension and obstructive hydrocephalus, such as headache and vomiting. A large cyst may act as a space-occupying lesion with variable effects according to site and size. Intraventricular and basilar cysts cause symptoms that are earlier in onset and more quickly progressing than parenchymal lesions. Basal subarachnoid neurocysticercosis in particular is progressive with a poor prognosis.

— Ophthalmic involvement occurs in only 1% to 3% of cysticercosis patients. Vision disturbances may occur from ocular involvement, but may also be related to cranial nerve impairment or other effects of neurocysticercosis.

— Subcutaneous cysticercosis causes small, movable, painless nodules, often located in the arms and chest.

Over months or years the nodules become inflamed and tender and then gradually disappear. Muscular cysticercosis produces small calcifications in the arms and thighs. These are of no significance except very rarely when massive loads result in muscular pseudohypertrophy. Often they are discovered as an incidental finding on plain films of the extremities. (Baily, 2003; Garcia et al., 2003a, 2003b; Schantz et al., 2000).

Complications

‾ Larger parasite loads and/or stronger host immune responses lead to more severe manifestations of neurocysticercosis. Psychiatric symptoms and motor deficits can occur. Other less common complications include stroke, spinal cord compression, and encephalitis, the latter being more common in children and teenagers.

Common Laboratory Findings

‾ CSF fluid may show lymphocytes or eosinophils, low glucose, and elevated protein (Garcia et al., 2003a).

Diagnosis

‾ The presence of *T. solium* proglottids or eggs in feces is diagnostic of taeniasis only. Because persons with taeniasis are at risk for developing cysticercosis through autoinfection, they should receive serologic testing as discussed later.

‾ Suspicion of cysticercosis is increased by a history of travel or residence in an endemic area. In developed countries, transmission may also occur from an immigrant household member infected by *T. solium.*

‾ The definitive diagnosis of cysticercosis is by the detection of cysticerci in tissue. But because of the risks of brain biopsy, neurocysticercosis is best diagnosed through neuroimaging and serology (Figure 77-1). Computed tomography (CT) is less expensive but less

sensitive than magnetic resonance imaging (MRI).
CT is better able to identify small calcifications, while
MRI is best at identifying the number, location, and
evolutionary stage of parasites, as well as the presence of
inflammation. Typically the lesions appear as multiple
unilocular cysts that may be enhancing.

The CDC's immunoblot assay with purified *T. solium*
antigens detects antibodies to one or more of seven
antigens and is the immunodiagnostic test of choice for
confirming the diagnosis of neurocysticercosis. However,
a negative test does not exclude the diagnosis for patients
with risk factors and characteristic neuroimaging findings
(CDC, 2002; Garcia et al., 2003a, 2004).

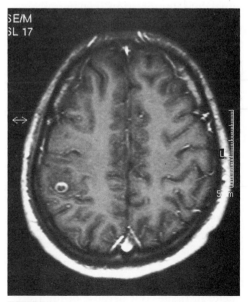

FIGURE 77–1

Cerebral cysticercosis shown by computed tomography. (*Source:* From
Peters, W., & Pasvol, G. [2002]. *Tropical medicine and parasitology*
[5th ed., p. 209]. Chicago: Mosby.)

Differential Diagnosis

— The differential diagnosis of neurocysticercosis includes
CNS neoplasm, tuberculosis, abscess, toxoplasmosis,
cytomegalovirus, echinococcosis, coenuriasis,
neuroschistosomiasis, paragonimiasis, angiostrongyliasis,
gnathostomiasis, and epilepsy (Evans, Garcia, & Gilman,
2000; Garcia et al., 2003a).

Treatment

— Taeniasis (and other intestinal tapeworm infections) may
be treated with praziquantel 5 to 10 mg/kg PO once.
Niclosamide is also used in a dose of 2 g PO once for
adults and 50 mg/kg PO once for children. Garcia et al.
(2003b) recommend laxatives and a modified diet to
improve recovery of the scolex, which confirms the
diagnosis and cure.

— Supportive treatment of neurocysticercosis includes
anticonvulsants for seizures, analgesics, and management
of intracranial hypertension including ventriculoperitoneal
shunting for obstructive hydrocephalus. Treatment of
intracranial hypertension should be urgent, taking
priority over antiparasitic therapy.

— Antiparasitic therapy for neurocysticercosis has long
been controversial, hampered by a dearth of good quality
evidence. However, in a recent double-blind
placebo-controlled trial in Peru, adults with parenchymal
neurocysticercosis (20 or fewer cysts) treated with 10 days
of albendazole 800 mg PO daily and dexamethasone
6 mg PO daily had a reduction in parasite load and a
67% reduction in generalized seizures compared to
placebo, with no difference in adverse effects except for
abdominal pain in the treatment group. Consequently,
antiparasitic therapy has been recommended as part of
the routine treatment of parenchymal neurocysticercosis.
Adults and children may be treated with albendazole
15 mg/kg PO daily for 8 to 10 days with simultaneous

steroids. An alternative is praziquantel 50 mg/kg PO daily for 15 days, also with steroids.

For other forms of neurocysticercosis, therapeutic decisions should be specific to the individual patient and based on the number, location, and viability of CNS parasites. In rare cases of massive brain infections, for example, the risks of severe side effects may outweigh potential benefits of antiparasitic therapy. Previous consensus guidelines (Garcia et al., 2002, 2003a, 2003b, 2004; Juan, Lopez Chegne, Gargala, & Favennec, 2002; *Medical Letter,* 2002) have recommended the following:

- Calcified cysticercosis should not be treated with antiparasitic drugs.
- Ventricular cysticercosis should be treated by neuroendoscopic removal where available.
- Subarachnoid cysts and chronic meningitis should be treated with antiparasitic drugs and steroids, and ventricular shunting if hydrocephalus is present.
- Cysticercotic encephalitis should be treated with high-dose steroids, osmotic diuretics, but not antiparasitic drugs.
- Hydrocephalus without visible cysts on neuroimaging should be treated with ventricular shunt, but not antiparasitic drugs.
- Spinal cysticercosis should usually be treated surgically.
- Ophthalmic cysticercosis should be treated surgically.

Prevention

Prevention of infection with *T. solium* (Chin, 2000; Garcia et al., 2003b) includes the following:

- Practice improved sanitation and disposal of feces.
- Encourage hand washing after defecation and before eating.
- Avoid the use of fresh feces or effluent as fertilizer.
- Thoroughly cook pork (and beef in the case of *T. saginata*).

- Prompt treatment and enteric precautions are indicated for people harboring adult *T. solium.*
- Encourage penned pig-raising (versus free foraging, which is common throughout the developing world). Swine should be kept away from latrines or other sources of human feces (which they will eat).
- Freeze meat at –5° C (23° F) for 4 days to kill cysticerci.
- Slaughterhouse meat inspection has worked well in the developed world.

In all cases, community education and cooperation are essential.

Reporting

The CDC does not consider tapeworm infection to be a nationally notifiable disease. The World Health Organization (WHO) considers tapeworm infection a Class 3C disease. See Appendix C for details and for upcoming changes in WHO reporting.

References

Baily, G.G. (2003). Other cestode infections: Intestinal cestodes, cysticercosis, other larval cestode infections. In G.C. Cook & A.I. Zumla (Eds.), *Manson's tropical diseases* (21st ed., pp. 1583-1597). Philadelphia: W.B. Saunders Company.

Centers for Disease Control and Prevention. (2002). *Cysticercosis.* Retrieved December 31, 2003, from *www.dpd.cdc.gov/dpdx/HTML/Cysticercosis.htm*

Chin, J. (Ed.). (2000). *Control of communicable diseases manual* (17th ed.). Washington, DC: American Public Health Association.

Evans, C.A.W., Garcia, H.H., & Gilman, R.H. (2000). Cysticercosis. In G.T. Strickland (Ed.), *Hunter's tropical medicine and emerging infectious diseases* (8th ed., pp. 862-866). Philadelphia: W.B. Saunders Company.

Garcia, H.H., Evans, C.A., Nash, T.E., Takayanagui, O.M., White, A.C., Botero, D., Rajshekhar, V., Tsang, V.C., Schantz, P.M., Allan, J.C., Flisser, A., Correa, D., Sarti, E., Friedland, J.S., Martinez, S.M., Gonzalez, A.E., Gilman, R.H., & Del Brutto, O.H. (2002). Current consensus guidelines for treatment of neurocysticercosis. *Clinical Microbiology Reviews, 15,* 747-756.

Garcia, H.H., Gonzalez, A.E., & Gilman, R.H., for The Cysticercosis Working Group in Peru. (2003a). Diagnosis, treatment and control of *Taenia solium* cysticercosis. *Current Opinion in Infectious Diseases, 16,* 411-419.

Garcia, H.H., Gonzalez, A.E., Evans, C.A.W., & Gilman, R.H. for The Cysticercosis Working Group in Peru. (2003b). *Taenia solium* cysticercosis. *The Lancet, 361,* 547-556.

Garcia, H.H., Pretell, E.J., Gilman, R.H., Martinez, S.M., Moulton, L.H., Del Brutto, O.H., Herrera, G., Evans, C.A., & Gonzalez, A.E. (2004). A trial of antiparasitic treatment to reduce the rate of seizures due to cerebral cysticercosis. *New England Journal of Medicine, 350,* 249-58.

Juan, J.O., Lopez Chegne, N., Gargala, G., & Favennec, L. (2002). Comparative clinical studies of nitazoxanide, albendazole and praziquantel in the treatment of ascariasis, trichuriasis and hymenolepiasis in children from Peru. *Transactions of the Royal Society of Tropical Medicine and Hygiene, 96,* 193-196.

Medical Letter. (2002). Drugs for parasitic infections. Retrieved October 30, 2003, from *www.medletter.com/freedocs/parasitic.pdf*

Peters, W., & Pasvol, G. (2002). *Tropical medicine and parasitology* (5th ed.). Chicago: Mosby.

Schantz, P.M., Tanowitz, H.B., & Wittner, M. (2000). General principles (of cestode infections). In G.T. Strickland (Ed.), *Hunter's tropical medicine and emerging infectious diseases* (8th ed., pp. 851-853). Philadelphia: W.B. Saunders Company.

78

TETANUS

Lockjaw

Geographic Distribution

Tetanus occurs worldwide, primarily in underdeveloped areas that lack universal immunization. Neonatal tetanus, the most common form, kills 270,000 to 500,000 infants yearly, most in tropical Africa and Asia (Arnon, 2004; Centers for Disease Control and Prevention [CDC], 2002).

Agent and Vector

Tetanus is caused by the bacillus *Clostridium tetani*, a slender, gram-positive anaerobic spore-forming rod found in soil and the alimentary tracts of numerous animals. Though the bacillus itself is sensitive to the environment, its hardy spores are able to resist boiling and many antiseptics. Infection occurs when the spores enter the body, usually through a wound, germinate under anaerobic conditions, and produce tetanus toxin (tetanospasmin). The toxin blocks the release of inhibitory neurotransmitters, resulting in unopposed muscle contractions and spasms. Tetanus toxin also destabilizes the autonomic nervous system.

In neonatal tetanus, infection occurs when birth and umbilical cord care are unhygienic and the mother is not immunized against tetanus. Most non-neonatal tetanus is the result of trauma, especially penetrating wounds such as those from a nail, splinter, or drug injection. Bites, burns, surgery, compound fractures, and other traumatic injuries may also result in tetanus (Arnon, 2004; CDC, 2002).

Incubation

— The incubation period is 3 to 21 days or longer, and averages around 10 days. A shorter incubation period is associated with heavier contamination and a poorer prognosis (Chin, 2000).

Clinical Findings and Treatment

Signs and Symptoms

— Tetanus may be either generalized or localized. *Generalized tetanus* is the most common form, accounting for 80% of reported cases. The most frequent presentation is descending, beginning with headache, restlessness, and irritability. These early symptoms are followed by trismus (masseter muscle spasm or lockjaw), and then stiff neck, dysphagia, rigidity of abdominal muscles, and involvement of lumbar, hip, and thigh muscles. Generalized muscle spasms last up to several minutes at the beginning of the illness and last longer as the illness progresses. Spasms are frequent and painful, and often precipitated by even minimal external stimuli such as sounds, light, touch, or movement. Characteristic features of the tetanic spasm are opisthotonus (severely arched back, neck extended, arms and legs rigidly flexed) and a grimacing or sardonic facial expression called *risus sardonicus*. Autonomic instability may occur, usually in the second week, causing fever, diaphoresis, labile hypertension, episodic tachycardia or arrhythmias, dysuria, diarrhea, and uncontrolled defecation. In general, when death does not occur the condition worsens in the first week, stabilizes in the second week, and improves during the next 3 to 6 weeks. The patient is often conscious and oriented throughout.

— *Neonatal tetanus* (or tetanus neonatorum) is a form of generalized tetanus that presents as an inability to suck between the third and tenth days of life after a period of normal sucking. The inability to suck progresses to dysphagia, spasms, stiffness, seizures, and often death. The umbilical stump may or may not show signs of contamination or infection.

— *Local tetanus* is an uncommon manifestation and in some cases precedes generalized tetanus. With local tetanus the patient has persistent painful contractions in the area around the wound lasting for up to several months. About 1% of cases are fatal.

— *Cephalic tetanus* is a rare variation of local tetanus and occurs as a result of wounds or infections involving the head, for example, chronic otitis media. It affects the cranial nerves, causing symptoms such as facial pain and stiffness, unilateral facial palsy (rarely bilateral), retracted eyelids, and deviated gaze.

— For all types of tetanus, complete recovery usually takes months (Al Azraqùi, Bollinger, & Ward, 2000; Arnon, 2004; CDC, 2002; Thwaites, Nga, & Smith, 2003).

Complications

— Bronchopneumonia, probably from aspiration, is a common complication and cause of death in neonatal tetanus. Laryngeal and/or respiratory muscle spasms may result in airway obstruction and respiratory failure. Severe spasms or convulsions can cause spine or long-bone fractures. Dehydration is common. Nosocomial infections occur among patients with prolonged hospitalization. Pulmonary embolism is most common in drug users and elderly patients.

— For unvaccinated persons the case fatality rate is around 22%. Survivors may have long-term sequelae such as limb deformities and contractures. Infants may suffer hypoxic encephalopathy and subsequent developmental delays (CDC, 2002; Stoll, 2004).

Common Laboratory Findings

There are no characteristic laboratory findings; mild polymorphonuclear leukocytosis may occur as a result of secondary wound infection or stress (Stoll, 2004).

Diagnosis

Diagnosis is usually made on the basis of clinical presentation, immunization status, and in most cases a history of trauma or unhygienic birth. The organism may be isolated from the wound in only 30% of cases. *C. tetani* forms terminal spores, giving the rod a "tennis racket" or "drumstick" appearance microscopically. Laboratory identification is based primarily on detection of toxin production in infected mice (CDC, 2002).

Differential Diagnosis

The differential diagnosis includes trismus from dental or other regional abscess, meningitis, or rabies. Strychnine poisoning is the condition most similar to tetanus. Other considerations include epileptic seizures, opioid withdrawal, dystonic reactions to neuroleptic drugs, hypocalcemia, and trichinosis (Al Azraqùi et al., 2000).

Treatment

The priorities of treatment are to stop the progression of disease and prevent complications. Tetanus immune globulin (TIG) in a single IM dose of 3000 to 5000 units should be given to neutralize unbound tetanus toxin, although it does not affect toxin that has already bound to nerve receptors. Infiltration of TIG around the wound was once practiced but is no longer recommended. Wound debridement and antibiotic treatment should be done immediately after the administration of TIG to stop further *C. tetani* multiplication and toxin production. The antibiotic of choice for adults is metronidazole 7.5 mg/kg IV qid for

10 to 14 days. For children, penicillin G is given 100,000 units/kg/24 hours IV divided q4-6h. Erythromycin and tetracycline (for children 8 years or older) are alternatives.

— Maintaining the patient's airway is a priority of supportive care. Spasm-inducing stimuli should be minimized by keeping the patient's room dark and quiet. Benzodiazepine treatment, often in large doses, helps decrease spasms and anxiety. If benzodiazepine treatment is not effective, paralysis with neuromuscular blocking agents and mechanical ventilation should be instituted. Pain control may require morphine, which is also useful for treating autonomic instability. Cardiovascular instability may also be treated with short-acting alpha-blocking or beta-blocking agents. Magnesium sulfate is sometimes used for both muscle spasms and autonomic instability.

— Neither infection with *C. tetani* nor treatment with TIG confers immunity, so all patients should be vaccinated (Arnon, 2004; CDC, 2002; Thwaites et al., 2003).

Prevention

— Tetanus is prevented by immunization with tetanus toxoid vaccine. The immunization schedule in the United States is a combined diphtheria toxoid-tetanus toxoid-acellular pertussis vaccine (DTaP) at 2, 4, 6, and 15 to 18 months, followed by a DTaP booster at 4 to 6 years and tetanus and diphtheria toxoids (Td) every 10 years thereafter. If an immunized patient has an unclean or major wound, Td should be given if more than 5 years has passed since the last booster.

— In addition to vaccination, community education about wound care and umbilical cord care is an integral part of prevention. The World Health Organization (WHO) and United Nations Children's Fund (UNICEF) are engaged in a maternal and neonatal tetanus elimination program that includes administering tetanus toxoid (TT) vaccinations and supplemental doses to women of childbearing age, TT vaccinations for pregnant women, increased DTaP immunization of children, clean birthing techniques and resources, and community education (Stoll, 2004; Thwaites et al., 2003; WHO, 2001).

Reporting

The CDC considers tetanus to be a nationally notifiable disease. The WHO considers tetanus a Class 2B disease. See Appendix C for details and for upcoming changes in WHO reporting.

References

Al Azraqùi, T., Bollinger, R.C., & Ward, B.J. (2000). Tetanus. In G.T. Strickland (Ed.), *Hunter's tropical medicine and emerging infectious diseases* (8th ed., pp. 379-381). Philadelphia: W.B. Saunders Company.

Arnon, S.S. (2004). Tetanus (*Clostridium tetani*). In R.E. Behrman, R.M. Kliegman, & H.B. Jenson (Eds.), *Nelson textbook of pediatrics* (17th ed., pp. 951-953). Philadelphia: W.B. Saunders Company.

Centers for Disease Control and Prevention. (2002). Tetanus. Retrieved January 5, 2004, from *www.cdc.gov/nip/publications/pink/tetanus.pdf*

Chin, J. (Ed.). (2000). *Control of communicable diseases manual* (17th ed., pp. 491-497). Washington, DC: American Public Health Association.

Stoll, B.J. (2004). Infections of the neonatal infant. In R.E. Behrman, R.M. Kliegman, & H.B. Jenson (Eds.), *Nelson textbook of pediatrics* (17th ed., pp. 623-640). Philadelphia: W.B. Saunders Company.

Thwaites, C.L., Nga, N.T.N., & Smith, M.D. (2003). Tetanus. In G.C. Cook & A.I. Zumla (Eds.), *Manson's tropical diseases* (21st ed., pp. 1119-1124). Philadelphia: W.B. Saunders Company.

World Health Organization. (2001). Maternal and neonatal tetanus elimination African region. Retrieved January 5, 2004, from *www.afro.who.int/nnt/planofaction.pdf*

79

Tinea

Dermatophytosis, ringworm

Geographic Distribution

— Dermatophytes are common causes of superficial skin infections worldwide; however, the prevalence is very high in tropical climates. The main infections seen in tropical countries include tinea corporis, tinea cruris, and tinea capitis (Hay, 2003).

Agent and Vector

— Pathogenic dermatophytes in humans consist of three genera, including *Microsporum*, *Trichophyton*, and *Epidermophyton*. They are able to cause infections within keratinized tissues, including skin, hair, and nails, by invading the epidermis, hair shaft, or nail plate. The main sources of infection are other humans (anthropophilic), animals (zoophilic), or soil (geophilic). Zoophilic tinea infections, such as those from cats and dogs *(Microsporum canis)*, cattle *(Trichophyton verrucosum)*, and rodents *(Trichophyton mentagrophytes* var. *mentagrophytes),* tend to elicit more of an acute infection with a brisk inflammatory reaction, as compared to the anthropophilic tinea infections, such as *T. rubrum*, *T. tonsurans*, *E. floccosum*, *T. mentagrophytes* var. *interdigitale*, or *T. concentricum*.

— *T. rubrum* is the most common dermatophyte worldwide and often causes tinea corporis, tinea cruris, tinea manuum, tinea pedis, and onychomycosis. *T. tonsurans* is a common cause of tinea corporis and tinea pedis in children and is the most common cause of tinea capitis in the United States. *M. canis* is the most common cause of tinea capitis worldwide. *T. concentricum* is endemic to areas in the South Pacific and South America, causing an entity known as tinea imbricata. *T. mentagrophytes* var. *interdigitale* is often associated with interdigital tinea pedis, tinea cruris, and white superficial onychomycosis. *E. floccosum* generally causes tinea cruris, tinea manum, and tinea pedis. *T. mentagrophytes* var. *mentagrophytes* tends to cause inflammatory tinea pedis or barbae. *T. verrucosum* also can cause inflammatory tinea barbae, which often mimics bacterial furunculosis.

— Tinea infections occur more frequently in postpubertal individuals, except tinea capitis, which is more common in children. Immunosuppressed people, such as those with HIV infection, do not have a higher incidence of dermatophyte infection; however, if they acquire tinea, the infection may be more severe, recurrent, or atypical in presentation (Arenas, 2001; Hay, 2003; Sobera & Elewski, 2003).

Incubation

— The incubation for dermatophytes is days to weeks.

Clinical Findings and Treatment

Signs and Symptoms

— Tinea corporis typically presents as erythematous annular plaques with an active scaly border, most commonly on the trunk and limbs (Figure 79-1). Infection spreads centrifugally, leading to annular lesions of varying sizes. Less common presentations include verrucous plaques, granulomatous nodules, and erythematous plaques with pustules at the active border, minimal scale (especially if corticosteroids have been used), or vesicles. Variants include tinea profunda (which is caused by an excessive inflammatory response and may resemble a deep fungal infection), Majocchi's granuloma (caused by *T. rubrum* and characterized by perifollicular pustules or papules), and tinea imbricata (which is a chronic infection caused by *T. concentricum*

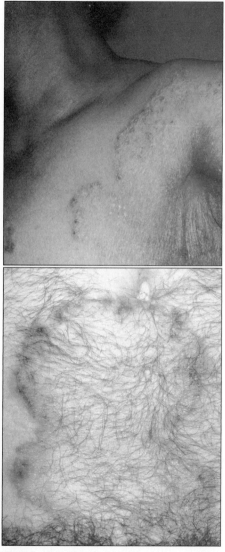

FIGURE 79–1

Tinea corporis. (*Source:* Courtesy of the University of Texas Southwestern Department of Dermatology.)

presenting as widespread concentric annular rings of scale).

— Tinea cruris presents as extremely pruritic erythematous plaques with a raised, scaly, active border in the groin area. This affects men more commonly than women, and other predisposing factors include obesity and excessive sweating. The most commonly involved area in men is between the scrotum and the inner thigh, with the scrotum itself generally being spared.

— Tinea capitis presents in different ways, depending on the causative organism. *T. tonsurans* causes an endothrix infection (the fungus is within the hair shaft) and presents as diffuse circumscribed, minimally scaly patches of alopecia with small black dots, representing short broken hair shafts. *M. canis* causes an inflammatory ectothrix tinea capitis infection (the fungus is outside the hair shaft), manifesting as scaly, pruritic, often crusted, areas of alopecia on the scalp. A highly inflammatory boggy plaque with pustules and abscesses, known as a kerion, may also form due to an exaggerated host immune response. Favus is a specific type of tinea capitis found only in specific areas of Africa, the Middle East, and South America, is caused by *T. schoenleinii*, and presents as large thick yellow matted crusts over the scalp. Patients with tinea capitis commonly present with posterior cervical or auricular lymphadenopathy (Hay, 2003; Sobera & Elewski, 2003).

Complications

— Permanent scarring alopecia may occur with kerion or favus formation. Patients who develop kerion infections may become systemically ill, developing fever, widespread lymphadenopathy, or bacterial superinfection (Brook, 2002; Sobera & Elewski, 2003).

Common Laboratory Findings

There are no laboratory findings commonly associated with tinea.

Diagnosis

The diagnosis of dermatophytosis is confirmed by visualization of fungal elements in skin scrapings, hair, or nail debris. Skin scrapings are collected with a scalpel from the scaling edge of the plaque. The ideal hair samples are plucked broken hairs from within the affected area on the scalp. Subungual debris can be scraped onto a slide using a pointed blade. Once the specimens are collected, they are mounted in 5% to 10% potassium hydroxide and then examined under the microscope for fungal elements. These same specimens may also be submitted for culture on Sabouraud agar in order to determine the causative species. Skin biopsies or nail clippings may also be sent for histologic examination with periodic acid-Schiff (PAS) staining in order to visualize the fungal elements. Tinea capitis caused by *T. tonsurans* and *M. canis* can be distinguished by fluorescing the affected area of the scalp with a Wood's lamp. Hairs infected with *M. canis* fluoresce yellow-green, whereas *T. tonsurans* does not fluoresce. This becomes important because the treatments are slightly different (Hay, 2003).

Differential Diagnosis

The differential diagnosis of tinea corporis includes eczema, psoriasis, subacute cutaneous lupus, leprosy, sarcoidosis, pityriasis rosea, granuloma annulare, figurate erythemas, and secondary syphilis. Tinea cruris may resemble intertrigo, candidiasis, seborrheic dermatitis, or inverse psoriasis. Tinea capitis may be confused with alopecia areata, trichotillomania, psoriasis, lichen planus, lupus erythematosus, or seborrheic dermatitis.

Inflammatory tinea capitis may be misdiagnosed
as a bacterial pyoderma infection (Weston, Lane, &
Morelli, 2002).

Treatment

Limited tinea corporis and tinea cruris can be treated
with topical antifungal creams, such as terbinafine,
miconazole, or clotrimazole, twice daily for 1 to 2 weeks.
Oral antifungals can be used for extensive or persistent
infections. Options include terbinafine 250 mg once
daily for 1 to 2 weeks, itraconazole 100 mg once daily
for 2 weeks or 200 mg daily for 1 week, or fluconazole
150 mg once weekly for 2 to 3 weeks.

Tinea capitis must be treated with oral antifungal
medications. Treatment options for *T. tonsurans*
infection include griseofulvin 20 mg/kg/day, up to
500 mg, for a minimum of 6 weeks or terbinafine
3 mg/kg/day, up to 250 mg, for 2 to 4 weeks. Treatment
options for *M. canis* infection include griseofulvin
20 mg/kg/day, up to 500 mg, for a minimum of 4 weeks
or itraconazole 5 mg/kg/day, up to 200 mg, for 2 weeks
(Budimulja et al., 2001; Lesher, 1999; Weston et al.,
2002).

Prevention

Prevention of tinea cruris may be possible by wearing
loose clothing, losing weight (in the case of obese
patients), keeping the area dry with the use of antifungal
powders, and cleaning contaminated clothing. Tinea
capitis can be prevented by eliminating or treating the
source. If *M. canis* is found, the source may be a family
pet, and the tinea on the animal needs to be treated.
If *T. tonsurans* is found, household contacts may be the
source, and the children need to avoid sharing brushes,
hats, or other items that may be transferring the fungus
(Sobera & Elewski, 2003; Weston et al., 2002).

Reporting

The U.S. Centers for Disease Control and Prevention (CDC) does not consider tinea to be a nationally notifiable disease. The World Health Organization (WHO) considers tinea a Class 4 disease. See Appendix C for details and for upcoming changes in WHO reporting.

References

Arenas, R. (2001). Dermatophytosis. In R. Arenas & R. Estrada, *Tropical dermatology* (pp. 2-11). Georgetown, TX: Landes Bioscience.

Brook, I. (2002). Secondary bacterial infections complicating skin lesions. *Journal of Medical Microbiology, 51,* 808-812.

Budimulja, U., Bramono, K., Urip, K.S., Basuki, S., Widodo, G., et al. (2001). Once daily treatment with terbinafine 1% cream (Lamisil) for one week is effective in the treatment of tinea corporis and cruris. A placebo-controlled study. *Mycoses, 44,* 300-306.

Hay, R.J. (2003). Fungal infections. In G.C. Cook & A.I. Zumla (Eds.), *Manson's tropical diseases* (21st ed., pp. 1173-1194). Philadelphia: W.B. Saunders Company.

Lesher, J.L. Jr. (1999). Oral therapy of common superficial fungal infections of the skin. *Journal of the American Academy of Dermatology, 40*(6 Pt 2), S31-S34.

Sobera, J.O., & Elewski, B.E. (2003). Fungal diseases. In J.L. Bolognia, J.L. Jorizzo, & R.P. Rapini (Eds.), *Dermatology* (pp. 1171-1198). Philadelphia: Mosby.

Weston, W.L., Lane, A.T., & Morelli, J.G. (2002). *Color textbook of pediatric dermatology* (3rd ed.). Philadelphia: Mosby.

Toxocariasis

Larva migrans visceralis, ocular larva migrans, Toxocara [canis] [cati] infection, visceral larva migrans

Geographic Distribution

— Toxocariasis occurs worldwide, with seroprevalences ranging from 0% to 4% in urban western Europe to more than 80% in some Caribbean populations. The illness is recognized primarily in children, but also occurs in adults (Chin, 2000).

Agent and Vector

— Toxocariasis is a zoonosis caused by nematodes (roundworms) commonly found in dogs *(Toxocara canis)* and cats *(T. cati)*. The most common sources of infection among humans are puppies and their lactating mothers, which harbor the parasite in their intestinal tract. There the female *T. canis* worms lay eggs, which are passed to the outside environment in feces. Humans, most commonly children, ingest the embryonated eggs when they are exposed to contaminated soil during play or other activities. Pica, the eating of nonfood items such as soil, increases the risk of exposure. Sandboxes and playgrounds are common environments of infection. Playing with puppies is not considered a risk for acquiring *T. canis* infection because the eggs take at least 2 weeks to embryonate and become infective. Occasionally, larvae may be ingested through eating raw liver from infected cattle, sheep, or chickens.

— In humans, the eggs hatch in the stomach, and the larvae (4 to 10 cm in length) penetrate stomach or intestinal mucosa. Some larvae enter the portal circulation and invade the liver where they are destroyed by the host's cell-mediated immunity. Other larvae enter the lungs, where some remain and others continue through the circulation. When migrating larvae encounter vessels that are too small to pass through, they enter adjacent tissue, commonly the brain, eyes, heart, kidneys, and striated muscle. Pathology is the result of the immediate or delayed hypersensitivity responses to dead or dying parasites, as well as granuloma formation in affected organs. Humans are accidental *Toxocara* hosts in whom the larvae are unable to continue their life cycle (Centers for Disease Control and Prevention [CDC], 2001, 2002; Chin, 2000; Gilles, 2003).

Incubation

- The incubation period is weeks to months, and in cases of eye involvement (ocular larva migrans) the illness may not manifest for as many as 10 years after the initial infection (Chin, 2000).

Clinical Findings and Treatment

Signs and Symptoms

- Most people infected with *Toxocara* are asymptomatic. There are two primary forms of symptomatic toxocariasis: visceral larva migrans and ocular larva migrans.
- Visceral larva migrans is most common among preschool children. Usual signs and symptoms include fever, anorexia, weight loss, wheezing, cough, abdominal pain, hepatomegaly, and splenomegaly. Less frequent are seizures, behavioral changes, chronic urticaria, nephrosis, and skin nodules.
- Ocular larva migrans is most common among older children. It can cause vision loss, which is often not recognized except for the development of strabismus or squinting. Leukocoria (white pupil) is sometimes seen. For patients with recent infection, ophthalmic exam may

reveal a mass, intraretinal tracks of larvae, vitreous haze, and/or cataract formation. Older infection may be manifested by a retinal scar (CDC, 2002; Gilles, 2003; McGavin, 2003; Schantz, 2000).

Complications

— With extensive liver, cardiac, pulmonary, or neurologic pathology, visceral larva migrans can cause death, but this is rare (CDC, 2002; Gilles, 2003).

Common Laboratory Findings

— Common laboratory findings include eosinophilia, leukocytosis, decreased albumin:globulin ratio and increased anti-*Toxocara* IgG, IgM, anti-A or anti-B isohemagglutinin titers (Gilles, 2003).

Diagnosis

— Diagnosis is often on the basis of clinical signs, a history of exposure to potentially contaminated soil, eosinophilia, and antibodies to *Toxocara*. Enzyme immunoassay with *Toxocara* excretory-secretory antigens is the preferred means of serologic confirmation. Human stool does not contain eggs, but the presence of other helminth eggs *(Ascaris* or *Trichuris)* increases the probability of *Toxocara* infection (CDC, 2002).

Differential Diagnosis

— The differential diagnosis for visceral larva migrans includes infection with other tissue-migrating helminths (ascarids, hookworm, filiariae, *Strongyloides stercoralis*, and *Trichinella spiralis*) as well as other causes of hypereosinophilia such as tropical pulmonary eosinophilia (TPE), fascioliasis, fasciolopsiasis, gnathostomiasis, loaiasis, onchocerciasis, paragonimiasis, and schistosomiasis. Some forms of visceral larva migrans are indistinguishable from asthma.

Ocular larva migrans may be mistaken for retinoblastoma, choroiditis secondary to toxoplasmosis, retinitis, trauma, and other eye infections (Gilles, 2003; Schantz, 2000).

Treatment

Adults and children with visceral larva migrans are treated with albendazole 400 mg PO bid usually for 5 days (and up to 20 days) or mebendazole 100 to 200 mg PO bid usually for 5 days (and up to 20 days). For severe symptoms or eye involvement, corticosteroids are added. Because ocular larva migrans is usually quiescent, it often is not treated except for management of inflammation; surgery is sometimes indicated (McGavin, 2003; *Medical Letter,* 2002).

Prevention

Because *Toxocara* are passed from the mother dog to puppies transplacentally, deworming fertile or lactating bitches helps in prevention. Children's play areas, especially sandboxes and dirt areas, should be protected from dogs and cats. Prompt disposal of dog stool should be practiced. Pica and the consumption of raw liver should be discouraged (Chin, 2000).

Reporting

The CDC does not consider toxocariasis to be a nationally notifiable disease. The World Health Organization (WHO) considers toxocariasis to be a Class 5 disease. See Appendix C for details and for upcoming changes in WHO reporting.

References

Centers for Disease Control and Prevention. (2001). Toxocariasis. Retrieved January 13, 2004, from *www.dpd.cdc.gov/dpdx/HTML/Toxocariasis.htm*

Centers for Disease Control and Prevention. (2002). Toxocariasis. Retrieved January 13, 2004, from *www.cdc.gov/ncidod/dpd/parasites/toxocara/factsht_toxocara.htm*

Chin, J. (Ed.). (2000). *Control of communicable diseases manual* (17th ed., pp. 497-499). Washington, DC: American Public Health Association.

Gilles, H.M. (2003). Soil-transmitted helminths (geohelminths). In G.C. Cook & A.I. Zumla (Eds.), *Manson's tropical diseases* (21st ed., pp. 1527-1560). Philadelphia: W.B. Saunders Company.

McGavin, D.D.M. (2003). Ophthalmology in the tropics and subtropics. In G.C. Cook & A.I. Zumla (Eds.), *Manson's tropical diseases* (21st ed., pp. 301-361). Philadelphia: W.B. Saunders Company.

Medical Letter. (2002). Drugs for parasitic infections. Retrieved October 30, 2003, from *www.medletter.com/freedocs/parasitic.pdf*

Schantz, P.M. (2000). Toxocariasis. In G.T. Strickland (Ed.), *Hunter's tropical medicine and emerging infectious diseases* (8th ed., pp. 787-790). Philadelphia: W.B. Saunders Company.

TOXOPLASMOSIS

Geographic Distribution

- The geographic distribution of *Toxoplasma gondii* is worldwide. Prevalence rates range from 12% to 90% in different populations, with most individuals infected asymptomatically. In recent years, scattered local epidemics have been identified in Panama, Canada, and Brazil; other unidentified epidemics have likely occurred elsewhere (Chin, 2000; Hegab & Al-Mutawa, 2003; Holland, 2003).

Agent and Vector

- *T. gondii* is an obligate intracellular coccidian protozoan whose definitive host is the cat. All mammals can be infected as can reptiles and fish. Humans acquire infection through ingestion of soil, vegetables, meat, water, and other materials contaminated with cat feces containing *T. gondii* oocysts. Once infected, hosts are infected for life, carrying cysts in tissues such as the central nervous system (CNS), skeletal muscle, and heart muscle. *Toxoplasmosis* refers to symptomatic infection from *T. gondii*. Immuno-compromised persons are at greatest risk of toxoplasmosis from either initial infection or reactivation of latent cysts.
- Congenital toxoplasmosis can occur when the mother acquires primary infection during pregnancy, especially late in the third trimester. Transplacental transmission rates are around 25% in the first trimester and 90% in the third. More severe congenital disease is associated with infection in early pregnancy. Regardless of the stage of pregnancy, the mother usually has unapparent infection.

Oocysts can remain viable in certain conditions such as warm, damp soil for up to a year. Risk behaviors for toxoplasmosis include gardening, handling cat litter, and handling or eating raw or incompletely cooked meat, especially pork or mutton (Centers for Disease Control and Prevention [CDC], 2003; Hegab & Al-Mutawa, 2003; McLeod & Remington, 2004).

Incubation

The incubation period is 5 to 23 days. However, clinically apparent illness may occur many years after the initial infection when an individual's immune system is compromised (Chin, 2000).

Clinical Findings and Treatment

Signs and Symptoms

Most people who are infected are asymptomatic or have mild symptoms. Among symptomatic immunocompetent patients with noncongenital infection, the most common manifestations are painless cervical lymphadenopathy, fatigue, anorexia, fever, headache, myalgia, arthralgia, and maculopapular rash sparing the palms and soles. A variety of other flu-like signs and symptoms may also occur. In most cases the illness resolves without treatment. In addition to immune deficiency, recurrences may occur during pregnancy or cataract surgery. Chorioretinitis occurs in 1% of acquired infection, causing blurred vision, photophobia, and other visual disturbances that are usually unilateral. Ocular disease can be progressive and recurrent, but in immunocompetent hosts is usually self-limiting over about 4 months.

For congenital toxoplasmosis, the classic triad of signs includes chorioretinitis, intracranial calcifications, and hydrocephalus. However, most infants infected transplacentally have no obvious early signs. In other cases, toxoplasmosis can cause hydrops fetalis, erythroblastosis, and perinatal death. Infected infants may be premature and small for gestational age with microcephaly and low Apgar scores. Diverse nonspecific manifestations may develop during the first month of life, including fever, persistent jaundice, seizures, hypotonia, and hepatosplenomegaly. In addition to chorioretinitis, congenital ocular toxoplasmosis may cause strabismus, microphthalmia, microcornea, cataracts, and nystagmus.

Immunocompromised patients include older persons with altered host defenses and persons with disease or treatment-related immune deficiency. Older patients recently infected with *T. gondii* tend to have a more symptomatic course of illness and more severe ocular disease. Patients with HIV/AIDS may have a high degree of inflammation, retinal destruction, and vision loss. Because such patients also commonly have toxoplasmosis encephalitis, current thinking is that the infection originates in the brain and spreads via the optic nerve to the eye. CNS involvement occurs in 30% to 50% of AIDS patients with toxoplasmosis. Common signs and symptoms of toxoplasmosis encephalitis include headache, fever, focal neurologic deficits, seizures, confusion, ataxia, lethargy, cranial nerve palsies, and vision changes (CDC, 2000; Collazos, 2003; Durlach, Kaufer, Carral, & Hirt, 2003; Hegab & Al-Mutawa, 2003; Holland, 2003; McLeod & Remington, 2004).

Complications

Untreated congenital toxoplasmosis leads to developmental delays, learning disabilities, and vision impairment by adolescence. In immunocompromised patients, ocular disease tends to be severe and is often bilateral, resulting in significant disability, including blindness. Disseminated toxoplasmosis may also occur in immunocompromised patients (Hegab & Al-Mutawa, 2003; Holland, 2003; Holliman, 2003; Rothova, 2003).

Common Laboratory Findings

— Cerebrospinal fluid (CSF) findings are usually nonspecific, but infants with congenital toxoplasmosis may have *T. gondii*-specific antibodies and/or may show elevated protein.

— Imaging can be useful in CNS toxoplasmosis. Intracranial calcifications in infected newborns are often detectable by plain films, ultrasonography, or computed tomography (CT). Patients with HIV/AIDS may have multiple ring-enhancing lesions seen by CT or magnetic resonance imaging (McLeod & Remington, 2004).

Diagnosis

— The diagnosis of toxoplasmosis may be made on the basis of serologic testing, polymerase chain reaction (PCR), identification of the organism in fluid or tissue samples, or isolation by tissue culture or intraperitoneal inoculation of mice.

— PCR testing of amniotic fluid is the best way to diagnose fetal infection, with a sensitivity of 81% and specificity of 96%. Combined with mouse inoculation, PCR has a sensitivity of 91%. By comparison, testing for *Toxoplasma*-specific immunoglobulin G (IgG) and immunoglobulin M (IgM) antibodies in fetal blood via cordocentesis has a sensitivity and specificity of less than 50%.

— Serologic testing is routinely used for diagnosis in other clinical situations. A high *Toxoplasma*-specific IgM antibody titer combined with a high IgG titer probably indicates an acute infection within the previous 3 months. A low to medium IgM titer and a high IgG titer may indicate an acute infection 3 to 6 months previously. Note, however, that IgM antibodies have been detected as long as 18 months after initial infection.

Serology cannot diagnosis active CNS infection in immunocompromised patients. In these patients, tissue and brain biopsy may be required to confirm the diagnosis (CDC, 2000; Foulon et al., 1999; Holliman, 2003).

Differential Diagnosis

The differential diagnosis of congenital toxoplasmosis includes erythroblastosis fetalis, cytomegalovirus (CMV), sepsis, aseptic meningitis, syphilis, or hemolytic disease. For ocular toxoplasmosis, the differential diagnosis includes colobomatous defect, intraocular hemorrhage, retinal vessel defect, retinoblastoma, and glioma. In patients with HIV/AIDS the differential diagnosis includes CMV infection, cryptococcal infection, bacterial CNS abscess, tuberculosis, and lymphoma (Holliman, 2003; McLeod & Remington, 2004).

Treatment

Except for congenital infection and patients with immune deficiency, toxoplasmosis is usually self-limited and treatment is not required. The use of corticosteroids is recommended by some experts, but is probably not indicated except when vision is threatened.

Pregnant women may be treated with spiramycin 3 g/day tid throughout the pregnancy. If fetal infection is confirmed, the mother may be treated with pyrimethamine 0.5 to 1.0 mg/kg daily (except for the first trimester, when pyrimethamine is contraindicated) plus sulfadiazine 50 to 100 mg/kg/day bid for 3 weeks and then spiramycin 3 grams/day tid for 3 weeks. These 3-week alternating courses are given until delivery.

Infants with congenital toxoplasmosis are treated for 12 months as follows: pyrimethamine 2 mg/kg/day PO for 2 days; then 1 mg/kg/day for 2 or 6 months; then 1 mg/kg/day on Mondays, Wednesdays, and Fridays for the duration of treatment plus sulfadiazine or triple sulfonamides 100 mg/kg/day PO divided bid plus folinic acid (calcium leucovorin) 5 to 10 mg/kg/day on Mondays, Wednesdays, and Fridays. Concurrent folinic acid decreases the (common) hematopoietic toxicity of pyrimethamine.

— Children may be treated with pyrimethamine 2 mg/kg/day (maximum 25 mg/day) for 3 days/week for 4 weeks plus sulfadiazine 100 to 200 mg/kg/day bid for 3 to 4 weeks. First-line treatment of adults is with pyrimethamine 25 to 100 mg/day PO plus sulfadiazine 1 to 1.5 g PO qid, both for 3 to 4 weeks.

— An alternative treatment is spiramycin 3 to 4 g/day tid for adults and 50 to 100 mg/kg/day tid for children, both for 3 to 4 weeks.

— For patients with HIV/AIDS, clinicians should consult infectious disease specialists and the most current literature for recommendations regarding acute treatment and maintenance therapy, which may be required for life (Collazos, 2003; Hegab & Al-Mutawa, 2003; Holliman, 2003; McLeod & Remington, 2004; *Medical Letter,* 2002).

Prevention

— Prevention is most important among pregnant and immunocompromised persons, and includes the following (Chin, 2000; CDC, 2000):
  • Cook pork, ground meat, and wild game to at least 160° F (internal temperature). Cook beef, lamb, and veal to at least 145° F before eating. Cook whole poultry to 180° F (measured in the thigh).
  • Peel or thoroughly wash fruits and vegetables.
  • Thoroughly clean cooking surfaces and utensils after they have contacted raw meat, poultry, seafood, or unwashed fruits or vegetables.
  • Pregnant women should avoid changing cat litter or, if handling the litter or litter container

is unavoidable, should change the litter daily, wear gloves, and then wash hands thoroughly.
- Pregnant women should not handle stray, unknown, or outside cats.
- Pregnant women should wear gloves when gardening or having contact with soil or sand. After gardening or contact with soil or sand, they should wash hands thoroughly.
- Protect sandboxes and play areas from cats.
- Do not feed cats raw or undercooked meat. Keeping cats inside helps decrease the acquisition of *Toxoplasma* from eating infected prey.
- HIV/AIDS patients with low CD4 counts should be on prophylactic cotrimoxazole or dapsone.

Community education is important, especially for pregnant or immunocompromised persons.

Reporting

The CDC does not consider toxoplasmosis to be a nationally notifiable disease. The World Health Organization (WHO) classifies toxoplasmosis as a Class 3C disease. See Appendix C for details and for upcoming changes in WHO reporting.

References

Centers for Disease Control and Prevention. (2000). Preventing congenital toxoplasmosis. *MMWR, 49 (RRO2)*. Retrieved January 19, 2004, from *www.cdc.gov/mmwr/preview/mmwrhtml/rr4902a5.htm*

Centers for Disease Control and Prevention. (2003). Toxoplasmosis. Retrieved January 20, 2004, from *www.cdc.gov/ncidod/dpd/parasites/toxoplasmosis/factsht_toxoplasmosis.htm.*

Chin, J. (Ed.). (2000). *Control of communicable diseases manual* (17th ed., pp. 500-503). Washington, DC: American Public Health Association.

Collazos, J. (2003). Opportunistic infections of the CNS in patients with AIDS. *CNS Drugs, 17,* 869-887.

Durlach, R.A., Kaufer, F., Carral, L., & Hirt, J. (2003). Toxoplasmic lymphadenitis—clinical and serologic profile. *Clinical Microbiology and Infection, 9,* 625-631.

Foulon, W., Pinon, J.M., Stray-Pedersen, B., Pollak, A., Lappalainen, M., et al. (1999). Prenatal diagnosis of congenital toxoplasmosis: A multicenter evaluation of different diagnostic parameters. *American Journal of Obstetric and Gynecology, 181*(4), 843-847.

Hegab, S.M., & Al-Mutawa, S.A. (2003). Immunopathogenesis of toxoplasmosis. *Clinical and Experimental Medicine, 3,* 84-105.

Holland, G.N. (2003). Ocular toxoplasmosis: A global reassessment. Part I: Epidemiology and course of disease. *American Journal of Ophthalmology, 136,* 973-988.

Holliman, R.E. (2003). Toxoplasmosis. In G.C. Cook & A.I. Zumla (Eds.), *Manson's tropical diseases* (21st ed., pp. 1365-1371). Philadelphia: W.B. Saunders Company.

McLeod, R., & Remington, J.S. (2004). Toxoplasmosis *(Toxoplasma gondii).* In R.E. Behrman, R.M. Kliegman, & H.B. Jenson (Eds.), *Nelson textbook of pediatrics* (17th ed., pp. 1144-1154). Philadelphia: W.B. Saunders Company.

Medical Letter. (2002). Drugs for parasitic infections. Retrieved October 30, 2003, from *www.medletter.com/freedocs/parasitic.pdf*

Rothova, A. (2003). Ocular manifestations of toxoplasmosis. *Current Opinion in Ophthalmology, 14,* 384-388.

82

TRACHOMA

Geographic Distribution

— Trachoma is the leading cause of preventable blindness worldwide. Although significant progress has been made toward eradicating the disease, blinding trachoma is hyperendemic in poor rural communities in the developing world, especially remote areas of north and sub-Saharan Africa, Southeast Asia, China, the Middle East, small pockets of Australia (among aboriginal people) and Latin America (Chin, 2000; West, 2003).

Agent and Vector

— Trachoma is a chronic keratoconjunctivitis caused by the obligate intracellular bacterium, *Chlamydia trachomatis*. *C. trachomatis* serovars A, B, Ba, and C cause ocular disease, while serotypes D through K cause genital tract infection. Person-to-person spread is from ocular and respiratory secretions via fingers, clothing, towels, and the like, with transmission usually occurring among close contacts, especially children ages 2 to 5. Spread may also occur by fluid-seeking flies. In addition, the serovars that cause genital infection may cause ocular infection when a newborn passes through the birth canal of an infected mother.

— Though infection is sometimes asymptomatic, the organism usually causes inflammation of the conjunctivae, particularly the superior tarsal surface. With repeated or severe infection, chronic inflammation and scarring result, causing the upper lid to shorten (entropion) and the eyelashes to turn inward (trichiasis) (Figure 82-1). The in-turned lashes cause painful corneal abrasions that, over time, lead to corneal edema, ulceration, scarring, opacity, and, finally, blindness. In advanced stages, the presence of abrasions and ulcers also facilitates the entry of sometimes severe secondary bacterial or fungal infections (Centers for Disease Control and Prevention [CDC], 2003; Mecaskey, Knirsch, Kumaresan, & Cook, 2003).

Incubation

The incubation period for an infection is 5 to 12 days. The onset of vision loss depends on the intensity and frequency of reinfection (Chin, 2000).

Clinical Findings and Treatment

Signs and Symptoms

The severity of ocular infection due to *C. trachomatis* depends on the serovar of the organism and the age of the host, with younger patients experiencing more severe manifestations. A single trachoma infection typically produces only a mild and self-limited mucopurulent conjunctivitis for which the patient often does not seek care. There may also be purulent nasal discharge, chronic serous otitis media, and productive cough.

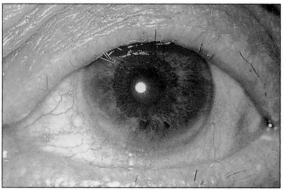

FIGURE 82–1

Entropion and trichiasis. (*Source:* From Peters, W., & Pasvol, G. [2002]. *Tropical medicine and parasitology* [5th ed., p. 242]. Chicago: Mosby.)

A secondary bacterial conjunctivitis may occur, manifested by more copious mucopurulent discharge. Examination of the superior tarsal conjunctivae by everting the upper eyelid may reveal papillary hypertrophy (seen as pinpoint red dots, not specific to trachoma) and subepithelial follicles (appearing as pale yellow-white or gray spots). The superior cornea may have characteristic pannus (scar tissue) formation, pitting, and opacification (Bailey, Mabey, & Taylor, 2000; Mabey, Soloman, & Foster, 2003; West, 2003).

Complications

The primary complications are trichiasis and blindness. Worldwide, approximately 11 million people develop trichiasis secondary to trachoma and 6 million people become blind each year from trachoma (CDC, 2003).

Common Laboratory Findings

There are no common specific laboratory findings.

Diagnosis

Diagnosis is generally on the basis of clinical examination, aided by community prevalence rates. Each eye should be examined separately using binocular loupes (2.5×), and classified according to the World Health Organization's (WHO's) simplified trachoma grading system:

- Follicular trachomatous inflammation with five or more follicles qualifies as follicular trachomatous inflammation (TF).
- Inflammation with pronounced inflammatory thickening obscuring more than half of the deep tarsal vessels is considered intense trachomatous inflammation (TI).

- Scarring of the tarsal conjunctiva is considered to be trachomatous scarring (TS).
- Trachomatous trichiasis (TT) is present when one or more eyelash rubs on the eyeball and/or there is evidence of recent removal of in-turned eyelashes.
- Corneal opacity (CO) is present when there is easily visible corneal opacity over the pupil, for example, the pupil margin is blurred when viewed through the opacity. Visual impairment will be present.

Trichiasis may also be classified as minor trichiasis (TT), in which only a few lashes contact the eye in the exterior quarter, and major trichiasis (TT+), in which many lashes touch the cornea.

For research and epidemiologic purposes, laboratory assays include examination of stained conjunctival scrapings, tissue culture, immunofluorescence, enzyme-linked immunosorbent assay (ELISA), and polymerase chain reaction (PCR) (Mabey et al., 2003; Mecaskey et al., 2003; WHO, 2004).

Differential Diagnosis

Acute infection may be mistaken for other bacterial or viral conjunctivitis, with viral conjunctivitis the most common cause of follicular conjunctivitis. Follicular conjunctivitis may also be caused by molluscum contagiosum, topical drugs, or allergy to eye cosmetics. The differential diagnosis further includes vernal conjunctivitis, Parinaud's oculoglandular syndrome (associated with syphilis, tuberculosis, tularemia, and lymphogranuloma venereum), inclusion conjunctivitis (due to chlamydial infection), Axenfeld's chronic follicular conjunctivitis, and Thygeson's chronic follicular keratoconjunctivitis—the latter two being probable forms of trachoma. Follicles are sometimes found in young children, but in the absence of inflammation or involvement of the superior tarsus are known as folliculosis (Bailey et al., 2000).

Treatment

— One of the more common and less expensive treatments is tetracycline ophthalmic ointment bid for 6 weeks. However the discomfort and duration of treatment result in poor adherence. The most effective treatment for active trachoma is a single oral 20 mg/kg dose of azithromycin, which has the additional advantage of eliminating extraocular reservoirs of chlamydia. Trichiasis can be treated with a variety of surgical procedures that rotate the in-turned eyelashes away from the cornea. The simplified WHO grading system described earlier may be used to guide treatment: TF, topical treatment; TI, topical treatment and consideration of systemic treatment; TT, refer for surgery.

Prevention

— Through the Global Elimination of Blinding Trachoma by 2020 (GET 2020) project, the WHO has implemented the SAFE strategy of treatment and prevention for individuals and communities. The SAFE strategy combines the following strategies, none of which is effective by itself:

- *Surgical management of trachomatis trichiasis.* The WHO has trained personnel to provide low-cost and widely available surgical treatment in some areas. However, there remains a low rate of utilization in some areas, especially in Africa. Recurrence rates range from 17% to 40%.
- *Antibiotics to reduce the prevalence of* Chlamydia *infection.* In addition to index cases, antibiotics may be used to prevent potential secondary cases. Options include all children in endemic areas, all persons in households where there is an active case, and all persons in defined areas of very high endemicity. There is no consensus on which strategy

is most effective, or with what frequency. In areas of very high endemicity, annual treatment is probably a minimal schedule.

- *Face washing to interrupt the transmission of trachoma.* Face washing on a regular basis, especially of children, significantly reduces the spread, severity, and auto-reinfection of trachoma.
- *Environmental change to interrupt the transmission of trachoma.* Poor living conditions tend to increase the incidence and prevalence of trachoma; trachoma, in turn, perpetuates poverty and poor living conditions. Areas identified as most important in environmental change include increasing the availability and use of clean water, reduction of flies through spraying and improved waste disposal, education in general and about trachoma in particular, reduction of crowding, and improving local economies.

Taken together, these measures show promise for the short- and long-term prevention and treatment of trachoma (Mabey et al., 2003; Mecaskey et al., 2003; West, 2003; WHO, 2004).

Reporting

The CDC does not consider trachoma to be a nationally notifiable disease. The WHO considers trachoma a Class 2B disease. See Appendix C for details and for upcoming changes in WHO reporting.

References

Bailey, R., Mabey, D.C.W., & Taylor, H.R. (2000). Trachoma and inclusion conjunctivitis. In G.T. Strickland (Ed.), *Hunter's tropical medicine and emerging infectious diseases* (8th ed., pp. 297-302). Philadelphia: W.B. Saunders Company.

Centers for Disease Control and Preventions. (2003). Trachoma. Retrieved January 29, 2004, from *www.cdc.gov/ncidod/dbmd/diseaseinfo/trachoma_t.htm*

Chin, J. (Ed.). (2000). *Control of communicable diseases manual* (17th ed., pp. 504-506). Washington, DC: American Public Health Association.

Mabey, D.C.W., Soloman, A.W., & Foster, A. (2003). Trachoma. *The Lancet, 362,* 223-229.

Mecaskey, J.W., Knirsch, C.A., Kumaresan, J.A., & Cook, J.A. (2003). The possibility of eliminating blinding trachoma. *The Lancet Infectious Diseases, 3,* 728-734.

West, S.K. (2003). Blinding trachoma: Prevention with the SAFE strategy. *American Journal of Tropical Medicine and Hygiene, 69*(Suppl 5), 18-23.

World Health Organization. (2004). Trachoma. Retrieved February 28, 2004, from *www.who.int/health_topics/trachoma/en/*

TREMATODES, HEPATIC

Liver flukes

Geographic Distribution

The trematode species that infect the liver each have
a distinct geographic distribution. *Opisthorchis viverrini*
is endemic in Thailand, Laos, and Cambodia with
a prevalence of 35% in those countries. *Opisthorchis
felineus* is found in Poland, Germany, Russia (especially
Siberia), and Kazakhstan. *Clonorchis sinensis* is endemic
in China, Korea, Vietnam, Japan, and Taiwan. *Fasciola
hepatica* is found worldwide, particularly in places where
people raise sheep or cattle or consume raw watercress.
Fasciola gigantica is less common and present in the
southern United States and Hawaii, Asia, the Middle
East, and Southeast Asia (Bunnag, Cross, & Bunnag,
2000).

Agent and Vector

Liver flukes have similar life cycles. Eggs in the feces
of infected animals are released into freshwater, where
they embryonate into miracidia that infect a snail
intermediate host. In the snail, the parasites mature into
cercariae that are again released into the water. For
Opisthorchis and *Clonorchis*, the cercariae then penetrate
freshwater fish and mature into metacercariae. Mammals
acquire the parasite when they consume infected fish.
In the case of *Fasciola,* the parasites encyst into
metacercariae as they deposit themselves on the leaves
of aquatic plants, infecting herbivores that eat the leaves
of the plants (for humans, this is commonly watercress).
In the duodenum of the mammalian host, the parasites
excyst, penetrate the intestinal wall into the peritoneal
space, invade the liver parenchyma, and migrate into the

biliary ducts. The adult *Opisthorchis* and *Clonorchis* worms live in the gallbladder, whereas *Fasciola* worms reside in the liver or bile ducts. There they mature and lay eggs to continue the cycle (Bunnag et al., 2000; Centers for Disease Control and Prevention [CDC], 2002a, 2002b; Hawn & Jong, 1999).

Incubation

The incubation period of liver flukes is variable, but symptoms often begin 1 to 4 weeks after consumption of infected fish. It takes approximately 1 month for *Clonorchis* and *Opisthorchis* to mature and migrate to the biliary tree, whereas *Fasciola* may take 3 to 4 months (CDC, 2002a, 2002b).

Clinical Findings and Treatment

Signs and Symptoms

Symptoms are usually mild or absent, especially for residents of endemic areas who are infected early in life. Acute illness is more common for travelers. When the parasites migrate from the duodenum into the biliary tree, they may cause fever, nausea, epigastric or right upper quadrant pain, and hepatomegaly. Urticaria is sometimes present. *O. felineus* can cause an illness similar to Katayama fever (see Schistosomiasis chapter) with facial edema, fever, lymphadenopathy, arthralgias, rash, and eosinophilia. Once the parasites are in the biliary tree, infection is usually asymptomatic, although some patients may have nonspecific gastrointestinal symptoms (CDC, 2002a; Hawn & Jong, 1999; Liu & Harinasuta, 1996).

Complications

Chronic heavy infections or large flukes can obstruct the common bile duct, causing jaundice and cholangitis. *Opisthorchis* and *Clonorchis* infections can lead to cholangiocarcinoma. Rarely, flukes may migrate to the lungs, skin, central nervous system, or intestinal wall, causing localized inflammatory nodules or abscesses (Hawn & Jong, 1999; Liu & Harinasuta, 1996).

Common Laboratory Findings

Marked eosinophilia is sometimes present. Serum immunoglobulin E (IgE) levels may also be elevated. Liver or biliary tree abnormalities can sometimes be seen by ultrasonography or computed tomography scan. Lesions from fascioliasis may resemble hypodense abscess-like nodules or hypodense branching patterns (Liu & Harinasuta, 1996).

Diagnosis

Microscopic detection of eggs in feces or duodenal aspirates is the most common method of diagnosing *Opisthorchis* and *Clonorchis* infection. *Fasciola* eggs can sometimes be detected in the stool or duodenal or biliary drainage, but not until 3 to 4 months after ingestion when the parasites have finished their migration and matured in the biliary tree. Even then, egg production is intermittent. Enzyme-linked immunosorbent assay (ELISA) tests for *Fasciola* antigens or antiparasite antibodies are specific and useful in the acute migratory stage. Antibodies may be present 2 to 4 weeks following ingestion. Similar tests for *Opisthorchis* and *Clonorchis* exist for research purposes but are not widely available (CDC, 2002a, 2002b; Hawn & Jong, 1999; Liu & Harinasuta, 1996).

Differential Diagnosis

Few diseases cause the combination of eosinophilia with liver lesions. Toxocariasis can cause eosinophilia with hepatomegaly but does not produce destructive lesions in the liver parenchyma (Freedman & Gotuzzo, 2003).

Treatment

For clonorchiasis and opisthorchiasis, the treatment of choice is praziquantel 75 mg/kg divided tid for 1 day. Clonorchis infections may also be treated with albendazole 10 mg/kg/day bid for 7 days. For fascioliasis, the only trematode infection not sensitive to praziquantel, the standard treatment is triclabendazole at 10 mg/kg in a single dose, with bithionol as an alternative at 30 to 50 mg/kg on alternate days for 10 to 15 doses. Antiparasite antibody levels fall to normal 6 to 12 months after successful therapy (CDC, 2002a, 2002b; *Medical Letter,* 2002).

Prevention

Prevention of liver fluke infection (Bunnag et al., 2000; Haswell-Elkins & Levri, 2003) includes the following:
- Cook freshwater plants (especially watercress), mollusks, and fish before consuming them.
- Avoid consuming untreated contaminated water or raw sheep liver.
- Promote hand washing after defecation and before contact with food.
- Treat and immunize dogs, cats, livestock, and other animals that contribute to maintaining the life cycle.
- Prohibit use of human, sheep, or swine excreta as pond fertilizer.
- Control snail populations where practical (though widespread use of molluscicide is seldom indicated).

Community education is important in the ongoing effort to decrease infection.

Reporting

The CDC does not consider liver fluke infection to be a nationally notifiable disease. The World Health Organization (WHO) considers liver fluke infections Class 3C (fasciolopsiasis) to Class 5 (fascioliasis) diseases.

See Appendix C for details and for upcoming changes in WHO reporting.

References

Bunnag, D., Cross, J.H., & Bunnag, T. (2000). Lung fluke infections. In G.T. Strickland (Ed.), *Hunter's tropical medicine and emerging infectious diseases* (8th ed., pp. 847-851). Philadelphia: W.B. Saunders Company.

Center for Disease Control and Prevention. (2002a). Fascioliasis. Retrieved February 5, 2004, from *www.dpd.cdc.gov/dpdx/HTML/Fascioliasis.htm*

Center for Disease Control and Prevention. (2002b). Opisthorchiasis. Retrieved February 5, 2004, from *www.dpd.cdc.gov/dpdx/HTML/Fascioliasis.htm*

Freedman, D.O., & Gotuzzo, E. (2003). Case 12: Diagnosis and discussion. Retrieved from *Tropical medicine cases from Peru* on February 5, 2004, from *www-cme.erep.uab.edu/onlineCourses/Gorgas03/Case12_03/CaseDiag12(03).htm*

Haswell-Elkins, M.R., & Levri, E. (2003). Food-borne trematodes. In G.C. Cook & A.I. Zumla (Eds.), *Manson's tropical diseases* (21st ed., pp. 1471-1486). Philadelphia: W.B. Saunders Company.

Hawn, T.R., & Jong E.C. (1999). Update on hepatobiliary and pulmonary flukes. *Current Infectious Disease Reports, 1,* 427-433.

Liu, L.X., & Harinasuta, K.T. (1996). Parasitic diseases of the liver and intestines. *Gastroenterology Clinics, 25,* 627-636.

Medical Letter. (2002). Drugs for parasitic infections. April, pp. 1-12.

Trematodes, Intestinal
Intestinal flukes
Geographic Distribution

There are more than 50 species of trematodes that infect the human gastrointestinal tract, but only a few that cause disease. *Fasciolopsis, Echinostoma,* and *Heterophyes* are the species responsible for most human infections. Fasciolopsiasis (from *F. buski*) is endemic in China, Taiwan, Southeast Asia, India, Bangladesh, and Indonesia. Echinostomiasis (from *E. ilocanum, E. malayanum, E. revolutum,* and *Hypoderaeum conoideum*) is common in Indonesia, the Philippines, Taiwan, and Thailand. Heterophyiasis (from *H. heterophyes* and *Metagonimus yokogawai*) is found in the Nile delta of Egypt and in Iran, Tunisia, Turkey, Japan, Korea, Taiwan, the Philippines, and Indonesia (Bunnag, Cross, & Bunnag, 2000; Liu & Harinasuta, 1996).

Agent and Vector

Intestinal trematodes are zoonoses for which humans are accidental hosts. Adult trematodes live in the intestines and lay eggs that are released into freshwater with feces. There they hatch into miracidia that infect the snail, the first intermediate host. In the snail, the parasites develop into cercariae that are again released into the water to develop into metacercariae.
The parasites proceed to infect a second intermediate host, which is different for each species. The *Fasciolopsis* metacercariae encyst on freshwater plants. *Echinostoma* cercariae encyst in other snails, fish, tadpoles, or vegetation. *Heterophyes* cercariae infect brackish or freshwater fish. Humans become infected when they

consume the raw or incompletely cooked second intermediate host. The metacercariae excyst in the human duodenum and attach themselves to the gastrointestinal mucosa where they mature into adult trematodes that lay eggs to continue the life cycle (Bunnag et al., 2000; Centers for Disease Control and Prevention [CDC], 2002a, 2002b; Liu & Harinasuta, 1996).

Incubation

Eggs may not appear in the stool until a few months following infection, but symptoms can begin as soon as 9 days after infection (Bunnag et al., 2000).

Clinical Findings and Treatment

Signs and Symptoms

Most infections are light and asymptomatic. Heavier infections commonly cause diarrhea and abdominal pain. The diarrhea may be intermittent or alternate with constipation. The abdominal pain is colicky or can resemble dyspepsia (Bunnag et al., 2000; Liu & Harinasuta, 1996).

Complications

Heavy *Fasciolopsis* infections can sometimes cause a protein-losing enteropathy, resulting in hypoalbuminemia and anasarca; intestinal obstruction can also occur. Rarely, *Heterophyes* eggs can migrate to extraintestinal sites such as the heart (causing myocarditis) or brain (Bunnag et al., 2000; CDC, 2002b; Liu & Harinasuta, 1996).

Common Laboratory Findings

Leukocytosis, marked eosinophilia, and anemia may be present in fasciolopsiasis (Liu & Harinasuta, 1996).

Diagnosis

Microscopic detection of eggs in stool is the primary method of diagnosis. Eggs are often difficult to distinguish between the trematodes. In some cases, the definitive diagnosis may be made by identifying the dead worms that are released into the stool following treatment (Bunnag et al., 2000; CDC, 2002a, 2002b).

Differential Diagnosis

Heavy infections can cause symptoms mimicking giardiasis or peptic ulcer disease. The edema from the chronic protein-losing enteropathy of severe fasciolopsiasis can resemble that of nephrotic syndrome or other causes of hypoproteinemia (Bunnag et al., 2000).

Treatment

For fasciolopsiasis, the treatment of choice for adults and children is a single 15 mg/kg dose of praziquantel taken at bedtime after supper. Niclosamide, either as a single 150 mg/kg dose or as 40 mg/kg/day for 2 days, is an alternative. Praziquantel has also been found to be effective for echinostomiasis (25 mg/kg in a single dose) and heterophyiasis (20 mg/kg/day for 1 day, or up to 3 days for heavy infections) (Bunnag et al., 2000; Liu & Harinasuta, 1996).

Prevention

Prevention of intestinal trematode infection (Bunnag et al., 2000; Haswell-Elkins & Levri, 2003) includes the following:

- Cook freshwater plants (especially watercress) and also mollusks and fish before consuming.
- Promote hand washing after defecation and before contact with food.
- Treat and immunize livestock and other herbivorous animals that contribute to maintaining the life cycle.

- Prohibit use of human or swine excreta as pond fertilizer.
- Control snail populations where practical (though widespread use of molluscicide is seldom indicated).

Community education is important in the ongoing effort to decrease infection.

Reporting

The CDC does not consider trematode infection to be a nationally notifiable disease. The World Health Organization (WHO) considers trematode infection to be a Class 3C disease. See Appendix C for details and for upcoming changes in WHO reporting.

References

Bunnag, D., Cross, J.H., & Bunnag, T. (2000). Intestinal fluke infections. In G.T. Strickland (Ed.), *Hunter's tropical medicine and emerging infectious diseases* (8th ed., pp. 832-840). Philadelphia: W.B. Saunders Company.

Centers for Disease Control and Prevention. (2002a). Fasciolopsiasis. Retrieved February 5, 2004, from *www.dpd.cdc.gov/dpdx/HTML/Fasciolopsiasis.htm*

Centers for Disease Control and Prevention. (2002b). Heterophyiasis. Retrieved February 5, 2004, from *www.dpd.cdc.gov/dpdx/HTML/Heterophyiasis.htm*

Haswell-Elkins, M.R., & Levri, E. (2003). Food-borne trematodes. In G.C. Cook & A.I. Zumla (Eds.), *Manson's tropical diseases* (21st ed., pp. 1471-1486). Philadelphia: W.B. Saunders Company.

Liu, L.X., & Harinasuta, K.T. (1996). Parasitic diseases of the liver and intestines. *Gastroenterology Clinics, 25,* 627-636.

TREMATODES, PULMONARY
Lung flukes, paragonimiasis
Geographic Distribution

Paragonimus infects an estimated 21 million people in the world, with endemic foci in Asia, Africa, and Central and South America. *P. westermani, P. skrjabini, P. miazakii,* and *P. heterotremus* are prevalent in Korea, China, Japan, and Taiwan as well as Southeast Asia. In Africa, *P. africanus* and *P. uterobilateralis* are present in Nigeria, Cameroon, Liberia, Guinea, and the Gambia. *P. mexicanus* is the principal species in Central and South America (Bunnag, Cross, & Bunnag, 2000).

Agent and Vector

Paragonimus has a life cycle similar to that of other trematodes. Eggs in the feces or sputum of infected animals are released into freshwater, where they embryonate into miracidia that infect the snail intermediate host. In the snail, the parasites mature into cercariae that are again released into the water. The parasites then infect freshwater crabs or crayfish, which are eaten by mammals. Once in the duodenum of the mammalian host, the parasites excyst, penetrate the intestinal wall into the peritoneal space, and invade the abdominal wall, where they develop into young flukes. The young flukes then migrate through the diaphragm and form pseudocapsules in the lung parenchyma. There they mature into adult flukes and lay eggs that are either coughed out in sputum or swallowed and passed in the feces to continue the life cycle (Bunnag et al., 2000; Centers for Disease Control and Prevention [CDC], 2002).

Incubation

Eggs may be detected in the sputum or feces as early as 8 to 10 weeks after infection. Flukes may survive for more than 20 years in the human host (Bunnag et al., 2000).

Clinical Findings and Treatment

Signs and Symptoms

Many patients have light infections and are asymptomatic. Even those with heavy infections may have only mild symptoms. The acute migratory phase can cause fever, abdominal pain, diarrhea, cough, and urticaria. In the chronic phase, the classic presentation resembles tuberculosis with the insidious onset of cough and hemoptysis. On examination, patients may have wheezing or rales, and occasionally digital clubbing. Those with skin involvement may have migratory tender subcutaneous nodules in the lower abdomen or inguinal areas (Bunnag et al., 2000; CDC, 2002; Hawn & Jong, 1999).

Complications

Rarely, the flukes may migrate to other parts of the body, causing cysts or granulomas. In the gastrointestinal tract, the parasites can cause nausea, vomiting, or bloody diarrhea; they may also form abscesses in the abdominal viscera. Central nervous system (CNS) involvement can mimic meningoencephalitis in the acute phase, causing seizures, headache, visual disturbances, cranial nerve abnormalities, and extremity weakness or paralysis (Bunnag et al., 2000; Hawn & Jong, 1999).

Common Laboratory Findings

Eosinophilia is sometimes present. Chest X-rays in the early stages may have ill-defined opacities. Later in the course of illness chest films may show cystic lesions, extensive nodular or linear infiltrates, pleural thickening, pleural effusions, multilocular cavities, or hilar enlargement. With CNS involvement, eosinophils may be present in cerebrospinal fluid, and cysts may be detected with computed tomography (Bunnag et al., 2000).

Diagnosis

The diagnosis of paragonimiasis should be suspected in patients with chronic cough and hemoptysis who live in endemic areas and have a history of eating raw crustaceans. Confirmation is by microscopic detection of eggs in feces or sputum. Sometimes, biopsy is required to confirm the diagnosis. In the acute phase or in patients with light infections, where eggs may not be detectable, antibody detection may be useful (CDC, 2002).

Differential Diagnosis

Clinicians should also consider pulmonary tuberculosis, echinococcosis, bacterial lung abscesses, chronic lung disease, or carcinoma. Patients with CNS involvement may have symptoms resembling those of tuberculomas, abscesses, cysticercosis, and other parasitic infections involving the brain or spinal cord.

Treatment

The treatment of choice is praziquantel 75 mg/kg/day divided tid for 2 days. Bithionol is an alternative at 30 to 50 mg/kg on alternate days for 10 to 15 doses (CDC, 2002; *Medical Letter,* 2002).

Prevention

Prevention of lung fluke infection (Bunnag et al., 2000; Chin, 2000; Haswell-Elkins & Levri, 2003) includes the following:
  • Cook freshwater mollusks, crustaceans, and fish before consuming.

- Promote hand washing after defecation and before contact with food.
- Prohibit use of human or swine excreta as pond fertilizer.
- Discourage spitting into freshwater.
- Control snail populations where practical (though widespread use of molluscicide is seldom indicated).

Community education is important in the ongoing effort to decrease infection.

Reporting

The CDC does not consider trematode infection to be a nationally notifiable disease. The World Health Organization (WHO) considers paragonimiasis a Class 5 disease. See Appendix C for details and for upcoming changes in WHO reporting.

References

Bunnag, D., Cross, J.H., & Bunnag, T. (2000). Lung fluke infections. In G.T. Strickland (Ed.), *Hunter's tropical medicine and emerging infectious diseases* (8th ed., pp. 847-851). Philadelphia: W.B. Saunders Company.

Centers for Disease Control and Prevention. (2002). Paragonimiasis. Retrieved February 19, 2004, from *www.dpd.cdc.gov/dpdx/HTML/Paragonimiasis.htm*

Haswell-Elkins, M.R., & Levri, E. (2003). Food-borne trematodes. In G.C. Cook & A.I. Zumla (Eds.), *Manson's tropical diseases* (21st ed., pp. 1471-1486). Philadelphia: W.B. Saunders Company.

Hawn, T.R., & Jong E.C. (1999). Update on hepatobiliary and pulmonary flukes. *Current Infectious Disease Reports, 1,* 427-433.

Medical Letter. (2002). *Drugs for parasitic infections*. April, pp. 1-12.

TRENCH FEVER

Five-day fever, Quintana fever, Wolhnyian fever

Geographic Distribution

Trench fever occurs in crowded, unhygienic conditions in most areas of the world except for Australia and Antarctica. In World War I, there were epidemics among soldiers living in trenches in Europe, but the incidence declined until around 1995 when there was a resurgence of the disease especially among homeless persons and persons with HIV/AIDS (Fournier, Ndihokubwayo, Guidran, Kelly, & Raoult, 2002; Ohl & Spach, 2001).

Agent and Vector

The agent of trench fever is *Bartonella quintana* (formerly *Rochalimaea quintana*), a fastidious, slow-growing gram-negative bacillus transmitted via an arthropod vector, the body louse *Pediculus humanus corporis*. *B. quintana* is shed in louse feces and enters the human host through breaks in the skin from a louse bite or when louse feces are rubbed into open skin lesions. Although there is no human-to-human spread, the (classic) indirect spread occurs when lice migrate as a result of changes in the human host's body temperature, either from fever or cooling down after death. In recent cases of "urban trench fever," found among homeless, urban, alcoholic persons, the means of spread is not well defined (Chin, 2000; Fournier et al., 2002; Jackson, 2000).

The pathogenesis of trench fever is poorly understood. *Bartonella* species are known to interact closely with host cells, including red blood cells, endothelial cells, and possibly bone marrow progenitor cells (Greub & Raoult, 2002).

Incubation

The incubation period is usually 7 to 9 days but can range from 5 to 20 days, depending on the means and degree of inoculation (Ohl & Spach, 2001; Scott & Wyllie, 2003).

Clinical Findings and Treatment

Signs and Symptoms

In classic trench fever there are four common clinical patterns: (1) asymptomatic or mild; (2) a single, acute illness lasting 3 to 4 (and up to 8) days; (3) periodic with a prolonged relapsing-remitting fever occurring at 5-day intervals; and (4) a continuous and prolonged typhoidal illness.

Presentation is nonspecific and variable, commonly including the acute onset of high fever, chills, sweating, malaise, conjunctival injection, retro-orbital headache, and pain in the lower extremities, especially anterior tibial pain. Most patients develop transient crops of erythematous macules or papules on the abdomen, chest, and back. Splenomegaly is common.

The course of urban trench fever is varied and commonly includes chronic bacteremia (usually lasting 1 to 8 weeks but sometimes more than a year) with subacute chronic fever, fatigue, and weight loss. Convalescence may last several months and, in some cases, symptoms may recur for many years (Chian, Arrese, & Piérard, 2002; Foucault, Barrau, Bronqui, & Raoult, 2002; Jackson, 2000; Scott & Wyllie, 2003).

Complications

Complications, more common among immunocompromised persons, include bacteremia, osteomyelitis, bacillary angiomatosis, endocarditis, and, rarely, pericardial effusion (Levy, Fournier, Carta, & Raoult, 2003).

Common Laboratory Findings

— There are no typical laboratory findings in trench fever.

Diagnosis

— Trench fever should be suspected in urban homeless individuals with a relapsing febrile illness, "culture-negative" endocarditis, or lesions compatible with bacillary angiomatosis (hemangioma-like skin lesions sometimes involving the lymphatics and viscera in immunocompromised patients).
— The organism can be isolated in blood, but growth may not be seen for as long as 5 to 6 weeks. Serologic tests are available but should be interpreted with caution because cross-reactivity has been described with *B. henselae, Coxiella burnetii,* and *Chlamydia* species. Because initial titers are often negative, paired acute and convalescent titers should be obtained. Most immunocompetent hosts will have a positive serology, with high titers (higher than 1:1600) among those with endocarditis. Direct polymerase chain reaction (PCR) detection of DNA from blood specimens can be used to differentiate among *Bartonella* species. PCR can also be used to identify infected lice (Agan & Dolan, 2002; Foucault, Raoult, & Brouqui, 2003; Fournier et al., 2002; Ohl & Spach, 2001).

Differential Diagnosis

— The differential diagnosis includes typhoid fever, typhus, malaria, and relapsing fever (Scott & Wyllie, 2003).

Treatment

— Data to guide therapy are limited. One open randomized trial demonstrated that bacteremia may be successfully

treated with a combination of gentamicin
3 mg/kg/24 hours IV for 14 days and doxycycline
200 mg/day PO for 28 days. Other regimens that have
been suggested include a 6-week course of doxycycline,
erythromycin (500 mg PO qid), or azithromycin
(500 mg PO daily). Endocarditis necessitates a 4- to
6-month course of therapy (Foucault et al., 2003;
Ohl & Spach, 2001).

Prevention

Good hygiene and sanitation are the keys to prevention.
Individual prevention in nonmass situations includes
washing clothing according to the guidelines given next.
Discarding or treating infested clothing and bathing
in hot water are sufficient to rid a person of body lice
because the lice live in the clothing as opposed to on
the body.

In mass population conditions favoring lice infestation,
such as refugee crises, Chin (2000) recommends that
residual insecticide powders be applied to the clothes
and bodies of persons at risk, such as 10% DDT
insufflating powder for clothing and 1% malathion
or 0.5% permethrin under clothing (Butler, 2000).
The U.S. military guidelines for prevention of
louse-borne diseases include (1) treatment of persons
infected with the disease(s), (2) bathing infested
persons, and (3) laundering all clothing with regimens
lethal to lice and eggs. Exposing clothing to water or
circulating air at a temperature of 140° F (60° C) for
15 min kills all stages of lice (Armed Forces Pest
Management Board, 2002; Butler, 2000; Centers for
Disease Control and Prevention [CDC], 2003;
Chin, 2000).

Reporting

The CDC does not consider trench fever to be a
nationally notifiable disease. The World Health

Organization (WHO) considers trench fever to be a Class 3B disease. See Appendix C for details and for upcoming changes in WHO reporting.

References

Agan, B.K., & Dolan, M.J. (2002). Laboratory diagnosis of *Bartonella* infections. *Clinics in Laboratory Medicine, 22,* 937-962.

Armed Forces Pest Management Board. (2002). Delousing procedures for the control of louse-borne disease during contingency. Retrieved December 26, 2003, from *www.afpmb.org/pubs/tims/TG6/TG6.pdf*

Butler, T. (2000). Relapsing fever. In G.T. Strickland (Ed.), *Hunter's tropical medicine and emerging infectious diseases* (8th ed., pp. 448-452). Philadelphia: W.B. Saunders Company.

Centers for Disease Control and Prevention. (2003). Rickettsial diseases. Retrieved March 19, 2004, from *www.cdc.gov/travel/diseases/rickettsial.htm*

Chian, C.A., Arrese, J.E., & Piérard, G.E. (2002). Skin manifestations of *Bartonella* infections. *International Journal of Dermatology, 41,* 461-466.

Chin, J. (Ed.). (2000). *Control of communicable diseases manual* (17th ed., pp. 506-508). Washington, DC: American Public Health Association.

Foucault, C., Barrau, K., Bronqui, P., & Raoult, D. (2002). *Bartonella quintana* bacteremia among homeless people. *Clinical Infectious Diseases, 35,* 684-689.

Foucault, C., Raoult, D., & Brouqui, P. (2003). Randomized open trial of gentamicin and doxycycline for eradication of *Bartonella quintana* from blood in patients with chronic bacteremia. *Antimicrobial Agents and Chemotherapy, 47,* 2204-2207.

Fournier, P.-E., Ndihokubwayo, J.-B., Guidran, J., Kelly, P.J., & Raoult, D. (2002). Human pathogens in body and head lice. *Emerging Infectious Diseases, 8,* 1515-1518.

Greub, G., & Raoult, D. (2002). Bartonella: New explanations for old diseases. *Journal of Medical Microbiology, 51,* 915-923.

Jackson, L.A. (2000). Trench fever. In G.T. Strickland (Ed.), *Hunter's tropical medicine and emerging infectious diseases* (8th ed., pp. 442-443). Philadelphia: W.B. Saunders Company.

Levy, P.Y., Fournier, P.E., Carta, M., & Raoult, D. (2003). Pericardial effusion in a homeless man due to *Bartonella quintana*. *Journal of Clinical Microbiology, 41,* 5291-5293.

Ohl, M.E., & Spach, D.H. (2001). *Bartonella quintana* and urban trench fever. *Clinical Infectious Diseases, 31,* 131-135.

Scott, G.M., & Wyllie, S.A. (2003). Bartonellosis, cat-scratch disease, trench fever, human ehrlichiosis, Whipple disease. In G.C. Cook & A.I. Zumla (Eds.), *Manson's tropical diseases* (21st ed., pp. 1095-1108). Philadelphia: W.B. Saunders Company.

87

TRICHINELLOSIS

Trichinella, trichiniasis, trichinosis

Geographic Distribution

— Trichinellosis occurs worldwide and is most common in Europe and the United States. The prevalence of trichinellosis is increasing worldwide (Centers for Disease Control and Prevention [CDC], 2002; Peters & Pasvol, 2002).

Agent and Vector

— Trichinellosis is caused by nematodes of the genus *Trichinella*, including the best known agent *T. spiralis* (found worldwide in carnivorous and omnivorous animals) and also *T. pseudospiralis, T. britovi, T. native,* and *T. nelsoni.* Animals are infected by eating the cyst-infected flesh of other animals, including prey, carrion, and garbage. Herbivores such as horses can become infected if they are given feed that contains or is contaminated with flesh (e.g., from rats). Humans are accidental hosts who often become infected by eating undercooked pork. However, in at least some locales, the consumption of horse meat, game meats, noncommercially raised animal meats, or exotic meats presents a greater risk than commercially processed pork (Roy, Lopez, & Schantz, 2003).

— Once ingested, *Trichinella* cysts pass to the small intestine where they excyst. The larvae then burrow into the intestinal mucosa where they molt, mature, and mate. After about 1 week, the female begins discharging live larvae and continues for 1 to 4 months. Larvae enter the lymphatics or bloodstream and migrate to skeletal (striated) muscle tissue where they encyst or encapsulate (except for *T. pseudospiralis*, which does not encapsulate)

and eventually calcify (CDC, 2002; Chin, 2000;
Peters & Pasvol, 2002).

Incubation

Gastrointestinal manifestations begin 1 to 2 days after
ingestion and systemic symptoms 1 to 8 weeks later
(CDC, 2003; Chin, 2000).

Clinical Findings and Treatment

Signs and Symptoms

Light infections are usually asymptomatic. There are
some differences in manifestations of infection according
to the parasite species. Symptomatic infections are
characterized by three stages of illness:

- *Enteric* (within the first week of ingestion). Larvae
  in the small intestine cause mild fever, colicky
  abdominal pain, nausea, vomiting, and sweating.
  A maculopapular rash may develop, as may headache,
  dizziness, pneumonitis, diarrhea, or constipation.
- *Migratory* (7 to 10 days after ingestion and lasting
  6 or more weeks when encapsulation begins).
  The cardinal features of trichinellosis occur in the
  migratory phase and include fever (high, remittent,
  typhoid-like), periorbital or facial edema, myalgia,
  and eosinophilia. Difficulty chewing, dysphagia,
  and dyspnea may also occur. These may be followed
  by conjunctivitis or conjunctival hemorrhage.
  Splinter hemorrhages under the nails may be
  found.
- *Encystment in the muscles* (beginning as early as
  14 days after infection and continuing for as long as
  a year). This stage is commonly characterized by
  myalgia and weakness, followed by decreased
  symptoms. In more severe cases there may be weight
  loss or cachexia, edema, dehydration, or lasting
  central nervous system (CNS) manifestations.

In mild to moderate infections, most symptoms subside within several months, although fatigue, weakness, and gastrointestinal distress may last for months after the initial illness (CDC, 2002; Dupouy-Camet, Kociecka, Bruschi, Bolas-Fernandez, & Pozio, 2002; Gilles, 2003; Peters & Pasvol, 2002).

Complications

Trichinella myocarditis can cause dysrhythmias 2 to 5 weeks after infection, congestive heart failure 4 to 8 weeks after infection, thromboembolisms, or pericardial effusion. Neurologic complications are a result of larvae passing through the CNS and may include meningitis, meningoencephalitis, vision disturbances, hearing impairment, ataxia, mental status changes, or coma. Respiratory muscle weakness and pneumonitis may occur. Death occurs through heart failure, dysrhythmia, renal failure, or toxemia (CDC, 2002; Gilles, 2003; Murrell, 2000).

Common Laboratory Findings

Common laboratory findings include a sometimes impressive eosinophilia that begins in week 2 or 3 and then decreases but remains persistently elevated. Muscle involvement may cause increased creatine phosphokinase levels. The erythrocyte sedimentation rate is usually normal. Hematuria and albuminuria are common. In the migratory phase larvae may be found in the cerebrospinal fluid, which may also have increased cell count and protein (CDC, 2002; Gilles, 2003).

Diagnosis

The three objectives in the detection of trichinellosis in humans are (1) recognizing the acute infection so that early anthelmintic therapy may begin, (2) making retrospective diagnosis, and (3) epidemiologic surveillance (Gamble et al., 2004). Trichinellosis should be suspected in a patient with the clinical features noted earlier and a history of ingesting undercooked meat. The possibility of infection is increased if other people eating the same meat have similar symptoms. Antibodies may become detectable at least 3 weeks following infection. The most sensitive serologic test is enzyme-linked immunosorbent assay (ELISA). Other serologic tests include indirect hemagglutination, bentonite flocculation, indirect immunofluorescence assay, and latex agglutination. Trichinoscopy, the microscopic examination of muscle tissue pressed between two slides, is useful only during the encystment phase (CDC, 2002; Gamble et al., 2004).

Differential Diagnosis

In early infection the differential diagnosis includes influenza and acute gastroenteritis. Later considerations include typhoid fever, encephalitis, myositis, tetanus, or other helminthic infections associated with eosinophilia (Gilles, 2003).

Treatment

Treatment is begun as soon as possible, usually based on clinical diagnosis and a high index of suspicion (Gamble et al., 2004). Steroids may be given for severe symptoms, though supporting evidence is equivocal. The treatment of choice is the same for adults and children: mebendazole 200 to 400 mg tid for 3 days, then 400 to 500 mg tid for 10 days. An alternative is albendazole 400 mg bid for 8 to 14 days (*Medical Letter,* 2002).

Prevention

Prevention of trichinellosis (CDC, 2003; Chin, 2000) includes the following:

- Governments should monitor meat processing facilities and test meats for the presence of *Trichinella.*

- Cook meat products until the juices run clear, the color of the meat changes from pink to gray, or an internal temperature of 170° F (77° C) is reached. Curing (salting), drying, smoking, or microwaving meat does not consistently kill infective worms.
- Freeze pork less than 6 inches thick for 20 days at 5° F (–15° C) to kill any worms.
- Cook wild game meat thoroughly. Unlike pork, freezing wild game meats even for long periods of time may not effectively kill all worms.
- Cook all meat fed to pigs or other wild animals.
- Do not allow hogs to eat garbage or the uncooked carcasses of other animals, including rats, which may be infected with *Trichinella*.
- Clean meat grinders thoroughly if you prepare your own ground meats.

Community education should be ongoing on these measures.

Reporting

The CDC considers trichinellosis to be a nationally notifiable disease. The World Health Organization (WHO) classifies trichinellosis as a Class 2B disease. See Appendix C for details and for upcoming changes in WHO reporting.

References

Centers for Disease Control and Prevention. (2002). Trichinellosis. Retrieved April 2, 2004, from *www.dpd.cdc.gov/dpdx/HTML/Trichinosis.htm*

Centers for Disease Control and Prevention. (2003). Trichinellosis. Retrieved April 2, 2004, from *www.cdc.gov/ncidod/dpd/parasites/trichinosis/factsht_trichinosis.htm*

Chin, J. (Ed.). (2000). *Control of communicable diseases manual* (17th ed.). Washington, DC: American Public Health Association.

Dupouy-Camet, J., Kociecka, W., Bruschi, F., Bolas-Fernandez, F., & Pozio, E. (2002). Opinion on the diagnosis and treatment of human trichinellosis. *Expert Opinion on Pharmacotherapy, 3*, 1117-1130.

Gamble, H.R., Pozio, E., Bruschi, F., Nöckler, K., Kapel, C.M.O., & Gajadhar, A.A. (2004). International Commission on Trichinellosis: Recommendations on the use of serological tests for the detection of *Trichinella* infections in animals and man. *Parasite, 11,* 3-13.

Gilles, H.M. (2003). Soil-transmitted helminths (geohelminths). In G.C. Cook & A.I. Zumla (Eds.), *Manson's tropical diseases* (21st ed., pp. 1527-1560). Philadelphia: W.B. Saunders Company.

Medical Letter. (2002). Drugs for parasitic infections. Retrieved October 30, 2003, from *www.medletter.com/freedocs/parasitic.pdf*

Murrell, K.D. (2000). Trichinosis. In G.T. Strickland (Ed.), *Hunter's tropical medicine and emerging infectious diseases* (8th ed., pp. 780-787). Philadelphia: W.B. Saunders Company.

Peters, W., & Pasvol, G. (2002). *Tropical medicine and parasitology* (5th ed.). Chicago: Mosby.

Roy, S.L., Lopez, A.S., & Schantz, P.M. (2003). Trichinellosis surveillance: United States, 1997-2001. *Morbidity and Mortality Weekly Report, 52*(SS06), 1-8.

88

Trichuriasis

Whipworm disease

Geographic Distribution

— Trichuriasis occurs worldwide, especially in warm, moist climates and in approximately the same geographic distribution as ascariasis. Close to 1 billion people are thought to be infected, slightly more than are infected with hookworm and slightly less than with *Ascaris* (Bundy & Cooper, 2000; Gilles, 2003).

Agent and Vector

— Trichuriasis is caused by the nematode (roundworm) *Trichuris trichiura*. Humans are the primary host, and infection usually occurs from ingestion of embryonated *Trichuris* eggs from vegetables or soil that is contaminated with human feces. The ingested eggs hatch in the small intestine, and the larvae pass directly to the cecum and ascending colon where they attach to the mucosa, mature, and continue the life cycle. Adult worms are slender and approximately 4 cm in length. They live in the colon for about 1 year. After about 3 months, females begin laying 3000 to 20,000 eggs daily. Concurrent infections with *Ascaris,* hookworm, or both are common (Centers for Disease Control and Prevention [CDC], 2002; Peters & Pasvol, 2002).

Incubation

— The incubation period is 2 to 3 months (Bundy & Cooper, 2000; CDC, 2002).

Clinical Findings and Treatment

Signs and Symptoms

— Manifestations of infection depend on the worm burden, with most infections light and asymptomatic. Burden and symptomatology tend to be heaviest in school-age children. Large numbers of worms, either *Trichuris* alone or combined with *Ascaris* or other parasites, can cause abdominal pain, nausea, vomiting, flatulence, chronic diarrhea (with blood and mucus sometimes present), weight loss, and anemia (CDC, 2002; Crompton & Nesheim, 2002; Gilles, 2003).

Complications

— Very heavy worm burdens sometimes result in rectal prolapse. Children with severe chronic infection may have clubbing, growth retardation, and possible cognitive delays.

Common Laboratory Findings

— Anemia and mild eosinophilia are sometimes present (Bundy & Cooper, 2000).

Diagnosis

— Diagnosis is through microscopic identification of eggs in feces. Stool concentration procedures (e.g., sedimentation) are recommended to detect light infections (CDC, 2002).

Differential Diagnosis

— In severe infection the differential diagnosis includes hookworm infection, acute abdomen, and amebiasis (Gilles, 2003).

Treatment

— Current treatment guidelines for adults and children are mebendazole 100 mg PO bid for 3 days (or 500 mg

once) or albendazole 400 mg PO for 3 days. In heavy
infections (more than 1000 eggs per gram of feces),
a 5- to 7-day regimen of albendazole produces an
improved cure rate. Another alternative is nitazoxanide
100 mg PO bid for 3 days (children ages 1 to 3) or
200 mg PO bid for 3 days (children ages 4 to 11).
Note that these medications are effective against both
Ascaris and hookworm. Pregnant women should not
be treated with these drugs in the first trimester
(Juan, Lopez Chegne, Gargala, & Favennec, 2002;
Medical Letter, 2002; Sirivichayakul et al., 2003).

Prevention

Prevention of trichuriasis (Chin, 2000; de Silva, 2003;
Gilles, 2003) includes the following:
- Wash hands after defecation and before contact
  with food.
- Wash vegetables before eating.
- Prevent infants and children from ingesting soil.
- When a sanitary water supply is unavailable, periodic
  deworming of school-age children with mebendazole
  or albendazole has been shown to decrease the overall
  worm burden in the community.

Community education is important in the ongoing effort
to decrease infection.

Reporting

The CDC does not consider trichuriasis to be a
nationally notifiable disease. The World Health
Organization (WHO) classifies trichuriasis as a
Class 5 disease. See Appendix C for details and for
upcoming changes in WHO reporting.

References

Bundy, D.A.P., & Cooper, E. (2000). Nematodes limited to the intestinal tract
(*Enterobius vermicularis, Trichuris trichiura,* and *Capillaria philippinensis*).

In G.T. Strickland (Ed.), *Hunter's tropical medicine and emerging infectious diseases* (8th ed., pp. 719-726). Philadelphia: W.B. Saunders Company.

Centers for Disease Control and Prevention. (2002). Trichuriasis. Retrieved April 30, 2004, from *www.dpd.cdc.gov/dpdx/HTML/Trichuriasis.htm*

Chin, J. (Ed.). (2000). *Control of communicable diseases manual* (17th ed., pp. 513-514). Washington, DC: American Public Health Association.

Crompton, D.W., & Nesheim, M.C. (2002). Nutritional impact of intestinal helminthiasis during the human life cycle. *Annual Review of Nutrition, 22,* 35-59.

de Silva, N.R. (2003). Impact of mass chemotherapy on the morbidity due to soil-transmitted nematodes. *Acta Tropical, 86,* 197-214.

Gilles, H.M. (2003). Soil-transmitted helminths (geohelminths). In G.C. Cook & A.I Zumla (Eds.), *Manson's tropical diseases* (21st ed., pp. 1527-1560). Philadelphia: W.B. Saunders Company.

Juan, J.O., Lopez Chegne, N., Gargala, G., & Favennec, L. (2002). Comparative clinical studies of nitazoxanide, albendazole and praziquantel in the treatment of ascariasis, trichuriasis and hymenolepiasis in children from Peru. *Transcripts of the Royal Society of Tropical Medicine and Hygiene, 96,* 193-196.

Medical Letter. (2002). Drugs for parasitic infections. Retrieved October 30, 2003, from *www.medletter.com/freedocs/parasitic.pdf*

Peters, W., & Pasvol, G. (2002). *Tropical medicine and parasitology* (5th ed.). Chicago: Mosby.

Sirivichayakul, C., Pojjaroen-Anant, C., Wisetsing, P., Praevanit, R., Chanthavanich, P., & Limkittikul, K. (2003). The effectiveness of 3, 5 or 7 days of albendazole for the treatment of *Trichuris trichiura* infection. *Annals of Tropical Medicine and Parasitology, 97,* 847-853.

TRYPANOSOMIASIS, AFRICAN
African sleeping sickness
Geographic Distribution

African trypanosomiasis is found north of the Kalahari desert in sub-Saharan Africa. The disease is endemic in 36 African countries, with most cases occurring in rural areas (Barrett et al., 2003).

Agent and Vector

Trypanosoma brucei is the protozoa that causes African trypanosomiasis. Two subspecies can produce disease in humans: *T. brucei gambiense* and *T. brucei rhodesiense*. *T. brucei gambiense* is transmitted by the riverine tsetse fly (*Glossina palpalis*), is distributed among western and central Africa, and has the highest incidence in the Congo, Angola, Sudan, and Uganda. The riverine tsetse flies are found most commonly in the vegetation around water holes and rivers, especially during dry weather. *T. brucei rhodesiense* is transmitted by the savanna tsetse fly (*G. morsitans*), which is found in eastern and southern Africa and has the highest incidence in Uganda, Tanzania, Mozambique, and Zambia. Savanna tsetse flies are found most commonly in the woodlands and savanna, especially when the bush has been recently cleared.

The life cycle of this protozoa involves only two hosts: humans as the definitive host and the tsetse fly as the intermediate host. In the blood, lymph, and spinal fluid of the infected human host, the organism exists as trypomastigotes, which are ingested during the blood meal of the tsetse fly. The organisms multiply in the midgut of the fly and migrate to the salivary gland, where they exist as epimastigotes. These multiply in the salivary gland, transform into infective metacyclic trypomastigotes, and are transmitted to the next host during a blood meal (Pepin, 2000).

Incubation

A chancre may develop at the site of inoculation 5 to 15 days after the bite; this is more likely to appear with *T. brucei rhodesiense* infection. The incubation period for *T. brucei gambiense* is approximately 2 to 3 weeks. *T. brucei rhodesiense* is a much more acute infection and parasitemia can appear hours to days after the chancre or 1 to 3 weeks after the bite (in the absence of a chancre) (Burri & Brun, 2003; Pepin, 2000).

Clinical Findings and Treatment

Signs and Symptoms

T. BRUCEI GAMBIENSE

In the early stage of infection with *T. brucei gambiense*, the first sign may be irregular cyclic fevers that do not respond to antimalarial medications. Affected individuals may also have lymphadenopathy, especially of the posterior cervical nodes (Winterbottom's sign), headache, myalgias, fatigue, hepatosplenomegaly, pruritus, transient facial edema, and a faint papular cutaneous eruption. As the disease progresses toward the second stage, parasites become more difficult to locate in the blood of the host, endocrine dysfunction (amenorrhea, loss of libido, spontaneous abortion) may appear, and severe anemia may develop.

The second stage occurs when trypanosomes invade the central nervous system (CNS), which may be several months to years after the initial infection. Affected people first develop intractable severe headaches, followed by impaired motor function, ataxia, slurred speech, abnormal Parkinsonian movements, and possibly personality changes or psychotic features, such as hallucinations or mania. Daytime somnolence develops, worsens with time, and may be associated with nighttime restlessness. These people typically become apathetic and disconnected from their surroundings. Several of these neurologic symptoms are reversible with treatment; however, many patients die without ever receiving the appropriate medications.

T. BRUCEI RHODESIENSE

The clinical features of this form of African trypanosomiasis are similar to *T. brucei gambiense;* however, it progresses much more rapidly. The incubation, first, and second phases of the disease, along with CNS involvement, occur over the course of a few weeks. The inoculation chancre occurs more often in this form (Figure 89-1), and systemic symptoms appear hours to days later. Cervical lymphadenopathy may develop but is less common than with *T. brucei gambiense.* The CNS symptoms are the same as with *T. brucei gambiense* infection; however, the rapid progression of disease can cause death within 1 to 3 months (Burri & Brun, 2003; Kennedy, 2004; Pepin, 2000; Stich, Abel, & Krishna, 2002).

Complications

Because of somnolence and inactivity during the second phase of the disease, many patients develop bed sores, secondary bacterial infections, wasting, and malnutrition. These and other complications, including aspiration pneumonia, seizures, and cerebral edema, may ultimately lead to death. Myocarditis is a rare complication but may result in arrhythmias, heart failure, or death (Burri & Brun, 2003; Kennedy, 2004).

Common Laboratory Findings

Nonspecific laboratory abnormalities may include anemia, thrombocytopenia, hypergammaglobulinemia,

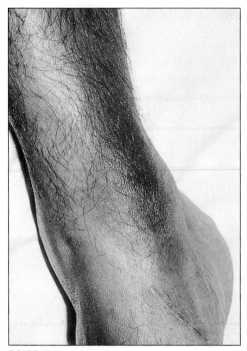

FIGURE 89–1

Trypanosomal chancre. (*Source:* From Peters, W., & Pasvol, G. [2002]. *Tropical medicine and parasitology* [5th ed., p. 51]. Chicago: Mosby.)

and an elevated sedimentation rate. Coagulation abnormalities and liver function elevations are seen more often with *T. brucei rhodesiense.* The lumbar puncture in the second stage of disease reveals lymphocytic pleocytosis and increased protein (40 to 200 mg/100 mL). The CNS leukocyte count may correlate with clinical symptoms: patients rarely have somnolence with less than 50/mm³, usually have debilitating somnolence with more than 100/mm³, and may have neck stiffness with more than 300/mm³ (Kennedy, 2004; Pepin, 2000).

Diagnosis

Wet and thick smears of the blood, as well as smears of lymph node aspirate fluid, may reveal trypanosomes. In *T. brucei gambiense*, the parasite count may be low and the yield of the smears can be improved by using hematocrit centrifugation (with analysis of the buffy coat) or the miniature anion-exchange centrifugation technique, which filters out the organisms. If an inoculation chancre is present, the organisms may be found in a wet smear of the wound exudate. If CNS disease is suspected, a lumbar puncture must be performed. The organism can be identified in the cerebrospinal fluid (CSF) in several ways: double centrifugation with microscopic analysis of the sediment, latex agglutination assay for immunoglobulin M (IgM) quantitation, and CSF polymerase chain reaction (PCR) to identify trypanosome DNA. Serology can be performed using the card agglutination test for trypanosomiasis (CATT) in order to identify *T. brucei gambiense*. This test is sensitive and can be performed in the field, but specificity is lacking due to cross-reactivity with animal trypanosomes. There are no serologic tests to identify *T. brucei rhodesiense* (Kennedy, 2004; Pepin, 2000).

Differential Diagnosis

Other infections with similar symptoms that may occur in these endemic areas need to be distinguished from African trypanosomiasis. They include malaria, tuberculosis, HIV infection, leishmaniasis, toxoplasmosis, typhoid, hookworm infection, syphilis, cryptococcus, and viral encephalitis (Kennedy, 2004; Pepin, 2000).

Treatment

To determine the proper treatment, the stage of disease and the organism need to be determined. CNS disease requires drugs that cross the blood-brain barrier and often have greater toxicity.

T. BRUCEI GAMBIENSE

The early stage of *T. brucei gambiense* can be treated with pentamidine 4 mg/kg/day IM daily to every other day in a series of 7 to 10 injections or diminazene aceturate series of one to three injections IM of 5 to 7 mg/kg over 2 days. Pentamidine is well tolerated, but possible side effects include reversible renal toxicity, hypotension, cardiac toxicity, pancreatic toxicity, hepatic impairment, and hematologic abnormalities. Diminazene has similar side effects to pentamidine but treatment is shorter, less painful when injected, and costs less. On the other hand, diminazene may have twice the failure rate of pentamidine and has demonstrated severe neurologic toxicity in animal models.

The late stage of disease can be treated with eflornithine 100 mg/kg in adults, 150 mg/kg in children, IV q6h for 14 days or melarsoprol. (For CSF leukocyte counts of less than 20/mm^3, give two series of three daily injections of 3.6 mg/kg each, up to 180 mg. For CSF leukocyte counts above 20 mm^3, give three series of three daily injections of the same dose.) Bone marrow toxicity is a common side effect of eflornithine, in addition to diarrhea, seizures, vomiting, and hearing loss. Neurotoxicity is most often seen with melarsoprol and can lead to fatal encephalopathy, with symptoms including seizures, impaired consciousness, status epilepticus, and coma. Other possible side effects of melarsoprol include peripheral thrombophlebitis, polyneuropathy, headache, agranulocytosis, cardiac, renal, and hepatic toxicity.

T. BRUCEI RHODESIENSE

Suramin 4 to 5 mg/kg as IV test dose, followed by IV injections of 20 mg/kg given on days 1, 3, 7, 14, and 21 is the first-line treatment in early disease and may be more effective than pentamidine. Side effects include nephrotoxicity, which is usually reversible, hypersensitivity reactions, hemolytic anemia, peripheral neuropathy, and bone marrow toxicity.

— Late disease can only be treated with melarsoprol, because eflornithine is ineffective even at twice the usual dose. Treatment-related encephalopathy and death are more common with *T. brucei rhodesiense*; therefore, the recommended regimen starts with small doses and increases gradually in order to minimize the risk. The regimen is 0.36 mg/kg (day 1), 0.72 mg/kg (day 2), 1.1 mg/kg (day 3), 1.8 mg/kg (days 10, 11, and 12), 2.2 mg/kg (day 19), 2.9 mg/kg (day 20), and 3.6 mg/kg (up to 180 mg) on days 21, 28, 29, and 30. Nifurtimox 5 mg/kg tid IV injection for 14 to 21 days can be used with melarsoprol in patients unresponsive to other treatments, those who relapse with CNS involvement, or those who live in an area with high relapse rates. Major side effects of nifurtimox are seizures, psychotic reactions, peripheral neuropathy, gastrointestinal disturbances, and generalized skin reactions.

— Prednisolone can be used to reduce the risk of encephalopathy with melarsoprol treatment and is given as 1 mg/kg/day (up to 40 mg), starting 2 days before the treatment and tapering after the last treatment over 3 days. If encephalopathy occurs, it may be treated with an anticonvulsant, dexamethasone, and subcutaneous epinephrine (Bouteille, Oukem, Bisser, & Dumas, 2003; Burri & Brun, 2003; Fairlamb, 2003; Pepin, 2000; Stich et al., 2002).

MONITORING

— Patients should be monitored for 2 years after treatment, and a lumbar puncture should be done every 6 months in *T. brucei gambiense* and every 3 months in *T. brucei rhodesiense*. Previous early-stage patients are considered in relapse if they have a CSF white cell count above

20 mm^3, and they should be treated with melarsoprol. For patients who previously had late-stage disease, a relapse (or reinfection) is suspected if the CSF white cell count is above 50 mm^3 or has doubled since the last examination. Retreatment with melarsoprol or drug combinations (such as melarsoprol plus nifurtimox) is recommended.

Prevention

- Prevention of African trypanosomiasis (Barrett, et al., 2003; Bouteille, et al., 2003; Burri & Brun, 2003) includes (1) health care and follow-up to prevent further transmission from infected persons and (2) vector control.
- Many tactics have been used to prevent African trypanosomiasis. Because patients are contagious long before the onset of CNS involvement, early identification and treatment of infected individuals can lead to decreased prevalence and transmission of disease. Once the affected individuals have CNS involvement, most are not parasitemic and do not pose a risk for transmission of the parasite. Ideally, endemic areas should be surveyed once a year, with treatment distributed to infected individuals. The CATT may be used to identify possible infections, and further diagnostic testing can be performed on those with positive reactions.
- Vector control includes the following (Robert, 2000):
    - Placing insecticide-impregnated tsetse fly traps with visual and olfactory attractants in high-risk areas near rivers. This helps decrease fly populations and the occurrence of new cases, but these regions still need surveillance for human reservoirs since the incubation period can be long, especially with *T. brucei gambiense* infection.

- Insecticide spraying of specific areas attractive to flies, for example, vegetation bordering streams and rivers or, in the case of savanna tsetse flies, only the parts of trees and vegetation attractive to resting flies.

— Community education of infected and noninfected persons is important in the ongoing prevention of human sleeping sickness.

Reporting

— The U.S. Centers for Disease Control and Prevention does not consider African trypanosomiasis to be a nationally notifiable disease. The World Health Organization (WHO) considers African trypanosomiasis to be a Class 3B disease. See Appendix C for details and for upcoming changes in WHO reporting.

References

Barrett, M.P., Burchmore, R.J., Stich, A., Lazzari, J.O., Frasch, A.C., et al., (2003). The trypanosomiases. *Lancet, 362,* 1469-1480.

Bouteille, B., Oukem, O., Bisser, S., & Dumas, M. (2003). Treatment perspectives for human African trypanosomiasis. *Fundamentals of Clinical Pharmacology, 17,* 171-181.

Burri, B., & Brun, R. (2003). Human African trypanosomiasis. In G.C. Cook & A.I. Zumla (Eds.), *Manson's tropical diseases* (21st ed., pp. 1303-1323). Philadelphia: W.B. Saunders Company.

Fairlamb, A.H. (2003). Chemotherapy of human African trypanosomiasis: Current and future prospects. *Trends in Parasitology, 19,* 488-494.

Kennedy, P.G. (2004). Human African trypanosomiasis of the CNS: Current issues and challenges. *Journal of Clinical Investigation, 113,* 496-504.

Pepin, J. (2000). African Trypanosomiasis. In G.T. Strickland (Ed.), *Hunter's tropical medicine and emerging infectious diseases* (8th ed., pp. 643-653). Philadelphia: W.B. Saunders Company.

Robert, L.L. (2000). Control of arthropods of medical importance. In G.T. Strickland (Ed.), *Hunter's tropical medicine and emerging infectious diseases* (8th ed., pp. 1019-1036). Philadelphia: W.B. Saunders Company.

Stich, A., Abel, P.M., & Krishna, S. (2002). Human African trypanosomiasis. *British Medical Journal, 325,* 203-206.

TUBERCULOSIS

Geographic Distribution

Tuberculosis (TB) occurs worldwide, with the highest incidence in Africa, but the highest fatality rate in Southeast Asia. The incidence of multidrug-resistant TB is highest in Eastern Europe and central Asia, with rates 10 times higher than in the rest of the world. About one-third of the world's population is infected with the TB bacillus. Worldwide, about 8.5 million new TB cases and 2 million deaths from TB occur annually (*Weekly Epidemiological Record,* 2004; World Health Organization [WHO], 2004).

Agent and Vector

TB is caused by the acid-fast bacillus *Mycobacterium tuberculosis*, for which humans are the primary reservoir. Other *Mycobacterium* complex agents include *M. africanum*, which is found in equatorial Africa, and *M. bovis*, which is found in cattle. Bovine TB is spread by ingestion of unpasteurized dairy products or airborne spread from cattle infected with *M. bovis*. *M. tuberculosis* is usually spread by airborne droplet nuclei (1 to 5 μm in size) produced by a person with active pulmonary or laryngeal TB, especially when coughing, and also when sneezing or singing (Figure 90-1). Droplet nuclei are small enough that they may remain suspended in the air for hours, especially in dark, poorly ventilated environments. Less common means of transmission include direct invasion through mucous membranes or breaks in the skin. Medical procedures such as intubation, bronchoscopy, and autopsy are relatively common means of transmission to health care workers.

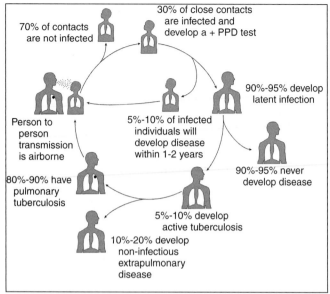

FIGURE 90–1

Tuberculosis transmission cycle. (*Source:* From Strickland, G.T. [2000]. *Hunter's tropical medicine and emerging infectious diseases* [8th ed., p. 495]. Philadelphia: W.B. Saunders Company.)

Primary infection occurs when one or more infectious particles are inhaled and deposited in terminal alveoli. The organisms are ingested by macrophages, in which they proliferate and spread locally. Additional blood-borne phagocytic cells aggregate around this local focus to form a foreign body granuloma that is known as the primary focus. Other bacilli spread to regional lymph nodes, resulting in lymphangitis and lymphadenitis, which, together with the primary focus, comprise the primary complex of TB. Hematogenous and lymphatic spread also occur, but in most cases (about 95%), the host immune response is successful in containing the initial infection, and the lung and lymph node lesions become fibrotic and later calcified.

However, within these dormant lesions, tubercle bacilli remain viable for years.
- Approximately 5% of infected patients develop primary clinical disease. This occurs through several mechanisms, including rupture of a primary focus or an involved lymph node, impingement of a lymph node on lung structures, or tissue destruction caused by progression of the primary lesion. Hematogenous dissemination may cause widespread disease, most often involving the central nervous system, kidneys, and bones (Centers for Disease Control and Prevention [CDC], 2002; Chin, 2000; Grange & Zumla, 2003; WHO, 2004).
- Postprimary clinical TB, occurring in 2% to 5% of patients with primary clinical disease, may result from progression of the primary lesion, from endogenous activation of the primary lesion, or from exogenous reinfection. Conditions that increase the risk of progression to active disease (CDC, 2000) include the following:
  - HIV infection
  - Very young or very old age
  - Substance abuse
  - Recent infection
  - Chest radiographic findings suggestive of previous TB
  - Diabetes mellitus
  - Silicosis
  - Prolonged corticosteroid therapy
  - Other immunosuppressive therapy
  - Cancer of the head or neck
  - Hematologic or reticuloendothelial diseases
  - End-stage renal disease
  - Intestinal bypass or gastrectomy
  - Chronic malabsorption syndromes
  - Low body weight (10% or more below the ideal)
- Postprimary pulmonary TB is characterized by large progressive upper-lobe lesions with necrotic material that resemble tumors (tuberculomas). The tuberculomas

cavitate and additional lesions develop in the lungs.
At this stage, the patient is highly infectious. Lesions
may also develop in the larynx and gastrointestinal
system.

Incubation

The incubation period for primary infection in otherwise
healthy persons ranges from 3 to 8 weeks for the
development of tuberculin positivity and/or the primary
complex. Postprimary disease can occur after a latency
period of several years. Immigrant communities from
high-incidence countries tend to have high incidence
rates even years after resettlement (Grange
& Zumla, 2003; Vos et al., 2004; WHO, 2004).

Clinical Findings and Treatment

Signs and Symptoms

The most common form of TB is pulmonary.
Extrapulmonary TB may affect any organ system and
is most common in children and persons with
immunodeficiency (Chin, 2000).

PULMONARY TB

Primary infection is usually asymptomatic but in some
cases causes mild and self-limited fever and fatigue.
Lymphadenopathy may rarely lead to airway obstruction,
cough, wheezing and/or atelectasis, especially in children.
Radiographic findings are often negative in primary
infection. Rarely, retrosternal pain or erythema
nodosum develop.

Early manifestations of primary pulmonary TB are
varied and may include constitutional symptoms of
fatigue, malaise, weight loss, low-grade fever, and night
sweats. Manifestations of later, advanced disease include
constitutional symptoms as well as cough (initially
nonproductive, sometimes primarily in the morning,
and later productive), chest pain, hemoptysis, and

hoarseness. Lower lobe infiltrates are common, as is hilar adenopathy. In some cases the only manifestations are weight loss and an appearance of chronic illness.
Manifestations of postprimary TB are similar, except that progressive worsening is experienced. Nodular infiltrates and cavities are frequently observed, but adenopathy is less common. Pulmonary fibrosis is a feature of continued progression (see Complications section).
Children most commonly develop illness as part of the initial infection with *M. tuberculosis* (primary TB). Primary TB in children is characterized by intrathoracic adenopathy, midlung and lower lung zone infiltrates, and the absence of cavitation. However, children and adolescents may also develop illness similar to that seen in adults (Grange & Zumla, 2003; WHO, 2004).

EXTRAPULMONARY TB

Extrapulmonary TB most commonly affects persons with HIV/AIDS or the very young or very old. The following are the most common extrapulmonary forms of TB:

- Tuberculous adenitis is the most common extrapulmonary form of TB and usually affects head and neck lymph nodes.
- Genitourinary TB usually affects the kidneys and is characterized by dysuria, urgency, and flank pain, and occasionally constitutional symptoms.
- Bone and joint TB occurs most often in children and usually affects the spine and joints of the lower or upper extremities. Spinal TB (Pott's disease) begins with chronic back pain and, because diagnosis is often delayed, leads to bone destruction and consequent kyphosis, disability, and neurologic sequelae.
- Central nervous system TB includes tuberculous meningitis, single space-occupying lesions,

or disseminated miliary (millet-seed shaped) lesions. Tuberculous meningitis occurs most often in infants and is an emergency characterized by a high mortality rate and high risk of disability in survivors.

- Miliary (disseminated) TB is characterized by numerous small lesions in the lungs and often elsewhere (especially kidneys and spleen). Miliary TB may be an acute and rapidly progressive disease, or chronic and insidious.
- Cryptic (disseminated) TB is primarily a disease of severely immunosuppressed persons, including the very old, and is characterized by progressive and severe constitutional symptoms, numerous lesions too small to be detected on X-ray, and death.
- Other forms of extrapulmonary TB include abdominal (intestinal and peritoneal), skin (Figures 90-2 and 90-3), pericardial, upper respiratory tract, ocular, and adrenal (Grange & Zumla, 2003; Small & Selcer, 2000; WHO, 2004).

Complications

Complications (in addition to those described earlier) are more common in postprimary TB and include pleural effusion, empyema, pneumothorax, and, in far advanced disease, chronic obstructive pulmonary disease (COPD) and cor pulmonale. Rarely, intestinal ulcers may occur. Complications increase with immunosuppression (Grange & Zumla, 2003; Small & Selcer, 2000; WHO, 2004).

Common Laboratory Findings

Common laboratory findings may include elevated lymphocyte count, raised erythrocyte sedimentation rate, elevated C-reactive protein levels, and mild anemia (Grange & Zumla, 2003).

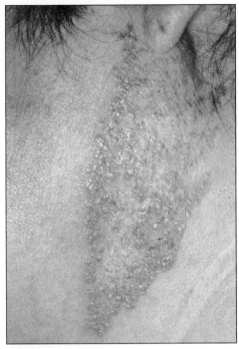

FIGURE 90–2

Verrucous tuberculosis. (*Source:* Courtesy of the University of Texas Southwestern Department of Dermatology.)

Diagnosis

The diagnosis of TB usually begins with clinical suspicion or screening of high-risk populations, such as refugees or immigrants from high-incidence countries or homeless persons (Table 90-1). The tuberculin skin test establishes whether a person has been infected, and active disease is confirmed by microscopic examination of sputum or other body fluids, isolation of *M. tuberculosis* on culture, radiologic studies, and/or molecular methods discussed later (CDC, 2000; Grange & Zumla, 2003; Small & Selcer, 2000; WHO, 2004).

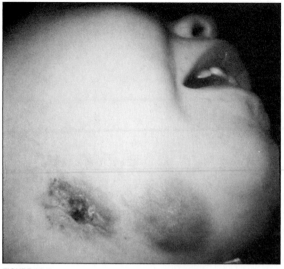

FIGURE 90–3

Scrofuloderma tuberculosis. (*Source:* Courtesy of the University of Texas Southwestern Department of Dermatology.)

TUBERCULIN SKIN TEST

Although not diagnostic, the tuberculin skin test identifies those who have been infected with the tubercle bacillus, but does not differentiate between those with active TB, past infection, or recipients of bacille Calmette-Guérin (BCG) vaccination. The most commonly used tuberculin skin test is the Mantoux test, in which 0.1 mL (1 international unit) of purified protein derivative (PPD) is injected intradermally into the volar surface of the forearm. Other tuberculin skin tests are the Heaf and tine tests. Reactivity to PPD in the Mantoux test is measured and positivity classified according to the area of induration (but not erythema) and the presence of risk factors as follows:

- Induration greater than 5 mm is classified as positive in persons who are HIV positive, who are recent

TABLE 90–1

Tuberculosis as Classified by the CDC

Class	Type	Description
0	No TB exposure Not infected	No history of exposure Negative reaction to tuberculin skin test
1	TB exposure No evidence of infection	History of exposure Negative reaction to tuberculin skin test
2	TB infection No disease (Latent)	Positive reaction to tuberculin skin test Negative bacteriologic studies (if done) No clinical, bacteriologic, or radiographic evidence of active TB
3	TB, clinically active	*M. tuberculosis* cultured (if done) Clinical, bacteriologic, or radiographic evidence of current disease
4	TB, not clinically active	History of episode(s) of TB or Abnormal but stable X-ray findings Positive reaction to the tuberculin skin test Negative bacteriologic studies (if done) and No clinical or X-ray evidence of current disease
5	TB suspected	Diagnosis pending

Source: Centers for Disease Control and Prevention. (2000). Core curriculum on tuberculosis. Retrieved May 12, 2004, from *www.cdc.gov/nchstp/tb/pubs/slidesets/core/default.htm*

contacts of a TB case, who have fibrotic changes on chest X-ray consistent with old, healed TB, or who have immunosuppression, such as organ transplant recipients.

- Induration greater than 10 mm is classified as positive in persons who are recent arrivals from high prevalence areas, who are injection drug users, who are residents or employees of high-risk congregate settings, who work with *M. tuberculosis* in laboratories, who have clinical conditions that place them at high risk (see earlier discussion), who are younger than 4 years old, or who are children or adolescents exposed to adults in high-risk categories.
- Induration greater than 15 mm is classified as positive in persons with no known risk factors for TB.

Targeted skin testing programs should be conducted only among high-risk groups. False-positive reactions may occur in persons with nontuberculous mycobacteria or who have had BCG vaccination. False-negative reaction may result from anergy secondary to HIV infection, overwhelming TB, severe or febrile illness, viral infection, live-virus vaccinations, or immunosuppressive therapy (CDC, 2003).

MICROSCOPY

Microscopic examination of sputum samples for acid-fast bacilli is the most common means of diagnosis. Three sputum specimens should be obtained 8 to 24 hours apart. In patients who are not producing sputum spontaneously, induction of sputum using aerosolized hypertonic saline or bronchoscopy (performed under infection control procedures) may be needed to obtain specimens. Positive smears are sufficient to begin therapy. Other body fluids may also contain acid-fast bacilli, including bronchoalveolar lavage, gastric washings (often used for young children who cannot produce sputum), cerebrospinal fluid, pleural aspirates, lymph node aspirates, bone marrow, and tissue biopsies.

CULTURE

— When possible, the diagnosis should be confirmed by isolation of *M. tuberculosis* on culture. If bacteriologic confirmation is not possible, active disease is still presumed if there is (1) a positive tuberculin skin test and (2) strong clinical evidence of TB by histologic or radiologic studies.

RADIOLOGIC STUDIES

— Plain radiography of the chest is the most common means of radiologic confirmation. Chest X-ray is sensitive, but not specific, and interpretation requires an experienced radiologist. Computed tomography scans, radioisotope scans, and magnetic resonance imaging are also used.

MOLECULAR METHODS

— Molecular methods of TB diagnosis include polymerase chain reaction (PCR), ligase chain reaction, and nucleic acid amplification.

Differential Diagnosis

— The differential diagnosis for pulmonary TB includes pneumonia, abscess, lung cancer, pulmonary Kaposi's sarcoma, pulmonary helminthic infection (hydatid, schistosomiasis, paragonimiasis), and COPD.
The differential diagnosis for other forms includes an enormous variety of diseases depending on the system and manifestations of infection (Grange & Zumla, 2003; Small & Selcer, 2000).

Treatment

— The treatment of TB is complex, and the authors recommend consulting a competent public health department when possible. TB is a reportable disease worldwide so, at minimum, public health authorities should be notified of new cases. Clinicians should also consult treatment guidelines that are periodically published and updated by the CDC and WHO. The goals of treatment are to (1) cure the patient and (2) minimize the risk of transmission of *M. tuberculosis* to others. Because of public health concerns, the health provider is responsible for the patient's successful completion of therapy. Directly observed therapy, in which patients are observed ingesting each dose, is the primary means of ensuring adherence to treatment. Treatment also may include other means of increasing adherence, such as social services, housing assistance, compliance rewards, and drug treatment (CDC, 2003).

In general, the regimens recommended for adults are also the regimens of choice for infants, children, and adolescents, with the exception that ethambutol is not used routinely in children. Medications and dosages recommended by the CDC (2003) are listed next. These are taken directly from the CDC, American Thoracic Society, and Infectious Diseases Society of America "Statement on the Treatment of Tuberculosis" published in the *MMWR*. Readers are encouraged to use that document for more comprehensive information, especially regarding drug toxicities, drug interactions, and the treatment of multidrug-resistant TB.

FIRST-LINE DRUGS

Isoniazid is a first-line agent for all TB known or presumed to be susceptible to it. The drug has early bactericidal activity against rapidly dividing cells. Dosing for adults is 5 mg/kg (up to 300 mg) daily; 15 mg/kg (up to 900 mg) one to three times per week. Dosing for children is 10 to 15 mg/kg (up to 300 mg) daily; 20 to 30 mg/kg (up to 900 mg) twice weekly.

Rifampin is a first-line agent for all TB known or presumed to be susceptible to it. The drug has activity against rapidly dividing organisms (early bactericidal to prevent emergence of rifampin resistance when primary resistance to isoniazid may be present. Ethambutol is generally not recommended for routine use in children when visual acuity cannot be monitored. However, if a child has adult-type or multidrug-resistant TB, ethambutol should be used. Dosing for adults is 15 to 20 mg/kg per day. Dosing for children is 15 to 20 mg/kg per day (up to 2.5 g); 50 mg/kg twice weekly (up to 2.5 g).

Two brand-name combination products are available in the United States as follows:

- *Rifamate* contains rifampin (300 mg) and isoniazid (150 mg).
- *Rifater* contains rifampin (120 mg), isoniazid (50 mg), and pyrazinamide (300 mg).

SECOND-LINE DRUGS

Cycloserine is used for treating patients with drug-resistant TB caused by organisms with known or presumed susceptibility to it. The drug may also be used temporarily for patients with acute hepatitis in combination with other nonhepatotoxic drugs. Dosing for adults is 10 to 15 mg/kg per day (up to 1 g). Usually 500 to 750 mg/day is given in two doses with the goal of achieving serum concentrations of 20 to 35 mg/mL. Dosing for children is 10 to 15 mg/kg per day (up to 1 g/day). Toxicity is more common at doses of more than 500 mg/day. There are no data to support intermittent administration.

Ethionamide is used for patients with drug-resistant TB caused by organisms that have demonstrated or presumed susceptibility to the drug. Dosing for adults is 15 to 20 mg/kg per day (up to 1 g/day), usually 500 to 750 mg/day in a single daily dose or two divided doses. Dosing for children is 15 to 20 mg/kg per day (up to 1 g/day). There are no data to support intermittent dosing.

activity) and against semidormant bacterial populations (sterilizing activity). Rifampin is an essential component of all short-course regimens. Dosing for adults is 10 mg/kg (up to 600 mg) daily or two to three times weekly. Dosing for children is 10 to 20 mg/kg (up to 600 mg) daily or twice weekly.

— *Rifabutin* is used as a substitute for rifampin for all forms of TB known or presumed to be susceptible to it. Rifabutin is generally used in patients taking medications with unacceptable interactions with rifampin or who cannot tolerate rifampin. Dosing for adults is 5 mg/kg (up to 300 mg) daily, or two to three times weekly. Dosage may be adjusted for patients who also take protease inhibitors or nonnucleoside reverse transcriptase inhibitors (see *www.cdc.gov*). Appropriate dosage for children is not known.

— *Rifapentine* may be used once weekly with isoniazid in the continuation phase of treatment for HIV-seronegative patients with noncavitary, drug-susceptible pulmonary TB who have negative sputum smears at completion of the initial phase of treatment. Dosing for adults is 10 mg/kg (up to 600 mg) once weekly during the continuation phase of treatment. Rifapentine is not approved for use in children.

— *Pyrazinamide* is a first-line agent for the treatment of all forms of TB caused by organisms with known or presumed susceptibility to it. Pyrazinamide is thought to exert greatest activity against dormant or semidormant organisms contained within macrophages or the acidic environment of caseous foci. Dosing for adults is 10 mg/kg (up to 600 mg) once daily, twice weekly, or three times weekly. Dosing for children is 10 to 20 mg/kg (up to 600 mg) once daily or twice weekly.

— *Ethambutol* is a first-line drug for treating all forms of TB. It is included in initial treatment regimens primarily

- *Streptomycin* and ethambutol are approximately equivalent when used in the initial phase of treatment with 6-month regimens, except that there is a relatively high rate of resistance among patients likely to have acquired *M. tuberculosis* in a high-incidence country. Dosing for adults is 15 mg/kg per day (up to 1 g/day) parenterally, usually given as a single daily dose (5 to 7 days/week) initially, and then two or three times a week after the first 2 to 4 months or after culture conversion, depending on the efficacy of the other drugs in the regimen. For persons older than age 59, the dose should be reduced to 10 mg/kg per day (up to 750 mg). The dosing frequency should be reduced (i.e., 12 to 15 mg/kg per dose two or three times per week) in persons with renal insufficiency. Dosing for children is 20 to 40 mg/kg per day (up to 1 g/day).
- *Amikacin* and *kanamycin* are closely related injectable drugs used for patients with drug-resistant TB whose isolate has demonstrated or has presumed susceptibility to them. There is nearly always complete cross-resistance between the two drugs, but most streptomycin-resistant strains are susceptible to both. Dosing for adults is 15 mg/kg per day (up to 1.0 g/day), IM or IV, usually given as a single daily dose (5 to 7 days/week) initially, and then reducing to two or three times a week after the first 2 to 4 months or after culture conversion, depending on the efficacy of the other drugs in the regimen. For persons older than age 59, the dose should be reduced to 10 mg/kg per day (up to 750 mg). The dosing frequency should be reduced (i.e., 12 to 15 mg/kg per dose, two or three times per week) in persons with renal insufficiency. Dosing for children is 15 to 30 mg/kg per day (up to 1 g/day) intramuscular or intravenous as a single daily dose.
- *Capreomycin* is a second-line injectable drug used for patients with drug-resistant TB caused by organisms that have known or presumed susceptibility to it.

Dosing for adults is 15 mg/kg per day (up to 1 g/day). It is usually given as a single daily dose five to seven times a week, and reduced to two or three times a week after the first 2 to 4 months or after culture conversion, depending on the efficacy of the other drugs in the regimen. For persons older than age 59, the dose should be reduced to 10 mg/kg per day (up to 750 mg). The dosing frequency should be reduced to 12 to 15 mg/kg two or three times per week in persons with renal insufficiency. Dosing for children is 15 to 30 mg/kg per day (up to 1 g/day) as a single daily or twice weekly dose.

p-*Aminosalicylic acid* is an oral drug used in treatment of drug-resistant TB caused by organisms that are susceptible to it. Dosing for adults is 8 to 12 g/day in two or three doses. For *p*-aminosalicylic acid granules, 4 g two to three times daily is the usual dosage. Dosing for children is 200 to 300 mg/kg per day in two to four divided doses.

Fluoroquinolones are used only for the treatment of drug-susceptible TB in patients who are intolerant of first-line drugs. Levofloxacin, moxifloxacin, and gatifloxacin have the most activity against *M. tuberculosis.* Levofloxacin is the preferred oral drug for treating drug-resistant TB caused by organisms known or presumed to be sensitive to this class of drugs, or when first-line drugs cannot be used because of intolerance. Data on long-term safety and tolerability of moxifloxacin and gatifloxacin, especially at doses above 400 mg/day, are limited. Cross-resistance has been demonstrated among ciprofloxacin, ofloxacin, and levofloxacin and presumably is a class effect. For levofloxacin, the dosing for adults is 500 to 1000 mg daily. Although long-term (more than several weeks) use of fluoroquinolones in children and adolescents has not been approved because of concerns about effects on bone and cartilage growth, most experts agree that the drug should be considered for children with multidrug-resistant TB. The optimal dose is not known.

Four basic regimens are recommended for treating adults with TB caused by organisms that are known or presumed to be susceptible to isoniazid, rifampin, pyrazinamide, and ethambutol. Children, depending on the circumstances, may not receive ethambutol in the initial phase of a 6-month regimen, but adult and child regimens are otherwise identical. Each regimen has an initial phase of 2 months, followed by a choice of several options for the continuation phase of either 4 or 7 months.

• *Six-month treatment regimen.* The current minimal acceptable duration of treatment for all children and adults with culture-positive TB is 6 months (26 weeks). The initial phase of a 6-month regimen for adults should consist of a 2-month period of isoniazid, rifampin, pyrazinamide, and ethambutol given daily throughout (56 doses) (Regimen 1), daily for 2 weeks (13 to 14 doses) followed by two times weekly for 6 weeks (12 doses) (Regimen 2), or three times weekly (24 doses) (Regimen 3). The continuation phase of treatment should consist of isoniazid and rifampin given for a minimum of 4 months (18 weeks). Patients should be treated until they have received the specified total number of doses for the treatment regimen (shown here in parentheses): daily (126 doses) (Regimen 1a), twice weekly (35 doses) (Regimens 1b and 2a), or three times weekly (54 doses) (Regimen 3a). The continuation phase should be extended for an additional 3 months for patients who have cavitation on the initial or follow-up chest X-ray and who are culture positive at the time of completion of the initial phase of treatment (2 months). Patients who are HIV negative, who do not have cavities on chest X-ray, and who have negative sputum acid-fast bacillus smears at completion of the initial phase of treatment may be treated with once weekly isoniazid and rifapentine in the continuation phase for 4 months. If the culture of the sputum obtained at 2 months is positive, observational data and expert opinion suggest that the continuation phase of once weekly isoniazid and rifapentine should be 7 months.

- *Nine-month treatment regimen.* If pyrazinamide cannot be included in the initial regimen, or if the isolate is determined to be resistant to pyrazinamide (more common in infection due to *M. bovis* and *M. bovis* var.), a regimen consisting of isoniazid, rifampin, and ethambutol should be given for the initial 2 months (56 doses) (Regimen 4) followed by isoniazid and rifampin for 7 months given either daily (217 doses) or twice weekly (62 doses) (Regimens 4a and 4b).

TREATMENT REGIMENS IN CULTURE-NEGATIVE TB

Note that treatment is initiated on a strong index of suspicion before sputum or other culture results are determined. If the cultures are negative, the tuberculin skin test is positive, and there is no response to treatment, the options are as follows:

- Stop treatment if rifampin and pyrazinamide have been given for at least 2 months; or
- Continue treatment with rifampin, with or without isoniazid, for a total of 4 months; or
- Continue treatment with isoniazid for a total of 9 months.

All three of these options provide adequate therapy for persons with prior TB once active disease has been excluded.

— If clinical suspicion for active TB is low, the options are to begin treatment with combination chemotherapy or to delay treatment until additional data are obtained. Even when the suspicion of active TB is low, treatment for latent TB infection with a single drug should not begin until active TB has been excluded.

— In low-suspicion patients not initially treated, if cultures remain negative, the PPD-tuberculin skin test is positive, and the chest X-ray is unchanged after 2 months, three treatment options are available. The preferred options are isoniazid for 9 months or rifampin, with or without isoniazid, for 4 months. Rifampin and pyrazinamide for a total of 2 months can be used for patients not likely to complete a longer regimen and who can be monitored closely. However, this last regimen has been associated with an increased risk of hepatotoxicity and should be used only in the limited circumstances described.

BASELINE AND FOLLOW-UP EVALUATIONS

— Patients suspected of having TB should have specimens collected for culture and microscopic examination. Susceptibility testing for isoniazid, rifampin, and ethambutol should be performed on an initial positive culture, regardless of the source. Second-line drug susceptibility testing should be done only in reference laboratories and be limited to specimens from patients who have had prior therapy, have been in contact with a patient with known drug resistance, have demonstrated resistance to rifampin or two other first-line drugs, or who have positive cultures after more than 3 months of treatment.

— When treatment begins, in addition to the microbiological examinations, it is recommended that all patients with TB have counseling and testing for HIV infection. Patients with epidemiologic factors suggesting a risk for hepatitis B or C (e.g., injection drug use, birth in Asia or Africa, or HIV infection) should have serologic tests for these viruses. HIV-infected patients should also undergo a CD4+ lymphocyte count measurement. Measurements of liver enzymes, bilirubin, alkaline phosphatase, and serum creatinine and a platelet count should be obtained for all adults. Testing of visual acuity and color vision should be performed when ethambutol is to be used.

– During treatment of patients with pulmonary TB, at a minimum, a sputum specimen for acid-fast bacillus smear and culture should be obtained at monthly intervals until two consecutive specimens are negative. As described subsequently, important decisions concerning the continuation-phase regimen hinge on the microbiological status at the end of the initial phase of treatment; obtaining sputum specimens is critical if sputum conversion to negative has not already occurred. For patients who had positive acid-fast bacillus smears at the time of diagnosis, follow-up smears may be obtained at more frequent intervals (e.g., every 2 weeks until two consecutive specimens are negative) to provide an early assessment of the response to treatment, especially when the risk of transmission is high. In some circumstances, acid-fact bacillus–positive sputum is culture negative, most commonly among patients with far advanced cavitary TB after the first months of treatment. It is thought that these organisms are dead and that their presence is not a sign of treatment failure, even if noted later in treatment. However, repeat cultures should be obtained to confirm that the earlier culture result was correct and not a false negative.

– Drug susceptibility tests should be repeated on isolates from patients who have positive cultures after 3 months of treatment (treatment failure). Patients who have positive cultures after 4 months of treatment should be considered as having failed treatment and be managed accordingly.

— For patients with extrapulmonary TB, the frequency and kinds of evaluations will depend on the sites involved and the ease with which specimens can be obtained.

— In addition to the microbiological evaluations, it is essential that patients have clinical evaluations at least monthly to identify possible adverse effects of the antituberculosis medications and to assess adherence.

— For patients with positive cultures at diagnosis, a repeat chest X-ray at the completion of 2 months of treatment may be useful but is not essential. A chest X-ray at completion of therapy provides a baseline against which subsequent examinations can be compared, but, as with the 2-month examination, it is not essential. When the initial sputum cultures are negative, a presumptive diagnosis can be made if radiographic improvement is noted, usually by the time 2 months of treatment have been completed. Generally, follow-up after completion of therapy is not necessary.

— It is not necessary to routinely monitor liver or renal function or platelet count for patients treated with first-line drugs unless there were abnormalities at baseline or there are symptoms of adverse effects. Patients who have stable abnormalities of hepatic or renal function at baseline should have repeat measurements early in the course of treatment, then less frequently, to ensure that there has not been worsening. Patients receiving ethambutol should be questioned regarding visual disturbances at monthly intervals; monthly repeat testing of visual acuity and color vision is recommended for patients receiving an ethambutol dose exceeding 15 to 20 mg/kg (the recommended range) and for patients receiving the drug for more than 2 months.

TREATMENT OF TB IN PATIENTS WITH HIV INFECTION

All patients with TB should be advised to undergo voluntary counseling and HIV testing. Recommendations for the treatment of TB in HIV-infected adults are, with two exceptions, identical to those for HIV-uninfected adults: a 6-month regimen consisting of an initial phase of isoniazid, rifampin, pyrazinamide, and ethambutol given for 2 months followed by isoniazid and rifampin for 4 months when the disease is caused by organisms that are known or presumed to be susceptible to the first-line drugs. This regimen may be given by daily or intermittent administration (CDC, 2003). However, on the basis of data showing an increased frequency of rifamycin resistance among patients having CD4+ cell counts of less than 100/μL, it is recommended that patients with advanced HIV disease be treated with daily or three times weekly therapy in the continuation phase. Twice weekly drug administration in the continuation phase should not be used in patients with CD4+ cell counts of less than 100/μL. Twice weekly therapy may be considered in patients with less advanced immunosuppression (CD4+ cell counts of 100/μL or above). Once weekly administration of isoniazid and rifapentine in the continuation phase should not be used in any patient with HIV infection.

Six months should be considered the minimum duration of treatment for adults with HIV infection, even with culture-negative TB. If there is evidence of a slow or suboptimal response (e.g., cultures are still positive after 2 months of therapy), prolongation of the continuation phase to 7 months (a total of 9 months of treatment) should be strongly considered. Direct-observation treatment and other adherence-promoting strategies should be used in all patients with HIV-related TB. The American Academy of Pediatrics recommends that for HIV-infected children the minimum duration of therapy be 9 months (CDC, 2003).

TREATMENT OF TB IN CHILDREN

– The lesions of primary TB have a smaller number of *M. tuberculosis* organisms than those of adult-type pulmonary TB, so treatment failure, relapse, and secondary resistance are uncommon among children who adhere to treatment.

– Children frequently swallow instead of expectorate sputum, making it more difficult to isolate *M. tuberculosis* from a child with pulmonary TB than from an adult. Sometimes it is necessary to rely on the results of culture and susceptibility tests of specimens from the person presumed to be the source of the infection in the child to guide the choice of drugs for the child. For children in whom drug resistance is suspected or for whom no source case isolate is available, attempts to isolate organisms via three early-morning gastric aspirations (optimally during hospitalization), bronchoalveolar lavage, or tissue biopsy must be considered.

– Because TB in infants and children younger than age 4 is more likely to disseminate, treatment should be started as soon as the diagnosis is suspected. Asymptomatic children with a positive PPD-tuberculin skin test and an abnormal chest X-ray should receive combination chemotherapy, usually with isoniazid, rifampin, and pyrazinamide as initial therapy.

– Six months of therapy with isoniazid and rifampin supplemented during the first 2 weeks to 2 months with pyrazinamide has been shown to be effective for hilar adenopathy and pulmonary disease caused by drug-susceptible organisms. This three-drug combination has a high success rate and a very low rate (less than 2%) of adverse effects.

Many experts prefer to treat children with three (rather than four) drugs in the initial phase because the bacillary population is low, because many infants and children cannot tolerate the pill burden of four oral drugs, and because of the difficulty in performing visual acuity tests in young children who are being treated with ethambutol. In children suspected or known to have been infected with an *M. tuberculosis* strain that is fully susceptible, the initial phase should consist of isoniazid, rifampin, and pyrazinamide. However, children and adolescents with adult-type pulmonary TB should be treated with the four-drug initial phase regimen, unless the infecting strain is known to be susceptible. When epidemiologic circumstances suggest an increased risk of drug-resistant organisms being present, ethambutol can be used safely in a dose of about 15 to 20 mg/kg per day, even in children too young for routine eye testing. Older children should have monthly evaluations of visual acuity and color discrimination while taking ethambutol. Streptomycin, kanamycin, or amikacin can be used as the fourth drug, when necessary.

Three times weekly therapy is not recommended for children. Pyridoxine is recommended for infants, children, and adolescents who are being treated with isoniazid and who have nutritional deficiencies, symptomatic HIV infection, or who are breast-feeding.

Direct-observation treatment should be used for all children with TB. The lack of pediatric dosage forms of most antituberculotics necessitates the use of crushed pills and suspensions. Even when drugs are given under direct observation, tolerance of the medications must be monitored closely. Parents should not be relied on to supervise direct-observation treatment.

— Because of the difficulties in isolating *M. tuberculosis* from children, bacteriologic examinations are less useful in evaluating the response to treatment, and clinical and radiographic examinations are of relatively greater importance. However, hilar adenopathy and resultant atelectasis may require 2 to 3 years to resolve, hence a persisting abnormality on chest radiographs is not necessarily a criterion for extending therapy. Recognition of treatment failure or relapse in a child is subject to the same difficulties as making a diagnosis. Thus, clinical and radiographic worsening may not be accompanied by positive acid-fast bacillus smears or mycobacterial cultures. A decision to modify the drug regimen should not be made lightly, but often must be made on clinical grounds.

— In general, extrapulmonary TB in children can be treated with the same regimens as pulmonary disease. Exceptions are disseminated disease and meningitis, for which 9 to 12 months of treatment is recommended because of inadequate data to support 6-month therapy. A fourth drug is recommended in the initial phase when there is disseminated TB.

— The optimal treatment of pulmonary TB in children and adolescents with HIV infection is unknown. The American Academy of Pediatrics recommends that initial therapy should include at least three drugs (isoniazid and rifampin, plus pyrazinamide for the first 2 months), and the total duration of therapy should be at least 9 months.

EXTRAPULMONARY TB

— The principles that guide treatment of pulmonary TB also apply to extrapulmonary forms of the disease. Generally among patients with extrapulmonary TB, a 6- to 9-month regimen (2 months of isoniazid, rifampin, pyrazinamide, and ethambutol followed by 4 to 7 months of isoniazid and rifampin)

is recommended as initial therapy unless the organisms
are known or strongly suspected of being resistant to
the first-line drugs. If pyrazinamide cannot be used
in the initial phase, the continuation phase must
be increased to 7 months, as described for
pulmonary TB.

— The exception to the recommendation for a 6- to
9-month regimen is tuberculous meningitis, for which
the optimal length of therapy has not been established,
but some experts recommend 9 to 12 months.

— Although in extrapulmonary TB there have not been
controlled trials of the various patterns of intermittent
drug administration, expert opinion suggests that
intermittent drug administration could be used, with
the exception of isoniazid-rifapentine once weekly in
the continuation phase. Given the lack of experience
with this regimen, it is not currently recommended
for treating extrapulmonary TB.

— Corticosteroid treatment is a useful adjunct in treating
some forms of extrapulmonary TB, specifically
meningitis and pericarditis caused by drug-susceptible
organisms.

DRUG-RESISTANT TB

— Guidelines for management of patients with TB caused
by drug-resistant organisms are based on the following
CDC guidelines:

  • A single new drug should never be added to a
    failing regimen.

  • When starting or revising therapy, always attempt
    to employ at least three previously unused drugs to
    which there is in vitro susceptibility. One of these
    should be injectable.

  • Do not limit the regimen to three drugs if other
    previously unused drugs that are likely to be active
    are available. In patients with multidrug-resistant
    organisms in whom there is resistance to first-line

agents in addition to isoniazid and rifampin,
regimens employing four to six medications appear
to be associated with better results.

- Patients should receive either hospital-based or home
direct-observation treatment. The implications of
treatment failure and further acquired patient and
community resistance are such that these cases
should receive highest priority for direct-observation
treatment.

- Intermittent therapy should not be used in treating
multidrug-resistant TB, except perhaps for injectable
drugs after an initial period (usually 2 to 3 months)
of daily therapy.

- Drugs to which there is demonstrated in vitro
resistance should not be used (assuming the test
results are accurate); usually, alternative medications
are available. However, the clinical significance and
effectiveness of the use of isoniazid in the setting
of low-level isoniazid resistance is unclear. Note that
the use of isoniazid was associated with better
survival rates in patients with the strain-W variety
of multidrug-resistant *M. tuberculosis* that was
susceptible to higher concentrations of isoniazid.

- Resistance to rifampin is associated in nearly all
instances with cross-resistance to rifabutin and
rifapentine. Rare strains with rifampin resistance
retain susceptibility to rifabutin; this is associated
with uncommon mutations of the RNA-polymerase
locus in the bacillus. However, unless in vitro
susceptibility to rifabutin is demonstrated, this
agent should not be employed in cases with
rifampin resistance.

- There is no cross-resistance between streptomycin
and the other injectable agents: amikacin,
kanamycin, and capreomycin (although resistance
to all may occur as independent events); however,
cross-resistance between amikacin and kanamycin

is universal. Simultaneous use of two injectable agents is not recommended due to the absence of proof of efficacy and potential amplification of drug toxicity.

- Determination of resistance to pyrazinamide is technically problematic and, thus, is not made in many laboratories. However, resistance to pyrazinamide is uncommon in the absence of resistance to other first-line drugs. If monoresistance to pyrazinamide is observed, consideration must be given to the possibility that the etiologic agent is *M. bovis*, not *M. tuberculosis* (*M. bovis* is genotypically resistant to pyrazinamide and is not distinguished from *M. tuberculosis* by nucleic acid hybridization-probe assays that are commonly used for identification).

Prevention

- The BCG vaccine is an attenuated strain of tubercle bacillus that is routinely administered to infants in many developing counties. BCG provides variable protection against disseminated primary TB, but it has little effect on postprimary pulmonary TB. Although false-positive PPD tests sometimes occur as a result of BCG received within the previous 5 years, tuberculin skin testing is still used for persons who have received BCG (CDC, 2003; WHO, 2004).

- The cornerstones of prevention are tuberculin skin testing for early identification of infected persons, and prompt and appropriate use of direct-observation treatment. Control of HIV is also essential to the control of TB. Social conditions that lead to transmission, such as overcrowding, should be ameliorated as much as is possible, especially where HIV-infected persons might congregate (e.g., hospitals, prisons, homeless shelters).

While community education is a part of prevention, the greater focus should be on enabling national programs (especially in high-risk areas) to provide (1) adequate testing of populations and (2) direct-observation treatment for all persons being treated (Elzinga, Raviglione, & Maher, 2004; Grange & Zumla, 2003; WHO, 2004).

Reporting

The CDC considers TB to be a nationally notifiable disease. The WHO considers TB to be a Class 2A disease. See Appendix C for details and for upcoming changes in WHO reporting.

References

Centers for Disease Control and Prevention. (2000). Core curriculum on tuberculosis. Retrieved May 12, 2004, from *www.cdc.gov/nchstp/tb/pubs/slidesets/core/default.htm*

Centers for Disease Control and Prevention. (2002). Questions and answers about TB. Retrieved May 4, 2004, from *www.cdc.gov/nchstp/tb/faqs/pdfs/qa.pdf*

Centers for Disease Control and Prevention. (2003). Treatment of tuberculosis. *MMWR, 52*(RR11), 1-77. Retrieved May 12, 2004, from *www.cdc.gov/mmwr/preview/mmwrhtml/rr5211a1.htm*

Chin, J. (Ed.). (2000). *Control of communicable diseases manual* (17th ed., pp. 521-532). Washington, DC: American Public Health Association.

Elzinga, G., Raviglione, M.C., & Maher, D. (2004). Scale up: Meeting targets in global tuberculosis control. *The Lancet, 363,* 814-819.

Grange, J.M., & Zumla, A. (2003). Tuberculosis. In G.C. Cook & A.I. Zumla (Eds.), *Manson's tropical diseases* (21st ed., pp. 995-1052). Philadelphia: W.B. Saunders Company.

Small, P.M., & Selcer, U.M. (2000). Tuberculosis. In G.T. Strickland (Ed.), *Hunter's tropical medicine and emerging infectious diseases* (8th ed., pp. 491-513). Philadelphia: W.B. Saunders Company.

Vos, A.M., Meima, A., Verver, S., Looman, C.W.N., Bos, V., et al. (2004). High incidence of pulmonary tuberculosis persists a decade after immigration, the Netherlands. *Emerging Infectious Diseases, 10,* 736-739.

Weekly Epidemiological Record. (2004). Drug resistant tuberculosis: Levels are ten times higher in eastern Europe and central Asia, *12,* 118-120.

World Health Organization. (2004). *Tuberculosis*. Retrieved May 11, 2004, from *www.who.int/mediacentre/factsheets/fs104/en/*

CHAPTER

91

TULAREMIA
*Deer-fly fever, Francis disease,
Ohara disease, rabbit fever*
Geographical Distribution

Tularemia is present throughout the temperate areas
of North America and Eurasia. Although it has been
reported in every state except Hawaii, most cases occur
in the western and midwestern states, especially
Missouri, Arkansas, Oklahoma, South Dakota, and
Montana. In Eurasia, most cases are reported from
Scandinavian countries and the former Soviet Union
(Dennis et al., 2001).

Agent and Vector

Tularemia is a bacterial zoonosis caused by the
gram-negative coccobacillus *Francisella tularensis*.
Mammals such as voles, squirrels, beavers, and hares
are its most important natural reservoir; humans are
accidental hosts. Infection is usually spread through
ticks and biting flies, but may also be from contact
with contaminated animal products, aerosol droplets,
contaminated mud and water, or animal bites.
Human-to-human transmission does not occur.
F. tularensis remains viable in the environment for
weeks in cool weather and is highly infectious, requiring
an inoculum of 10 or fewer organisms to cause illness.
After inoculation, the organisms spread to regional
lymph nodes where they multiply before disseminating
through blood and lymph to target organs (lymph
nodes, lungs, spleen, liver, and kidney). There are
two strains of *F. tularensis*, with type A being the most
virulent and the most likely to be weaponized
(Box 91-1).

BIOTERRORISM CONSIDERATIONS   BOX 91-1

Tularemia is considered by the CDC to be a Category A
critical biological agent. Category A agents have the
greatest potential for mass casualties and a moderate to
high potential for large-scale dissemination. The most
likely application of tularemia would be as an aerosol.
Japan studied the biological weapon of *F. tularensis* during
World War II, and during the Cold War both the United
States and Soviet Union stockpiled *F. tularensis* weapons,
including strains resistant to antibiotics and vaccines. The
World Health Organization (WHO) has estimated that the
release of 50 kg of *F. tularensis* under ideal conditions
over a city of 5 million people would result in about
250,000 incapacitating casualties, including 19,000 deaths
(Cross & Penn, 2000; Dennis et al., 2001; Rotz, Khan,
Lillibridge, Ostroff, & Hughes, 2002; WHO, 1970).

Incubation

The usual incubation period is 3 to 5 days with a range
of 1 to 14 days depending on the virulence of the
infecting strain, as well as the size and site of inoculum
(Chin, 2000; Dennis et al., 2001).

Clinical Findings and Treatment

Signs and Symptoms

The presentation of tularemia depends on the route of
introduction and the virulence of the agent. The major
disease presentations are classified as typhoidal, septic,
pneumonic, oropharyngeal, ulceroglandular, glandular,
and oculoglandular, although there may be overlap
between these entities.

Typhoidal tularemia is a systemic illness without signs
of inoculation or organ localization. Patients have abrupt
onset of fever, headache, chills, myalgias, coryza, and

sore throat. Nausea, vomiting, abdominal pain, and diarrhea may occur. Relative bradycardia is present in around 40% of patients. Hepatosplenomegaly may not be present early in the illness, but can develop in later stages. Gastrointestinal symptoms are more severe in children.

- *Septic tularemia* presents similarly to typhoidal tularemia initially with fever, abdominal pain, diarrhea, vomiting, and toxicity. Patients may develop confusion and coma. Untreated, the illness may progress to include disseminated intravascular coagulation, acute respiratory distress syndrome, and multiple-system organ failure.

- *Pneumonic tularemia* may occur from aerosol exposure or hematogenous spread from a primary site. Manifestations include pharyngitis, bronchiolitis, pneumonitis, pleural effusion, and hilar lymphadenopathy. Often the systemic signs and symptoms are more prominent than respiratory. Radiographic signs may be absent or minimal, with one or more small discrete infiltrates or granulomatous lesions. In other cases the pneumonia is severe, leading to respiratory failure and death.

- *Oropharyngeal tularemia* results from ingesting contaminated food or water and is characterized by severe throat pain. On examination, patients may have an exudative pharyngitis, tonsillitis, and oral ulcers. Cervical or retropharyngeal lymphadenopathy may occur, sometimes with abscess formation.

- *Ulceroglandular tularemia* is the most often recognized form of tularemia, resulting from tick bites or handling materials from infected animals. Tender, localized adenopathy is often the presenting symptom. A red, painful papule in the area draining to the lymph node may occur either simultaneously or several days afterward. The papule then ulcerates, sometimes taking weeks to heal (Figure 91-1).

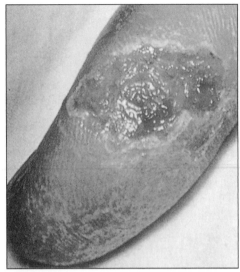

FIGURE 91–1

Primary ulcer of tularemia. (*Source:* From Peters, W., & Pasvol, G. [2002]. *Tropical medicine and parasitology* [5th ed., p. 24]. Chicago: Mosby.)

Glandular tularemia usually is a result of an infected insect bite and is similar to the ulceroglandular version except no skin lesion is identified.

Oculoglandular tularemia occurs when the conjunctivae are inoculated either by contaminated hands or from splashes or aerosols of contaminated fluids. Patients have photophobia, excessive tearing, and swollen eyelids. Preauricular, submandibular, or cervical lymphadenopathy may be present (Cross & Penn, 2000; Dennis et al., 2001).

Complications

Affected lymph nodes may suppurate, even after antibiotic treatment. Pneumonic tularemia usually does not have permanent sequelae, though fibrosis and calcifications can occur. Severe disease may be complicated by coagulopathy, renal failure, hepatitis, and rhabdomyolysis. Without treatment, fever may last for weeks. Recovery may be marked by months of debility, adenopathy, and weight loss (Cross & Penn, 2000).

Common Laboratory Findings

Tularemia does not have specific findings on routine laboratory tests. Leukocytosis, elevated sedimentation rate, thrombocytopenia, hyponatremia, elevated liver enzymes, increased creatine phosphokinase, myoglobinuria, and pyuria have been described (Cross & Penn, 2000).

Diagnosis

Suspicion of a tularemia attack should be aroused by a cluster of otherwise healthy patients with the sudden onset of an acute febrile illness with severe respiratory symptoms. The development of similar illness among laboratory personnel would increase suspicion.

Serologic tests are probably the most common way to confirm the diagnosis of tularemia. An elevated titer of anti–*F. tularensis* antigen in a person without a history of tularemia vaccination is presumptive evidence of infection. A fourfold or greater rise in titer between acute and convalescent specimens is confirmatory.

Infection also may be identified through direct fluorescent antibody or immunohistochemical stains of secretions, aspirated fluids, or biopsy specimens. These rapid diagnostic procedures are available through the National Public Health Laboratory Network. Definitive diagnosis is by culture, which may be positive within 24 to 48 hours but may take as long as 10 days. Some research or reference laboratories are able to perform antigen detection assays, polymerase chain reaction (PCR), immunoblotting, and other specialized techniques (Centers for Disease Control and Prevention [CDC], 2003; Chin, 2000; Dennis et al., 2001).

Differential Diagnosis

Typhoidal tularemia has signs and symptoms similar to typhoid fever, brucellosis, Q fever, disseminated tuberculosis, rickettsioses, malaria, and endocarditis. The differential diagnosis for pneumonic tularemia includes atypical pneumonias (e.g., from *Mycoplasma*, *Legionella*, *Chlamydia*), psittacosis, and tuberculosis. Patients with ulceroglandular or glandular disease may have an illness resembling cat scratch disease, bacterial abscess, atypical mycobacterial infection, or syphilis among others (Cross & Penn, 2000).

Treatment

In a contained casualty situation, parenteral antibiotics should be given (Dennis et al., 2001):

- *Adults:* Streptomycin 1 g IM twice daily for 10 days, or gentamicin 5 mg/kg/24 hours IM or IV once daily for 10 days. Alternatives include doxycycline, chloramphenicol, and ciprofloxacin.
- *Children:* Streptomycin 15 mg/kg IM every 12 hours (up to 2 g/24 hours) or gentamicin 2.5 mg/kg IM or IV q8h for 10 days. Alternatives include intravenous doxycycline (which may cause tooth discoloration in children under 8 years old), chloramphenicol, or ciprofloxacin for 14 to 21 days (Dennis et al., 2001).

In a mass casualty situation and for postexposure prophylaxis, oral antibiotics are recommended. Because human-to-human transmission is not known to occur, postexposure prophylaxis is not necessary for close contacts of tularemia patients (Dennis et al., 2001).

- *Adults:* Doxycycline 100 mg PO bid or ciprofloxacin 500 mg PO twice daily.
- *Children:* If weighing 45 kg or more, give

doxycycline 100 mg PO bid. If less than 45 kg, give doxycycline 2.2 mg/kg PO bid. An alternative (not FDA-approved) is ciprofloxacin 15 mg/kg PO bid not to exceed 1 g/24 hours.

Prevention

— Isolation of persons with tularemia is not necessary. Laboratory procedures should be conducted in biological safety level (BSL) 2 conditions. Contaminated clothing and linen and bodies of deceased patients should be handled using standard precautions. A live attenuated tularemia vaccine is available only for personnel who routinely work with *F. tularensis* in the laboratory (CDC, 2003; Dennis et al., 2001).

— Naturally occurring tularemia may be prevented in areas where infection exists among wild or domestic animals (CDC, 2003; Dennis et al., 2001) as follows:
  - Use DEET repellent and permethrin-treated clothing to avoid tick, fly, or mosquito bites.
  - Avoid drinking, bathing, or swimming in untreated water.
  - Avoid handling animal carcasses, and wash hands with soap and water following exposure to animal tissues. Wear heavy rubber gloves if exposure is unavoidable. Wash gloved hands after contact and, after removing gloves, wash ungloved hands.
  - Consume only properly cooked foods.
  - Veterinarians should be consulted regarding ill pets or livestock.

— Community education on these measures is part of ongoing prevention efforts.

Reporting

— The CDC considers tularemia to be a nationally notifiable disease. The WHO considers tularemia to be a Class 3B disease. See Appendix C for details and for upcoming changes in WHO reporting.

References

Centers for Disease Control and Prevention. (2003). Tularemia. Retrieved March 17, 2004, from *www.bt.cdc.gov/agent/tularemia/*

Chin, J. (Ed.) (2000). *Control of communicable diseases manual* (17th ed., pp. 532-535). Washington, DC: American Public Health Association.

Cross, J.T., & Penn, R.L. (2000). *Francisella tularensis* (tularemia). In G. Mandell, J. Bennett, & R. Dolin (Eds.), *Principles and practice of infectious diseases* (5th ed., pp. 2393). New York: Churchill Livingstone.

Dennis, D.T., Inglesby, T.V., Henderson, D.A., Bartlett, J.G., Ascher, M.S., et al. (2001). Tularemia as a biological weapon: Medical and public health management. *JAMA, 285,* 2763-2773.

Rotz, L.D., Khan, A.S., Lillibridge, S.R., Ostroff, S.M., & Hughes, J.M. (2002). Public health assessment of potential biological terrorism agents. *Emerging Infectious Diseases, 8,* 225-230.

World Health Organization Group of Consultants. (1970). *Health aspects of chemical and biological weapons.* Geneva; pp. 105-107.

92

TUNGIASIS
Chigoe infestation
Geographic Distribution

— Tungiasis is endemic to Central and South America, the Caribbean, and Africa, but is also found sporadically in India, Pakistan, and Madagascar (Heukelbach, de Oliveira, Hesse, & Feldmeier, 2001; Vega-Lopez & Chopra, 2003).

Agent and Vector

— Tungiasis is caused by the burrowing flea, or sandflea, *Tunga penetrans*. Larvae are found in sand or dry soil and, once mature, the adult female flea penetrates human skin in order to obtain a blood meal. The flea remains within the skin for weeks while laying eggs. Once this process is complete, the female flea dies and is sloughed from the skin, leaving the eggs behind (Feldmeier, Eisele, Saboia-Moura, & Heukelbach, 2003; Heukelbach et al., 2001; Vega-Lopez & Chopra, 2003).

Incubation

— The initial burrow, erythema, and edema may be evident within the first few days; however, the characteristic crateriform nodule is present 3 to 4 weeks after inoculation (Vega-Lopez & Chopra, 2003).

Clinical Findings and Treatment

Signs and Symptoms

— The flea typically penetrates the sole of the foot, toe web spaces, or periungual region, although young children may develop lesions on other areas, such as the hands, neck, and genitals. The site of entry becomes painful within a few days, and local erythema and edema may develop. The lesion becomes pruritic, and scratching the area helps to release eggs into the skin. After all the eggs are laid, the flea dies and is expelled. The characteristic crateriform nodule (Figure 92-1) with a central hemorrhagic punctum develops within 3 to 4 weeks (Heukelbach et al., 2001; Vega-Lopez & Chopra, 2003).

Complications

The crateriform nodule may be a portal of entry for other infections if not properly treated. Patients may develop impetigo, ecthyma, cellulitis, phagedenic (rapidly spreading and sloughing) ulcers, or gangrene at the site of infection. Those with periungual lesions commonly develop nail deformities or loss of the nail. In children, tetanus is a common complication.

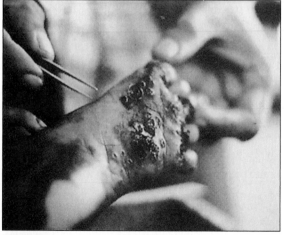

FIGURE 92–1

Tungiasis in a foot. (*Source:* From Peters, W., & Pasvol, G. [2002]. *Tropical medicine and parasitology* [5th ed., p. 269]. Chicago: Mosby.).)

More severe, but less common, complications include lymphedema, auto-amputation of the digit, sepsis, and loss of the entire limb. Rarely, individuals can be infected with multiple fleas at the same time, increasing the risk of complication and making treatment more difficult (Feldmeier et al., 2003; Heukelbach et al., 2001; Vega-Lopez & Chopra, 2003).

Common Laboratory Findings

There are no common laboratory findings in patients with tungiasis.

Diagnosis

Diagnosis is often made clinically, especially in endemic areas. Within several days of the initial infection, the flea can be seen in the lesion as a white area with a black dot in the center. Once the flea dies, a crust develops over the nodule, and eggs can occasionally be found on the skin nearby. A skin biopsy can also be taken in order to visualize the flea or eggs microscopically (Heukelbach et al., 2001).

Differential Diagnosis

Tungiasis may resemble skin lesions caused by scabies, cutaneous myiasis, cutaneous larva migrans, plantar warts, and possibly acral melanoma (Vega-Lopez & Chopra, 2003).

Treatment

The treatment of tungiasis includes removal of the flea and eggs with a sterile needle, surgical excision of the lesion, or cryotherapy. Antibiotic ointment should be applied following these procedures in order to prevent secondary infection. Some evidence suggests that topical ivermectin, thiabendazole, or metrifonate may reduce the number of lesions, however, further studies are needed

(Heukelbach et al., 2001; Heukelbach, Eisele, Jackson, & Feldmeier, 2003; Vega-Lopez & Chopra, 2003).

Prevention

The prevention of tungiasis (Heukelbach et al., 2001; Schwalfenberg, Witt, Kehr, Feldmeier, & Heukelbach, 2004) includes the following:

- Wear shoes in endemic areas, especially around pig-raising areas and in sandy soil.
- Inspect the feet and exposed areas of young children daily. Fleas may then be extracted before eggs are laid. Adults should also be inspected and fleas removed.
- Treat endemic areas and domestic animals with insecticides to reduce the reservoir of the fleas.

Community education is part of the ongoing prevention of tungiasis.

Reporting

The U.S. Centers for Disease Control and Prevention (CDC) does not consider tungiasis to be a nationally notifiable disease. The World Health Organization (WHO) considers tungiasis to be a Class 5 disease. See Appendix C for details and for upcoming changes in WHO reporting.

References

Feldmeier, H., Eisele, M., Saboia-Moura, R.C., & Heukelbach, J. (2003). Severe tungiasis in underprivileged communities: Case series from Brazil. *Emerging Infectious Diseases, 9,* 949-955.

Heukelbach, J., de Oliveira, F.A., Hesse, G., & Feldmeier, H. (2001). Tungiasis: A neglected health problem of poor communities. *Tropical Medicine and International Health, 6,* 267-272.

Heukelbach, J., Eisele, M., Jackson, A., & Feldmeier, H. (2003). Topical treatment of tungiasis: A randomized, controlled trial. *Annals of Tropical Medicine and Parasitology, 97,* 743-749.

Schwalfenberg, S., Witt, L.H., Kehr, J.D., Feldmeier, H., & Heukelbach, J. (2004). Prevention of tungiasis using a biological repellent: A small case series. *Annals of Tropical Medicine and Parasitology, 98,* 89-94.

Vega-Lopez, F., & Chopra, S. (2003). Dermatological problems. In G.C. Cook & A.I. Zumla (Eds.), *Manson's tropical diseases* (21st ed., pp. 363-400). Philadelphia: W.B. Saunders Company.

TYPHOID AND PARATYPHOID FEVERS

Enteric fever, typhus abdominalis

Geographic Distribution

— Typhoid and paratyphoid fevers are endemic in many areas of Asia, Africa, the Middle East, and Latin America. Paratyphoid fever occurs to a lesser extent in southern and Eastern Europe. Worldwide, each year there are an estimated 16 million cases of typhoid fever and 200,000 to 600,000 deaths (Gillespie, 2003; Parry, 2004).

Agent and Vector

— Typhoid fever and paratyphoid fever are caused by the gram-negative, flagellated, facultative anaerobes *Salmonella enterica* serovar Typhi and *S. enterica* serovar Paratyphi, respectively. Formerly these were designated *S. typhi* and *S. paratyphi*. They differ primarily in that typhoid fever is a more severe illness than paratyphoid fever.

— Typhoid and paratyphoid fevers affect only humans (Box 93-1). Transmission is usually by ingestion of food or water that has been contaminated with infected feces or urine. Important sources of infection include shellfish living in contaminated water, vegetables fertilized with human waste, infected food handlers, ice cream or ice drinks from street vendors, and close contacts who are *S. enterica* carriers.

— The primary bacterial illness occurs when ingested bacteria multiply in the intestinal lumen and penetrate the mucosa. Infectivity depends on the number of organisms ingested, gastric acidity (which decreases the numbers of organisms entering the intestine), and whether the organisms possess the Vi antigen (which

---

BIOTERRORISM CONSIDERATIONS | BOX 93–1

Salmonella species are classified by the CDC as Category B biological warfare agents because they "have some potential large-scale dissemination with resultant illness, but generally cause less illness and death" (than Category A agents such as anthrax) (Rotz, Khan, Lillibridge, Ostroff, & Hughes, 2002, p. 226).

---

confers increased virulence). In the intestine, organisms penetrate the Peyer's patches and pass into regional lymphatics before causing a transient primary bacteremia. A secondary bacteremia then occurs after organisms in the liver and spleen further multiply and enter the bloodstream in large numbers, disseminating to multiple organs. Necrosis and ulceration of Peyer's patches sometimes leads to gastrointestinal bleeding (Centers for Disease Control and Prevention [CDC], 2003; Gillespie, 2003; Parry, 2004; World Health Organization [WHO], 2001).

Incubation

The incubation period depends on the number of infecting organisms and the factors just noted. For typhoid fever the incubation period ranges from 3 to 30 days (typically 8 to 14 days), and for paratyphoid fever the incubation period is 1 to 10 days (Chin, 2000).

Clinical Findings and Treatment

Signs and Symptoms

The onset of typhoid fever is insidious with few distinguishing clinical features. Manifestations range from mild to severe. In the first week manifestations include remitting fever, chills, malaise, headache, constipation or diarrhea, and myalgia. In the second week, the fever increases and is sustained. Relative bradycardia is sometimes seen. Diarrhea and/or mild vomiting occur in some cases. Rose spots, which are blanching pink papules 2 to 4 mm in diameter, occur on the chest and abdomen in the second week in about 50% of cases. Splenomegaly and diffuse abdominal tenderness are common.

In the third week of untreated severe illness, the patient appears toxic, weak, and very ill. High fever (39° to 40° C, or 102° to 104° F) persists and the patient may become delirious ("typhoid state"). Splenomegaly progresses to abdominal distention and bowel sounds decrease. Diarrhea, sometimes bloody, with foul-smelling greenish-yellow stools is common in the third week. The pulse weakens and the patient becomes dyspneic. Weight loss is common and it is at this stage that the patient may die from toxemia, myocarditis, intestinal hemorrhage, or perforation.

Without treatment, 10% to 20% of patients die. Those who survive experience gradual improvement and a lengthy convalescence. Among treated patients, about 1% die and 10% to 20% experience relapse 1 to 7 weeks after treatment stops. Approximately 5% of infected people become chronic carriers.

Paratyphoid fever has features similar to typhoid fever but is generally a milder disease (CDC, 2003; Gillespie, 2003; Parry, 2004; WHO, 2001).

Complications

Gastrointestinal complications include hemorrhage and potentially life-threatening perforation, which is often difficult to diagnose because many patients with perforation do not have classic peritoneal findings, and many patients without perforation have severe abdominal pain and tenderness. Gallbladder involvement and preexisting gallbladder disease may result in chronic biliary infection and a chronic carrier state. Myocarditis is a common cause of death in endemic areas. Neurologic complications include delirium, which occurs most often in the late stages but sometimes is present through most of the illness, meningitis, encephalitis, and seizures. Other possible complications include pneumonia, glomerulonephritis, hemolytic-uremic syndrome, disseminated intravascular coagulation, osteomyelitis, miscarriage, and focal abscesses (Lee & Hoffman, 2000).

Common Laboratory Findings

Early in the infection, mild leukocytosis is usually present. With progression of the illness, leukopenia, neutropenia, and anemia may develop. Mild thrombocytopenia, elevated serum transaminases, and proteinuria are common (Gillespie, 2003).

Diagnosis

The diagnosis of *S. enterica* infection may be made by culture of blood or bone marrow, and occasionally of stool or urine. Of these, bone marrow aspirate is the most sensitive. The most common serologic test is the Widal test; however, this test cross-reacts with other *Salmonella* species and lacks the sensitivity and specificity of the newer rapid dipstick and dot enzyme immunoassays (Lee & Hoffman, 2000; Olsen et al., 2004; Parry, 2004).

Differential Diagnosis

The differential diagnosis includes numerous bacterial (e.g., endocarditis, leptospirosis, tuberculosis, tularemia, abscesses), rickettsial (e.g., typhus), protozoal (e.g., malaria, amebiasis, visceral leishmaniasis), viral (e.g., influenza, infectious mononucleosis), and noninfectious diseases (e.g., connective tissue diseases and lymphoproliferative disorders) (Lee & Hoffman, 2000).

Treatment

— The treatment of typhoid and paratyphoid fevers is complicated by widespread multiple-drug resistance to traditional antibiotics (such as chloramphenicol, ampicillin, and trimethoprim-sulfamethoxazole) and decreased susceptibility to fluoroquinolones. Antibiotic therapy must therefore be based on local resistance patterns as well as the severity of illness.

— Table 93-1 (WHO, 2003) summarizes antibiotic therapy for uncomplicated typhoid fever. In general, fluoroquinolones are considered first-line therapy. However, alternatives are used in areas where fluoroquinolones are too expensive or quinolone resistance is prevalent. Whether fluoroquinolones are superior to less expensive alternatives in areas without resistance is debated. Though fluoroquinolones are relatively contraindicated for children because of animal experiments demonstrating articular cartilage damage in growing beagles, their demonstrated benefits in typhoid fever outcomes in children are generally thought to outweigh the theoretical risk.

— Antibiotic guidelines for severe typhoid fever (characterized by delirium, obtundation, stupor, coma, or shock) are summarized in Table 93-2 (WHO, 2003). For both adults and children with severe typhoid fever, corticosteroids started promptly after the first dose of antibiotic can decrease the risk of mortality. Dexamethasone may be administered at a dose of 3 mg/kg infused slowly over 30 min, followed by 1 mg/kg q6h for eight additional doses.

— Supportive measures for typhoid fever include oral or intravenous fluid support, antipyretics, nutrition, and blood transfusions if indicated. Any patient with

TABLE 93-1 Treatment of Uncomplicated Typhoid Fever

Susceptibility	Optimal therapy			Alternative effective drugs		
	Antibiotic	Daily dose mg/kg	Days	Antibiotic	Daily dose mg/kg	Days
Fully sensitive	Fluoroquinolone e.g. ofloxacin or ciprofloxacin	15	5–7[a]	Chloramphenicol Amoxicillin TMP-SMX	50–75 75–100 8–40	14–21 14 14
Multidrug resistance	Fluoroquinolone or cefixime	15 15–20	5–7 7–14	Azithromycin	8–10	7
Quinolone resistance[b]	Azithromycin or ceftriaxone	8–10 75	7 10–14	Cefixime	20	7–14

Source: World Health Organization. (2003). Background document: The diagnosis, treatment, and prevention of typhoid fever. Retrieved May 24, 2004, from *www.who.int/vaccine-documents/DocsPDF03/www740.pdf*

[a]Three-day courses are also effective and are particularly so in epidemic containment.

[b]The optimum treatment for quinolone-resistant typhoid fever has not been determined. Azithromycin, the third-generation cephalosporins, or a 10–14 day course of high-dose fluoroquinolones, is effective. Combinations of these are now being evaluated.

TABLE 93-2 Treatment of Severe Typhoid Fever

Susceptibility	Optimal parenteral drug			Alternative effective parenteral drugs		
	Antibiotic	Daily dose mg/kg	Days	Antibiotic	Daily dose mg/kg	Days
Fully sensitive	Fluoroquinolone e.g. ofloxacin	15	10–14	Chloramphenicol Amoxicillin TMP-SMX	100 100 8–40	14–21 14 14
Multidrug resistant	Fluoroquinolone	15	10–14	Ceftriaxone or cefotaxime	60 80	10–14
Quinolone resistant	Ceftriaxone or cefotaxime	60 80	10–14	Fluoroquinolone	20	7–14

Source: World Health Organization. (2003). Background document: The diagnosis, treatment, and prevention of typhoid fever. Retrieved May 24, 2004, from *www.who.int/vaccines-documents/DocsPDF03/www/740.pdf*

a possible intestinal perforation should be evaluated by a surgeon immediately.
- The treatment of chronic carriers is challenging, especially in the presence of chronic gallbladder disease. A 28-day course of a fluoroquinolone at maximum dose is probably the best option. Chronic urinary carriers should be evaluated for urinary tract abnormalities or schistosomiasis (Chandel, Chaudhry, Dhawan, Pandey, & Dey, 2000; Gillespie, 2003; Parry, 2004; WHO, 2003).

Prevention

- Typhoid vaccines are effective but often are not available in endemic areas. An oral four-dose Ty21a vaccine may be used by adults and children older than age 6, whereas a single-dose intramuscular Vi vaccine is available for children older than age 2. Because Ty21a is a live attenuated vaccine, it should not be given to persons who are immunocompromised or taking antibiotics. Booster doses are required every 5 years for Ty21a recipients, and every 2 years for Vi vaccine recipients. Vaccination should be offered to travelers to endemic areas, household contacts of carriers, and laboratory personnel working with *S. enterica*. Vaccination programs may also prevent epidemics among disaster victims or refugee camp populations (Chin, 2000; Parry, 2004; WHO, 2001).
- Personal protection and public health interventions to prevent enteric fevers (Chin, 2000; Parry, 2004; WHO, 2001) include the following:
  - Treat water through chlorination of community supplies or household boiling.
  - Dispose of human waste in a sanitary manner.
  - Exclude *Salmonella* carriers from food handling.
  - Control flies through the use of insecticides, improved community hygiene, and screens on windows and doors.

- Cook shellfish for at least 10 min. Peel or wash vegetables and fruits in clean water.
- Use enteric precautions around patients.
- Breastfeed infants.

Public education is important, especially on personal hygiene and regarding hand washing after toilet use and before food preparation.

Reporting

The CDC considers typhoid fever to be a nationally notifiable disease. The WHO considers typhoid to be a Class 2A disease. See Appendix C for details and for upcoming changes in WHO reporting.

References

Centers for Disease Control and Prevention. (2003). Typhoid fever. Retrieved May 1, 2004, from *www.cdc.gov/ncidod/dbmd/diseaseinfo/typhoidfever_t.htm*

Chandel, D.S., Chaudhry, R., Dhawan, B., Pandey, A. & Dey, A.B. (2000). Drug-resistant *Salmonella enterica* serotype Paratyphi A in India. *Emerging Infectious Diseases, 6,* 420-421.

Chin, J. (Ed.). (2000). *Control of communicable diseases manual* (17th ed., pp. 535-541). Washington, DC: American Public Health Association.

Gillespie, S. (2003). *Salmonella* infections. In G.C. Cook & A.I. Zumla (Eds.), *Manson's tropical diseases* (21st ed., pp. 937-961). Philadelphia: W.B. Saunders Company.

Lee, T.P., & Hoffman, S.L. (2000). Typhoid fever. In G.T. Strickland (Ed.), *Hunter's tropical medicine and emerging infectious diseases* (8th ed., pp. 471-483). Philadelphia: W.B. Saunders Company.

Olsen, S.J., Pruckler, J., Bibb, W., Thanh, N.T., Trinh, T.M., et al. (2004). Evaluation of rapid diagnostic tests for typhoid fever. *Clinical Microbiology, 42,* 1885-1889.

Parry, C.M. (2004). Typhoid fever. *Current Infectious Disease Reports, 6,* 27-33.

Rotz, L.D., Khan, A.S., Lillibridge, S.R., Ostroff, S.M., & Hughes. J.M. (2002). Public health assessment of potential biological terrorism agents. *Emerging Infectious Diseases, 8,* 225-230.

World Health Organization. (2001). Typhoid and paratyphoid enteric fevers. Retrieved May 1, 2004, from *www.who.int/water_sanitation_health/diseases/typhoid/en/*

World Health Organization. (2003). Background document: The diagnosis, treatment, and prevention of typhoid fever. Retrieved May 24, 2004, from *www.who.int/vaccines-documents/DocsPDF03/www740.pdf*

94

TYPHUS

Geographic Distribution

— Epidemic louse-borne typhus (louse-borne typhus, typhus exanthematicus, classic typhus fever) is most prevalent in cooler, mountainous areas of Africa, Asia, and Latin America. Scrub typhus (Tsutsugamushi disease, mite-borne typhus) is found in south Asia (Pakistan, India), East Asia (Japan, China, Korea, and parts of Russia), and the western Pacific (Australia). Endemic murine typhus (endemic flea-borne typhus, shop typhus) is found worldwide, especially in temperate and subtropical coastal regions (Centers for Disease Control and Prevention [CDC], 2003).

Agent and Vector

— The typhus group of illnesses are caused by *Rickettsiae*, gram-negative obligate intracellular bacteria transmitted by the bites of infected arthropods or exposure to their feces. Typhus is one of several rickettsioses that include the spotted fever group of illnesses (Rocky Mountain spotted fever, Boutonneuse fever, North Asian tick typhus, and rickettsial pox), Q fever, trench fever, and ehrlichiosis. The typhus group includes epidemic louse-borne typhus, scrub typhus, and endemic (murine) typhus.

— Epidemic louse-borne typhus is caused by *Rickettsia prowazekii*, which is transmitted from person to person by the body louse. Its spread is facilitated by infrequent bathing, infrequent changes of clothing, and by crowded, unsanitary living conditions such as concentration camps or refugee camps, especially in cold climates (Saah, 2000a).

— Scrub typhus, from *Orientia tsutsugamushi,* is transmitted by the bite of infected chiggers, the larval stage of mites.

These vectors live not only in scrub vegetation but also in sandy beaches and semiarid areas. The mites are also probably the main reservoir for the bacteria. Humans, who are accidental hosts, are often exposed to the mites in areas that have been recently cleared of vegetation (CDC, 2003; Saah, 2000b).

Murine typhus is caused by *R. typhi* and is transmitted from its rat reservoir by fleas. Humans can be directly infected by flea bites, but inoculation is usually by flea feces contaminating the bite wounds. In an outbreak on the Thai-Cambodian border, 70% of Cambodian refugees with unexplained fever had murine typhus (Dumler & Walker, 2000).

Incubation

The incubation period is variable, but typically is approximately 7 days in epidemic louse-borne typhus, 6 to 18 days for scrub typhus, and 8 to 16 days for murine typhus (CDC, 2003).

Clinical Findings and Treatment

Signs and Symptoms

The early symptoms of the typhus group of illnesses, as for all rickettsial diseases, are nonspecific: fever, headache, and malaise, with most patients developing an exanthem.

Epidemic louse-borne typhus is characterized by a prodrome of headache and constitutional symptoms, then the abrupt onset of high fever, chills, and prostration. By the fifth day an erythematous macular rash appears in the axillary folds and upper trunk and spreads centrifugally, sparing only the face, palms, and soles. The rash becomes maculopapular and petechial, and may become hemorrhagic and necrotic. Other common manifestations are delirium, conjunctival injection, photophobia, eye pain, flushed facies, hearing loss, hypotension, pulmonary involvement, renal insufficiency, and splenomegaly. Recovery may be spontaneous with the fever remitting after 2 weeks, though full recovery from weakness may take a few months. Elderly patients have the highest mortality, while children usually have a mild illness.

— The symptoms of scrub typhus range from mild to severe, and include the gradual onset of fever, chills, headache, myalgias (backache), cough, nausea, and abdominal pain. Patients develop an eschar at the site of the infecting bite. Travelers from outside endemic areas commonly develop regional lymphadenopathy and an erythematous rash, which is initially macular and becomes papular. Indigenous people usually do not develop these manifestations. In untreated cases the fever resolves after 2 weeks.

— Murine typhus is characterized by several days of prodromal constitutional symptoms, followed by the abrupt onset of fever, chills, and nausea and vomiting. Pulmonary involvement is common and may include interstitial pneumonia, pleural effusion, and/or pulmonary edema. Only half of patients develop an erythematous macular rash, and of those with a rash only 10% are petechial. The disease is rarely fatal (Dumler & Walker, 2000; Saah, 2000a, 2000b; Sirisanthana, Puthanakit, & Sirisanthana, 2003).

Complications

— Potentially life-threatening complications of epidemic louse-borne typhus include pneumonia, shock, myocarditis, and uremia. A recrudescent mild form of epidemic typhus (Brill-Zinsser disease) may develop many years after recovery. Severe scrub typhus is characterized by encephalitis and pneumonia. Murine typhus may be complicated by central nervous system (CNS) involvement, respiratory failure, renal insufficiency, or liver failure (Singh-Behl, La Rosa, & Tomecki, 2003; Sirisanthana et al., 2003).

Common Laboratory Findings

Patients may have early leukopenia followed by
leukocytosis. Mild to moderate elevations in serum
transaminases may also be seen. Those with CNS
findings may have a moderate cerebrospinal fluid
pleocytosis. Hypoalbuminemia, hyponatremia,
hypocalcemia, and uremia may also be present
(Dumler & Walker, 2000; Saah, 2000b).

Diagnosis

The diagnosis of the typhus group of illnesses is similar
to other rickettsial diseases, requiring two or more of the
following: (1) a travel or exposure history and symptoms
consistent with the disease, (2) development of specific
antibodies (e.g., by indirect immunofluorescence assay or
enzyme immunoassay) to a given organism or antigenic
group, (3) a positive polymerase chain reaction (PCR)
test, or (4) isolation of the organism. Serologic tests are
currently unable to distinguish between different
rickettsial species (CDC, 2003).

Differential Diagnosis

Because the clinical features are nonspecific, the
differential diagnosis for typhus group illnesses
is extensive, including meningococcemia, measles,
bacterial or viral meningitides, leptospirosis, infectious
mononucleosis, toxic shock syndrome, anthrax, and
Kawasaki disease.

Treatment

Antibiotic therapy should be started when a typhus
group illness is suspected without waiting for
confirmatory test results. Murine typhus may be treated
with a single 200-mg dose of doxycycline (100 mg for
children). For epidemic typhus and scrub typhus,
doxycycline at a dose of 2.2 mg/kg/dose to a maximum

of 100 mg PO or IV bid should be given until the patient is afebrile for more than 72 hours. Typically, antibiotics are given for 7 to 10 days. A second cycle of treatment is sometimes necessary for scrub typhus. Because of the potential for serious illness, doxycycline is the preferred treatment for children despite the risk of tooth staining for those younger than age 8. If a patient has had a life-threatening reaction to doxycycline in the past, chloramphenicol may be used at a dose of 12.5 mg/kg/dose q6h. Those responding poorly to doxycycline and chloramphenicol may respond to rifampin. Ciprofloxacin has also been used in adults and roxithromycin (a macrolide available in Europe and Latin America) in children (Dasch & McQuiston, 2003; Lee, Lee, Hong, Hur, & Whang, 2003).

Prevention

- No commercially licensed vaccines for typhus are available. Individual prevention in nonmass situations includes washing clothing according to the guidelines given next. Discarding or treating infested clothing (see next paragraph) and bathing in hot water are sufficient to rid an individual of body lice because the lice live in the clothing as opposed to on the body.
- In mass population conditions that favor lice infestation, for example, in refugee crises, Chin (2000) recommends that residual insecticide powders be applied to the clothes and bodies of persons at risk, such as 10% DDT insufflating powder for clothing and 1% malathion or 0.5% permethrin under clothing (Butler, 2000). The U.S. military guidelines for prevention of louse-borne diseases include (1) treatment of persons infected with the disease(s), (2) bathing infested persons, and (3) laundering all clothing with regimens lethal to lice and eggs. Exposing clothing to water or circulating air at a temperature of 140° F (60° C) for 15 min kills all stages of lice. Individuals may also reduce their risk

by using DEET-containing repellents and permethrin-treated clothing to prevent fleas and mites. Avoiding exposure to rodents can reduce the risk of murine typhus (Armed Forces Pest Management Board, 2002; Butler, 2000; CDC, 2003; Dash & McQuiston, 2003).

Reporting

The CDC does not consider typhus to be a nationally notifiable disease. The World Health Organization (WHO) considers louse-borne typhus to be a Class 1 disease. See Appendix C for details and for upcoming changes in WHO reporting.

References

Armed Forces Pest Management Board. (2002). Delousing procedures for the control of louse-borne disease during contingency. Retrieved December 26, 2003, from *www.afpmb.org/pubs/tims/TG6/TG6.pdf*

Butler, T. (2000). Relapsing fever. In G.T. Strickland (Ed.), *Hunter's tropical medicine and emerging infectious diseases* (8th ed., pp. 448-452). Philadelphia: W.B. Saunders Company.

Centers for Disease Control and Prevention. (2003). Rickettsial diseases. Downloaded March 19, 2004, from *www.cdc.gov/travel/diseases/rickettsial.htm*

Chin, J. (Ed.). (2000). *Control of communicable diseases manual* (17th ed., pp. 541-545). Washington, DC: American Public Health Association.

Dasch, G.A., & McQuiston, J.H. (2003). Other *Rickettsia* species. In S. Long, L. Pickering, C.G. Prober (Eds.), *Principles and practice of pediatric infectious diseases* (2nd ed., pp. 946-951). Philadelphia: Churchill Livingstone.

Dumler, J.S., & Walker, D.H. (2000). *Rickettsia typhi* (murine typhus). In G. Mandell, J. Bennett, & R. Dolin (Eds.), *Principles and practice of infectious diseases* (5th ed., pp. 2053-2055). New York: Churchill Livingstone.

Lee, K.-Y., Lee, H.-S., Hong, J.-H., Hur, J.-K., & Whang, K.-T. (2003). Roxithromycin treatment of scrub typhus (Tsutsugamushi disease) in children. *Pediatric Infectious Disease Journal, 22,* 130-133.

Saah, A.J. (2000a). *Rickettsia prowazekii* (epidemic or louse-borne typhus). In G. Mandell, J. Bennett, & R. Dolin (Eds.), *Principles and practice of infectious diseases* (5th ed., pp. 2050-2053). New York: Churchill Livingstone.

Saah, A.J. (2000b). *Orientia tsutsugamushi* (scrub typhus). In G. Mandell, J. Bennett, & R. Dolin (Eds.), *Principles and practice of infectious diseases* (5th ed., pp. 2056-2057). New York: Churchill Livingstone.

Singh-Behl, D., La Rosa, S.P., & Tomecki, K.J. (2003). Tick-borne infections. *Dermatologic Clinics, 21,* 237-244.

Sirisanthana, V., Puthanakit, T., & Sirisanthana, T. (2003). Epidemiologic, clinical and laboratory features of scrub typhus in thirty Thai children. *Pediatric Infectious Disease Journal, 22,* 341-345.

Yaws

Framboesia tropica, pian, buba, parangi
Geographic Distribution

— Yaws is primarily found in tropical rural areas with high humidity and rainfall, including equatorial Africa, Central and South America, India, Thailand, Indonesia, and Papua New Guinea (Perine & Bell, 2000).

Agent and Vector

— Yaws is an endemic nonvenereal infection related to syphilis that is caused by *Treponema pallidum pertenue*. Yaws occurs in underdeveloped rural areas where sanitation, medical care, and living conditions are poor. The infection is transmitted by direct contact with open purulent skin lesions. Inoculation is facilitated by skin barriers that have been compromised by scratching or trauma. Indirect inoculation may also take place by transmission of the bacteria on fomites or insects. Most cases occur in children before the age of 15 (Antal, Lukehart, & Meheus, 2002; Kapembwa, 2003; Perine & Bell, 2000).

Incubation

— The first skin manifestation of infection occurs 2 to 8 weeks after inoculation (Perine & Bell, 2000).

Clinical Findings and Treatment

Signs and Symptoms

— The initial skin lesion, or the "mother yaw," appears at the site of inoculation and usually occurs on exposed areas. This primary lesion starts as an erythematous scaly papule, progresses to a large papilloma, often several centimeters in diameter, and heals after 3 to 6 months.

Regional lymphadenopathy may be present at this stage. The primary lesion contains a high number of treponemes and is highly infectious.

Secondary lesions, which are also highly infectious, appear in crops several weeks to years after the primary lesion and may occur with fever and generalized lymphadenopathy (Figure 95-1). They can occur locally around the area of the primary lesion or may be widely disseminated. The most characteristic secondary lesions are papules and papillomas; however, other manifestations include annular or irregularly shaped plaques, palmar-plantar hyperkeratosis (crab yaws), and moist papules and plaques around the nose and mouth, which resemble condyloma lata of secondary syphilis. The skin lesions continue to appear in crops for up to 6 months, and relapses may occur for up to 5 years (Antal et al., 2002; Kapembwa, 2003; Perine & Bell, 2000).

Complications

Bone involvement can occur with the secondary lesions and manifests as painful osteitis or periostitis of the arms,

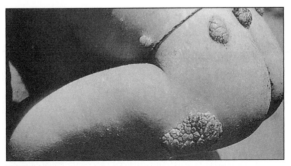

FIGURE 95–1

Secondary framboesiform yaws. (*Source:* From Peters, W., & Pasvol, G. [2002]. *Tropical medicine and parasitology* [5th ed., p. 252]. Chicago: Mosby.)

legs, or fingers. Chronic periostitis of the tibia may occur, resulting in saber tibia deformities. Periostitis of the fingers can lead to polydactylitis. Rarely, hypertrophic osteitis of the maxilla can cause severe swelling along the bridge of the nose *(goundou)* and can cause nasal obstruction.

Late yaws occurs in approximately 10% of cases and manifests as destructive gummatous lesions of the skin, bones, and overlying tissue. Affected individuals may also develop chronic mutilating skin ulcerations of the face and extremities, hyperkeratosis and fissuring of the palms and soles, juxtaarticular nodules, bursitis, and ulceration and perforation of the nasal septum *(gangosa)* and pharynx. Congenital transmission does not occur, as it does with venereal syphilis (Antal et al., 2002; Kapembwa, 2003; Perine & Bell, 2000).

Common Laboratory Findings

There are no common laboratory findings in patients with yaws.

Diagnosis

Treponemes can be demonstrated by examining the exudate from skin lesions with dark-field microscopy; however, this does not distinguish yaws from other treponemal infections. Nontreponemal and treponemal antigen tests (see the Syphilis chapter for further details) facilitate the diagnosis of a treponemal infection, but they are also incapable of speciation and subspeciation. The diagnosis may be made clinically in characteristic cases in endemic areas (Kapembwa, 2003; Perine & Bell, 2000).

Differential Diagnosis

Endemic and venereal syphilis are sometimes indistinguishable from yaws. Primary and secondary lesions of yaws may resemble scabies, cutaneous fungal infections, impetigo, or psoriasis. Gummatous lesions may be confused with a tropical ulcer, Buruli ulcer, other cutaneous mycobacterial infections, leishmania, or a neoplastic process (Kapembwa, 2003).

Treatment

Benzathine penicillin G in a single IM dose (2.4 million units in adults, 1.2 million units in children ages 6 to 15, and 600,000 units for children younger than age 6) is the treatment of choice. Penicillin-allergic patients may take tetracycline if they are older than age 8: 500 mg qid for 14 days for adults; 250 mg qid for 14 days for those ages 8 to 15. Or, they may take erythromycin if they are younger than age 8: 10 mg/kg qid for 14 days. Treatment will cure early lesions and prevent relapses; however the destruction caused by late lesions is permanent.

Prevention

A sharp decline in the prevalence of the endemic treponematoses was brought about by mass treatment campaigns with penicillin under the guidance of the World Health Organization (WHO) and with support from UNICEF in the 1950s and 1960s. Although these were initially very successful, lack of integration of control measures into rural health services allowed resurgence of the disease and its reservoirs. Recently, long-term community-based surveillance programs and follow-up treatment have been successful in eradicating the disease in Ecuador, thus giving hope for eradication in other countries. Personal hygiene is critical to the prevention of yaws (Anselmi, Moreira, Caicedo, Guderian, & Tognoni, 2003; Meheus & Antal, 1992).

Reporting

The U.S. Centers for Disease Control and Prevention does not consider yaws to be a nationally notifiable disease. The WHO classifies it as a Class 3B disease.

See Appendix C for details and for upcoming changes in WHO reporting.

References

Anselmi, M., Moreira, J.M., Caicedo, C., Guderian, R., & Tognoni, G. (2003). Community participation eliminates yaws in Ecuador. *Tropical Medicine and International Health, 8,* 634-638.

Antal, G.M., Lukehart, S.A., & Meheus, A.Z. (2002). The endemic treponematoses. *Microbes and Infection, 4,* 83-94.

Kapembwa, M. (2003). Endemic treponematoses. In G.C. Cook & A.I. Zumla (Eds.), *Manson's tropical diseases* (21st ed., pp. 1143-1148). Philadelphia: W.B. Saunders Company.

Meheus, A., & Antal, G.M. (1992). The endemic treponematoses: Not yet eradicated. *World Health Statistics Quarterly, 45,* 228-237.

Perine, P.L., & Bell, T.A. (2000). Syphilis and the endemic treponematoses. In G. Strickland (Ed.), *Hunter's tropical medicine and emerging infectious diseases* (8th ed., pp. 354-364). Philadelphia: W.B. Saunders Company.

YELLOW FEVER

Geographic Distribution

— Yellow fever occurs in tropical South America and sub-Saharan Africa. In South America, most cases are from occupational exposure in forested or transitional areas. Each year as many as 200,000 people contract yellow fever (Centers for Disease Control and Prevention [CDC], 2004; Monath, 2001).

Agent and Vector

— Yellow fever is a single-stranded RNA arbovirus in the *Flaviviridae* family. Its natural reservoir is nonhuman primates. In South American jungles, yellow fever is transmitted from animal to animal or from animals to humans by *Haemagogus* mosquitoes, whereas in Africa the vector is the *Aedes* species. These mosquitoes are diurnally active and breed primarily in jungle tree holes. *A. aegypti* breeds in collections of water in urban areas and is responsible for human-to-human transmission in South America and Africa. Yellow fever is the original viral hemorrhagic fever, causing 1000 times more illness and death than Ebola virus, with the potential for explosive outbreaks in urban populations. Countries in Asia and North America that are outside the endemic zones but infested with *Aedes* mosquitoes may also be at risk (Monath, 2001; Robertson et al., 1996; Tomori, 1999).

Incubation

— Symptoms appear 3 to 6 days after a bite from an infected mosquito (Chin, 2000).

Clinical Findings and Treatment

Signs and Symptoms

Most patients with yellow fever experience the sudden onset of nonspecific flu-like symptoms that are self-limited. Some infections are asymptomatic. In both mild and severe yellow fever, the illness sometimes has two stages with a short intervening remission. The first stage has the sudden onset of fever, chills, intense headache, lumbosacral back pain, myalgia, nausea and vomiting, conjunctival injection, and dark urine. The fever lasts an average of 3.3 days, and may be associated with relative bradycardia. During this time, patients may transmit the virus to biting mosquitoes. After several days, there is a period of remission characterized by decreased temperature, no headache, and general improvement. This lasts up to 24 hours, but in 15% to 25% of patients is followed by an "intoxication" or hepatorenal stage that features the reemergence of fever, increased nausea and vomiting, abdominal pain, jaundice, renal failure, and hemorrhagic symptoms. The hemorrhagic manifestations may include hematemesis, melena, metrorrhagia, petechiae, ecchymosis, and bleeding from mucous membranes. Though patients may have encephalopathy, encephalitis is rare (CDC, 2004; Monath, 2001).

Complications

Yellow fever has a relatively high case fatality rate of 5% to 10%. Of patients with hemorrhagic symptoms, 20% to 50% die. Death occurs 7 to 10 days after the onset of symptoms and may be preceded by hypotension, delirium, coma, metabolic acidosis, electrolyte abnormalities, and cerebral edema. Those who survive the acute illness may have secondary infections (sepsis or pneumonia) or renal failure. Full recovery from weakness and fatigue may take several weeks (CDC, 2004; Monath, 2001).

Common Laboratory Findings

During the initial fever, leukopenia and neutropenia may be present. Serum transaminases often rise 48 to 72 hours before the onset of jaundice, with aspartate aminotransferase (AST) levels greater than alanine aminotransferase (ALT). In one study, fatal cases had a mean AST of 2766 international units/L, while survivors with jaundice had a mean AST of 929 international units/L. In survivors, transaminase levels may take up to 2 months to return to normal. Laboratory abnormalities during the hemorrhagic phase include thrombocytopenia, increased clotting and prothrombin times, and decreased fibrinogen (Broom, Smith, Hall, Johansen, & Mackenzie, 2003; Monath, 2001).

Diagnosis

In endemic areas, the diagnosis is usually clinical. Confirmatory tests are available only in specialized laboratories. Serologic diagnosis of yellow fever may be accomplished by the detection of immunoglobulin M (IgM) antibodies by enzyme-linked immunosorbent assay (ELISA), or by a fourfold increase in antibody titers between acute and convalescent sera. These tests may cross-react with other flaviviruses, however. Viral antigen may be detectable by immunostaining. The virus may be also be isolated in culture, but the polymerase chain reaction (PCR) procedure is more sensitive (Monath, 2001).

Differential Diagnosis

Mild yellow fever resembles many other common viral illnesses. Early (anicteric) stages of severe yellow fever resemble malaria (which may coexist), typhoid fever, rickettsial infections (typhus, Rocky Mountain spotted fever, Boutonneuse fever, trench fever, Q fever, ehrlichiosis), viral encephalitis, other arboviral fevers (dengue fever and other viral hemorrhagic fevers), and influenza. For patients with hemorrhagic features or hepatorenal dysfunction, the differential diagnosis includes viral hepatitis, leptospirosis, and other viral hemorrhagic fevers (dengue fever, Lassa fever, Marburg fever, Ebola fever, Crimean-Congo fever, Rift Valley fever, and hemorrhagic fever with renal syndrome) (Broom et al., 2003; Monath, 2001).

Treatment

There is no specific treatment for yellow fever. Supportive measures include fluid and electrolyte maintenance, nasogastric suctioning to prevent gastric distention and aspiration, intravenous H_2 blockers to prevent gastric bleeding, oxygen, and fresh frozen plasma for patients with hemorrhagic symptoms. Hypotension may be treated by intravenous fluids and vasopressors, but patients with yellow fever often do not respond as expected to fluid replacement (Broom et al., 2003; Monath, 2001).

Prevention

Preventive measures in endemic areas (Chin, 2000; Koren, Matsui, & Bailey, 2003; White, 2003) include the following:
- Kill adult mosquitoes by spraying inside and outside human habitations and surrounding areas with residual insecticides. The goal is to kill as many female mosquitoes as possible, thus decreasing the likelihood of disease transmission. See Appendix D.
- Kill larvae and eliminate breeding areas as much as possible. Elimination of breeding areas includes

draining standing water such as swamps, emptying open water-filled containers and used tires, and reducing the number of plants that hold standing water, for example, bromeliads.

Personal protection includes the following:

- Screen living and working quarters.
- Use a residual insecticide inside homes and work areas. See Appendix D.
- Use insecticide-impregnated mosquito netting over beds. Nets must be retreated with insecticide annually. See Appendix D.
- Stay inside as much as possible during hours when mosquitoes are biting, which, in the case of *Aedes* mosquitoes, is primarily during the day with peaks during midmorning and late afternoon.
- Use DEET repellant on skin and permethrin on clothing when outside during biting hours. DEET may be used to protect pregnant and lactating women traveling to endemic areas. Formulations with concentrations of 30% or less can be used safely in children and infants older than 2 months. Long-acting repellents in which DEET is bound in a polymer have the advantages of longer duration and decreased systemic absorption.

Provide ongoing community education regarding the preceding measures.

Travelers to endemic areas who are older than 9 months should receive live attenuated yellow fever vaccine, even if the country of destination does not officially report yellow fever. The dose is 0.5 mL given subcutaneously with boosters every 10 years, although studies suggest that immunity probably lasts more than 30 years. Some countries may require travelers from or transiting through endemic countries to provide proof of vaccination. Because of the risk of encephalitis from the vaccine, infants younger than age 6 months should not be given the vaccine, and those ages 6 to 8 months only in situations where exposure to mosquito vectors is unavoidable. Severe and usually fatal vaccine-associated viscerotropic disease has been documented with an estimated incidence in the United States of 1/400,000 doses. Individuals age 65 and older may be at increased risk for such adverse reactions. Because of these risks, the vaccine should only be administered to travelers truly at risk of exposure (Advisory Committee on Immunization Practices, 2002; CDC, 2004; Chin, 2000).

Reporting

The CDC considers yellow fever to be a nationally notifiable disease. The World Health Organization (WHO) considers it to be a Class 1 disease. See Appendix C for details and for upcoming changes in WHO reporting.

References

Advisory Committee on Immunization Practices. (2002). *Mortality and Morbidity Weekly Reports, 51*(RR-17): 1-11.

Broom, A.K., Smith, D.W., Hall, R.A., Johansen, C.A., & Mackenzie, J.S. (2003). Arbovirus infections. In G.C. Cook & A.I. Zumla (Eds.), *Manson's tropical diseases* (21st ed., pp. 725-764). Philadelphia: W.B. Saunders Company.

Centers for Disease Control and Prevention. (2004). Yellow fever. Downloaded March 24, 2004, from *www.cdc.gov/travel/diseases/yellowfever.htm*

Chin, J. (Ed.). (2000). *Control of communicable diseases manual* (17th ed.). Washington, DC: American Public Health Association.

Koren, G., Matsui, D., & Bailey, B. (2003). DEET-based insect repellents: Safety implications for children and pregnant and lactating women. *Canadian Medical Association Journal.* Retrieved November 27, 2003, from *www.cmaj.ca/pdfs/deet-koren.pdf*

Monath, T.P. (2001). Yellow fever: An update. *The Lancet Infectious Diseases, 1,* 11-20.

Robertson, S.E., Hull, B.P., Tomori, O., Bele, O., LeDuc, J.W., & Esteves, K. (1996). Yellow fever: A decade of reemergence. *Journal of the American Medical Association, 276,* 1157-1162.

Tomori, O. (1999). Impact of yellow fever on the developing world. *Advances in Virus Research, 53,* 5-34.

White, N.J. (2003). Malaria. In G.C. Cook & A.I. Zumla (Eds.), *Manson's tropical diseases* (21st ed., pp. 1205-1295). Philadelphia: W.B. Saunders Company.

A DIFFERENTIAL DIAGNOSIS OF DISEASES BY SIGNS, SYMPTOMS, AND GEOGRAPHY

INTRODUCTION

This appendix presents a framework for forming the preliminary differential diagnosis of tropical and emerging infectious diseases in immigrants or travelers. The first part lists diseases according to major and/or presenting signs and symptoms; the second part lists diseases according to geography. Applying these two sections together to the case of a patient from Southeast Asia who has anemia, for example, one would generate this initial list of possible etiologies: HIV, hookworm, leishmaniasis, malaria, schistosomiasis, trichuriasis, or tuberculosis. Other signs and symptoms in this patient would then help narrow the differential diagnosis.

Readers will note that listings do not include some of the common diseases with which most practitioners are familiar. The purpose here is not to list what diagnoses are most likely for a given sign or symptom; rather, it is to stimulate thinking about diagnoses beyond what is ordinarily encountered. Listings also do not include all signs and symptoms of diseases, and absence from a listing does not necessarily mean that a disease is not associated with a particular sign, symptom, or region. Opportunistic infections among immunocompromised patients may be found in areas other than the regions listed here. In the cases of internally displaced people, refugees, undocumented immigrants, migrant workers, trafficked persons, the poor, and other marginalized groups, the role of malnutrition should be considered.

There is repetition in this appendix. Given the choice of repetition or referring readers from section to section, repetition seemed the better choice. We would welcome your feedback to refine this appendix for future editions.

PART 1: MAJOR OR PRESENTING SIGNS AND SYMPTOMS

Fever

Acute Fever

Amebiasis
Arboviral encephalitides (dengue, Eastern equine, Japanese, Venezuelan, Western equine, West Nile, and others)
Bartonellosis
Influenza and other common viral infections
Hepatitis A, B
HIV (acute infection)
Leptospirosis
Malaria
Schistosomiasis (Katayama fever)
Trypanosomiasis (African trypanosomiasis, Chagas disease)
Typhoid
Typhus
Viral hemorrhagic fevers

Chronic or Recurring Fever

Amebic liver abscess
Brucellosis
Hepatitis A, B
HIV/AIDS
Leishmaniasis (visceral)
Leptospirosis
Malaria
Relapsing fever (louse-borne, tick-borne)

Trench fever
Tuberculosis
Typhus (endemic, epidemic, scrub)
Yellow fever

Fever and Rash

Dengue
Leptospirosis
Measles
Meningococcemia
Rickettsial diseases (e.g., Rocky Mountain spotted fever,
  typhus, and others)
Rubella
Smallpox
Varicella
Viral hemorrhagic fevers

Fever with Respiratory Distress

Anthrax
Community-acquired bacterial pneumonia
Hantavirus
Legionella
Melioidosis
Plague (pneumonic)
Q-fever
SARS
Tularemia

Fever with Neurological Signs

Arboviral encephalitides (dengue, Eastern equine,
  Japanese, Venezuelan, Western equine, West Nile,
  and others)
Meningitis (meningococcus and other bacteria)
Meningoencephalitis (amebic, Lyme, and others)
Viral meningitis (enteroviruses and others)
Yellow fever

Fever with Hemorrhage or Shock

Dengue hemorrhagic fever or dengue shock syndrome
Ebola and other viral hemorrhagic fevers
Hantavirus hemorrhagic fever with renal syndrome
Leptospirosis
Meningococcemia
Plague (septicemic)
Typhoid fever

Respiratory

Pharyngitis

Chikungunya fever
Diphtheria
Ebola and Marburg hemorrhagic fevers
Lassa fever
Tularemia

Hemoptysis

Echinococcosis with ruptured cyst
Hantavirus hemorrhagic fever with renal syndrome
Histoplasmosis
Lassa fever
Leptospirosis
Melioidosis (chronic)
Paragonimiasis
Plague (pneumonic)
Sporotrichosis (pulmonary)
Tuberculosis
Viral hemorrhagic fevers

Pneumonia

Aspergillosis
Blastomycosis
Coccidioidomycosis
Community-acquired bacterial pneumonia
Cryptococcosis
Histoplasmosis

Legionella
Melioidosis
Paracoccidioidomycosis
Plague (pneumonic)
Pneumocystis
Psittacosis
Q fever
SARS
Tuberculosis
Tularemia
Typhus (murine)

Distinctive Chest X-Ray Findings

Anthrax—widened mediastinum
Histoplasmosis—enlarged mediastinal lymph nodes
Melioidosis—upper lobe infiltrates, cavitations
SARS—ground-glass appearance with underlying opacities
Tuberculosis—hilar adenopathy, cavitations, miliary pattern

Cardiovascular
Bradycardia (Including Relative Bradycardia with Fever)

Chagas' disease or American trypanosomiasis
Dengue
Hantavirus pulmonary syndrome
Lassa fever
Legionella in elderly patients
Psittacosis
South American hemorrhagic fever
Tularemia
Typhoid and paratyphoid fever
Viral hemorrhagic fevers
Yellow fever

High-Output Heart Failure

Hookworm with severe anemia

Myocarditis

Chagas' disease or American trypanosomiasis
Diphtheria
Leptospirosis
Relapsing fever (Borreliosis)
Trichinellosis
Typhoid and paratyphoid fever
Typhus (epidemic louse-borne)

Gastrointestinal

Acute Abdomen or Intestinal Obstruction

Actinomycosis
Amebiasis
Anisakidosis
Ascariasis
Brucellosis
Chagas' disease or American trypanosomiasis (chronic)
Fascioliasis
Parastrongyliasis
Schistosomiasis (intestinal)
Typhoid and paratyphoid fever

Gastrointestinal Bleeding

Amebiasis
Anthrax (gastrointestinal)
Chikungunya fever
Dengue hemorrhagic fever
Hantavirus hemorrhagic fever with renal syndrome
Hookworm—in infants
Schistosomiasis—with portal hypertension
Typhoid and paratyphoid fever
Viral hemorrhagic fevers

Acute Diarrhea

Amebiasis
Campylobacter
Cholera

Clostridium (C. botulinum, C. perfringens)
Cryptosporidiosis
Cyclosporiasis
Escherichia coli
Giardiasis
Salmonella
Shigella
Staphylococcus aureus
Viral gastroenteritis (e.g., rotavirus)
Yersinia enterocolitica

Chronic Diarrhea

Amebiasis
Campylobacter
Clonorchiasis
Clostridium difficile
Cryptosporidiosis
Cyclosporiasis
Giardiasis
Salmonella
Schistosomiasis
Strongyloidiasis
Trichuriasis
Tropical sprue
Tuberculosis (intestinal)
Yersinia

Hepatomegaly

Amebic liver abscess
Babesiosis
Bartonellosis
Brucellosis
Chagas' disease or American trypanosomiasis
Echinococcosis
Gnathostomiasis
Leptospirosis
Malaria

Paracoccidioidomycosis
Relapsing fever (louse-borne, tick-borne)
Schistosomiasis
Toxocariasis
Toxoplasmosis
Trematodes (Clonorchis, Fasciola, Opisthorchis)
Trypanosomiasis
Tuberculosis
Viral hepatitis

Splenomegaly

Babesiosis
Bartonellosis
Brucellosis
Chagas' disease or American trypanosomiasis
Hepatitis A, B (especially chronic)
Leishmaniasis
Leptospirosis
Malaria
Paracoccidioidomycosis
Psittacosis
Relapsing fever (louse-borne, tick-borne)
Schistosomiasis
Toxocariasis
Toxoplasmosis
Trench fever
Trypanosomiasis
Tuberculosis
Typhoid and paratyphoid fever
Typhus
Viral hepatitis

Jaundice

Babesiosis
Echinococcosis
Leptospirosis
Malaria
Melioidosis

Relapsing fever (louse-borne, tick-borne)
Toxoplasmosis (congenital)
Trematodes (Clonorchis, Fasciola, Opisthorchis)
Viral hemorrhagic fevers
Viral hepatitis
Yellow fever

Renal and Genitourinary
Hematuria

Filariasis
Hantavirus hemorrhagic fever with renal syndrome
Leptospirosis
Malaria
Q fever (chronic)
Relapsing fever (louse-borne, tick-borne)
Schistosomiasis
Trichinellosis
Viral hemorrhagic fevers

Nephrotic Syndrome

Filariasis
Hepatitis B
Leprosy or Hansen's disease with secondary amyloidosis
Malaria (P. malariae)
Schistosomiasis (S. mansoni)
Toxocariasis

Acute Renal Failure

Cholera
Leprosy or Hansen's disease
Leptospirosis
Malaria
Melioidosis
Salmonella
Schistosomiasis (S. mansoni, S. haematobium)
Scrub typhus
Shigella
Tetanus

Genital Lesions

Chancroid
Granuloma inguinale
Herpes simplex virus
Lymphogranuloma venereum
Scabies
Schistosomiasis
Syphilis
Tuberculosis

Skin

Note that in some disorders lesions change with time and that more than one feature may be present.

Analgesia

Leprosy or Hansen's disease

Pruritus

Cutaneous larva migrans
Enterobiasis or pinworm infection
Fungal infections (superficial)
Larva currens, in acute Strongyloides infection
Leishmaniasis, cutaneous
Onchocerciasis or river blindness with
  "leopard skin" (filariasis)
Scabies
Schistosomiasis (swimmer's itch)
Toxocariasis
Trichuriasis
Trypanosomiasis (African)
Tungiasis

Macules

Bejel or nonvenereal endemic syphilis
Lyme disease
Malnutrition especially pellagra
Onchocerciasis or river blindness with "leopard skin"

Pinta or mal de pinto or carate
Syphilis
Yaws or frambesia

Papules

Bejel or nonvenereal endemic syphilis
Candidiasis
Cutaneous larva migrans
Cutaneous tuberculosis
Fungal infections (deep)
Kaposi's sarcoma (human herpes virus 8)
Leishmaniasis, cutaneous
Leprosy or Hansen's disease
Lyme disease
Myiasis
Onchocerciasis or river blindness with "leopard skin"
Scabies
Staphylococcus
Superficial fungal infections
Syphilis
Tungiasis
Varicella
Yaws or frambesia

Plaques

Chromomycosis
Coccidioidomycosis
Cutaneous leishmaniasis
Kaposi's sarcoma (human herpes virus 8)
Leprosy or Hansen's disease
Lobomycosis
Lyme disease
Malnutrition (e.g. pellagra)
Mycobacterium infections
Onchocerciasis or river blindness with "leopard skin"
Paracoccidioidomycosis
Sporotrichosis

Superficial fungal infections
Syphilis
Tuberculosis, cutaneous
Yaws or frambesia

Vesicles

Anthrax, cutaneous
Cutaneous larva migrans
Herpes
Onchocerciasis (in areas of edema) or river blindness
  with "leopard skin"
Pemphigus disorders, for example, foliaceus, vulgaris
Scabies
Varicella

Urticaria

Ascariasis
Chagas' disease or American trypanosomiasis
Cutaneous larva migrans
Dracunculiasis or Guinea worm disease
Fascioliasis
Filariasis
Schistosomiasis
Strongyloidiasis
Trichinellosis

Nodules

Bartonellosis or Oroya fever
Bejel or nonvenereal endemic syphilis
Boutonneuse fever or African tick fever
  or Marseilles fever or tick typhus
Chikungunya fever
Chromomycosis
Cutaneous tuberculosis
Cysticercosis
Dengue fever
Enterovirus exanthems
Granuloma inguinale or Donovanosis

Kaposi's sarcoma (human herpes virus 8)
Leishmaniasis, cutaneous
Leprosy or Hansen's disease
Lobomycosis
Mycetoma or maduromycosis or Madura foot; related
  infections include eumycetoma and actinomycetoma
Mycobacterium infections
Myiasis
Prototheosis
Sporotrichosis
Staphylococcus
Syphilis
Trypanosomiasis (African) or African sleeping sickness
Tungiasis
Yaws or frambesia

Swelling or Erythematous Lesions

Chagas' disease or American trypanosomiasis
Gnathostomiasis
Leprosy or Hansen's disease
Loiasis or loa loa
Lyme disease
Onchocerciasis or river blindness with "leopard skin"
  (filariasis)
Pinta or mal de pinto or carate
Trypanosomiasis (African) or African sleeping sickness

Ulcer/Pustule/Abscess

Actinomycosis
Amebiasis, cutaneous, affecting genitals
Anthrax
Bartonellosis or Oroya fever
Bejel or nonvenereal endemic syphilis
Buruli ulcer (Africa, Australia)
Cancrum oris or gangrenous stomatitis or noma
Candidiasis
Chagas' disease or American trypanosomiasis
Chancroid

Coccidioidomycosis
Cutaneous leishmaniasis
Dracunculiasis or Guinea worm disease
Granuloma inguinale or Donovanosis
Herpes
Leishmaniasis, cutaneous
Leprosy or Hansen's disease
Lymphogranuloma venereum
Mycetoma
Mycobacterium other than tuberculosis
Myiasis
Paracoccidioidomycosis
Scabies
Sporotrichosis
Staphylococcus
Streptococcus
Syphilis
Trypanosomiasis (African) or African sleeping sickness
Tuberculosis, cutaneous
Tularemia
Typhus group (endemic murine, epidemic louse borne, scrub), eschar with erythematous margins
Yaws or frambesia (tropical areas worldwide)

Lymphedema/Lymphadenitis

Anthrax
Bartonellosis or Oroya fever
Cat scratch disease
Filariasis (Bancroftian, Malayan, onchocerciasis, and others)
Kaposi's sarcoma (human herpes virus 8)
Leishmaniasis, cutaneous
Loiasis—transient wrist or ankle swelling
Melioidosis
Mycobacteria (atypical and tuberculosis)
Pinta or mal de pinto or carate
Plague
Schistosomiasis or bilharzia

Sporotrichosis
Trypanosomiasis, African—transient hand and foot
  edema
Tuberculosis

Hematologic
Anemia of Chronic Disease

Amebiasis
Giardiasis
Hemoglobinopathies
HIV
Hookworm
Leishmaniasis
Malaria
Malnutrition
Schistosomiasis
Trichuriasis
Tuberculosis

Anemia from Hemolysis

Babesiosis
Bartonellosis
Lassa fever and other viral hemorrhagic fevers
Malaria
Schistosomiasis—with portal hypertension
Trypanosomiasis
Typhoid and paratyphoid fever—hemolytic uremic
  syndrome

Anemia from Hemorrhage or Coagulopathy

Dengue fever
Hantavirus hemorrhagic fever with renal syndrome
Hepatitis A, B—with liver failure
Leptospirosis
Melioidosis
Meningococcemia
Sepsis from other bacterial causes
Smallpox

Tularemia
Viral hemorrhagic fevers

Eosinophilia

Angiostrongyliasis
Ascariasis
Coccidioidomycosis
Filariasis
Gnathostomiasis
Hookworm
Paragonimiasis
Schistosomiasis (Katayama fever)
Strongyloidiasis
Toxocariasis
Trematodes (Clonorchis, Fasciola, Opisthorchis)
Trichinosis
Tuberculosis (chronic)
Whipworm

Leukopenia

Brucellosis
Dengue
HIV/AIDS
Leishmaniasis
Malaria
Measles
Meningococcemia
Q fever
Typhus
Viral hemorrhagic fevers
Yellow fever

Thrombocytopenia

Babesiosis
Bartonellosis
Brucellosis
Dengue

Hantavirus hemorrhagic fever with renal syndrome
Hantavirus pulmonary syndrome
Leishmaniasis
Leptospirosis
Malaria
Meningococcemia
Q fever—in acute phase, thrombocytosis in recovery phase
SARS
Trypanosomiasis, African
Tularemia
Typhoid and paratyphoid fever—mild
Viral hemorrhagic fevers
Yellow fever

Musculoskeletal
Arthritis

Arboviruses
Filariasis
Hepatitis B
Lyme disease
Malaria
Reactive arthritis (Campylobacter, Salmonella, Shigella, Yersinia)
Relapsing fever (tick-borne)
Schistosomiasis
Septic arthritis (Brucellosis, Staphylococcus, Salmonella, Gonococcal, Tuberculosis)

Myalgia

Brucellosis
Dengue
Leptospirosis
Malaria
Plague
Q fever
Schistosomiasis (Katayama fever)—in acute stage
Typhoid and paratyphoid fever

Typhus (endemic, epidemic, and scrub)
Viral hemorrhagic fevers

Central Nervous System

Altered Mental Status

African trypanosomiasis
Arboviral encephalitides (dengue, Eastern equine,
 Japanese, Venezuelan, Western equine, West Nile,
 and others)
Bartonellosis
HIV encephalopathy
Typhoid fever

Cranial Nerve Deficits

Cryptococcal meningitis
Diphtheria
Lyme meningoencephalitis
Neurocysticercosis
Parastrongyliasis meningitis
Poliomyelitis (bulbar)
Tetanus (cephalic)
Toxoplasmosis encephalitis

Meningitis

Angiostrongyliasis (Eosinophilic meningitis)
Cryptococcosis
Meningococcus and other bacteria
Neurocysticercosis
Parastrongyliasis
Tuberculosis

Paralysis

Arboviral encephalitides
Botulism
LaCrosse encephalitis
Poliomyelitis
Tick-borne encephalitis
West Nile virus

Seizures

Amebiasis
Arboviral encephalitides
Echinococcosis
HIV/AIDS with opportunistic CNS infection
Measles
Meningitis (see previous entry)
Neurocysticercosis
Paragonimiasis
Schistosomiasis
Toxocariasis
Toxoplasmosis
Trichinosis
Trypanosomiasis

Eye
Conjunctivitis

Anthrax
Chikungunya fever
Chlamydia trachomatis
Community-acquired viral and bacterial causes
Diphtheria
Measles
Onchocerciasis
Tularemia
Typhus
Viral hemorrhagic fevers

Vision loss

Chlamydia trachomatis
Leprosy or Hansen's disease
Malaria (cerebral)
Onchocerciasis
Toxocara (ocular larva migrans)

Other Eye Findings

Chagas' disease or American trypanosomiasis—unilateral
  eyelid edema or Romana's sign

Gnathostomiasis—lid edema, chemosis
Leprosy or Hansen's disease—lagophthalmos
Leptospirosis—conjunctival suffusion
Filariasis, especially loiasis—subconjunctival worm
Toxocara—leukocoria
Trichinosis—bilateral eyelid edema
Trypanosomiasis, African—eyelid edema
Typhoid fever—conjunctival rose spots

PART 2: GEOGRAPHIC DISTRIBUTION, ARRANGED ALPHABETICALLY BY CONTINENT OR REGION

Global

Be aware of the following illnesses in travelers and immigrants worldwide, and vaccinate when appropriate.

Amebiasis
Ascariasis
Botulism
Echinococcosis
Fascioliasis
Giardiasis
Hepatitis A, B
HIV/AIDS
Leptospirosis
Measles
Pertussis
Plague
Q fever
Rabies
Scabies
Tetanus
Toxocariasis
Trachoma
Traveler's diarrhea (E. coli, Salmonella, Shigella, and other viral and bacterial causes)

Trench fever
Trichinellosis
Trichuriasis
Tuberculosis
Typhoid
Typhus (endemic murine)

Africa
North Africa

Anthrax
Brucellosis
Chikungunya fever
Cholera
Cutaneous larva migrans
Cysticercosis
Dengue
Filariasis (lymphatic)
Heterophyiasis
Hookworm (Ancylostoma duodenale)
Leishmaniasis
Leprosy or Hansen's disease
Malaria
Mycetoma or maduromycosis
Myiasis
Onchocerciasis
Paragonimiasis
Plague
Poliomyelitis
Relapsing fever (tick-borne endemic)
Rift Valley fever
Schistosomiasis
Sporotrichosis
Strongyloidiasis
Tungiasis
West Nile fever
Yaws

East, West, and Central Africa

Anthrax
Buruli ulcer
Cholera
Cutaneous larva migrans
Cysticercosis
Dengue
Filariasis (dracunculiasis, loiasis, lymphatic)
Hookworm (Necator americanus)
Lassa fever
Leishmaniasis
Leprosy or Hansen's disease
Malaria
Mycetoma or maduromycosis
Myiasis
Measles
Meningococcemia
Onchocerciasis
Paragonimiasis
Plague
Poliomyelitis
Relapsing fever (louse-borne or tick-borne epidemic)
Rift Valley fever
Schistosomiasis
Sporotrichosis
Strongyloidiasis
Trypanosomiasis
Tungiasis
Typhus (epidemic louse-borne)
Viral hemorrhagic fever (Marburg, Ebola)
Yaws
Yellow fever

Southern Africa

Anthrax
Cholera
Chromoblastomycosis
Cutaneous larva migrans

Cysticercosis
Dengue
Filariasis (lymphatic)
Granuloma inguinale
Hookworm (Necator americanus)
Leishmaniasis
Leprosy or Hansen's disease
Malaria
Measles
Mycetoma or maduromycosis
Onchocerciasis
Paragonimiasis
Plague
Rift Valley fever
Schistosomiasis
Sporotrichosis
Strongyloidiasis
Trypanosomiasis
Tungiasis
Yellow fever

America
Mexico and Central America

Anisakidosis
Anthrax
Bartonellosis
Brucellosis
Buruli ulcer
Chagas' disease or American trypanosomiasis
Cholera
Chromoblastomycosis
Coccidioidomycosis
Cutaneous larva migrans
Cysticercosis
Dengue
Eastern equine encephalomyelitis
Filariasis (lymphatic)

Fogo selvagem (endemic foliaceus pemphigus)
Gnathostomiasis
Hantavirus pulmonary syndrome
Histoplasmosis
Hymenolepiasis
Leishmaniasis
Malaria
Mycetoma or maduromycosis
Myiasis
Onchocerciasis
Paracoccidioidomycosis
Paragonimiasis
Parastrongyliasis
Pinta
Relapsing fever (tick-borne endemic)
Sporotrichosis
Strongyloidiasis
Tungiasis
Typhus (epidemic louse-borne)
Venezuelan equine encephalitis
Western equine encephalitis
Yaws

North America

Anisakidosis
Arboviral encephalitides
Babesiosis
Blastomycosis
Coccidioidomycosis
Cutaneous larva migrans
Eastern equine encephalomyelitis
Hantavirus pulmonary syndrome
Histoplasmosis
Lyme disease
Plague
Rabies
Relapsing fever (tick-borne endemic)

St. Louis encephalitis
Strongyloidiasis
Tularemia
Venezuelan equine encephalitis
West Nile fever
Western equine encephalitis

South America, Temperate

Anthrax
Brucellosis
Chagas' disease or American trypanosomiasis
Cysticercosis
Dengue
Fogo selvagem (endemic foliaceus pemphigus)
Hantavirus pulmonary syndrome
Histoplasmosis
Leishmaniasis
Leprosy or Hansen's disease
Malaria
Mycetoma or maduromycosis
Paragonimiasis
Relapsing fever (louse-borne epidemic)
Sporotrichosis
Strongyloidiasis
Tungiasis
Typhus (epidemic louse-borne)
Western equine encephalitis
Yellow fever

South America, Tropical

Brucellosis
Chagas' disease or American trypanosomiasis
Cholera
Chromoblastomycosis
Coccidioidomycosis
Cutaneous larva migrans
Cysticercosis

Dengue
Eastern equine encephalomyelitis
Filariasis (lymphatic)
Fogo selvagem (endemic foliaceus pemphigus)
Gnathostomiasis
Granuloma inguinale
Hantavirus pulmonary syndrome
Histoplasmosis
Leishmaniasis
Leprosy or Hansen's disease
Malaria
Mycetoma or maduromycosis
Myiasis
Onchocerciasis
Paracoccidioidomycosis
Paragonimiasis
Parastrongyliasis
Pinta
Relapsing fever (louse-borne or tick-borne epidemic)
Sporotrichosis
Strongyloidiasis
Tungiasis
Typhus (epidemic louse-borne)
Venezuelan equine encephalitis
Western equine encephalitis
Yaws
Yellow fever

Asia
East Asia

Anisakidosis
Anthrax
Capillariasis
Chromoblastomycosis
Clonorchiasis
Dengue
Fasciolopsiasis
Filariasis (Lymphatic)

Gnathostomiasis
Hantavirus hemorrhagic fever with renal syndrome
Heterophyiasis
Hookworm (Ancylostoma duodenale)
Japanese encephalitis
Leishmaniasis
Leprosy or Hansen's disease
Malaria
Myiasis
Paragonimiasis
Parastrongyliasis
Plague
SARS
Sporotrichosis
Strongyloidiasis
Tularemia
Typhus (epidemic louse-borne and scrub)

South Asia

Brucellosis
Chikungunya fever
Cholera
Dengue
Fasciolopsiasis
Filariasis (Lymphatic)
Granuloma inguinale
Hookworm (Ancylostoma duodenale)
Hookworm (Necator americanus)
Hymenolepiasis
Japanese encephalitis
Kyasanur forest disease
Leishmaniasis
Malaria
Mycetoma or maduromycosis
Paragonimiasis
Plague
Poliomyelitis
Relapsing fever (tick-borne endemic)

Strongyloidiasis
Tungiasis
Typhus (scrub)
Yaws

Southeast Asia

Buruli ulcer
Capillariasis
Chikungunya fever
Chromoblastomycosis
Clonorchiasis
Dengue
Echinostomiasis
Fasciolopsiasis
Filariasis
Gnathostomiasis
Heterophyiasis
Japanese encephalitis
Kunjin fever
Leishmaniasis
Leprosy or Hansen's disease
Malaria
Melioidosis
Myiasis
Opisthorchiasis
Paragonimiasis
Parastrongyliasis
Plague
SARS
Schistosomiasis
Strongyloidiasis
Typhus (scrub)
Yaws

Australia and South Pacific

Buruli ulcer
Dengue

Filariasis (lymphatic)
Granuloma inguinale
Hookworm (Necator americanus)
Leprosy or Hansen's disease
Japanese encephalitis
Kunjin fever
Malaria
Murray Valley encephalitis
Parastrongyliasis
Ross River virus
Typhus (scrub)
Yaws

Caribbean

Cutaneous larva migrans
Eastern equine encephalomyelitis
Dengue
Filariasis (lymphatic)
Hookworm (Necator americanus)
Leishmaniasis
Malaria
Parastrongyliasis
Schistosomiasis
St. Louis encephalitis
Tungiasis

Europe
Eastern Europe and Russia

Anthrax
Brucellosis
Cholera
Diphtheria
Hantavirus hemorrhagic fever with renal syndrome
Hookworm (Ancylostoma duodenale)
Lyme disease
Opisthorchiasis
Relapsing fever (louse-borne or tick-borne epidemic)

Tick-borne encephalitis
Tularemia
West Nile fever

Western Europe

Anisakidosis
Babesiosis
Hantavirus hemorrhagic fever and renal syndrome
Hymenolepiasis
Louping ill (arboviral encephalitis)
Lyme disease
Myiasis
Relapsing fever (louse-borne epidemic)
Tick-borne encephalitis
Tularemia
West Nile fever

Middle East

Brucellosis
Capillariasis (rare)
Chikungunya fever
Dengue
Filariasis (lymphatic)
Heterophyiasis
Hymenolepiasis
Leishmaniasis
Malaria
Meningococcemia—especially travelers to Mecca
Onchocerciasis
Plague
Poliomyelitis
Relapsing fever (tick-borne endemic)
Schistosomiasis
West Nile fever

B DIARRHEA

Table B-1 expands on the "approach to the patient with diarrhea" section of Chapter 3. The format is based loosely on that of the disease chapters. Most of the differential diagnosis of infectious diarrhea is summarized in this table. Readers will note that several of the diseases are discussed at greater length in separate chapters.

The table lists unique clinical features of each illness. Not included are the many aspects that all diarrhea illnesses share in common. Electrolyte imbalance, dehydration, and shock are always potential complications. Treatment for all diarrheal infections includes correcting fluid deficits and electrolyte imbalances and maintaining hydration (see Chapter 3). For children, encourage oral rehydration and avoid antimotility drugs. Some bacterial gastrointestinal infections should be treated with antibiotics, while for others antibiotics either are ineffective or carry increased risks (e.g., potential for hemolytic uremic syndrome from *E. coli* 0157 in children). Specific recommendations are summarized in the table.

Prevention for almost all gastrointestinal infections includes personal hygiene (especially hand washing), using clean water for drinking and food preparation, breast-feeding infants, washing and cooking foods thoroughly, avoiding sexual practices that may permit fecal-oral transmission, properly disposing human and animal waste, protecting water systems from contamination, and private and governmental monitoring of food handling and production. Health care workers should practice enteric precautions around all patients, because some may be asymptomatically infected with diarrheal pathogens. In many gastrointestinal infections, the patient remains a carrier for weeks or longer after resolution of signs and symptoms.

TABLE B-1 Diarrheal Diseases

Pathogen	Epidemiology (CSO = common source outbreak; S = sporadic)	Transmission and pathogenesis	Incubation	Signs and symptoms	Complications	Common laboratory findings	Diagnostic tests	Treatment
Bacillus cereus	Worldwide; A source of two types of "food poisoning": emetic and diarrheal; CSO	Soil, decaying organic matter, vegetables, water; spore-forming rod with preformed enterotoxin; diarrheal illness associated with contaminated meat or vegetables	1-6 hours in emetic illness; 10-12 hours in diarrheal	Emetic illness: upper GI distress, nausea and vomiting sometimes lasting less than 12 hours Diarrheal illness: Abdominal pain and cramps, profuse watery, nonbloody diarrhea lasting up to 48 hours; self-limiting	Rarely liver failure	None	Usually not necessary; in outbreaks may test food or stool for toxin	Supportive

Organism	Distribution	Mechanism/Transmission	Incubation	Clinical Features	Complications	Prevention	Diagnosis	Treatment
Campylobacter jejuni (also C. coli, C. lari, C. upsaliensis)	Worldwide; a cause of traveler's diarrhea; CSO, S	Fecal-oral, human to human, animal to human (commonly pets), food (especially commercially raised poultry), water, and milk; gram-negative bacteria producing inflammatory and noninflammatory diarrhea possibly by preformed toxin or toxin production	2-5 days	Range from mild, noninflammatory without blood or fever to acute colitis with severe, massive, and grossly bloody stools (10 or more per day), fever, cramping abdominal pain relieved by defecation; often prodrome of malaise, fever, headache, myalgia; lasting 2-10 days	Bacteremia (usually with risk factors such as malnutrition, hepatic dysfunction, cancer, diabetes); reactive arthritis; Guillain-Barré syndrome (2-3 weeks after onset of illness); pseudo-appendicitis	None	Stool culture, sometimes blood culture; direct exam of feces by dark-field or phase-contrast microscopy	Erythromycin; or azithromycin; alternatives include quinolones, tetracycline, clindamycin; antimotility agents may prolong illness

continued

TABLE B-1 Diarrheal Diseases—cont'd

Pathogen	Epidemiology	Transmission	Incubation	Symptoms	Complications	Lab	Diagnosis	Treatment
Clostridium botulinum (botulism)	Worldwide; Category A biological warfare agent; CSO (even one case a public health emergency);	Food-borne acquired by ingesting preformed neurotoxin (especially in inadequately preserved or cooked canned foods) from spore-forming obligate anaerobe found in soil. Intestinal botulism results when infants ingest spores from contaminated food (such as honey) or soil; spores.	Food-borne: usually 12-36 hours and ranging from 2 hours to 8 days. Intestinal (infant): 2-4 weeks.	Afebrile, vomiting, diarrhea, symmetric neurologic manifestations such as bulbar palsies, descending flaccid paralysis, but no sensory deficits, clear sensorium	Paralysis, respiratory failure, death	None	Confirmation through specialized laboratory testing for culture and toxin in stool, blood, food	Early treatment essential; passive immunization with antitoxin; ventilatory support and other supportive care

Clostridium difficile	Worldwide; S	germinate in the colon and produce neurotoxin; Causes antibiotic associated diarrhea and pseudomembranous colitis through actions of two intestinal toxins following antibiotic therapy	Begins during or weeks after antibiotic therapy	Ranges from mild, self-limited diarrhea to profuse watery diarrhea with mucus, occult blood, fever, abdominal cramps and pain, nausea and vomiting; asymptomatic carriage can occur in infants	Bacteremia and abscess formation; intestinal perforation(s); relapse(s)	Leukocytosis, fecal leukocytes	Enzyme assay to identify toxin in stool; stool culture	Metronidazole; vancomycin if metronidazole fails or disease is severe; discontinue offending antibiotic
Clostridium perfringens types A and C	Worldwide; CSO	Type A causes mild diarrheal illness. Type C is part of	Type A food poisoning: 7-15 hours	Type A: watery diarrhea, abdominal cramping,	Type A: fatalities unusual	Peripheral neutrophilic leuko-cytosis;	Type A: culture food, test stool for	Type A: Self-limited Type C:

continued

TABLE B-1 Diarrheal Diseases—cont'd

Pathogen	Epidemiology	Transmission	Incubation	Symptoms	Complications	Lab	Diagnosis	Treatment
Clostridium perfringens types A and C—cont'd		normal intestinal flora and is found in soil, produces severe necrotic enteritis by unknown mechanism, possibly due to β toxin that may overgrow after ingestion of contaminated meat in persons with protein deficiency.	Type C enteritis necroticans: 2 days, range 1-7 days, usually	resolution within 6-24 hours Type C: Severe upper abdominal pain, vomiting, distention, small bowel obstruction.	Type C: bowel obstruction, perforation, severe recurrent bleeding	fecal blood and leukocytes	enterotoxin Type C: Fluorescent antibody; cultures hard to interpret because of high asymptomatic carriage rates	antibiotics may include metronidazole, ampicillin, chloramphenicol, or penicillin; surgical intervention for intestinal obstruction, perforation, bleeding
Enterotoxigenic *Escherichia coli* (ETEC)	Worldwide, year-round, more common in wet season; second to	Fecal-oral, food or water; human to human; colonize small	24-48 hours	Voluminous, explosive watery cholera-like stool, 10×	None	None	Stool culture; PCR, ELISA	Supportive; traveler's diarrhea may be treated by

	rotavirus as cause of gastroenteritis; most common cause of traveler's diarrhea; CSO, S	intestine, release toxins		day; usually no fever; self-limiting 1-5 days in healthy persons	None			fluoroquinolones
Entero-invasive *E. coli* (EIEC)	Worldwide; less common; CSO, S	Fecal-oral, food or water; human to human; colonize small intestine, mucosal invasion and inflammation	24-48 hours	Fever, watery stools, similar to shigellosis but less severe, sometimes bloody/mucoid with cramps, tenesmus, urgency	None	Fecal leukocytes present	Stool culture; DNA hybridization, PCR, ELISA	Fluoroquinolones; resistance to TMP-SMX common
Entero-pathogenic *E. coli* (EPEC)	Worldwide; CSO, S; a cause of traveler's diarrhea; chronic diarrhea in infants	Fecal-oral, food or water; creates "attaching effacement" intestinal mucosa seen by electron microscopy	24-48 hours	Usually acute, profuse, watery nonbloody, mucoid; vomiting, fever common; may remit and relapse	Sometimes leads to chronic diarrhea, malnutrition	None	Stool culture, DNA probe	TMP-SMX, but increasing resistance, fluoroquinolones

continued

TABLE B-1 Diarrheal Diseases—cont'd

Pathogen	Epidemiology	Transmission	Incubation	Symptoms	Complications	Lab	Diagnosis	Treatment
Enterohemorrhagic *E. coli* (EHEC) or Shigatoxin-producing (STEC); serotype 0157:H7 most common	Worldwide; at-risk populations are age 6 months to 10 years and the elderly; CSO; Category B biological warfare agent	Animal feces, incompletely cooked foods such as hamburger; less frequently, human-to-human. Verocytotoxins (shiga-like) cause inflammatory hemorrhagic colitis and hemolytic uremic syndrome	3-4 days	Hemorrhagic colitis, abdominal cramps, watery diarrhea followed by large amounts of blood; fever rare; may be asymptomatic	Hemolytic uremic syndrome: acute renal failure, coagulopathy, anemia	May have elevated leukocyte count with left shift; thrombocytopenia, elevated BUN and creatinine	Stool culture must be specifically requested; ELISA, PCR	Antibiotics possibly increase risk of hemolytic uremic syndrome; dialysis for renal failure
Enteroaggregative *E. coli* (EAggEC) or adherent	Worldwide; found in infants and travelers; AIDS-associated diarrhea; S	Fecal-oral; food; mucous film on intestinal mucosa, hemorrhagic	24-48 hours	Secretory, watery, mucoid; less than half of patients with grossly bloody	Chronic diarrhea		Stool culture, PCR	In travelers, ciprofloxacin may be useful

Organism	Epidemiology	Pathophysiology	Incubation	Clinical	Complications	Stool findings	Diagnosis	Treatment
		necrosis, inflammatory; toxin production		stools; low-grade fever, no nausea; acute or persistent				
Salmonella spp. with multiple serotypes (non-typhoidal)	Worldwide; a cause of traveler's diarrhea; CSO; Category B biological warfare agent	Spread is usually animal to human, especially poultry and eggs, but also mammals, reptiles; *Salmonella* (and in some species, an enterotoxin) causes acute enterocolitis with mucosal inflammation, edema, and sometimes erosions; after infection, humans carry	6-72 hours, usually 24 hours	Acute-onset nausea, vomiting, abdominal cramps (often RLQ), then mild to severe watery diarrhea (sometimes with blood and mucus), fever. Neonates, infants, and patients with immuno-suppression have higher risk of severe disease, illness lasts	Bacteremia, especially in immuno-suppressed patients and patients with sickle cell disease; extra-intestinal focal infections, especially of bone, meninges, heart. Patients with inflammatory bowel disease may develop toxic megacolon. Patients with schistosomiasis have persistent infection	Stool with polymorpho-nuclear leukocytes and occult blood; mild leukocytosis	Stool culture, latex agglutination, fluorescent antibody	Fluoroquinolones, third-generation cephalosporins; antibiotics prolong carrier state and are reserved for bacteremia or serious underlying disease (e.g., AIDS), infants under 3 months, or extraintestinal focal infection. Antimotility drugs contraindicated

continued

TABLE B-1 Diarrheal Diseases—cont'd

Pathogen	Epidemiology	Transmission	Incubation	Symptoms	Complications	Lab	Diagnosis	Treatment
Salmonella—cont'd		*Salmonella* for 5 weeks or longer		2-7 days in healthy patients				
Salmonella typhi or *paratyphi*, other serotypes (typhoid, paratyphoid, or enteric fever)	Primarily developing nations; CSO, S; Category B biological warfare agent	Human to human; fecal (or urine)-oral, water or food; penetration of intestinal wall and invasion of lymph and spleen, then bacteremia and localization of infection in small intestine with ulceration	Typhoid: average 10-20 days; range 3-56 days; paratyphoid range 1-10 days	Malaise, headache, and rising and remitting fever, abdominal pain, hepatomegaly, splenomegaly, rose spots, mental status changes; paratyphoid similar to typhoid but less severe	Toxemia, myocarditis, intestinal hemorrhage or perforation, hepatitis; long-term carriage increased for women, biliary abnormalities, Schistosoma bladder infection	Mild leukocytosis early, leukopenia and neutropenia, anemia, mild thrombocytopenia, elevated serum transaminases, mild proteinuria	Isolation of organism from blood or bone marrow; stool culture; serologic tests and PCR available	Fluoroquinolones, third-generation cephalosporin; others depending on local resistance patterns; corticosteroids possibly helpful for severely ill patients

Shigella dysenteriae, other spp. (bacillary dysentery)	Worldwide, especially tropics, developing nations; especially among children; a cause of traveler's diarrhea; CSO, S	Human to human; fecal-oral; direct; food, water; invades mucosal cells of terminal ileum and colon causing edema, ulceration; *S. dysenteriae* produces shiga toxin	Usually 1-4 days; may be 6-8 days for *S. dysenteriae* type I	Varies from mild watery diarrhea to profuse, frequent, bloody mucoid stools, up to 30 per day; malaise, fever headache, severe abdominal pain, nausea and vomiting, tenesmus; untreated lasts 1-2 weeks	Bacteremia, toxic megacolon, hemolytic uremic syndrome, seizures, encephalopathy, Reiter syndrome	Leukocytosis with left shift	Stool and rectal culture; blood culture; enzyme immunoassay for shiga toxin	Fluoroquinolone; third-generation cephalosporin; azithromycin; narrower depending on susceptibility of isolate
Staphylococcus aureus	Worldwide; CSO, S	Commonly from contaminated foods (custard, meats) in which organisms multiply and	2-7 hours	Sudden onset salivation, vomiting (primary manifestation), abdominal cramps, watery			Isolation of organism in stool, food, food handler	Supportive

continued

TABLE B-1 Diarrheal Diseases—cont'd

Pathogen	Epidemiology	Transmission	Incubation	Symptoms	Complications	Lab	Diagnosis	Treatment
Staphylococcus aureus—cont'd		produce enterotoxin; human to human (nasopharyngeal colonization) via food; rarely overgrowth resulting from antibiotic therapy		diarrhea, fever absent or low; duration about 8 hours				
Vibrio cholerae (cholera)	Developing nations; 7 pandemics since 1817; CSO, S; Caterogry B biological warfare agent	Fecal (or vomitus)-oral; food- and water-borne; bacteria colonizes small intestine and produces enterotoxin responsible	Usually 2-3 days; as short as a few hours	Some asymptomatic; abrupt onset profuse watery "rice water" diarrhea, often nausea and vomiting	Coma, seizures, other sequelae of hypoglycemia and electrolyte imbalance; renal failure; sometimes aspiration pneumonia from vomiting	Leukocytosis in severe disease	Clinical diagnosis in epidemics; stool microscopy; culture; biotyping and serotyping	Aggressive oral or intravenous rehydration; doxycycline, TMP-ZMX, erythromycin, fluoroquinolone; vaccines available outside United States

Organism	Distribution	Source/Transmission	Incubation	Clinical	Complications	Fecal leukocytes	Culture	Treatment
Vibrio parahaemolyticus	Worldwide, part of normal marine flora; a cause of traveler's diarrhea; CSO, S	Ingestion of raw or undercooked shellfish; inflammatory reaction to saltwater *Vibrio* and, to lesser extent, toxin	Usually 24 hours or less	Abrupt onset profuse watery diarrhea, abdominal cramps sometimes low-grade fever, chills, headache; symptoms resolve in 2-5 days	Rarely bacteremia; skin infections in immunocompromised patients	Fecal leukocytes	Stool culture	Supportive only for severe diarrhea
Yersinia enterocolitica	Worldwide, especially northern Europe; most patients are children <5 years of age; uncommon; CSO, S	Animal feces; food-borne, person to person; also contaminated blood; mucosal ulceration in terminal ileum, enlargement of mesenteric lymph nodes	3-7 days	Fever, abdominal pain, diarrhea (sometimes bloody) lasting 1-3 weeks; mesenteric adenitis causes fever, RLQ pain mimicking appendicitis	Septicemia, polyarthritis, erythema nodosum	Fecal leukocytes; leukocytosis	Stool, blood culture, mesenteric lymph node or peritoneal fluid culture	Antibiotics not indicated for uncomplicated illness; gentamicin or chloramphenicol for septicemia

continued

TABLE B-1 Diarrheal Diseases—cont'd

Pathogen	Epidemiology	Transmission	Incubation	Symptoms	Complications	Lab	Diagnosis	Treatment
Viruses								
Adenovirus serotypes 40, 41	Worldwide; illness most common for children under 2 years of age; S	Fecal-oral, food; invades small intestine mucosal cells	3-10 days	Usually begins with profuse vomiting, followed in some patients by diarrhea, low-grade fever; less severe than rotavirus, but may last 1-2 weeks	None	None	Antigen detection	Supportive
Astrovirus	Worldwide; illness most common young ages; S	Fecal-oral, food, invades small intestine mucosal cells	24-48 hours	Usually begins with vomiting, followed in some patients by diarrhea, low-grade fever; less severe than	None	None	Antigen detection, usually used only for research purposes	Supportive

				...rotavirus; lasts 4-5 days				
Norwalk-like viruses (human caliciviruses)	Worldwide; illness most common young ages; a cause of traveler's diarrhea, especially on cruise ships; CSO	Fecal-oral, food, human to human; invades small intestine mucosal cells	1-2 days	Usually begins with profuse vomiting, followed in some patients by diarrhea, abdominal pain, low-grade fever; lasts 2-3 days	None	None	Antigen detection, PCR; electron microscopy and serology used to investigate outbreaks	Supportive
Rotavirus	Worldwide; illness most common ages 4 months to 3 years; leading cause of dehydrating gastroenteritis worldwide; S	Fecal-oral, human to human; invades small intestine mucosal cells	1-3 days	Varies from mild diarrhea to severe gastroenteritis; usually begins with vomiting, followed by pale loose to watery stools; lasts 2-23 days, median 6 days	Intussusception; rarely extraintestinal, e.g., acute myositis, hemophagocytic lymphohistiocytosis, paralysis, encephalitis		Stool antigen detection, RT-PCR, viral culture	Supportive

continued

TABLE B-1　Diarrheal Diseases—cont'd

Pathogen	Epidemiology	Transmission	Incubation	Symptoms	Complications	Lab	Diagnosis	Treatment
Parasites								
Entamoeba histolytica	Worldwide; CSO, S	Fecal-oral, food, water; inflammation and invasion of colonic mucosa	1-4 weeks; hepatic amebiasis 2-5 months	90% asymptomatic; intestinal infection: fever, colicky abdominal pain, increased stools, often mucoid and bloody, anorexia, jaundice, tenesmus; extraintestinal (usually hepatic): fever, malaise, RUQ pain, hepatomegaly, nausea and vomiting	Megacolon, necrotizing colitis	Leukocytosis, eosinophilia	Trophozoites in stool, antigen detection, DNA tests	Dehydroemetine, emetine, and metronidazole act on amebas in bowel wall; diloxanide furoate, iodoquinol and paromomycin act on amebas in lumen. Tetracycline inhibits growth in both the bowel wall and lumen

Giardia lamblia (giardiasis)	Worldwide, greater prevalence in warmer areas; a cause of traveler's diarrhea; CSO, S	Fecal-oral, water or food; protozoan flagellate colonizes and sometimes invades small intestine	1-3 weeks or longer	Many asymptomatic cases; gradual onset diarrhea with wide range of severity; often mucoid, pale, frothy, steatorrheic, and foul-smelling stools; nausea, vomiting	Chronic infection causes weight loss, failure to thrive		Microscopy; ELISA, IFA	Metronidazole, paromomycin, tinidazole (not available in the United States)
Trichinella spiralis	Worldwide, greater in Americas and Europe	From under-cooked animal flesh (muscle), typically pork; larvae travel from GI system via lymphatics and blood to heart, lungs, and striated muscle	7-21 days	Enteric phase characterized primarily by nausea and vomiting, also diarrhea; migratory phase includes periorbital edema, high fever, dysphagia, dyspnea,	Myocarditis, pneumonia, meningitis, meningo-encephalitis, other neurologic compli-cations in very heavy infection	Eosino-philia, hematuria, albumi-nuria	Antibody detection; muscle biopsy rarely necessary	Albendazole, thiabendazole; prednisone may be helpful for critically ill patients

continued

TABLE B-1 Diarrheal Diseases—cont'd

Pathogen	Epidemiology	Transmission	Incubation	Symptoms	Complications	Lab	Diagnosis	Treatment
Trichinella spiralis—cont'd				myalgia, sometimes paralysis of extremities				
Cryptosporidium spp. (cryptosporidiosis)	Worldwide; a source of traveler's diarrhea; serious illness in immunocompromised persons; Category B biological warfare agent; S	Fecal-oral, water, human to human; colonization	1-12 days	Diarrhea ranging from mild to profuse, watery, mucoid, abdominal cramping; less commonly malaise, fever, nausea and vomiting, myalgia; lasts 4-14 days, may wax and wane	Biliary tract infection	None in otherwise healthy persons	Immunofluorescent assay; enzyme immunoassay; stool microscopy with acid fast stain	Nitazoxanide

Cyclospora cayetanensis	Probably worldwide	Fecal-oral, water; organism colonizes small intestine causing inflammation	12 hours–11 days	Diarrhea lasting 1-8 weeks; sometimes abdominal pain, gas, bloating, nausea, vomiting, anorexia, weight loss	Guillain-Barré syndrome	None	Light microscopy to identify oocysts	TMP-SMX
Hymeno-lepis nana (dwarf tapeworm)	Worldwide, especially warm, dry climates	Fecal-oral, water, food; tapeworm colonizes intestine causing mucosal damage	Variable onset symptoms, worms mature in about 2 weeks	Enteritis with or without diarrhea, abdominal pain, anorexia, weight loss, weakness	None	Eosino-philia	Microscopy	Praziquantel 25 mg/kg once (adults and children), niclosamide

Bibliography

Bennet, R.G. (1999). Acute gastroenteritis and associated conditions. In L.R. Barker, J.R. Burton, & P.D. Zieve (Eds.), *Principles of ambulatory medicine* (5th ed., pp. 319-330). Baltimore: Williams & Wilkins.

Blaser, M.J. (2000). *Campylobacter jejuni* and related species. In G. Mandell, J. Bennett, & R. Dolin (Eds.), *Principles and practice of infectious diseases* (5th ed., pp 2276-2285). New York: Churchill Livingstone.

Butler, T. (2000). *Yersinia* species, including plague. In G. Mandell, J. Bennett, & R. Dolin (Eds.), *Principles and practice of infectious diseases* (5th ed., pp 2406-2414). New York: Churchill Livingstone.

Centers for Disease Control and Prevention. (2003). Parasites and health: Amebiasis. Retrieved July 12, 2003, from *www.dpd.cdc.gov/dpdx/HTML/Amebiasis.htm*

Chappell, C.L., & Okhuysen, P.C. (2002). Cryptosporidiosis. *Current Opinion in Infectious Diseases, 15,* 523-527.

Chin, J. (2000). *Control of communicable diseases manual* (17th ed.). Washington, DC: American Public Health Association.

Cleary, T.G. (2004). Shigella. In R.E. Behrman, R.M. Kliegman, & H.B. Jenson (Eds.), *Nelson textbook of pediatrics* (17th ed., pp. 919-921). Philadelphia: W.B. Saunders Company.

Diaz, E., Mondragon, J., Ramirez, E., & Bernal, R. (2003). Epidemiology and control of intestinal parasites with nitazoxanide in children in Mexico. *American Journal of Tropical Medicine and Hygiene, 68,* 382-383.

Fisher, M.C. (2004). *Clostridium difficile*-associated diarrhea. In R.E. Behrman, R.M. Kliegman, & H.B. Jenson (Eds.), *Nelson textbook of pediatrics* (17th ed., pp. 953-954). Philadelphia: W.B. Saunders Company.

Gillespie, S. (2003). Salmonella infections. In G.C. Cook & A.I. Zumla (Eds.), *Manson's tropical diseases* (21st ed., pp. 937-949). Philadelphia: W.B. Saunders Company.

Hart, C.A., & Shears, P. (2003). Gastrointestinal bacteria. In G.C. Cook & A.I. Zumla (Eds.), *Manson's tropical diseases* (21st ed., pp. 915-935). Philadelphia: W.B. Saunders Company.

Mirdha, B.R., & Samantray, J.C. (2002). Hymenolepis nana: A common cause of paediatric diarrhea in urban slum dwellers in India. *Journal of Tropical Pediatrics, 48,* 331-334.

Narayan, N. (2001). Adenovirus. Retrieved December 30, 2003, from *www.med.sc.edu:85/pdf-vir/adeno.pdf*

Nimri, L.F. (2003). *Cyclospora cayetanensis* and other intestinal parasites associated with diarrhea in a rural area of Jordan. *International Microbiology, 6,* 131-135.

Rotz, L.D., Khan, A.S., Lillibridge, S.R., Ostroff, S.M., & Hughes. J.M. (2002). Public health assessment of potential biological terrorism agents. *Emerging Infectious Diseases, 8,* 225-230.

Todd, J.K. (2004). Staphylococcus. In R.E. Behrman, R.M. Kliegman, & H.B. Jenson (Eds.), *Nelson textbook of pediatrics* (17th ed., pp. 861-867). Philadelphia: W.B. Saunders Company.

White, A.C. (2003). Nitazoxanide: An important advance in anti-parasitic therapy. *American Journal of Tropical Medicine and Hygiene, 68,* 382-383.

C NOTIFIABLE DISEASES

"The first step in the control of any communicable disease ... is prompt recognition and identification" (Chin, 2000, p. xxv).

Each chapter in this text on a specific disease ends with information on the notification status of that disease. As this work is written, the International Health Regulations (IHR) document of the World Health Organization (WHO) classifies diseases as follows (Chin, 2000; WHO, 1969/1995):

Class 1: Case report universally required by IHR as a disease under surveillance by WHO

1. Diseases *subject to international quarantine* include cholera, plague, yellow fever.

1A. Diseases *under surveillance* by the WHO include louse-borne typhus, relapsing fever, paralytic poliomyelitis, malaria, and influenza.

Class 2: Case report regularly required wherever the disease occurs

2A. Diseases for which case reports should be made to local authorities by telephone or other rapid means include typhoid fever and diphtheria as well as diseases that may be used by bioterrorists such as anthrax, botulism, plague, smallpox, tularemia, and others.

2B. Diseases for which case reports should be made by the most practicable means include brucellosis and leprosy.

Class 3: Selectively reportable in recognized endemic areas

3A. Diseases for which case reports should be made by rapid means in specified areas where the disease ranks in importance with Class 2A include scrub typhus and arenaviral hemorrhagic fever.

3B. Diseases for which case reports should be made as a collective report weekly or monthly include bartonellosis and coccidioidomycosis.

3C. Diseases for which case reports should be made at intervals ranging from weekly to annually include fasciolopsiasis and schistosomiasis.

Class 4: Obligatory report of epidemics; no case report required

Outbreaks of public health importance require rapid notification, regardless of other classification status, for example, an unidentified syndrome.

Class 5: Official report not ordinarily justifiable

Illnesses such as the common cold require no notification.

There are several avenues of notification:

- The WHO and cooperating organizations maintain a Communicable Disease Surveillance & Response website, the Weekly Epidemiological Record (WER), and the Global Public Health Intelligence Network (GPHIN). These and other services work in cooperation with the 191 member states of the WHO and other sources to monitor disease outbreaks. Under current International Health Regulations, member states are legally obligated to report only cholera, yellow fever, and plague. The IHRs were expected to be changed in 2005 so that any disease outbreak will be risk assessed and reported if the outbreak meets more than one of the following considerations: serious public health impact (including high morbidity or mortality) or unusual event (including unknown cause or suspected intentional release) that requires international assistance, international spread, or interferes with international travel or trade. If there is an actual or suspected outbreak of a disease of public health importance, notification should be made through the WHO Global Outbreak Alert and Response Team (*outbreak@who.int*),

WHO regional or national office, the national institute of public health of the member state, and any key nongovernmental organizations (NGOs). We suggest using several avenues of notification because communications may be delayed or overlooked under some circumstances (Grein et al., 2000; Shindo, 2004; WHO, 2003).

- The U.S. Centers for Disease Control and Prevention (CDC) should be notified of outbreaks or occurrences of diseases in the United States. The CDC phone number is (404)489-6150 and the fax number is (404)489-6255. The CDC e-mail is *soib@cdc.gov*. Reports may be made via the Internet through the CDC website at *www.cdc.gov/epo/dphsi/phs/infdis2004.htm*.
- Although the WHO covers most nations and areas, some circumstances and areas require different reporting practices. War, famine, and refugee situations, for example, are particularly prone to outbreaks of unusual diseases. Under some circumstances, notification might go through a military body or NGO.

Lists of reportable diseases from the WHO (2003) and CDC (2004) follow. Readers should be aware that these listings are based on information available at the time this book was written. Suspicion of a disease with the potential for high morbidity or mortality, whether on these lists or not, should always be reported.

WORLD HEALTH ORGANIZATION COMMUNICABLE DISEASE SURVEILLANCE & RESPONSE (CSR) LISTING OF DISEASES

- Acute diarrheal syndrome
- Acute febrile syndrome

- Acute hemorrhagic fever syndrome
- Acute neurologic syndrome
- Acute respiratory syndrome
- Acute watery diarrheal syndrome
- Anthrax
- Buffalopox
- Cholera
- Coccidioidomycosis
- Creutzfeldt-Jakob disease
- Crimean-Congo hemorrhagic fever
- Dengue fever
- Ebola hemorrhagic fever
- Encephalitis, Saint Louis
- Enterohemorrhagic *E. coli* infection
- Enterohemorrhagic *E. coli* (O157:H7)
- Enterovirus
- Food-borne diseases
- Hantavirus pulmonary syndrome
- Hemorrhagic fever with renal syndrome
- HIV/AIDS
- Influenza
- Japanese encephalitis
- Lassa fever
- Legionellosis
- Leptospirosis
- Listeriosis
- Louse-borne typhus
- Malaria
- Measles
- Meningococcal disease
- Monkeypox
- Myocarditis
- Nipah virus
- O'nyong-nyong fever
- Pertussis
- Plague
- Poliomyelitis

- Rabies (animal and human)
- Relapsing fever
- Rift Valley fever
- Severe acute respiratory syndrome–associated coronavirus (SARS-CoV) disease
- Shigellosis
- Smallpox
- Staphylococcal food intoxication
- Tuberculosis
- Tularemia
- Typhoid fever
- West Nile fever
- Yellow fever

CENTERS FOR DISEASE CONTROL AND PREVENTION NATIONALLY NOTIFIABLE INFECTIOUS DISEASES

- Acquired immunodeficiency syndrome (AIDS)
- Anthrax
- Botulism (food-borne, infant, wound, and unspecified)
- Brucellosis
- Chancroid
- *Chlamydia trachomatis* genital infection
- Cholera
- Coccidioidomycosis
- Cryptosporidiosis
- Cyclosporiasis
- Diphtheria
- Ehrlichiosis
- Encephalitis/meningitis, arboviral (all types)
- Enterohemorrhagic *Escherichia coli* (0157:H7, shiga toxin positive, serogroup non-0157, and shiga toxin+ [not serogrouped])
- Giardiasis
- Gonorrhea

- *Haemophilus influenzae,* invasive disease
- Hansen disease (leprosy)
- Hantavirus pulmonary syndrome
- Hemolytic uremic syndrome, postdiarrheal
- Hemorrhagic fevers, all types
- Hepatitis, viral, acute
- Hepatitis, viral, chronic
- HIV infection
- Legionellosis
- Listeriosis
- Lyme disease
- Malaria
- Measles
- Meningococcal disease
- Mumps
- Pertussis
- Plague
- Poliomyelitis, paralytic
- Psittacosis
- Q fever
- Rabies (animal and human)
- Rocky Mountain spotted fever
- Rubella
- Rubella, congenital syndrome
- Salmonellosis
- Severe acute respiratory syndrome–associated coronavirus (SARS-CoV) disease
- Shigellosis
- Smallpox
- Streptococcal disease, invasive, Group A
- Streptococcal toxic shock syndrome
- *Streptococcus pneumoniae,* drug resistant, invasive disease
- *Streptococcus pneumoniae,* invasive in children <5 years
- Syphilis (all stages and types, including syphilitic stillbirth)

- Tetanus
- Toxic shock syndrome
- Trichinosis
- Tuberculosis
- Tularemia
- Typhoid fever
- Vancomycin, intermediate *Staphylococcus aureus* (VISA)
- Vancomycin, resistant *Staphylococcus aureus* (VRSA)
- Varicella
- Yellow fever

References

Centers for Disease Control and Prevention. (2004). Nationally notifiable infectious diseases—United States 2004. Retrieved June 7, 2004, from *www.cdc.gov/epo/dphsi/phs/infdis2004.htm*

Chin, J. (Ed.). (2000). *Control of communicable diseases manual* (17th ed.). Washington, DC: American Public Health Association.

Grein, T.W., Kamara, K-B.O., Rodier, G., Plant, A.J., Bovier, P., et al. (2000). Rumors of disease in the global village: Outbreak verification. *Emerging Infectious Diseases, 6,* 97-102.

Shindo, N. (2004, June 14). Personal communication. Dr. Shindo is the medical officer for the WHO Global Outbreak Alert and Response Team.

World Health Organization. (1969/1995). International health regulations. Retrieved June 12, 2004, from *www.who.int/csr/ihr/en/*

World Health Organization. (2003). Communicable disease surveillance & response. Retrieved June 2, 2004, from *www.who.int/csr/don/en/*

D VECTOR CONTROL

INSECTS

Repellents and Other Personal Protection

Personal protection from most insects includes permethrin-impregnated bed netting and protective clothing, and application of insect repellents, especially those containing N,N-diethylmetatoluamide (DEET) to exposed skin. DEET can be used to protect pregnant and lactating women who are traveling to malarial and other disease-endemic areas (Centers for Disease Control and Prevention [CDC], 2003). Formulations with concentrations of 30% or less can be used safely in children and infants older than 2 months (American Academy of Pediatrics, 2003). Long-acting repellents in which DEET is bound in a polymer have the advantages of longer duration and decreased systemic absorption. Other effective repellents are those containing picaridin, also known as KBR 3023, which may be comparable with DEET products of similar concentration. Repellents containing picaradin are widely available in Europe, Australia, Latin America, and Asia. Oil of lemon eucalyptus, also known as *p*-menthane 3,8-diol or PMD, may provide protection time similar to low concentration DEET products (CDC, 2005).

In most cases, light-colored clothing is better than dark because some insects are attracted to dark clothing and most insects are easier to detect on light-colored clothing. Protection against ticks and biting flies may require headgear. Minimize skin exposure by wearing long pants and long sleeves—especially when outside at times when vectors are known to feed. For example, *Aedes* mosquitoes (chikungunya fever, dengue fever) usually feed during the day as opposed to *Anopheles* mosquitoes (malaria), which feed mostly at dusk or dawn. When possible, stay in screened or air-conditioned rooms.

After leaving tick-infested areas, check the entire body, including creases, for ticks and remove them. Removal of a feeding tick is accomplished by using blunt-tipped forceps to grasp the tick as close to the skin as possible, then lifting away from the skin with steady, straight traction; take care not to leave the head embedded in the skin. Wear gloves or wash hands after touching ticks, and thoroughly wash the attachment site with antiseptic solution.

Insecticides

In general, the use of insecticides for vector control should be part of an integrated pest management plan that includes surveillance, source reduction (e.g., draining standing water such as swamps, emptying open water-filled containers, disposing of used tires, and reducing the number of plants such as bromeliads that hold standing water), larvicide, biological control, and public relations and education. The selection of insecticide is based on several factors, including insect habits, insect resistance to insecticide, risk of harm to the environment (including people and animals), cost of insecticide, ability to apply the insecticide, and other factors. Insect resistance should be determined before mass or extensive application is instituted. The means of application may affect efficacy and toxicity (Rose, 2001; White, 2003; World Health Organization [WHO], 2002).

Rodents

Personal and Habitat Protection Measures

Controlling rodents requires ongoing individual and community effort. Measures to control rodents include (CDC, 1993; Painter et al., 2004):

- Store food and food products, including pet food and animal feed, in rodent-proof metal or thick plastic containers with tight-fitting lids.
- Store garbage inside homes in rodent-proof metal or thick plastic containers with tight-fitting lids
- Wash dishes and cooking and serving utensils immediately after use.
- Remove all spilled food.
- Dispose of trash and clutter.
- Use spring-loaded (as opposed to live) rodent traps in the home continuously.
- Use rodenticide (see later discussion) with bait according to product instructions. It is essential to protect humans (and also domestic or desirable wild animals) from accidental ingestion. Always precede rodenticide use with insecticide for flea control.
- Wear heavy rubber or plastic gloves to handle rodent carcasses. Place carcasses in a plastic bag with enough disinfectant to thoroughly wet the carcass. Bury in a 2- to 3-foot-deep hole or burn. Wash gloved hands in a disinfectant (e.g., hypochlorite solution of 50 mL bleach/gallon of water) before removing gloves and wash hands with soap and water after removing gloves.
- Seal all openings (equal to or more than 1/4 inch in diameter) into the home (including cellar, roof, porches, and other attached or nonliving areas) with steel wool or cement. Rodents are able to enter openings significantly smaller than their apparent body size.

- Place metal roof flashing as a rodent barrier around the base of wooden, earthen, or adobe dwellings up to a height of at least 12 inches and buried in the soil to a depth of at least 6 inches.
- Place 3 inches of gravel under the base of homes or under temporary dwellings to discourage burrowing.
- Reduce rodent shelter and food sources within 100 feet of the home by removing woodpiles or raising them at least 12 inches off the ground.
- Remove trash, abandoned vehicles, old tires, and other potential rodent shelters.
- Store hay on pallets and use rodenticides continuously to keep hay free of rodents.
- Dispose of garbage in rodent-proof containers that are located at least 12 inches off the ground.
- Cut grass, brush, and dense shrubbery within 100 feet of the home.
- Prevent rodents from entering habitations

Rodenticides

The most commonly used rodenticides, anticoagulants, are relatively safe to humans. For example, in 2003 there were 20,000 human exposures to rodenticides (of which 80% were anticoagulants) but only 2 deaths reported. More than 75% of the exposures were to children under 6 years old. Rodenticides currently in use (Marcus, 2001; Painter et al., 2004) include the following:

- Warfarin-type anticoagulants and long-acting brodifacoum anticoagulants prevent the activation of vitamin K and thus inhibit coagulation. Death occurs from hemorrhage.
- Red squill rat poison, a powder made from the bulb of the red squill, contains a cardiac glycoside that when ingested produces glycoside intoxication and pulmonary edema. Theoretically, red squill is safe

for humans and toxic to rodents because humans reflexively vomit the poison, whereas rats lack this ability. Red squill has become less common as more effective poisons have become available.

- Strychnine excites the central nervous system, producing seizures and vomiting.
- Thallium is a heavy metal that is absorbed through the skin and also ingested. Its effects include convulsions and a variety of other neurologic and systemic manifestations.
- Arsenic was in wide use as a rodenticide until recently. It causes vomiting, seizures, and kidney failure. Contamination of farm buildings with arsenic is relatively common and is long lasting.
- *Salmonella*-based rodenticides produce salmonellosis in rodents.

Because of their toxicity, strychnine, thallium, arsenic, and *Salmonella*-based rodenticides are seldom used in the developed world, but may be common in some developing countries. Other rodenticides include barium-containing rodenticides, cholecalciferol-containing rodenticides, yellow phosphorus, alpha naphthyl thiourea, ANTU, sodium monofluoroacetate, *N*-3-pyridylmethyl-*Np*-nitrophenyl urea, PNU, Vacor, zinc phosphide, bromethalin, and norbormide.

References

American Academy of Pediatrics. (2003). Follow safety precautions when using DEET on children. Retrieved December 7, 2003, from *www.aap.org/family/wnv-jun03.htm.*

Centers for Disease Control and Prevention. (1993). Hantavirus infection—Southwestern United States: Interim recommendations for risk reduction. *MMWR, 42*(RR-11). 1-13. Retrieved June 8, 2004, from *www.cdc.gov/epo/mmwr/preview/mmwrhtml/00030643.htm*

Centers for Disease Control and Prevention. (2003). Malaria. Retrieved November 3, 2003, from *www.cdc.gov/travel/diseases/malaria/index.htm*

Centers for Disease Control and Prevention. (2005). CDC adopts new repellent guidance for upcoming mosquito season. Retrieved April 28, 2005, from *www.cdc.gov/od/oc/media/pressrel/r050428.htm*

Marcus, S. (2001). Toxicity, rodenticide. *EMedicine*. Retrieved June 25, 2004, from *www.emedicine.com/emerg/topic511.htm*

Painter, J.A., Mølbak, K., Sonne-Hansen, J., Barrett, T., Well, J.G., & Tauxe, R. (2004). Salmonella-based rodenticides and public health. *Emerging Infectious Diseases, 10,* 985-987.

Rose, R.I. (2001). Pesticides and public health: Integrated methods of mosquito management. *Emerging Infectious Diseases, 7,* 17-23.

White, G.B. (2003). Mosquitoes. In G.C. Cook & A.I. Zumla (Eds.), *Manson's tropical diseases* (21st ed., pp. 1741-1772). Philadelphia: W.B. Saunders Company.

World Health Organization. (2002). The WHO recommended classification of pesticides by hazard and guidelines to classification 2000-2002. Retrieved May 28, 2004, from *www.who.int/pcs/docs/Classif_Pestic_2000-02.pdf*

E DIAGNOSIS AND TREATMENT OF HUMAN IMMUNODEFICIENCY VIRUS/ACQUIRED IMMUNODEFICIENCY SYNDROME IN RESOURCE-LIMITED SETTINGS

INTRODUCTION

— Human immunodeficiency virus (HIV), the etiology of acquired immunodeficiency syndrome (AIDS), is a global pandemic. Of the estimated 39.4 million people infected, 25.4 million live in sub-Saharan Africa and 7.1 million live in south and southeast Asia. Women account for 17.6 million cases, and children under 15 years 2.2 million. In 2004, an average of more than 8000 people died of AIDS each day (World Health Organization [WHO], 2004a).

— A complete discussion of the diagnosis, treatment, prevention, and ethical dimensions of HIV/AIDS is beyond the scope of this book. When possible, patients with AIDS should be referred for evaluation to infectious disease specialists or health care facilities experienced with AIDS. Treatment should be consistent with standardized regimens recommended by local or national public health authorities. The purpose of this appendix is to present the rationale underlying the diagnosis and treatment of HIV/AIDS in resource-limited settings, and to provide readers with references with further information that can be downloaded from the Internet.

PATHOGENESIS

HIV, a retrovirus spread through the exchange of blood and body fluids, was identified as the cause of AIDS in the 1980s. Retroviruses are widely distributed in nature, infecting many mammalian species. Simian immunodeficiency virus (SIV), which causes an AIDS-like disease in certain monkey and ape species in Africa, is thought to be the probable origin of HIV. Of the two strains of HIV, HIV-1 causes most infections, whereas HIV-2 cases are concentrated in certain areas of the world. The first clusters of patients in the AIDS epidemic were homosexual men in the United States, but HIV/AIDS has since grown into a disease that is spread primarily through heterosexual contact. After gaining entry into the body, HIV produces an intense viremia during which millions of copies of viral RNA can be detected in a single milliliter of blood. During acute infection the number of peripheral CD4 T cells, the primary targets of the virus, falls precipitously then stabilizes 3 to 4 weeks later. Over the ensuing years, gradual depletion of CD4 cells continues as CD8 T cells attempt to control viral replication by killing infected CD4 cells. Patients are generally asymptomatic until CD4 counts fall below 500. They then develop mild disease, which may include recurrent herpes simplex virus (HSV), varicella zoster, oral candidiasis, recurrent diarrhea, fever, unexplained weight loss, and recurrent bacterial infections such as sinusitis or pneumonia. As CD4 levels drop below 200, patients develop the hallmarks of AIDS: opportunistic infections such as *Pneumocystis carinii* pneumonia, esophageal candidiasis, tuberculosis, *Toxoplasma gondii* encephalitis, cryptosporidiosis, and isosporiasis. The median time from infection to the development of AIDS is 8 to 10 years, but 20% of infected individuals have AIDS within 5 years.

In the advanced stages of disease, as CD4 counts fall below 50, other opportunistic infections commonly occur, such as *Mycobacterium avium* complex, cryptococcal meningitis, and disseminated forms of coccidioidomycosis, aspergillosis, and histoplasmosis. End-stage central nervous system manifestations may include lymphoma or progressive multifocal leukoencephalopathy (Apetrei, 2004; Vergis & Mellors, 2000).

DIAGNOSIS OF AIDS

The diagnosis of HIV/AIDS may be confirmed by detecting any of the following: antibodies to HIV, HIV p24 antigen, HIV RNA or DNA, or HIV in viral culture. Antibodies are usually detectable 4 to 6 weeks after the initial infection, and are almost always present by 6 months. Infants born to HIV-infected mothers may have a false-positive test because of maternal antibodies that can persist in the infant's circulation for up to 18 months. In resource-limited settings where laboratory facilities are either unavailable or unaffordable, rapid tests for antibodies to HIV in serum or plasma are the most practical method of testing. Today's rapid tests have greater than 99% sensitivity and specificity, use finger-stick whole-blood samples, give a visual result within 30 min that does not require sophisticated equipment or electricity, and cost around $2 per test. The WHO suggests the algorithm shown in Figure E-1 for using rapid HIV tests. Before testing, informed consent must be obtained to ensure that the patient understands the purpose of the testing, is aware of treatment and support available after the test result, and freely decides whether to be tested or not. Pretest counseling should also include information on HIV transmission and prevention, the testing process, benefits and risks of testing, and the implications of positive and

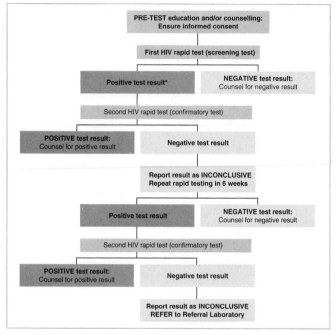

*In the context of labour in an MTCT-prevention setting, it is advised to offer a single dose of nevirapine on the basis of a single positive rapid test. This should then be confirmed after delivery. In late pregnancy in MTCT-prevention settings the use of a third rapid test as a tiebreaker may exceptionally be considered after inconclusive results where the need to start short-course ARV prophylaxis must be decided without delay.

FIGURE E–1

Algorithm for use of rapid HIV tests in testing and counseling services. (*Source:* World Health Organizations. [2004b]. "Flow Chart 1" [p. 21]. Retrieved from *www.who.int/entity/hiv/pub/vct/en/rapidhivtestsen.pdf*)

negative test results. If a second rapid test is required, ideally it should be for antibodies to a different antigen than the first test. When used for the purpose of reducing the risk of mother-to-child transmission for a woman in labor, it is recommended that antiretroviral medication be given to the mother on the basis of a single positive test, with confirmatory testing performed after delivery (WHO, 2004b, 2004c). In HIV-infected persons, the CD4 count is usually used along with clinical criteria to determine the stage

WHO Staging System for HIV Infection in Adults and Adolescents

Clinical Stage I
1. Asymptomatic
2. Generalized lymphadenopathy
   Performance scale 1: asymptomatic, normal activity

Clinical Stage II
3. Weight loss <10% of body weight
4. Minor mucocutaneous manifestations (seborrhoeic dermatitis, prurigo, fungal nail infections, recurrent oral ulcerations, angular cheilitis)
5. Herpes zoster within the last five years
6. Recurrent upper respiratory tract infections (i.e. bacterial sinusitis)
   And/or performance scale 2: symptomatic, normal activity

Clinical Stage III
7. Weight loss >10% of body weight
8. Unexplained chronic diarrhea, >1 month
9. Unexplained prolonged fever (intermittent or constant), >1 month
10. Oral candidiasis (thrush)
11. Oral hairy leucoplakia
12. Pulmonary tuberculosis
13. Severe bacterial infections (i.e. pneumonia, pyomyositis)
    And/or performance scale 3: bedridden <50% of the day during last month

Clinical Stage IV:
14. HIV wasting syndrome[a]
15. *Pneumocystic* carinii pneumonia
16. Toxoplasmosis of the brain
17. Cryptosporidiosis with diarrhea >1 month
18. Cryptococcosis, extrapulmonary
19. Cytomegalovirus disease of an organ other than liver, spleen or lymph node (e.g. retinitis)
20. Herpes simplex virus infection, mucocutaneous (>1month) or visceral
21. Progressive multifocal leukoencephalopathy
22. Any disseminated endemic mycosis
23. Candidiasis of esophagus, trachea, bronchi
24. Atypical mycobacteriosis, disseminated or pulmonary
25. Non-typhoid Salmonella septicemia
26. Extrapulmonary tuberculosis
27. Lymphoma
28. Kaposi's sarcoma
29. HIV encephalopathy[b]
And/or performance scale 4: bedridden >50% of the day during last month

Source: World Health Organization. (2004). Annex E. WHO staging system for HIV infection and disease in adults and adolescents (p. 61). Retrieved April 27, 2005, from *www.who.int/hiv/pub/prev_care/en/arvrevision2003en.pdf*
[a]*HIV wasting syndrome: weight loss of >10% of body weight, plus either unexplained chronic diarrhea (>1 month) or chronic weakness and unexplained prolonged fever (>1 month).*
[b]*HIV encephalopathy: clinical findings of disabling cognitive and/or motor dysfunction interfering with activities of daily living, progressing over weeks to months, in the absence of a concurrent illness or condition, other than HIV infection, which could explain the findings.*

of infection. Because such T-cell subset tests are not available in resource-limited settings, the WHO has developed a clinical staging system that does not require laboratory tests (Table E-1). Separate criteria have been developed for children (Table E-2). Though the staging criteria are several years old, they are used in current treatment guidelines for HIV/AIDS in low-resource settings (WHO, 2004d).

TABLE E–2

WHO Staging System for HIV Infection in Children

Clinical Stage I:
1. Asymptomatic
2. Generalized lymphadenopathy

Clinical Stage II:
3. Chronic diarrhea >30 days duration in absence of known etiology
4. Severe persistent or recurrent candidiasis outside the neonatal period
5. Weight loss or failure to thrive in the absence of known etiology
6. Persistent fever >30 days duration in the absence of known etiology
7. Recurrent severe bacterial infections other than septicaemia or meningitis (e.g. osteomyelitis, bacterial [non-TB] pneumonia, abscesses)

Clinical Stage III:
8. AIDS-defining opportunistic infections
9. Severe failure to thrive (wasting) in the absence of known etiology[a]
10. Progressive encephalopathy
11. Malignancy
12. Recurrent septicaemia or meningitis

[a]Peristent weight loss > 10% of baseline or less than 5th percentile on weight for height chart on 2 consecutive measurements more than 1 month apart in the absence of another etiology or concurrent illness.

Source: World Health Organization. (2004). Annex E. WHO staging system for HIV infection and disease in children (p. 62). Retrieved April 27, 2005, from *www.who.int/hiv/pub/prev_care/en/arvrevision2003en.pdf*

TREATMENT

- When possible, refer patients with AIDS to infectious disease specialists or health care facilities with experience in treating HIV/AIDS. Treatment should be consistent with standardized treatment guidelines recommended by local or national public health authorities.
- The three main categories of antiretroviral medications are as follows (Hare, 2004):
  - Reverse transcriptase inhibitors block the enzyme that converts viral RNA into DNA before the virus enters the nucleus of an infected cell; the two types are nucleoside analog and non-nucleoside reverse transcriptase inhibitors (NNRTI).
  - Protease inhibitors block viral enzymes that are necessary for viral maturation, causing the virus to create copies of itself that are incapable of infecting other cells.
  - Fusion inhibitors attach themselves to the outside of the virus and prevent it from fusing with the host cell membrane, a necessary step for the virus to infect a cell.
- Tables E-3 and E-4 list antiretroviral medications used in WHO treatment guidelines, and Table E-5 lists examples of first-line antiretroviral regimens (WHO, 2004d). Again, readers should consult local or national public health authorities for the specific regimens recommended for their area.
- One of the first steps in the treatment of AIDS is deciding whom to offer antiretroviral therapy. The decision-making process is an attempt to balance the desire to reduce morbidity and mortality for all infected individuals against the potential adverse effects of therapy and the need to conserve limited resources for those who may benefit from treatment the most.

In resource-limited settings, the WHO recommends that antiretroviral therapy be offered to adults and adolescents with confirmed HIV infection and either:

- WHO Stage IV disease, irrespective of CD4 count, or
- WHO Stage III disease with consideration of using CD4 counts of less than 350/mm^3 to guide decision making, or
- WHO Stage I or II disease with consideration of using CD4 counts of less than or equal to 200/mm^3 to guide decision making

When CD4 testing is not available, the total lymphocyte count may be used as a proxy. Although the total

TABLE E-3

Dosages of Antiretroviral Drugs for Adults and Adolescents

Drug class/drug	Dose[a]
Nucleoside RTIs	
Abacavir (ABC)	300 mg twice daily
Didanosine (ddI)	400 mg once daily (250 mg once daily if <60 kg) (250 mg once daily if administered with TDF)
Lamivudine (3TC)	150 mg twice daily or 300 mg once daily
Stavudine (d4T)	40 mg twice daily (30 mg twice daily if <60 kg)
Zidovudine (ZDV)	300 mg twice daily
Nucleotide RTI	
Tenofovir (TDF)	300 mg once daily (Note: drug interaction with ddI necessitates dose reduction of latter)
Non-nucleoside RTIs	
Efavirenz (EFV)	600 mg once daily[b]

continued ➲

Table E–3 continued

Nevirapine (NVP)	200 mg once daily for 14 days, then 200 mg twice daily
Protease inhibitors	
Indinavir/ritonavir (IDV/r)	800 mg/100 mg twice daily[c,d]
Lopinavir/ritonavir (LPV/r)	400 mg/100 mg twice daily[b] (533 mg/133 mg twice daily when Combined with EFV or NVP)
Nelfinavir (NFV)	1250 mg twice daily
Saquinavir/ritonavir (SQV/r)	1000 mg/100 mg twice daily or 1600 mg/200 mg once daily[b,d,e]

Source: World Health Organization. (2004). Dosages of antiretroviral drugs for adults and adolescents (pp. 48-49). Retrieved April 27, 2005, from *www.who.int/hiv/pub/prev_care/en/arvrevision2003en.pdf*

[a] *These dosages are in common clinical use. The dosages featured in this table were selected on the basis of the best available clinical evidence. Dosages that can be given once daily or twice daily were preferred in order to enhance adherence to therapy. The doses listed are those for individuals with normal renal and hepatic function. Product-specific information should be consulted for dose adjustments that may be indicated with renal or hepatic dysfunction or for potential drug interactions with other HIV and non-HIV medications.*

[b] *See TB section for other specific TB dosing.*

[c] *This dosage regimen is in common clinical use. Other IDV/r dosage regimens that range from 800 mg/200 mg bid to 400 mg/100 mg bid are also in clinical use.*

[d] *Dosage adjustment when combined with an NNRTI is indicated but a formal recommendation cannot be made at this time. One consideration is to increase the RTV component to 200 mg bid when EFV or NVP is used concomitantly. More drug interaction data are needed.*

[e] *Both the hard-gel and soft-gel capsule formulations can be used when SQV is combined with RTV.*

lymphocyte count correlates poorly with CD4 counts in asymptomatic individuals, it does have prognostic value for those with symptomatic HIV disease. Specifically, the WHO recommends that antiretroviral therapy be offered to adults and adolescents with:

- WHO Stage III or IV disease, irrespective of the total lymphocyte count, or

Text continued on p. 781

TABLE E–4 Dosages of Antiretroviral Drugs for Children

Name of drug	Formulations	Pharmaco-kinetic data available	Age (weight), dose and dose frequency	Other comment
Nucleoside analogue reverse transcriptase inhibitors				
Zidovudine (ZDV)	• Syrup: 10 mg/ml • Capsules: 100 mg; 250 mg • Tablet: 300 mg	• All ages	• <4 weeks: 4 mg/kg/dose twice daily • 4 weeks to 13 years: 180 mg/m²/dose twice daily • Maximum dose: ≥13 years: 300 mg/dose twice daily	• Large volume of syrup not well tolerated in older children • Syrup needs storage in glass jars and is light-sensitive • Can be given with food • Doses of 600 mg/m² per day required for HIV encephalopathy • Capsule can be opened and contents dispersed or tablet crushed and contents mixed with small amount of water or food and immediately taken (solution is stable at room temperature) • Do not use with d4T (antagonistic antiretroviral effect)

Lamivudine (3TC)	• Oral solution: 10 mg/ml • Tablet: 150 mg	• All ages	• <30 days: 2 mg/kg/dose twice daily • ≥ 30 days or <60 kg: 4 mg/kg/dose twice daily • Maximum dose: >60 kg: 150 mg/dose twice daily	• Well tolerated • Can be given with food • Store solution at room temperature (use within one month of opening) • Tablet can be crushed and contents mixed with small amount water or food and immediately taken
Fixed-dose combination of ZDV plus 3TC	• No liquid available • Tablet: 300 mg ZDV plus 150 mg 3TC	• Adolescents and adults	• Maximum dose: >13 years or >60 kg: 1 tablet/dose twice daily (should not be given if weight <30 kg)	• Preferably tablet should not be split • Tablet can be crushed and contents mixed with small amount of water or food and immediately taken • At weight <30 kg, ZDV and 3TC cannot be dosed accurately in tablet form

continued

TABLE E-4 Dosages of Antiretroviral Drugs for Children—cont'd

Name of drug	Formulations	Pharmaco-kinetic data available	Age (weight), dose and dose frequency	Other comment
Nucleoside analogue reverse transcriptase inhibitors—cont'd				
Stavudine (d4T)	• Oral solution: 1 mg/ml • Capsules: 15 mg, 20 mg, 30 mg, 40 mg	• All ages	• <30 kg: 1 mg/kg dose twice daily • 30 to 60 kg: 30 mg/dose twice daily • Maximum dose: >60 kg: 40 mg/dose twice daily	• Large volume of solution • Keep solution refrigerated; stable for 30 days; must be well shaken and stored in glass bottles • Capsules can be opened and mixed with small amount of food or water (stable in solution for 24 hours if kept refrigerated) • Do not use with AZT (antagonistic antiretroviral effect)
Fixed-dose combination of d4T plus 3TC	• No liquid available • Tablet: d4T 30 mg plus 3TC 150 mg; d4T 40 mg plus 3TC 150 mg	• Adolescents and adults	• Maximum dose: 30–60 kg: one 30-mg d4T- based tablet twice daily • ≥60 kg: one 40-mg d4T-based tablet twice daily	• Preferably, tablet should not be split • See comments under individual drug components

Didanosine (ddI, dideoxyinosine)	• Oral suspension pediatric • Powder/water: 10 mg/ml; in many countries needs to be made up with additional antacid • Chewable tablets: 25 mg; 50 mg; 100 mg; 150 mg; 200 mg • Enteric-coated beadlets in capsules: 125 mg; 200 mg; 250 mg; 400 mg	• All ages	• <3 months: 50 mg/m^2/dose twice daily • 3 months to <13 years: 90–120 mg/m^2/dose twice daily or 240 mg/m^2/dose once daily • Maximum dose: ≥13 years of >60 kg: 200 mg/dose twice daily or 400 mg once daily	• Keep suspension refrigerated; stable for 30 days; must be well shaken • Administer on empty stomach, at least 30 minutes before or 2 hours after eating • If tablets dispersed in water, at least 2 tablets of appropriate strength should be dissolved for adequate buffering • Enteric-coated beadlets in capsules can be opened and sprinkled on small amount of food

continued

TABLE E-4 Dosages of Antiretroviral Drugs for Children—cont'd

Name of drug	Formulations	Pharmaco-kinetic data available	Age (weight), dose and dose frequency	Other comment
Nucleoside analogue reverse transcriptase inhibitors—cont'd				
Abacavir (ABC)	• Oral solution: 20 mg/ml • Tablet: 300 mg	• Over age of 3 months	• <16 years or <37.5 kg: 8 mg/kg/dose twice daily • Maximum dose: <16 years of ≥37.5 kg: 300 mg/dose twice daily	• Can be given with food • Tablet can be crushed and contents mixed with small amount water or food and immediately ingested • PARENTS MUST BE WARNED ABOUT HYPERSENSITIVITY REACTION • ABC should be stopped permanently if hypersensitivity reaction occurs
Fixed-dose Combination of ZDV plus 3TC plus ABC	• No liquid available • Tablet: ZDV 300 mg plus 3TC 150 mg plus ABC 300 mg	• Adolescents and adults	• Maximum dose: >40 kg: 1 tablet/dose twice daily	• Preferably, tablet should not be split • At weight <30 kg, ZDV/3TC/ABC cannot be dosed accurately in tablet form • MUST WARN PARENTS ABOUT HYPERSENSITIVITY REACTION.

					• ZDV/3TC/ABC should be stopped permanently if hypersensitivity reaction occur

Non-nucleoside reverse transcriptase inhibitors

| Nevirapine (NVP) | • Oral suspension: 10 mg/ml
• Tablet: 200 mg | | • All ages | | • 15 to 30 days:
  5 mg/kg/dose once daily X 2 weeks, then 120 mg/m²/dose twice daily x 2 weeks, then 200 mg/m²/dose twice daily[a]
• >30 days to 13 years: 120 mg/m²/dose once daily for 2 weeks, then 120-200 mg/m²/dose twice daily[a]
• Maximum dose: >13 yrs: 200 mg/dose once daily for first 2 weeks, then 200 mg/dose twice daily | • If rifampicin coadministration, avoid use (see TB section)
• Store suspension at room temperature; must be well shaken
• Can be given with food
• Tablets are scored and can be divided into two equal parts to give a 100 mg dose; can be crushed and combined with a small amount of water or food and immediately administered
• PARENTS MUST BE WARNED ABOUT RASH
• Do not escalate dose if rash occurs (if mild/moderate |

continued

TABLE E-4 Dosages of Antiretroviral Drugs for Children—cont'd

Name of drug	Formulations	Pharmaco-kinetic data available	Age (weight), dose and dose frequency	Other comment
Non-nucleoside reverse transcriptase inhibitors—cont'd				
Nevirapine (NVP)—cont'd				rash, hold drug; when rash has cleared, restart dosing from beginning of dose escalation, if severe rash, discontinue drug) • Drug interactions
Efavirenz (EFV)	• Syrup: 30 mg/ml (note: syrup requires higher doses than capsules; see dosing chart) • Capsules: 50 mg, 100 mg, 200 mg	• Only for children over 3 years of age	• Capsule (liquid) dose for >3 years: 10 to 15 kg: 200 mg (270 mg = 9 ml) once daily • 15 to <20 kg: 250 mg (300 mg = 10 ml) once daily • 20 to <25 kg: 300 mg (360 mg = 12 ml) only daily	• Capsules may be opened and added to food but have very peppery taste; however, can be mixed with sweet foods or jam to disguise taste • Can be given with food (but avoid after high-fat meals, which increase absorption by 50%); best given at bedtime, especially first 2 weeks, to reduce CNS side-effects • Drug interactions

			• 25 to <33 kg: 350 mg (450 mg = 15 ml) once daily • 33 to <40 kg: 400 mg (510 mg = 17 ml) once daily • Maximum dose: ≥40 kg: 600 mg once daily	
Fixed-dose combination of d4T plus 3TC plus NVP	• No liquid available • Tablet: 30 mg d4T/150 mg 3TC/200 mg NVP; 40 mg D4T/150 mg 3TC/200 mg NVP	• Adults and adolescents	• Maximum dose: 30–60 kg: one 30 mg d4T-based tablet twice daily • ≥60 kg: one 40 mg d4T-based tablet twice daily	• Preferably, tablet should not be split • At weight <30 kg, d4T/3TC/NVP cannot be dosed accurately in tablet form; if tablets are split, NVP dose requirements will be inadequate for very young children and additional NVP is needed to give total of 200 mg/m^2/dose twice daily

continued

TABLE E-4 Dosages of Antiretroviral Drugs for Children—cont'd

Name of drug	Formulations	Pharmaco-kinetic data available	Age (weight), dose and dose frequency	Other comment
Non-nucleoside reverse transcriptase inhibitors—cont'd				
Fixed-dose—cont'd				• Contains NVP, therefore dose escalation required (see NVP dosing recommendations) • See comments under individual drug components
Protease inhibitors				
Nelfinavir (NFV)	• Powder for oral suspension (mix with liquid): 200 mg per level teaspoon (50 mg per 1.25 ml per 5 ml scoop): 5 ml • Tablet: 250 mg (tablets can be halved; can be crushed and added to food or	• All ages • However extensive pharmacokinetic variability in infants, with requirement for very high doses in infants <1 year	• <1 year: 50 mg/kg/dose three times daily or 75 mg/kg/dose twice daily • >1 year to <13 years: 55 to 65 mg/kg/dose twice daily • Maximum dose: ≥13 years: 1250 mg/dose twice daily	• Powder is sweet, faintly bitter but gritty and hard to dissolve; must bereconstituted immediately before administration in water, milk, formula, pudding etc.; do not use acidic food or juice (which increase bitter taste); solution stable for 6 hours • Because of difficulties with use of powder, use of crushed tablets preferred (even for infants) if appropriate dose can be given

Lopinavir/ ritonavir, (LPV/r)	• Oral solution: 80mg/ml lopinavir plus 20 mg/ml ritonavir • Capsules: 133.3 mg lopinavir plus 33.3 mg ritonavir	• 6 months of age or older	• >6 months to 13 years: 225 mg/m² LPV/ 57.5 mg/m² ritonavir twice daily[a] or weight-based dosing: 7–15 kg: 12mg/kg LPV/ 3 mg/kg ritonavir/ dose twice daily 15–40 kg: 10 mg/kg lopinavir/2.5 mg/kg ritonavir twice daily • Maximum dose: >40 kg: 400 mg LPV/100 mg ritonavir (3 capsules or 5 ml) twice daily	• Preferably, oral solution and capsules should be refrigerated; however, can be stored at room temperature up to 25 °C (77 of) for 2 months; attemperature > 25 °C (77 °F) the drug degrades more rapidly • Liquid formulation has low volume but bitter taste • Capsules large • Capsules should not be crushed or opened but must be swallowed whole • Should be taken with food • Drug interactions
	dissolved in water)			• Powder and tablets can be stored at room temperature • Take with food • Drug interactions (less than ritonavir-containing protease inhibitors)

Source: World Health Organization. (2004). Summary of Paediatric drug formulations and doses (pp. 50-59). Retrieved April 27, 2005, from *www.who.int/hiv/pub/prev_care/en/arvrevision2003en.pdf*

[a] *Meter² body surface area calculation: square root of (height in centimetres times weight in kilograms divided by 3600).*

Potential Toxicities of First-Line Antiretroviral Regimens and Recommended Drug Substitutions

Regimen	Toxicity	Drug substitution
d4T/3TC/NVP	• d4T-related neuropathy or pancreatitis • d4T-related lipoatrophy • NVP-related severe hepatotoxicity • NVP-related severe rash (but not life-threatening) • NVP-related life-threatening rash (Stevens-Johnson syndrome)	• Switch d4T ZDV • Switch d4T TDF or ABC[a] • Switch NVP EFV (except in pregnancy) • Switch NVP EFV • Switch NVP PI[b]
ZDV/3TC/NVP	• ZDV-related persistent GI intolerance or severe haematological toxicity • NVP-related severe hepatotoxicity • NVP-related severe rash (but not life-threatening • NVP-related life-threatening rash (Stevens-Johnson syndrome)	• Switch ZDV d4T • Switch NVP EFV (except in pregnancy; in this situation switch to NFV, LPV/r or ABC) • Switch NVP EFV • Switch NVP PI[b]
d4T/3TC/EFV	• d4T-related neuropathy or pancreatitis • d4T-related lipoatrophy • EFV-related persistent CNS toxicity	• Switch d4T ZDV • Switch d4T TDF or ABC[a] • Switch EFV NVP
ZDV/3TC/EFV	• ZDV-related persistent GI intolerance or severe haematological toxicity • EFV-related persistent CNS toxicity	• Switch ZDV d4T • Switch EFV NVP

Source: World Health Organization. (2004). Table C. Major potential toxicities of first-line ARV regimens and recommended drug substitutions (p. 22). Retrieved April 27, 2005, from *www.who.int/hiv/pub/prev_care/en/arvrevision2003en.pdf*
[a]*Switiching off d4T typically does not reverse lipotrophy but may slow its progression. TDF and ABC can be considered as alternatives but availability is currently limited in resource-constrained settings. In the absence of TDF or ABC availability, ddl or ZDV are additional alternatives to consider.*
[b]*PI can be LPV/r or SQV/r. IDV/r or NFV can be considered as alternatives (see text).*

- • WHO Stage II disease with consideration of using a total lymphocyte count of less than or equal to 1200/mm^3 to guide decision making
– For infants and children in areas where CD4 testing is not available, the WHO recommends offering antiretroviral therapy to those who are:
  - • Under 18 months old with a positive HIV virology test (HIV DNA polymerase chain reaction test, HIV RNA amplification assay, or p24 antigen assay) and
    - • WHO Pediatric Stage III, or
    - • WHO Pediatric Stage II with consideration of using a total lymphocyte count of less than 2500/mm^3 to guide decision making
  - • 18 months or older with a positive HIV antibody test and
    - • WHO Pediatric Stage III, or
    - • WHO Pediatric Stage II with consideration of using a total lymphocyte count of less than 1500/mm^3 to guide decision making
– In areas where HIV virology tests are not available, the WHO does not recommend offering antiretroviral treatment to infants under 18 months old who have a positive HIV antibody test, because the positive test may reflect maternal antibodies rather than actual infection (WHO, 2004d).
– While on antiretroviral treatment, patients should be monitored for adherence to therapy, possible adverse effects of medication, and treatment failure. Monitoring may consist of a schedule of clinical and laboratory assessments, depending on the treatment regimen being used. Adverse effects can sometimes be ameliorated by a drug substitution. Table E-5 lists potential toxicities seen with some treatment regimens and recommended substitutions (WHO, 2004d).
– In developed countries, health care providers assess the success or failure of treatment by monitoring clinical disease progression, viral load, and CD4 counts.

For resource-limited settings where sophisticated laboratory facilities are lacking, treatment failure must be detected by clinical signs alone. These signs include the occurrence of new opportunistic infections or malignancies, recurrence of previous opportunistic infections (except for tuberculosis, which can reinfect patients even though they are responding to therapy), and the onset or recurrence of conditions satisfying WHO Stage III criteria (for example, wasting syndrome, chronic diarrhea, chronic fever without source, recurrent invasive bacterial infections, and mucosal candidiasis). For children, growth and neurodevelopment are additional indicators of treatment success. A child who initially responds and grows with treatment and then experiences a deceleration or cessation of growth may be failing treatment. Encephalopathy and regression of developmental milestones are other ominous signs of treatment failure in children.

During the first few weeks of starting antiretroviral therapy, some patients with advanced disease may develop an immune reconstitution syndrome that can be confused for treatment failure. As part of this syndrome, patients may appear to have an opportunistic infection, but in fact the signs and symptoms are caused by the recovering body's inflammatory response to a previously subclinical opportunistic infection that was present prior to starting antiretroviral therapy (WHO, 2004d).

Many aspects of the treatment and diagnosis of HIV/AIDS have been omitted from this appendix for the sake of brevity. For more complete and current information on the management of HIV/AIDS, access the WHO website (*www.who.int/hiv*), where many publications and technical briefs can be downloaded for free. Readers working with nongovernmental organizations or community-based organizations who are interested in learning from the knowledge and experience of other organizations in the treatment of HIV/AIDS may also wish to visit the website of the International HIV/AIDS Alliance (*www.aidsalliance.org*). In addition to having many resources online, the International HIV/AIDS Alliance has a CD-ROM containing all of their publications that can be ordered without charge from their website.

References

Apetrei, C. (2004). The evolution of HIV and its consequences. *Infectious Disease Clinics of North America, 18,* 369-394.

Hare, C.B. (2004). Clinical overview of HIV disease. Retrieved April 29, 2005, from *http://hivinsite.ucsf.edu/InSite?page=kb-03*

Vergis, E.N., & Mellors, J.W. (2000). Natural history of HIV-1 infection. *Infectious Disease Clinics of North America, 14,* 809-825.

World Health Organization. (2004a). AIDS epidemic update 2004. Retrieved April 27, 2005, from *www.unaids.org/wad2004/report.html*

World Health Organization. (2004b). Antiretroviral drugs for treating pregnant women and preventing HIV infection in infants. Retrieved May 1, 2005, from *www.who.int/hiv/pub/mtct/en/arvdrugswomenguidelinesfinal.pdf*

World Health Organization. (2004c). Rapid HIV tests: Guidelines for use in HIV testing and counseling services in resource-constrained settings. Retrieved April 28, 2005, from *www.who.int/entity/hiv/pub/vct/en/rapidhivtestsen.pdf*

World Health Organization. (2004d). Scaling up antiretroviral therapy in resource limited settings: Treatment guidelines for a public health approach. Retrieved April 27, 2005, from *www.who.int/hiv/pub/prev_care/en/arvrevision2003en.pdf*

INDEX

Page numbers with "t" denote tables; those with "f" denote figures; and those with "b" denote boxes